AWARDS

BENJAMIN FRANKLIN AWARD
Top national award for Education / Teaching / Academic Textbooks
Presented by The Publishers Marketing Association, April, 1999

BENJAMIN FRANKLIN AWARD NOMINEE
Top three national finalist for Professional / Technical Reference
Presented by The Publishers Merketing Association, April, 1999

BENJAMIN FRANKLIN AWARD NOMINEE
Top three national finalist for Interior Design Using 3 or More Colors
Presented by The Publishers Merketing Association, April, 1999

ENTERPRISE AWARD FOR EDUCATION / MULTI-MEDIA PRODUCTS
Top national award in the equine industry
Presented by EQUITANA U.S.A., June, 1999

NEW AND INNOVATIVE PRODUCT AWARD IN EDUCATION
Top international award in the equine industry
Presented by Spruce Meadows Equi-Fair ,
Calgary, Alberta, Canada, September, 1999

Illustrated Atlas of
Clinical Equine Anatomy and Common Disorders of the Horse

Ronald J. Riegel, D.V.M.
Susan E. Hakola, B.S., R.N., C.M.I.

Illustrated By:
Jeffrey B. Dirig, B.S.
Susan E. Hakola, B.S., R.N., C.M.I.

Volume Two
Reproduction, Internal Medicine, and Skin

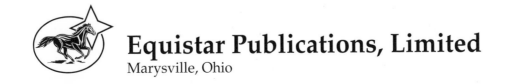

Equistar Publications, Limited
Marysville, Ohio

Equistar Publications, Ltd.
P.O. Box 311
Marysville, Ohio U.S.A. 43040

(800)440-8064 Toll-free in U.S.A. & Canada
(937)642-1055
(937)642-1054 Facsimile

Visit our website: www.equistarpub.com

First Edition 1999
Second Printing: January, 2000
Third Printing: November, 2002

Library of Congress Cataloging in Publication Data

Riegel, Ronald J.
Hakola, Susan E.

Illustrated Atlas of Clinical Equine Anatomy and
Common Disorders of the Horse, Volume Two:
Reproduction, Internal Medicine, and Skin

Bibliography: p.
Includes index.
  1. Equine anatomy   2. Horse diseases
  3. Equine Internal Medicine
  II. Title.

96-085764
ISBN 0-9654461-1-5

The information contained in this text is believed to
be true and accurate at the time of production.
Neither the authors, the illustrators, nor the
publisher can accept any legal responsibility for
any errors or omissions that may be made. The
authors, illustrators, and publisher make no
guarantee, express or implied, with respect to the
material contained within this text.

PRINTED IN THE UNITED STATES OF AMERICA

Text printed on 80# Mead gloss
Cover printed on .035 Classic Quality Poly

Art Director:
Susan E. Hakola, B.S., R.N., C.M.I.

Illustrators:
Jeffrey B. Dirig, B.S.
Susan E. Hakola, B.S., R.N., C.M.I.

Cover Design:
Jeffrey B. Dirig, B.S.

Layout Design:
Jeffrey B. Dirig, B.S.
Susan E. Hakola, B.S., R.N., C.M.I.

Editorial Staff:
June A. Hakola
Marcia L. Leonino

Typography Services:
David L. Ritchie
Chrystal Schrock

Printing Facility:
Rod Owens, Project Coordinator
Bindery & Specialties Pressworks
351 W. Bigelow
Plain City, Ohio U. S. A. 43064
1-800-562-2382

Color Prepress Services:
Larry Mason, Electronic Prepress Director
Bindery & Specialties Pressworks
351 W. Bigelow
Plain City, Ohio U. S. A. 43064
1-800-562-2382

Website Design and Technical Assistance:
Steve Brady, Brady Design, Columbus, Ohio

DEDICATIONS

I believe each individual is blessed. I have been blessed by having loving, guiding, and supportive parents; children, who have provided me with the most important task of my life; a lifemate, without whose love and support would have left my life without meaning; and friends who have seen me through some very difficult times. My life and this text are dedicated to them all.

My entire life I have been in awe of the horse. The motivation for this book has always rested in the idea that in some small way, I have provided a higher quality of life for this animal through the knowledge that I possess. This knowledge has been gained through my own horses and through every single one of my patients. These animals have been tolerant of my inadequacies and have left me with a greater understanding of the species each new day. It would be remiss not to include them in the dedication and thank them for enriching my life.

To Sue, my friend and partner in this endeavor, without her perseverance, creativity, and support, this would have never reached completion. As I say to all: "Anyone could have written this text, but I was lucky enough to know the best illustrator for the work." Thank you for all of your tolerances.

R.J.R.

To my husband Jeff, without whose loving support this text would never have come to fruition. Your encouragement, guidance, and uncanny common sense kept me focused and motivated. Thank you for your understanding, hard work, humility, all of your sacrifices, and for your quiet sense of humor. This is my opportunity to voice to the entire world that you are the best. I love you.

In loving memory of my parents, Earnest and Corinne Ritchie, and my grandparents. I like to think you all would be very proud of our family and this endeavor. I was certainly blessed to have had you as my guiding lights for the too few years that we had together. We all miss you.

To Sherwin, Bonnie, Bethany, Dirk, Steve, Pam, David, Paula, Corrine, and Emmalee. Your contributions through sweat equity, encouraging mental support, and organizational skills cannot be acknowledged enough. Thank you. To Bob and June Hakola, the greatest in-laws anyone could ever hope to have. Thanks for everything you both have done for Jeff and me over the years. To Russ, Carol, Timothy, Scott, Christopher, Matthew, Heather, and Derek. This is for all of you, the best family with which I could be blessed.

To Neil Riley, who was the first in my artistic instruction to express belief in my talents. You opened my eyes and my future and restored long buried dreams. To Gordon Lee, Walt King, and Larry Pointer for your teachings. And to Steve Moon, Ruth Krabach, and Bob Hummel, I say, "Thank you," for without the education I received under your tutelage, I would not have my medical illustration career.

Thanks to the membership of the Association of Medical Illustrators for the additional educational and growth opportunities you have given me.

And lastly, to the O.R. staff at Riverside Methodist Hospital. You all gave me the chance to pursue my dreams. Your ongoing support, encouragement, and heartfelt praise are very big reasons why I am in the position that I am today. I feel you are a part of this project. My thanks to you all.

S.E.H.

To the lovely Dr. Kelly Dirig, my wife, for always standing beside me. For being my strongest critic and keeping me honest. I love you.

To Pat and Tom, my parents, for always being there to stand behind me in my endeavors. For giving me the strength to move in new directions and to never stop challenging myself.

To Diane Seeling, for teaching me to see the world.

J.B.D.

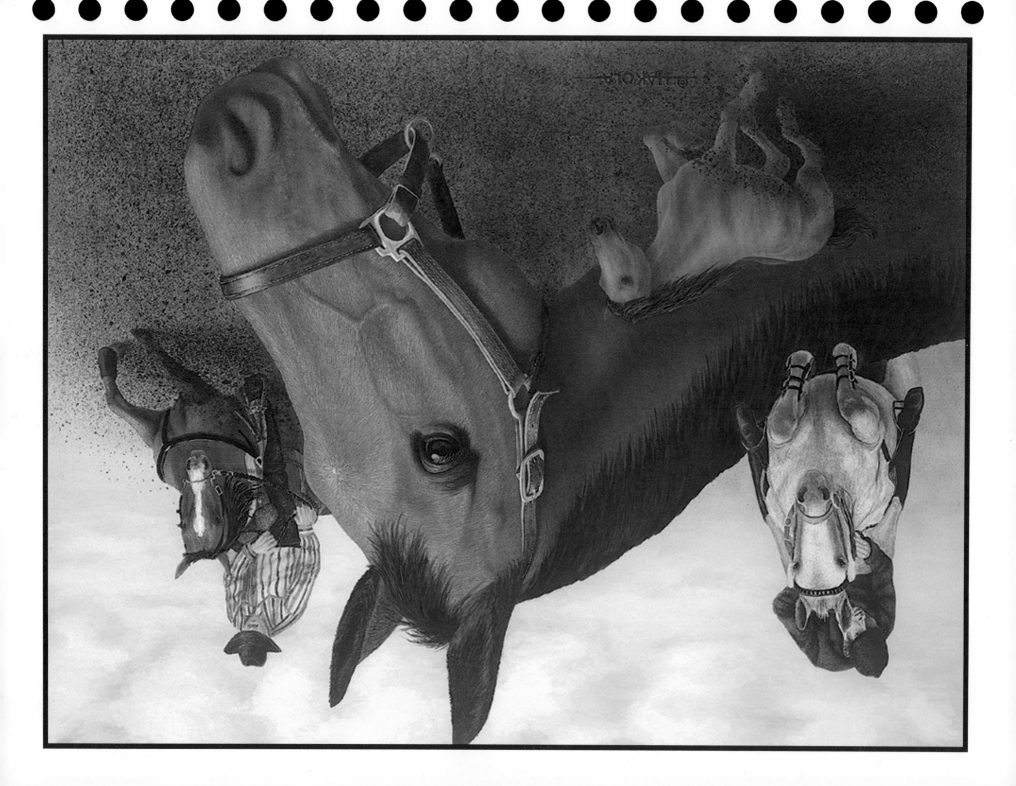

PREFACE

It was frustrating, as a young veterinary student, to try and understand all the basic concepts involved with the equine species. Years later, it was equally frustrating to try and educate my clients using rudimentary artistic skills as a basis for their education in respect to the problems involved with their horses. This text is intended to help fill this void for the horse owner, trainer, equine professional, and both the veterinary student and practicing veterinarian.

This book is structured in its own unique way, originating with all of the basic anatomy leading to the significant physiology, pathogenesis, and logical pathways of diagnosis, and finally the current treatment protocols of the most commonly seen equine disorders. Accurate, detailed illustrations will depict each area for clarification. Numerous times, these illustrations could stand alone in their explanation of a specific area of interest. Often times photographs, and especially radiographs are difficult to interpret and contain extraneous material that does not correlate with the text. Illustrations are utilized not only because they are aesthetically pleasing, but because they serve as a medium to define an area of interest.

Complex and difficult terms could not be avoided in the creation of the text. To include the interest of the specialist and the novice, this was unavoidable. The detailed glossary hopefully includes all of the current nomenclature and their respective definitions.

In years of experience within the equine industry, most of the information that is conveyed is unfortunately misinformation. This text is to educate and clarify, to define and illustrate, and to expand each individual's horizon of the equine species. Maybe most importantly, it will result in better care and a better quality of life for our horses.

INTRODUCTION

When one views the beauty of the horse, a realization is made as to the creation of a biomechanically balanced, structurally massive, and evolutionary perfected animal. We ask this animal to perform a myriad of tasks for us that range from strenuous athletic events to simply being the gentle companion in the complex human-animal bond.

The majority of the people involved in the equine industry invest an enormous amount of time and thought into achieving a high standard in the quality of life for their horses. The purpose of this book is to promote a clearer understanding and comprehension of the anatomy and disorders within the internal systems of the horse. A foundation of basic knowledge is presented along a system-based line. The reader can then build on this foundation through the investigation of the different disorders within that system. This approach will allow the reader a greater understanding of the problems that confront them and allow them the knowledge needed to reach intelligent solutions concerning these problems.

We have witnessed huge amounts of new knowledge concerning the health care of the horse within the last ten years. Equine owners, breeders, and trainers are faced with new concepts and information on a regular basis. Basic understanding of this information is essential in establishing a common knowledge base with your veterinarian, trainer, farrier, or breeder in order to increase the level of care that the animal receives.

We ask the horse to perform innumerable tasks from pleasurable trail riding, to working long hours on a ranch or farm, to racing and eventing. This responsibility requires us to have a high level of knowledge concerning the horse's health care. The goal of this text is to provide the knowledge and understanding that is essential to the health and quality of life for the horse.

TABLE OF CONTENTS

Preface & Introduction

Chapter One: The Stallion

Chapter Two: The Mare

Chapter Three: Foal Disorders

Chapter Four: The Oral Cavity

Chapter Five: The Digestive System

This page intentionally left blank

This page intentionally left blank

Artwork by S. Hakola / J. Dirig
Copyright Equistar Publications, Ltd.

Ventral View of Inguinal Region with Right Testis Exposed

Male Reproductive Tract Right Lateral View

Layers of the Scrotum

1

The Stallion

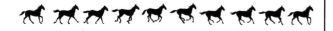

REPRODUCTIVE ANATOMY AND PHYSIOLOGY

The general anatomy of the stallion consists of two testicles with all their coverings and appendages which include the epididymides contained within a scrotum, the paired deferent ducts, the seminal vesicles, a musculoglandular prostate, the paired bulbourethral glands, the urethra, and a musculocavernous penis with its protective prepuce. The accessory sexual glands: the seminal vesicles, the prostate, and the bulbourethral glands discharge their respective secretions into the urethra where the secretions are mixed with fluid secreted by the testicles. This composite fluid of spermatozoa and secretions from the testicles, the excurrent duct system, and the accessory genital glands is called semen.

The Scrotum

The scrotum, which contains the testicles and the corresponding distal parts of the spermatic cord, is situated high between the hind limbs. The scrotum is slightly pendulous and has a globular shape. There is a distinct longitudinal indentation ventrally which is termed the scrotal or median raphe. This groove is representative of the most ventral portion of the scrotal septum and divides the scrotum into two distinct pouches. Commonly, the scrotum is asymmetrical since one testicle, most often the left, is larger, more dependent, and placed slightly caudally when compared to the right testicle.

The function of this scrotum is to protect its contents: the testicles, the epididymides, the spermatic cords, and the cremaster muscles. This outpouching of skin also plays a vital role in testicular and epididymis thermoregulation.

There are four layers to the wall of the scrotum. The outside layer is basically skin which contains an unusually large number of sweat and sebaceous glands. Just beneath the skin and its associating connective tissue is the tunica dartos muscle. This layer of smooth muscle fibers is intermingled with connective tissue that provides contractile

properties to the scrotum. Along the median raphe, this second layer forms the septum scroti which divides the scrotum into two pouches. The scrotal ligament consists of fibers of the tunica dartos muscle closely intertwined with the tunica vaginalis. The tunica dartos layer contracts and relaxes to change the size, shape, and position of the testis to aid in the control of testicular and epididymal temperature.

The third layer consists of loose connective tissue called the scrotal fascia. This layer functions to allow the testis significant vertical and horizontal movement within the scrotal sack. This loose connective tissue also prevents one hundred and eighty degree rotation of the testicles within the scrotal sack.

The inner most layer of the scrotum is the parietal vaginal tunic. This is a fibroserous sack which is continuous with the parietal peritoneum of the abdomen originating at the internal inguinal ring. This parietal vaginal tunic covers the testis and epididymis and also contributes to the spermatic cord. The space that is created within the vaginal cavity between the parietal vaginal tunic and the visceral vaginal tunic (the outer most covering around the testicle and epididymis) contains a fluid which serves as a lubricant and facilitates movement of the testis within the sack formed by the parietal vaginal tunic.

The blood supply to the scrotum is derived from the external pudic artery. The veins drain chiefly to the external pudic vein. Neurological supply is derived from the ventral branches from the second and third lumbar nerves.

The Testes

The testicles or testes are paired and are situated in the prepubic region enclosed within the scrotal structures. "Testes," rather than "testicles," is the correct term for the primary male reproductive organs. Testicle literally means "small testis" and is a synonym for testis. The testes are ovoid in shape and compressed when viewed from side to side. Normally, their long axis is directed horizontally, but when the testis is retracted, the long axis becomes more vertical so that the caudal

THE STALLION

Anatomy of the Testes

Artwork by S. Hakola / J. Dirig
Copyright Equistar Publications, Ltd.

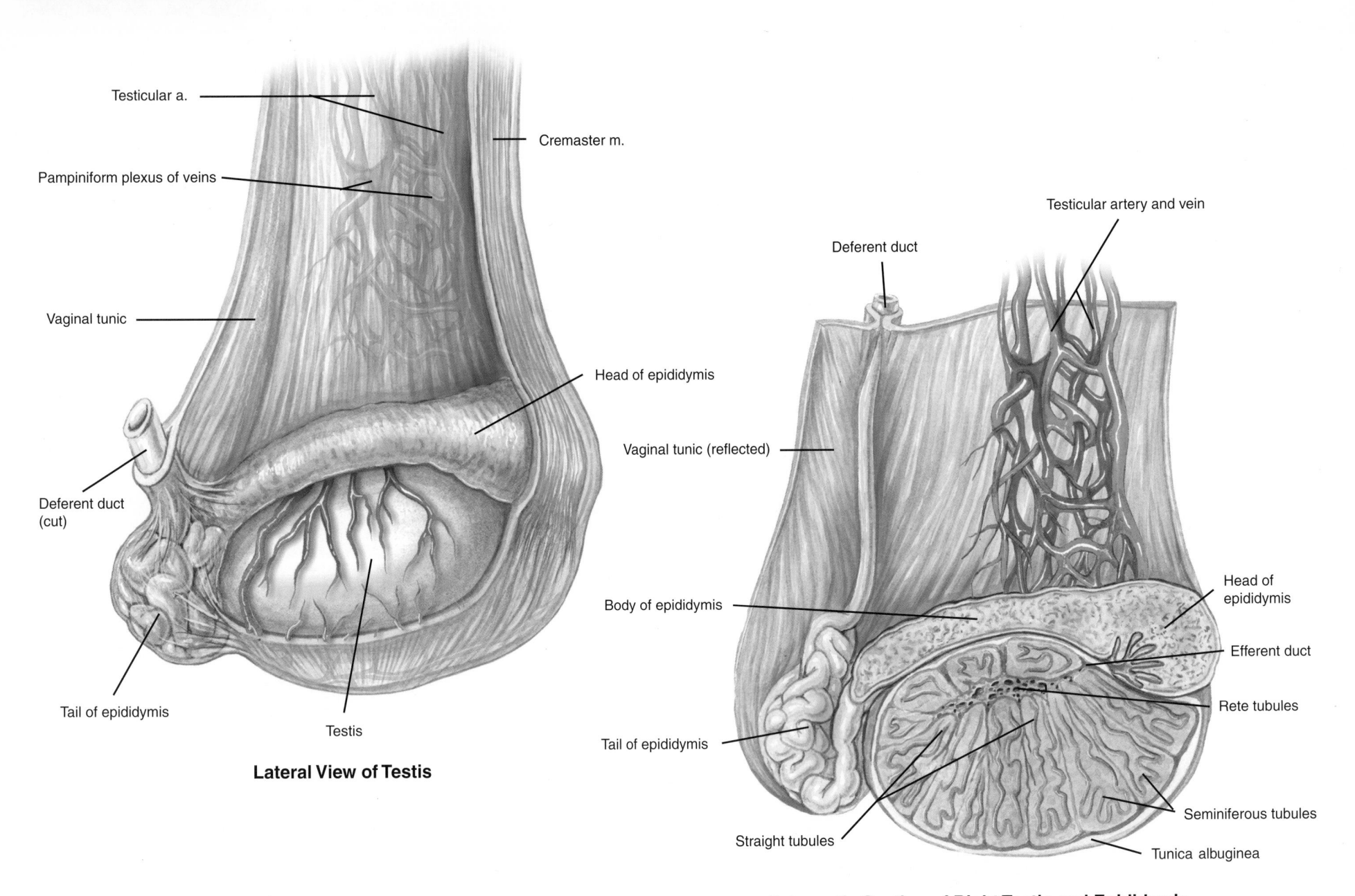

Lateral View of Testis

Testicular a.

Cremaster m.

Pampiniform plexus of veins

Vaginal tunic

Head of epididymis

Deferent duct (cut)

Tail of epididymis

Testis

Schematic Section of Right Testis and Epididymis

Deferent duct

Testicular artery and vein

Vaginal tunic (reflected)

Body of epididymis

Head of epididymis

Efferent duct

Rete tubules

Tail of epididymis

Seminiferous tubules

Straight tubules

Tunica albuginea

epididymis becomes ventrally oriented rather than caudally located. The average testis of a postpubertal stallion will measure between eighty to one hundred and forty millimeters in length by fifty to eighty millimeters in width and weigh approximately two hundred and twenty-five grams. The stallion's age and the season of the year greatly effects testis weight and size. Testes perform both an exocrine and endocrine function. Spermatogenesis (the production of male gametes) is the exocrine function. Hormones that are important in spermatogenesis, sexual differentiation, the development of secondary sexual characteristics and sex drive are the endocrine functions of the testes.

In the stallion, as with other mammals, the testes descend from the abdominal cavity into a scrotum. The epididymides are located dorsally or caudomedially on the testes depending on the position of the gonads within the scrotal pouch. The epididymis will be lateral and the ductus deferens will be found medially. The testis is enclosed by a peritoneum, or tunica vaginalis, in a network of small blood vessels and delicate areolar tissue. The testis itself is composed of testicular parenchyma encapsulated by a thick fibrous tissue termed the "tunica albuginea." This fibrous tunica albuginea actually penetrates the underlying testicular parenchyma and divides it into numerous lobules. The outermost portion of this tunica albuginea is intimately adhered to the visceral layer of the vaginal tunic.

The parenchyma occupies nearly ninety percent of the mass of the total testis. Seventy percent of this mass is the seminiferous tubules. The interstitial tissues of the testis are located between the seminiferous tubules and comprises the remainder of the parenchyma. Leydig cells comprise approximately fifteen percent of the testicular parenchyma. Other interstitial cells such as fibroblasts, lymphocytes, and mast cells account for 1% and blood vessels, lymphatic vessels, and other noncellular components comprise the remaining fifteen percent.

The seminiferous tubules are small convoluted tubules that are composed of a lumen surrounded by seminiferous epithelium. This epithelium consists of Sertoli cells and germ cells that are then surrounded by myoid cells in boundary tissues. Testicular germ cells (spermatogoniae, spermatocytes, and spermatids) are interspersed between the Sertoli cells. Myoid cells maintain the integrity of the seminiferous tubules. Their rhythmic contractions help move spermatozoa and fluids through the seminiferous tubules.

Sertoli cells function in coordinating germinal cell differentiation. They produce several proteins needed to carry vitamin A, iron, and copper to developing germ cells. They also produce a number of proteins involved in regulating formation of spermatozoa. Sertoli cells secrete luminal fluid and lactate as a germ cell energy source. These cells respond to stimulation by the follicle stimulating hormone and testosterone.

Leydig cells function to support spermatogenesis and the maintenance of secondary sex characteristics and sexual drive. These cells are stimulated by luteinizing hormone to produce testosterone. The Leydig cells are located in the interstitium adjacent to the seminiferous tubules. There is a wide range of seasonal variation in the total volume of Leydig cells per testis. The number of Leydig cells per testis is greater in the summer than it is in the winter. Age is also a factor. The older the animal, the volume density as well as the number of Leydig cells per testicle changes as the animal increases with age.

Thermoregulation of the Testes

For normal spermatogenesis to occur, the testes and epididymides of the stallion require a temperature below that of normal core body temperature. There are three anatomical structures whose combined actions provide a suitable temperature for sperm production. These three anatomical structures are the scrotum, the pampiniform plexus, and the cremaster muscle.

The scrotum allows the testes and epididymis to be situated outside of the body proper. Within the structure of the scrotum, the tunica dartos muscle relaxes in warm weather. This allows the testes and the epididymis to distance themselves further from the body wall. The tunica dartos muscle relaxation also allows for a more pendulous structure which in turn provides more surface area for evaporative cooling from the numerous sweat glands that are contained within the scrotal skin.

The testicular vein forms the pampiniform plexus as it leaves each testis and divides to form many intercommunicating vessels that intertwine around the testicular artery en route to the testes. The temperature of the blood in the superficial branches of this venous plexus is, therefore, lower than body temperature because of the loss of heat by evaporative cooling. This cooled venous blood enters the pampiniform plexus which serves as the heat exchange area between it and the testicular artery. The heat is transferred from the warm testicular artery to the cooler pampiniform plexus allowing the reduction of the temperature of the arterial blood several degrees before it enters the testis.

Lastly, the cremaster muscles can contract to raise the testis near to the body wall. Complete relaxation of these muscles permits the testis to assume a more distal scrotal position away from the body wall which facilitates the cooling of these tissues.

Spermatogenesis

The process of spermatogenesis occurs in the convoluted portions of the seminiferous tubules which constitute most of the mass of the testicular parenchyma. Spermatogenesis is the chronological order of germ cell divisions and transformations within these seminiferous tubules that results in the formation of spermatozoa. Spermatogonia cell division produces a normal stem-cell population which results in primary spermatocytes. These divide through meiosis to produce haploid spermatids that differentiate into the spermatozoa.

There are three phases in spermatogenesis: spermatocytogenesis, meiosis, and spermiogenesis. Each one of these phases is specific for one of the three major germ cell types. These three major germ cell types are spermatogonia, spermatocytes, and spermatids.

Artwork by S. Hakola / J. Dirig
Copyright Equistar Publications, Ltd.

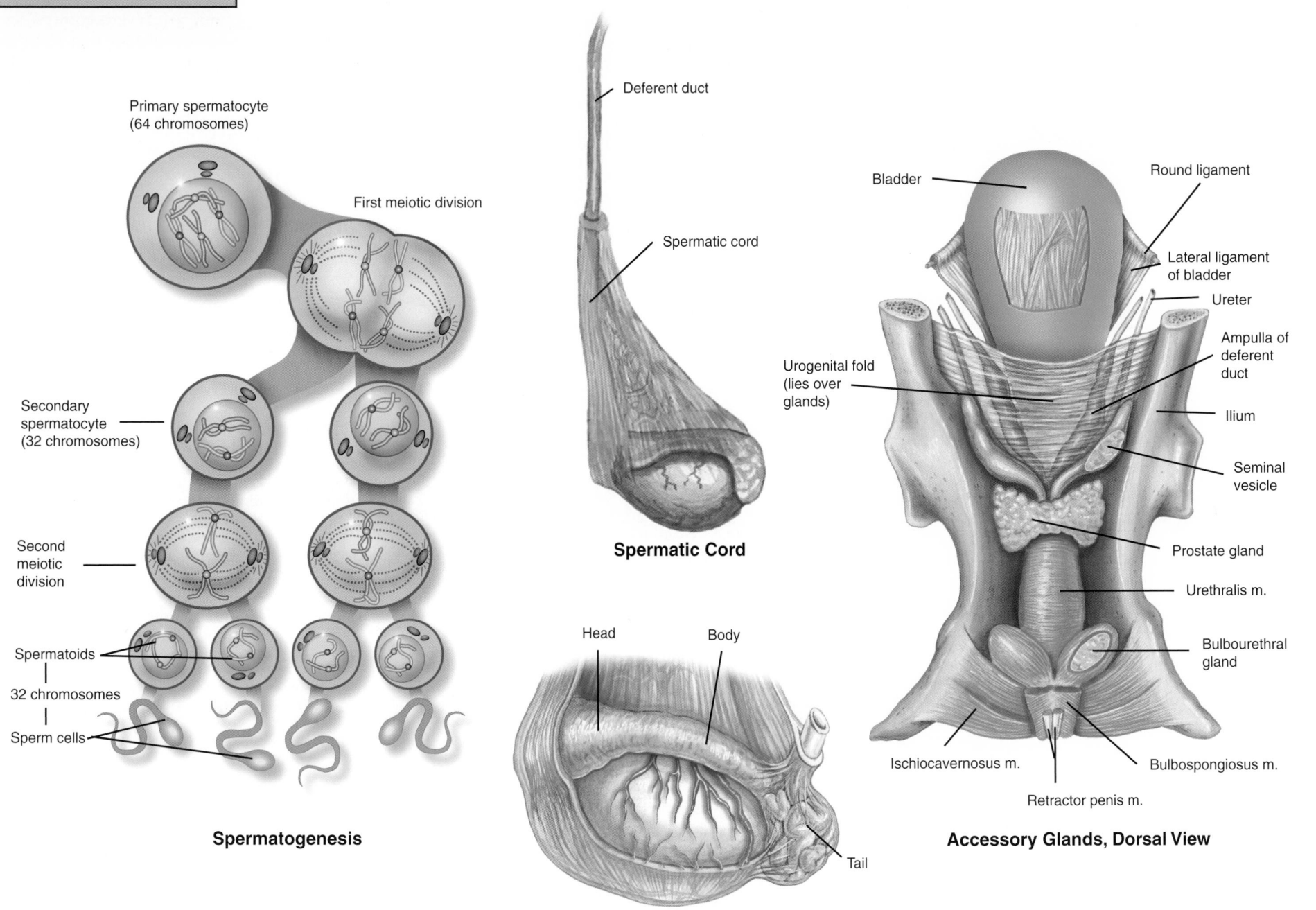

Spermatogenesis

Primary spermatocyte (64 chromosomes)

First meiotic division

Secondary spermatocyte (32 chromosomes)

Second meiotic division

Spermatoids

32 chromosomes

Sperm cells

Spermatic Cord

Deferent duct

Spermatic cord

Epididymis

Head

Body

Tail

Accessory Glands, Dorsal View

Bladder

Round ligament

Lateral ligament of bladder

Ureter

Ampulla of deferent duct

Urogenital fold (lies over glands)

Ilium

Seminal vesicle

Prostate gland

Urethralis m.

Bulbourethral gland

Ischiocavernosus m.

Retractor penis m.

Bulbospongiosus m.

The first phase (which is spermatocytogenesis) lasts for about one third of the duration of spermatogenesis. It is during this phase of spermatogenesis that spermatogonia mitotically divide to produce other stem cells and primary spermatocytes.

The meiosis phase of spermatogenesis begins with the production of primary spermatocytes from the division of spermatogonia. The division of secondary spermatocytes to produce spermatids indicates the end of this phase of spermatogenesis. It is during this phase where chromosomes are duplicated, and there is an exchange of genetic material between paired homologous chromosomes.

The final phase of spermatogenesis is spermiogenesis. This phase follows the meiosis phase. It is during this time that flagellum equipped spermatozoa, with condensed elongated heads and overlying acrosomal caps, are transformed from basic spherical spermatids with spherical nuclei.

Epididymides

Each epididymis is attached to the border of the testicle on the dorsolateral surface. The head is the enlarged cranial portion, whereas the slightly enlarged tail is situated posteriorly. Between the head and the tail is the intermediate narrow part called the body. The head of the epididymis is closely connected to the testis by the efferent ducts, connective tissue, and serous membranes. The body is more loosely attached by the serous covering. The tail is continued by the ductis deferens.

Actually the epididymis is a singular tortuous duct that is seventy to eighty meters long in the stallion. This duct serves as a conduit for spermatozoa. It also functions to concentrate these cells and provides a special milieu that enables sperm to mature and achieve a fertilizing capacity. Rhythmic smooth muscle contractions within the epididymal wall allow sperm to be transported through the head and body of the epididymis. These cells then accumulate in the tail of the

epididymis until the smooth muscle and the epididymis contract during ejaculation. Therefore, the tail of the epididymis actually serves as a storage site for mature spermatozoa.

Deferent Ducts (Ductus Deferens)

These two tubes extend from the tail of the epididymis to the pelvic part of the urethra. They serve as a passageway for mature spermatozoa. These long ducts are highly muscular and ascend through their respective spermatic cords through the vaginal rings and into the abdominal cavity. They then pass caudally through the peritoneum to enter the pelvic cavity. The ducts terminate as small orifices on the seminal colliculus located on the dorsal surface on the pelvic urethra.

In order to facilitate this long transfer of spermatozoa, the wall of the deferent duct consists of thick longitudinal and circular muscle fibers. The entire structure is covered with peritoneum except for the last few inches of its course. The lumen is very small and the tube appears almost like a piece of string when viewed externally.

Spermatic Cord

The spermatic cord extends from the vaginal ring to the attached border of each testis. The entire cord is enclosed by the parietal layer of the vaginal tunic and contains within it the following structures: the testicular artery, the network of convoluted small veins known as the pampiniform plexus, the ductis deferens, lymph vessels, nerves, and bundles of smooth muscle, The external cremaster muscle, which is a striated muscle, originates on the abdominal wall and attaches to the lateral and caudal borders of each spermatic cord.

Accessory Genital Glands

The accessory glands in a stallion include the seminal vesicles, the bilobed prostate gland, the paired ampullae, the paired bulbourethral glands, and the disseminate urethral glands. These accessory genital glands provide secretions as a vehicle for the transportation of spermatozoa from the male to the female reproductive tract during ejaculation. Many functions of the secretory products from these different accessory glands still remains undetermined.

At the end of the deferent ducts there are enlarged structures referred to as the ampullae. They are 1 - 2 cm. in diameter and are located near the midline on the pelvic floor.

Partially enclosed in the genital fold are the two elongated seminal vesicles. These lay on each side of the posterior portion of the dorsal surface of the bladder. Their long axes are parallel to the deferent ducts. The seminal vesicles are usually six to eight inches long and approximately two inches in diameter. The excretory duct of these glands lay beneath the prostate and open up in common with or along the side of the ductus deferens in the pouch of the mucous membrane on the side of the seminal colliculus. Each seminal vesicular gland expands greatly during sexual stimulation due to the secretory products that it produces.

The prostate gland is a lobulated gland which lies on the neck of the bladder at the beginning of the urethra ventral to the rectum. It consists of two lobes lateral to the pelvic urethra and connecting isthmus. Each lobe is approximately five to eight centimeters long, two to three centimeters wide, and one to two centimeters thick. The isthmus is a thin transverse band about two centimeters wide that courses over the dorsal surface of the pelvic urethra at the level of the seminal colliculus. There are fifteen to twenty prostatic ducts on either side which perforate the urethra and open up laterally to the seminal colliculus.

The two bulbourethral glands are located on the dorsolateral surface of the pelvic urethra near the ischial arch caudal to the prostate gland. They are ovoid in shape and are three to

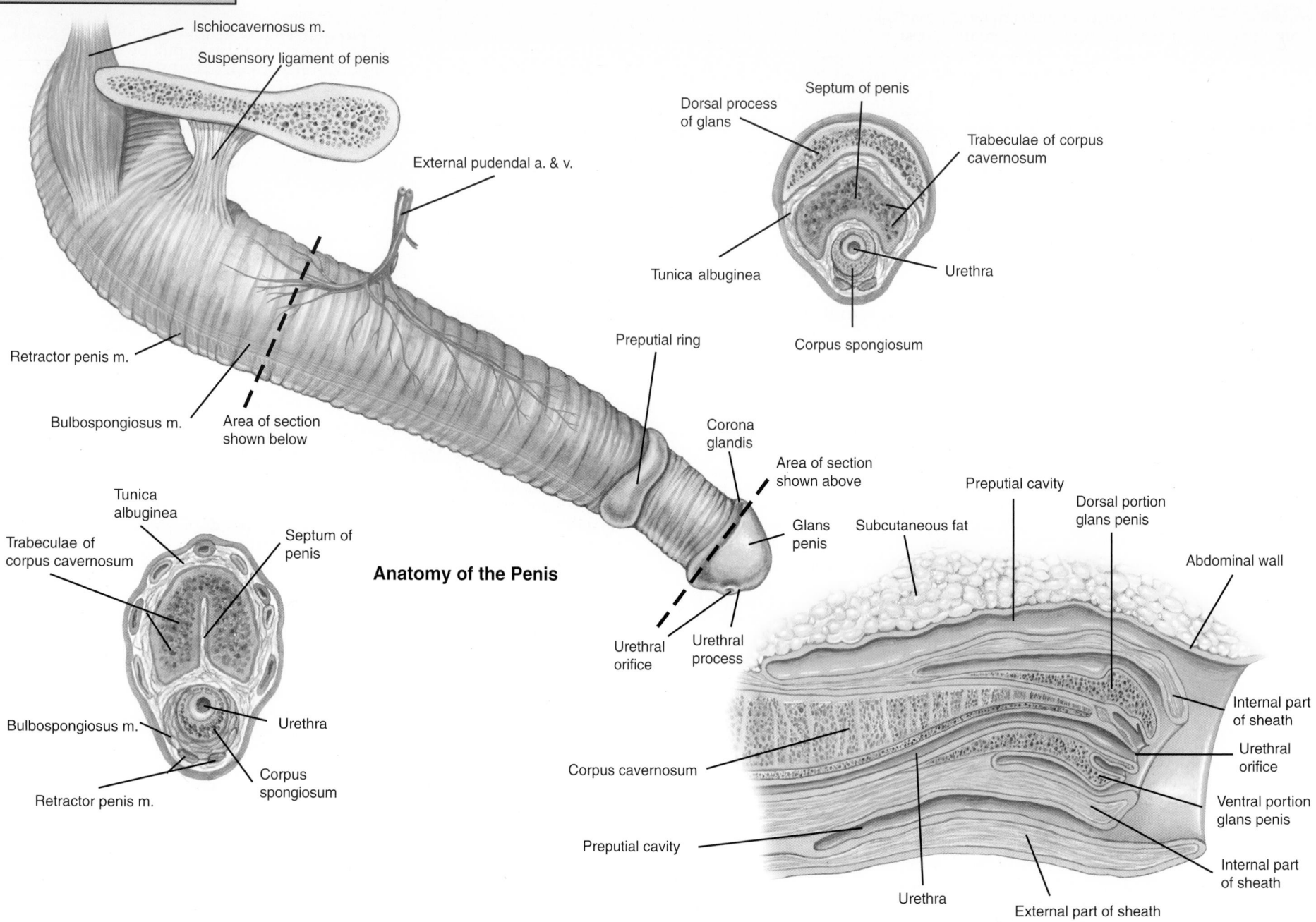

Ischiocavernosus m.

Suspensory ligament of penis

External pudendal a. & v.

Retractor penis m.

Bulbospongiosus m.

Area of section shown below

Dorsal process of glans

Septum of penis

Trabeculae of corpus cavernosum

Tunica albuginea

Urethra

Corpus spongiosum

Preputial ring

Corona glandis

Area of section shown above

Glans penis

Urethral orifice

Urethral process

Anatomy of the Penis

Tunica albuginea

Trabeculae of corpus cavernosum

Septum of penis

Bulbospongiosus m.

Urethra

Retractor penis m.

Corpus spongiosum

Subcutaneous fat

Preputial cavity

Dorsal portion glans penis

Abdominal wall

Internal part of sheath

Urethral orifice

Ventral portion glans penis

Internal part of sheath

Corpus cavernosum

Preputial cavity

Urethra

External part of sheath

Longitudinal Section of Prepuce

four centimeters long and two to two and a half centimeters wide with their long axis directed obliquely forward and outward. They resemble the prostate in general structure but the interstitial tissue is much less abundant. They are not as distinctly lobular and the parenchyma consists of large collecting tubules. There are several excretory ducts from these glands that enter the urethral lumen distal to the seminal colliculus near the dorsal midline.

The Urethra

The urethra serves as a passageway for both urine and semen. It is a long membranous canal which extends from the bladder to the glans penis. It transverses backwards on the floor of the pelvis, turns around the ischial arch forming a sharp bend, and passes forward as a part of the penis. The portion within the penis is enclosed by the corpus spongiosum penis. The pelvic portion of the urethra is surrounded by a layer of erectile tissue called the corpus cavernosum, which itself is enveloped by the thick striated urethralis muscle. The pelvic part is four to five inches long and at its origin is not distinguishable from the neck of the bladder. It runs behind the prostate near the ischial arch between the bulbourethral glands. It is related dorsally to the rectum and the prostate and laterally to the bulbourethral glands. This pelvic urethra is entirely enclosed by urethral muscle except at its origin on the bladder. The urethra in the stallion is unique because it actually secretes mucus into both the urine and the seminal ejaculate. The urethra ends in a free extension termed the urethral process.

The Penis

The erectile copulatory male organ of the stallion is called the penis and is composed essentially of erectile tissue which encloses the extrapelvic portion of the urethra. It consists of three regions: the root, which is that portion attached directly to the skeletal system; the body or shaft, which is the main portion of the penis; and the glans, which is the enlarged free end of the penis. The root of the penis, which is called the radix penis, is attached to the lateral parts of the ischial arch by two

ligamentous crura. The two crura fuse at the root of the penis and extend distally along the body of the penis as part of the corpus cavernosum penis. The urethra passes over the ischial arch between these crura and then courses sharply forward to become incorporated within the penis. The body of the penis, or corpus penis, begins at the junction of these crura and constitutes the bulk of the organ. The cranial surface of the glans penis contains a deep depression called the fossa glandis. The urethral process originates here. The fossa glandis contains two ventrolateral recesses and a large dorsal diverticulum. This diverticulum is sometimes filled with a caseous mass of sebaceous matter and epithelial debris. This is commonly referred to as smegma or a "bean."

The structure of the penis itself is essentially three erectile bodies: the corpus cavernosum penis, the corpus spongiosum penis, and the corpus spongiosum glandis. This is in contrast to the fibroelastic penis of most male ruminents. Forming the main component of the body of the penis and spanning the entire length of the penis is the corpus cavernosum penis. It is composed of spongy erectile tissue which is continuous with veins draining the penis. Its surface is covered by a thick tunic albuginea. When the stallion is first sexually stimulated, the precopulatory erection is achieved through the engorgement of the corpus cavernosum penis. On the ventral surface, there is a longitudual groove within the corpus cavernosum penis which shields and protects the penile urethra. The corpus spongiosum penis surrounds the penile urethra along its entire length but is not enclosed by the tunica albuginea. The cavernous tissue which comprises this portion is an extension of the erectile stratum cavernosum which surrounds the pelvic urethra. The bulb of the penis at the proximal end of the ischial arch is an enlargement of the corpus spongiosum of the penis. The corpus spongiosum penis becomes the corpus spongiosum glandis located within the glans penis. This is richly endowed with nerve endings and with sexual excitement becomes engorged with blood during erection. The corpus spongiosum glandis expands to form the "belling" or "flowering" of the glans penis during coitus.

The nonerect penis is about fifty centimeters long

by two and a half to five centimeters in diameter. Approximately fifteen to twenty centimeters of this structure is free within the prepuce. The erection of the stallion increases the length and diameter of the penis by approximately fifty percent. The glans penis itself increases about three hundred to four hundred percent in diameter when it becomes engorged through stimulation.

The internal and external pudic, obturator, and expudic arteries all supply blood to the penis. The internal pudic artery enters the root of the penis as the artery of the bulb and breaks up within the bulb into numerous branches. The obturator artery supplies blood to the corpus cavernosum penis whereas the external pudic artery gives off the dorsal arteries of the penis. Branches of the external pudic pass through the tunica albuginea. There is a rich plexus dorsally and laterally on the penis which is drained by the external pudendal and obturator veins. The blood draining from the root of the penis is carried away by the internal pudic veins. Neurological supply is derived from the pudic nerves and the pelvic plexus of the sympathetic system.

There are two muscles that function to aid in the movement of the penile tissue. The ischio-cavernosus muscle is a paired muscle which arises from the tuber ischii and the adjacent part of the sacrosciatic ligament. This muscle inserts on the crus and adjacent part of the body of the penis. It functions to pull the penis against the pelvis and assists in producing and maintaining erection by compressing the dorsal veins of the penis. The retractor penis muscle is a nonstriated muscle which is continuous with the suspensory ligaments of the anus. It arises on the ventral surface of the first and second coccygeal vertebrae and passes downward over the sides of the rectum to meet below the anus. This forms a suspensory apparatus for the posterior part of the rectum and the anus. It passes along the ventral surface of the penis where it is loosely attached. As it approaches the glans penis, the retractor penis splits into bundles which pass through the cavernosus areas to attach on the tunica albuginea. On the lateral sides of the penis, the right and left muscles are adherent to each other. They function to withdraw the penis into the sheath after protrusion.

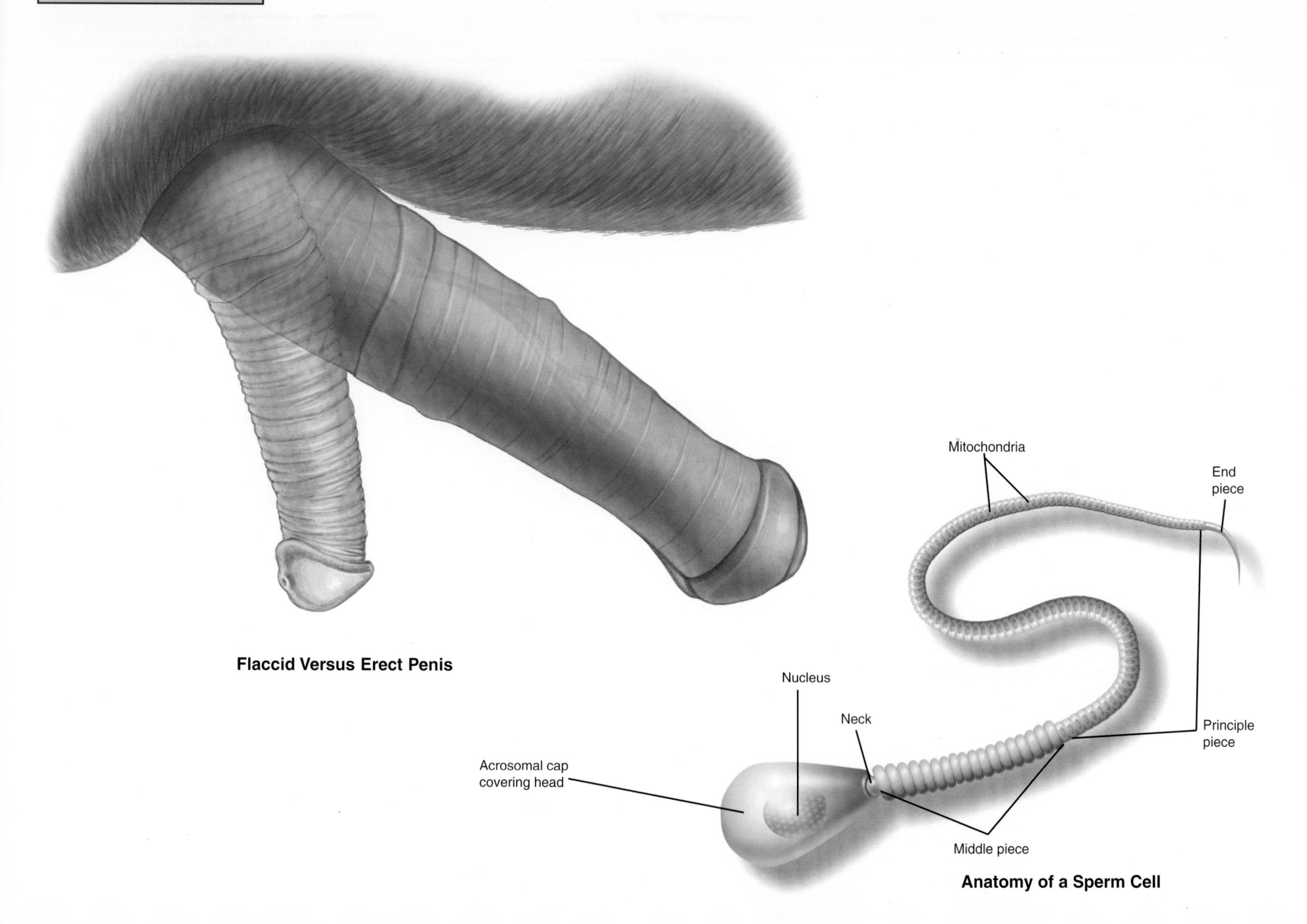

Flaccid Versus Erect Penis

Mitochondria

End piece

Nucleus

Neck

Principle piece

Acrosomal cap covering head

Middle piece

Anatomy of a Sperm Cell

The Prepuce

The prepuce of the stallion is unlike that of other domestic species in that it telescopes around the nonerect penis to form two distinct folds. This forms the external and internal prepuce. Its primary function is to shield the nonerect penis. The external prepuce consists of external and internal lamina that meet at the preputial orifice. When the penis is not erect, only the external lamina of the external prepuce is exposed.

The internal lamina does not attach directly to the penis in the stallion but continues as the internal prepuce. The external and internal lamina of the internal prepuce meet at a second orifice called the preputial ring. The internal prepuce separates the preputial cavity into two distinct compartments. This creates an external and internal prepucial cavity. The internal lamina of the internal prepuce reflects onto the body of the penis at the fornix of the internal preputial cavity.

Erection

The penis must attain a rigid erection in order to deposit semen within the reproductive tract of the mare. This occurs through stimulation of the central nervous system which results in a circulatory change within the penis. When a mare in heat or other sexual stimulation is presented to the stallion, there is a psychic stimulation within the cerebral cortex of the stallion's brain. This induces muscles at the root of the penis to contract and pulls the body of the penis up against the pelvic bone. This results in pressure on the penis and eliminates the venous drainage from the penis. The arteries of the penis become dilated due to the stimulation from the central nervous system and the sensory nerves within the penis itself. This allows blood to engorge the sinuses within the corpus cavernosum penis and the corpus cavernosus urethra. Surrounding these cavernous structures are fibroelastic capsules which allow the penis to become rigid without a great increase in diameter. However, the length of the penis increases approximately fifty percent.

Ejaculation

The expulsion of semen from the penis is termed ejaculation and is caused by stimulation of nerves within the base of the penis and special stimuli from the brain. Neurologically stimulated muscles within the walls of the accessory sex glands and the epididymis contract to expel sperm and fluid into the urethra. When the semen from the duct system moves into the urethra, it is referred to as emission. When ejaculation occurs, it is contraction of muscles within the penis and urethra which causes the actual release of semen from the male copulatory organ during the breeding process. Ejaculation itself consists of about ten pulsations that occur at approximately one second intervals. The first three or four pulsations of spurting fluid contain about seventy-five percent of the total sperm present in that particular ejaculate.

Semen

Semen is a mixture of sperm cells, or spermatozoa, and secretions from the testes, the accessory genital glands, and the excurrent duct system that is expelled into the female genital tract during ejaculation. The spermatozoa carry the stallion's genetic contribution to the offspring and is essential for the propagation of the species. There is a complex reproductive duct system that produces seminal fluid to help as a transport medium for the spermatozoa. When measuring a stallion's fertility, the quality of the semen is an important characteristic. Semen is usually contaminated with exfoliated epithelial cells and bacteria from the distal urethra and exterior surface of the penis. In order to evaluate the semen quality from the stallion, a breeder should have a basic knowledge of what comprises a normal semen sample.

Each spermatogonium has the potential of producing numerous spermatozoa depending on the number of cell divisions that occur through mitosis and meiosis. The maturation process produces a sperm cell that has the ability to locate, fuse with, and penetrate an oocyte at fertilization. The head of the sperm is approximately six by three by one microns in size and appears as a

flattened egg in shape. The head is composed of a nucleus and an overlying acrosomal cap. The nucleus itself contains the haploid complement of genetic material that will unite with the female haploid compliment at fertilization to form a zygote. The acrosome appears as a "bathing cap" over the cranial aspect of the sperm nucleus and contains enzymes that are necessary to break down the protective membranes of the ovum upon contact. The tail, or flagellum, of the spermatozoa is connected to the head by a small neck which is divided into a middle piece, principle piece, and end piece. The middle piece contains the mitochondrial supply for energy which is required for cellular processes and spermatozoa motility. The long axis of the tail should be parallel with the long axis of the head. When the tail has its whip-like movement, the sperm head rotates on its long axis from left to right and moves forward in a wave-like pattern.

There is a wide range to the normal volume of ejaculate from a stallion. The average is sixty to seventy millimeters but can be as little as twenty and as much as two hundred and fifty millimeters. This volume of ejaculate is determined by the frequency of ejaculation, the intensity and length of precopulatory sexual stimulation, and the season of the year. The actual spermatozoal concentration within the ejaculated semen averages one hundred and twenty to one hundred and eighty million sperm per milliliter but it also can have a wide range of as little as twenty to as many as six hundred million sperm per milliliter. Spermatozoa concentration within the ejaculate is inversely proportional to the ejaculate volume. The larger the seminal volume, the smaller the spermatozoa concentration.

The ejaculate of the stallion is characterized by four continuous but recognizable parts: A "presperm" fraction, a "sperm-rich" fraction, a "postsperm" fraction, and a "tail-end" fraction. These different fractions originate in different anatomical areas of the reproductive tract and reflect accessory sex gland and epididymal activity.

When the stallion is first sexually stimulated, the initial clear fluid that is dribbled from the end of the stallion's penis is termed the "presperm"

Artwork By S. Hakola / J. Dirig
Copyright Equistar Publications, Ltd.

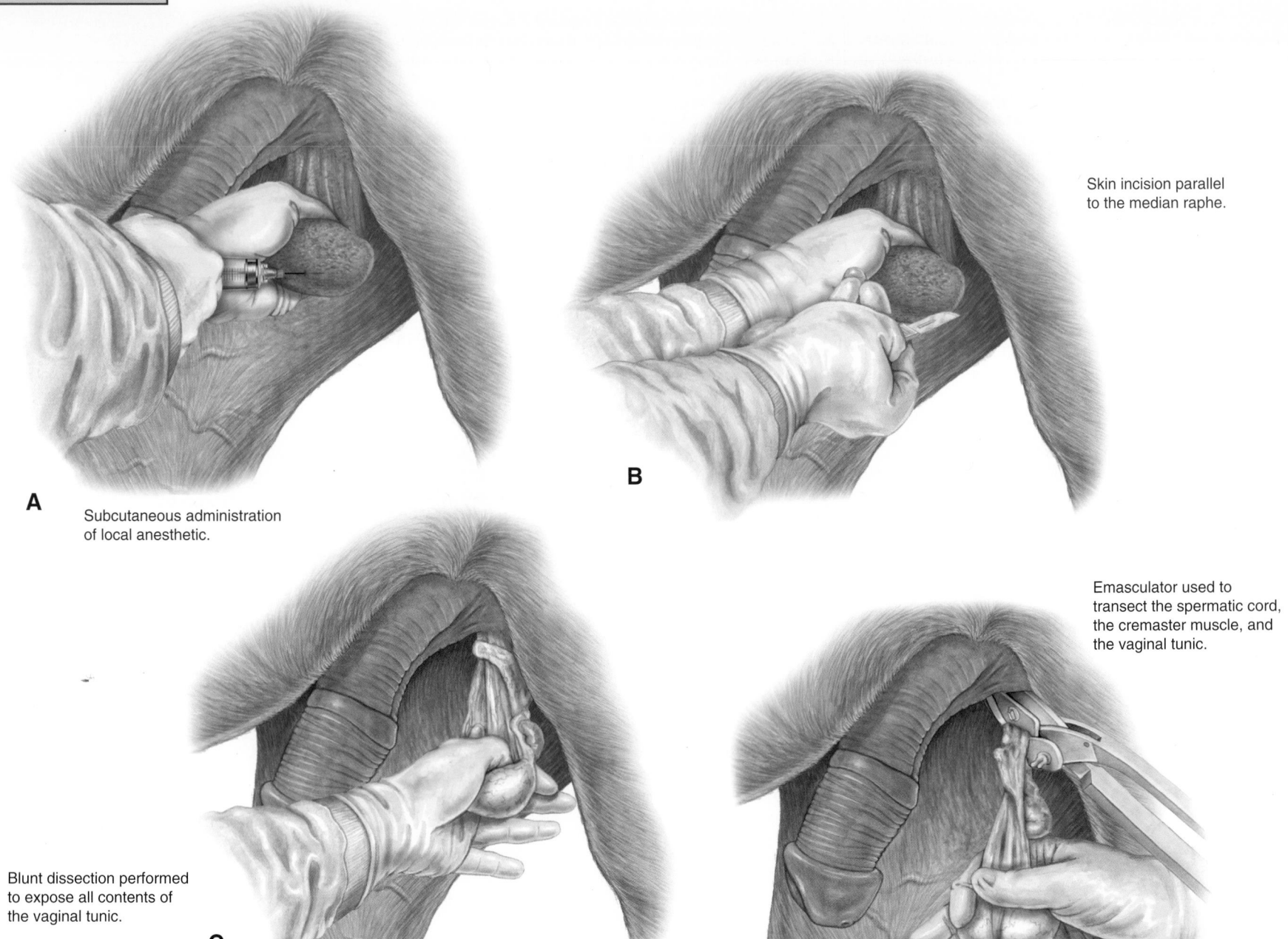

A Subcutaneous administration of local anesthetic.

B Skin incision parallel to the median raphe.

C Blunt dissection performed to expose all contents of the vaginal tunic.

D Emasculator used to transect the spermatic cord, the cremaster muscle, and the vaginal tunic.

fraction. This secretion is usually free from spermatozoa and averages about ten cubic centimeters in volume. The function of this fraction is to clean and lubricate the urethra prior to the ejaculation. Urine and debris are removed and the pH of the urethra is adjusted; therefore, a more suitable environment is available for the passage of sperm. When studied under a microscope, this presperm fraction contains the greatest concentration of bacteria and it should be discarded when collections are being made for artificial insemination purposes. It has been theorized that this fraction is secreted by the bulbourethral glands in addition to the prostate and vesicular glands.

The sperm rich fraction of ejaculate occurs when the glans penis swells to seal off the vagina. The volume of this fraction is usually about thirty to seventy-five cubic centimeters and contains about eighty to ninety percent of the total number of spermatozoa within the ejaculate. Most of the fluid within this secretion is secreted by the ampulla. The sperm rich fraction of the stallion also contains a high concentration of ergothionine which is a chemical agent that protects the sperm from the detrimental effects of chemical oxidation which occur within the semen. There are also two sugars, inositol and sorbitol, present within this fraction to support the energy supply to the sperm.

The sticky gel that is secreted by the seminal vesicles is noticeable when the penis collapses after ejaculation or after the stallion dismounts. This is called the "postsperm" fraction. This fraction will vary in volume from eight to eighty-five milliliters or may even be nonexistent in some samples. In other samples it is so extensive that it forms over twenty percent of the total ejaculate. This difference in volume is determined by several factors. One factor is a breed characteristic. Some breeds produce a greater gel fraction than other breeds. The second factor that involves the volume of the postsperm fraction is that of individuals with high libido. Lastly, the season of the year has a great influence on gel production. The postsperm or gel fraction is usually slightly more alkaline than the sperm rich fraction and contains a high level of citric acid. The gel fraction will contain about twelve to twenty percent of the total sperm cells, a

fact that should be considered when the gel fraction is filtered out for semen evaluation or artificial insemination. It is important to note that this gel fraction is usually filtered out when collecting for artificial insemination purposes. Studies have shown that the sperm survival is lower when the gel fractions are frozen with the sample than when gel-free samples are frozen for storage.

The tail end fraction results from an accesory sex gland secretion and contains very little gel and few, if any, sperm. Removal of this fraction upon collection improves the pregnancy rates with artificial insemination.

CASTRATION TECHNIQUES

There are many terms for the surgical removal of the testes. This surgical removal is referred to as castration, emasculation, gelding, cutting, and orchiectomy. Castration is one of the most commonly performed equine surgical procedures and its goal is to prevent or decrease aggressive temperament, sexual behavior, or reproduction by inferior stallions. During the castration procedure, not only are the testes removed but also eliminated are a major source of the circulating androgens responsible for male sexual behavior. Stallions may be gelded at any age and it is usually determined by a matter of convenience than by a specific chronological age. The period of time between one and two years of age is usually when the horses are castrated because this is when objectionable sexual behavior emerges. Some owners feel that the ideal time to castrate a stallion is when they are only a few weeks to a few months old. This is to avoid the nuisance of masculine behavior as the animal becomes more sexually mature. The time during the stallion's life when castration is performed is purely subjective.

When a stallion is being referred to as having been proud cut, a reference is made that the castration was not done properly; therefore, the gelding still exhibits some male sexual behavior. This sexual behavior may be exhibited as mounting with the

capability of copulation and ejaculation. Studies have been completed where geldings were compared after castration. No signigicant difference was noted between sexual and aggressive behaviors whether the stallions were gelded at less than two years of age or greater than three years of age. There are, however, a certain percentage of geldings that display a stallion-like sexual behavior and aggression toward other horses. This may be related to steroid metabolites originating from other sources in their body. When castrating a horse, it is difficult not to remove the entire testis and epididymis. The epididymis itself is incapable of producing testosterone in proud cut horses which means the epididymal tissue that is left in the horse could not produce any testosterone. The most logical theory in these cases is that the horses that are referred to as "proud cut" are possibly the result of a unilateral cryptorchiectomy rather than the result of a specific type of castration technique.

After castration, many geldings are still fertile. This is due to the fact that spermatozoa may remain in the ampulla and ductus deferens for some period of time after the surgical technique was performed. This fertility, however, is usually very low since most ejaculations that are collected within a week after castration are usually nonmotile samples.

Standing Castration Techniques

In order to perform a standing castration, a combination of sedation and local anesthesia must be utilized. Sedation or tranquilization should be performed with one or a combination of the following drugs: xylazine, acepromazine maleate, butorphanol tartrate, and/or detomide hydrochloride. After the surgical site is prepped, the area is anesthetized by subcutaneous infiltration of fifteen to twenty milliliters of a local anesthetic such as two percent lidocaine HCl. This is followed by a second administration of ten to fifteen milliliters into each spermatic cord. Some people advocate an administration of twenty to thirty milliliters of two percent lidocaine HCl directly into the parenchyma of each testes. The theory behind this is to allow a diffusion of the anesthetic agent proximally up the entire cord. This administration is usually more

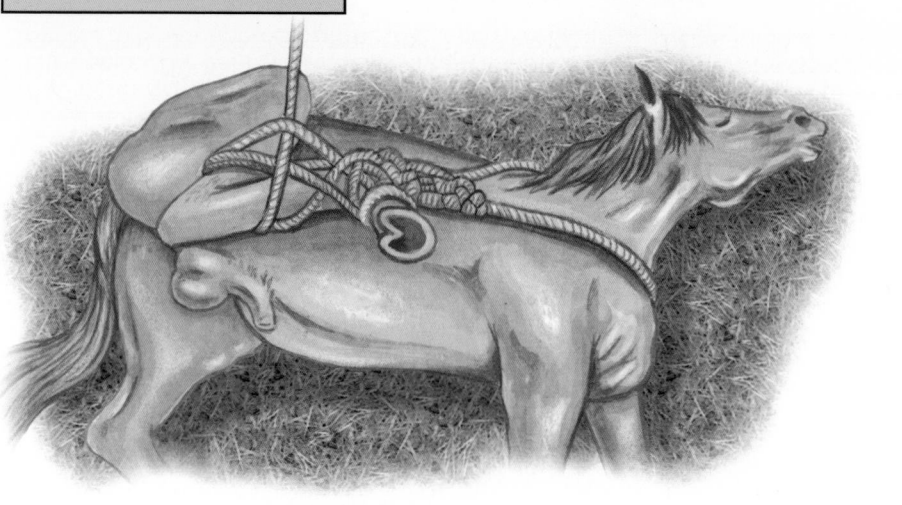

Anesthesized horse in lateral recumbent position.

Dual incisions are made in the scrotal sac equally parallel to the median raphe.

A

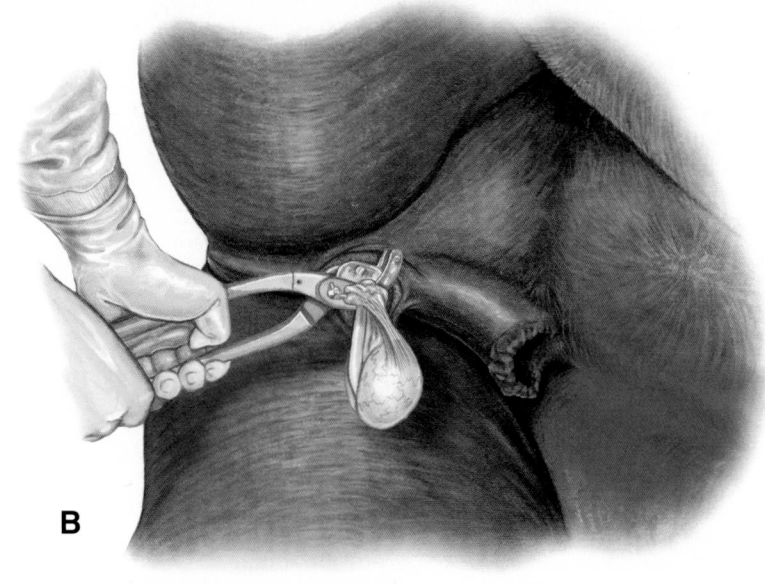

B

Use of the emasculator to transect the contents of the vaginal tunic.

C

Removal of the scrotal septum to provide better postoperative drainage.

difficult than that where the anesthetic agent is administered directly into the spermatic cord at a specific location. A twitch is usually applied, even though the animal is under tranquilization, while the administrations of these subcutaneous and inner spermatic cord anesthetics are accomplished.

To allow time for the local anesthetics to infiltrate the tissues, a more thorough and final surgical scrub is performed on the scrotal and inguinal areas. At least fifteen minutes should be allowed for the local anesthetic to infiltrate these tissues and to provide good analgesic action. The surgeon usually approaches from the left side and leans into the horse's side to avoid any type of sudden kicking by the stallion. The twitch is again applied, and it is important for the horse to be on good solid footing so that any sudden movement would not result in a loss of balance or falling.

It is at this point where a thorough exam can be performed of the testicles and spermatic cords to check for any possible abnormalities or inguinal hernias. Both testicles should be evident and immobilized by grasping with the left hand and squeezing them toward the base of the scrotum. Two parallel incisions are made at equal distances from the median raphe over the length of the entire testicle. These incisions are usually ten to fifteen centimeters long depending on the size of the testis. The incision is made through the skin, the tunica dartos, and the underlying scrotal fascia. If one chooses to perform an "open" castration, the common vaginal tunic is also incised. The caudal ligament of the epididymis which fixes the common vaginal tunic to the epididymal tail and attached testicle is then severed. The spermatic cord is transected close to the superficial inguinal ring with the use of an emasculator. The common vaginal tunic is not removed when an open castration is performed.

If a surgeon chooses to perform a "closed" castration, the common vaginal tunic is not incised except at the point of spermatic cord transection. All of the contents of the common vaginal tunic: the testicle, the epididymis, the spermatic cord, and the attached external cremaster muscle, are freed from the surrounding fascia by blunt dissection and are removed by transection close to the

superficial inguinal ring with an emasculator. There is a modification of this closed technique where a three to four centimeter longitudinal incision is made in the vaginal tunic proximal to each testicle. The left thumb is placed through the incision in the vaginal cavity and ventral traction is applied while the fingers of the hand force the epididymis and testicle through the incision. The testis and epididymis are exteriorized through this small incision and then transected with an emasculator near the superficial inguinal ring. The reason for this modification is that this technique allows observation of all the enclosed structures within the vaginal tunic.

During a closed castration procedure, the vaginal tunic and all associated structures are removed and the likelihood of an infection or a hydrocele is greatly decreased. If a scrotal or inguinal hernia becomes evident during the castration procedure, when using the closed technique of castration, simply placing a ligature around the spermatic cord proximal to the site of transection reduces the complication of exteriorizing the bowel.

Castration Technique in Lateral Recumbency

A variety of anesthetic agents can be used for this procedure. The animal is initially tranquilized with xylazine, acepromazine maleate, or detomide hydrochloride. After the animal is exhibiting signs of tranquilization and muscle relaxation, an IV administration of an ultrashort acting barbiturate or ketamine HCl provides good analgesia with smooth induction and recovery. Ketamine HCl will provide general anesthesia for approximately fifteen minutes.

Once general anesthesia is achieved, the animal is positioned in a lateral recumbency. The right handed surgeon would want, if possible, the horse to be in a left lateral recumbency. The assistant, during this procedure is usually up by the animal's head providing moderate pressure on the animal's neck and monitoring the animal's pulse and respiration rates.

The scrotal and inguinal areas are prepared aseptically by numerous applications of scrub and rinses of clean water. Before any incision is made, a thorough palpation should be initiated to check for any abnormalities or hernias. The neck of the scrotum is grasped with the left hand and both testicles are teased distally into the base of the scrotum. Two parallel incisions are made at equal distances from the median raphe in the same manner as that for a standing castration. An "open," "closed," or "modified closed" technique is utilized for the emasculator transection of the tissues. The scrotal septum is usually removed after the procedure is completed to provide better postoperative drainage.

Postoperative Care

Immediately before or after castration, the administration of both tetanus antitoxin and tetanus toxoid should be given to all animals not previously immunized with tetanus toxoid. Theriogenologists argue the point as to whether systemic antibiotics are necessary in this procedure. Years of practice has taught us that it is important to administer systemic antibiotics immediately before and for several days after the castration procedure. It is also important to administer analgesic agents such as phenylbutazone at least for the first few days of postoperative care. In addition to these recommendations, it is important that the animal receive a good amount of exercise. The stalls should be cleaned and the animals should be rested at least twelve to twenty-four hours post surgery. Thereafter, the animal should be exercised twice a day if possible to assist in drainage of the surgical area and prevent excessive edema within the scrotal and preputial tissues. The new gelding should be isolated from mares for at least three to four weeks after castration.

Artwork By S. Hakola / J. Dirig
Copyright Equistar Publications, Ltd.

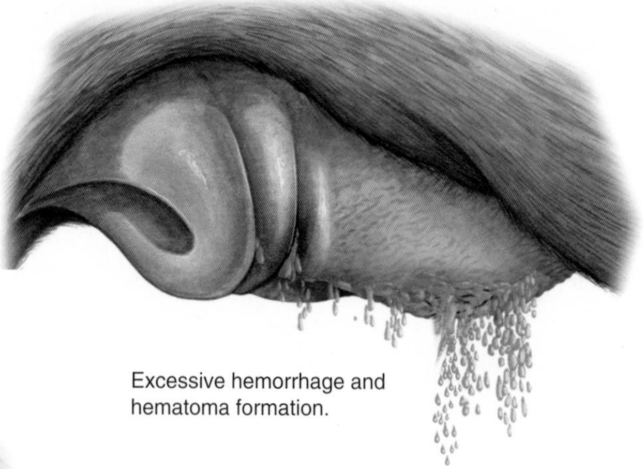

Excessive hemorrhage and
hematoma formation.

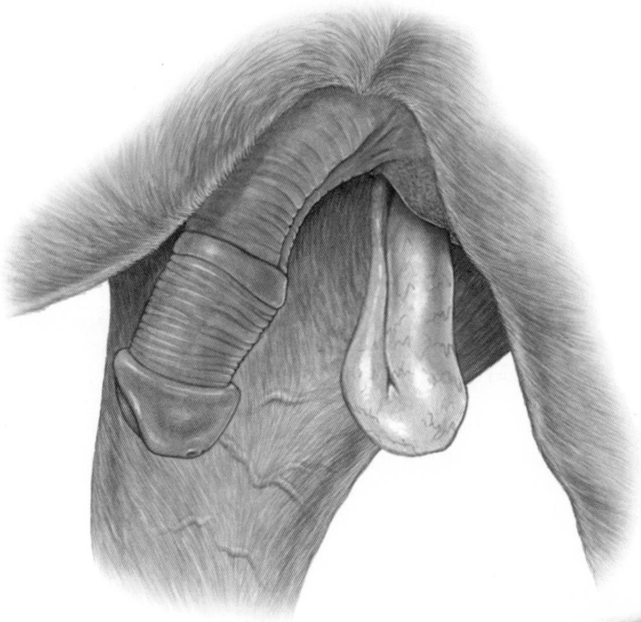

Evisceration of
intestine.

**Complications of
Castration**

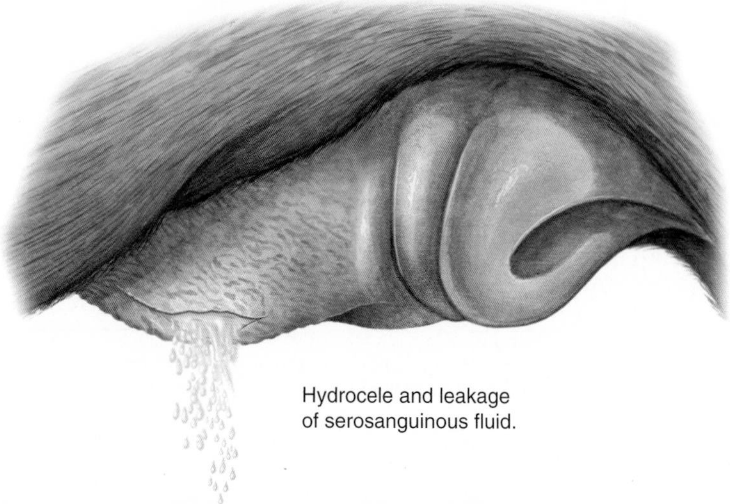

Hydrocele and leakage
of serosanguinous fluid.

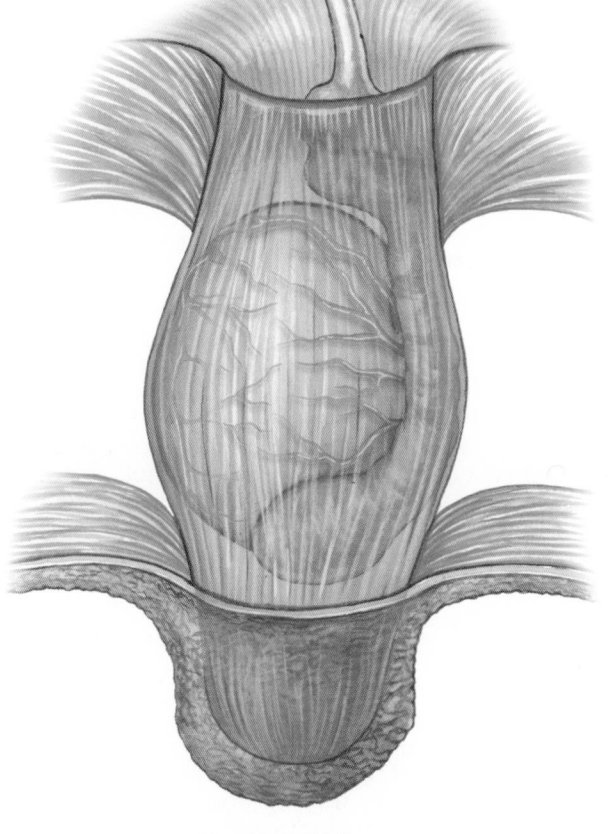

Cryptorchidism

Testis has passed through the internal
inguinal ring but not through the external
inguinal ring and scrotum.

Postoperative Castration Complications

Complications involved with castration include hemorrhage, edema, infection, hydrocele, varicocele, peritonitis, and evisceration.

The most common postoperative complication of castration is excessive hemorrhage. This is due to an improperly applied or a malfunctioning emasculator. The most significant source of this hemorrhage is the testicular artery; however, hemorrhage may come from the scrotal skin or the large pudendal vessels that occur in this area. If the origination of this hemorrhage is the testicular artery, it is necessary to reanesthetize the animal and provide hemostasis. If the source of the hemorrhage is from the scrotal vessels, this hemorrhage usually stops spontaneously.

It has been a traditional practice in the case of excessive hemorrhage to pack sterile gauze into the scrotal incision and up into the inguinal and scrotal cavities to facilitate hemostasis. This pack is then removed the following day if hemostasis is achieved. This procedure involves the complication of allowing infection to invade through this packing.

Edematous swelling of the prepuce and scrotum is expected following castration. There is usually no cause for alarm if it is not excessive. The cause of this edema is usually insufficient exercise after castration which results in poor drainage from the open scrotal incisions. If excessive swelling does occur, manual massage of the area or hydrotherapy will prevent the wounds from resealing prematurely and will decrease the swelling in the scrotum and the prepuce.

In some cases, postoperative swelling or edema is caused by bacterial infection. This infection is treated like any local wound. The area is rescrubbed, washed thoroughly, and drainage induced. The administration of local and systemic antibiotics are indicated with infections. These medications, along with physical hydrotherapy, will usually correct the problem.

Evisceration following castration is uncommon but when it does occur, it is usually fatal. This complication can occur up to one week postcastration but usually happens within a few hours of the operation. It is caused by a preexisting inguinal hernia that has gone undetected. If an intestine appears in the scrotal incision following castration, the horse should immediately be reanesthetized and repaired post haste. Before the intestine is replaced back into the abdomen, it should be thoroughly cleaned with copius amounts of normal saline solutions and replaced with great care. Ligatures should be transfixed to the edges of the superficial inguinal ring with absorbable suture. Systemic antimicrobial treatment should be initiated immediately to prevent peritonitis. Peritoneal taps should be obtained twenty-four to forty-eight hours later and evaluated for the development for possible septic peritonitis.

A hydrocele is a fluid-filled painless swelling in the scrotum. The fluid is a sterile amber-colored fluid that can be aspirated by a needle and examined. In most cases, the fluid fills the vaginal tunic and can become quite large in size. The condition of hydrocele occurs in just castrated horses as well as intact stallions. The technique of "open" castration predisposes this condition as the vaginal tunic is not removed during the open castration method. The only correction for this condition is to reanesthetize the animal and surgically remove the vaginal tunic.

A chronically infected spermatic cord stump is called a scirrhous cord and can be caused by any number of bacteria or fungi. This scirrhous cord adheres to the scrotal skin and usually includes many drainage tracts. It is painful upon palpation and may be the cause of a hindlimb lameness. The only treatment for this is surgical removal. The animal is usually placed under general anesthesia in a dorsal recumbency. The cord is isolated and totally removed. The wound is left open to heal by second intention and postoperative care is the same as that for a routine castration.

CRYPTORCHIDISM

In a stallion where one or both testes are in a location other than the scrotum, this, by definition, is a cryptorchid. The common term for this disorder among horsemen is "ridgling." A "high flanker" refers to a condition when the testis has passed through the vaginal ring but is not within the abdomen. "Abdominal cryptorchidism" is when the testis remains in the abdominal cavity.

The clinical history of these animals can vary a great deal. The animal may visually appear as a gelding but have no history of having been castrated. This is usually accompanied by an animal with a very difficult disposition.

Clinical examination of the horse's scrotal area can be difficult to perform. Visual examination alone is inadequate because a stallion can temporarily retract the testes into the inguinal region through a contraction of the cremaster muscles.

It is often useful to tranquilize the animal before external palpation is attempted. Both testicles should be readily palpable within the scrotum. If a testis is absent on a particular side, the superficial inguinal ring should be located and explored digitally to locate this testis. The deep inguinal ring can be palpated rectally just beyond and lateral to the pelvic rim.

Ultrasonography offers a diagnostic technique helpful in the diagnosis of incomplete retention and positive location of an abdominal testis. Transcrotal scanning will determine the location of the testis within the canal whereas transrectal scanning will provide positive identification of a testicle within the abdomen.

There are many theories as to the causes of cryptorchidism. The descent of the testis is a very complex process which offers a great variation in its final result. Theories include the following: overstretching of the gubernacular cord, an inadequate growth of the gubernaculum and related structures (such as the vaginal ring and the inguinal canal), and

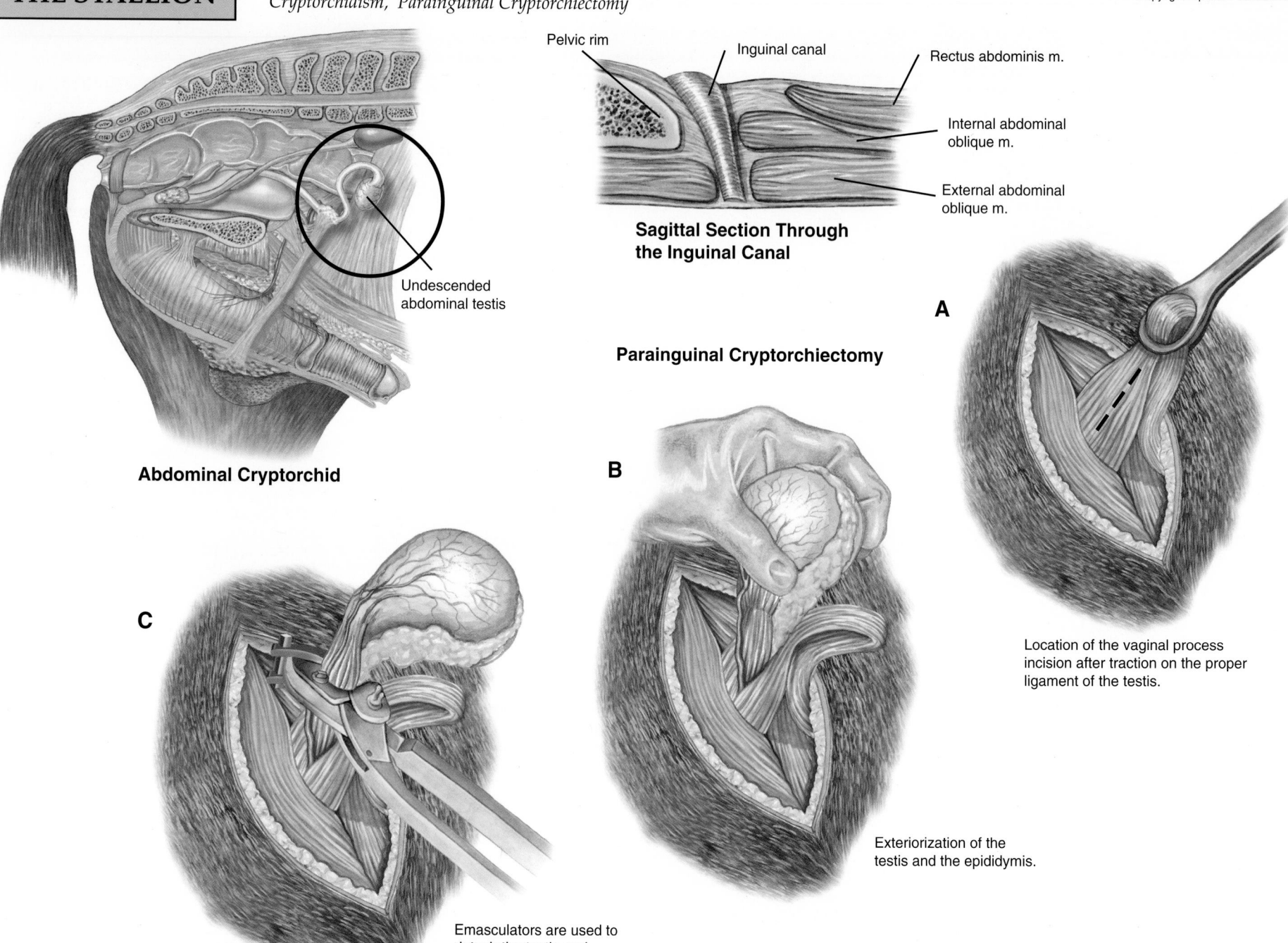

Pelvic rim

Inguinal canal

Rectus abdominis m.

Internal abdominal oblique m.

External abdominal oblique m.

Sagittal Section Through the Inguinal Canal

Undescended abdominal testis

Abdominal Cryptorchid

Parainguinal Cryptorchiectomy

A

Location of the vaginal process incision after traction on the proper ligament of the testis.

B

Exteriorization of the testis and the epididymis.

C

Emasculators are used to detach the testis and the epididymis.

displacement of the testis in the pelvic cavity.

A genetic basis for cryptorchidism has been reported numerous times in scientific research literature. There have been studies to indicate that this trait is transmitted by an autosomal dominate gene and an autosomal recessive gene. It has been suggested that the condition of cryptorchidism has resulted from abnormal sex chromosome complements. In each and every case, the data that has been provided so far does not provide a clear cut inheritance pattern for cryptorchidism in stallions. It is quite conceivable that more than one pattern of inheritance exists genetically as well as mechanically.

Diagnosis Through Blood Tests

By determining the testosterone concentration within a serum sample, a tentative diagnosis of cryptorchidism can be established. This procedure is accomplished with a pair of blood samples. One is initially obtained and another approximately two hours after the intravenous injection of six thousand international units of human chorionic gonadotropin. True geldings have concentrations of testosterone less than forty pg/ml whereas cryptorchids have concentrations of testosterone in excess of one hundred pg/ml. Care must be taken to use a good laboratory for these analyses because such small amounts of testosterone are being measured. It would be very easy to have a result fall in the middle of the range of data, which creates a false positive.

The only treatment for cryptorchidism is the removal of the retained testis through surgery. The animal should be placed in dorsal recumbency with the hind legs covered but left completely free. When the animal is in this position, it is easy to examine the inguinal region for the presence of scars which may indicate that a previous incision has been made. The location of the scar may indicate what surgical procedures have been previously attempted.

Under general anesthesia, palpation of the inguinal region is possible through digital manipulation. It is also possible to lie behind the animal and perform a rectal palpation that was not possible while the animal was in a standing position.

Surgical Technique for an Inguinal Cryptorchid

The inguinal and scrotal area of the horse is surgically prepped for sterility. The surgeon either stands or kneels directly behind the horse with the hind legs of the horse on each side. An incision is made through the skin in the area where the scrotum should be (directly over the superficial inguinal ring.) Blunt dissection is then used to exteriorize the vaginal process through the inguinal fascia to the superficial inguinal ring. Care must be taken to avoid the external pudendal vein which is in this area. This approach will result in less hemorrhage from the skin vessels and the inguinal fat does not have to be displaced or incised to reach the superficial inguinal ring. The testis is usually found within the inguinal ring and enveloped by the tunica vaginalis. All the structures should be exteriorized and then removed with an emasculator in a technique similar to that of a closed castration. If the testis on this side has previously been removed, the surgeon will find the partially incised spermatic cord within the inguinal canal. Care should be taken to examine this spermatic cord for any epididymal or testicular tissue that was left behind during the previous operation.

In a case of a partial abdominal cryptorchid, often times the vaginal process and a closed epididymis are found in the inguinal canal. Using an inguinal approach, these structures can be identified for surgical removal. The proper ligament of the testis can be identified where it attaches to the epididymal tail. This can be isolated through surgical instrumentation and then traction applied to this ligament while dilation to the vaginal ring is applied digitally. In this case, the testis is gradually retracted through the vaginal ring and into the inguinal canal. Here it can be exteriorized along with its attached epididymis and be emasculated.

In the case of a complete abdominal cryptorchid, the vaginal process is usually completely within the abdomen, but there are times when traction can be applied to the gubernaculum and cause its eversion into the inguinal canal. After the gubernaculum is identified, traction upon this structure with surgical instrumentation could aid in everting the vaginal process, much like a winding wench. Once exteriorized, the vaginal process can be incised and the epididymis and attached testis can be emasculated.

If all of these techniques fail, a finger can be inserted into the abdomen through the internal abdominal oblique muscle and peritoneum cranial to the vaginal ring. This area is then explored for the proper ligament of the testis or the scrotal ligament. If this ligament can be hooked with a finger, again traction can be used to exteriorize the structures needing removal.

If all of the above techniques fail, the parainguinal approach is necessary. Whenever the superficial inguinal ring or peritoneal opening has been stretched and manipulated greater than an inch in diameter, sutures should be placed within these structures to prevent evisceration.

Surgical Approach to an Abdominal Cryptorchid

The parainguinal approach utilizes a skin incision made medial and parallel to the superficial inguinal ring. The aponeurosis of the external abdominal oblique muscle is incised medial to the vaginal ring along the ring's cranial aspect. The next structure encountered will be the internal abdominal oblique muscle which is separated, in the direction of its fibers, to allow one to two fingers into the abdomen. The peritoneum is then incised and the region around the vaginal ring is explored for the gubernaculum, epididymis, or deferent duct. These structures are all connected to the testis by the proper ligament of the testis. Traction placed on these structures will lead the surgeon to the testis and allow exteriorization. In utilizing any abdominal procedure for cryptorchid surgery, the smallest possible opening should be made in order to prevent complications within the abdomen. In extreme cases, it is necessary to enlarge the incision to allow the entrance of the entire hand within the abdomen. After removal of

Artwork By S. Hakola / J. Dirig
Copyright Equistar Publications, Ltd.

Scrotal Trauma

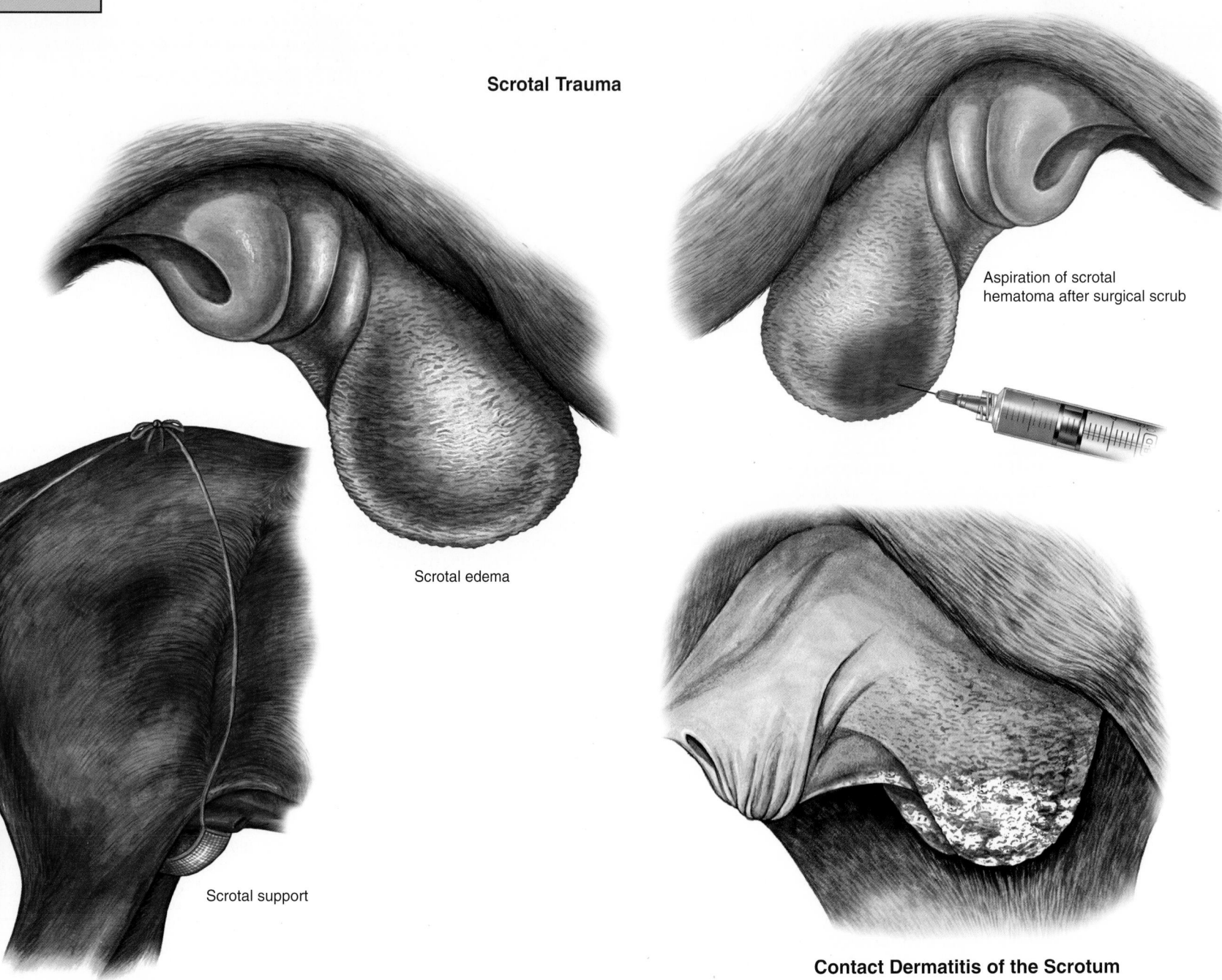

Scrotal edema

Scrotal support

Aspiration of scrotal
hematoma after surgical scrub

Contact Dermatitis of the Scrotum

the testis and epididymis, each layer is closed routinely in whatever suture pattern the surgeon so desires.

Flank and suprapubic paramedian approaches for the removal of cryptorchid testes have been described. These approaches may be necessary when there is an unusually large abdominal testis such as one affected by neoplasia. A standing flank approach is a possibility when general anesthesia is not feasible. In almost all cases, the inguinal or parainguinal approach provides a successful avenue for this surgery.

SCROTAL DISORDERS

The scrotum of the equine is well concealed between the hind limbs. Anatomically, this provides protection from physical injury except during copulation. Examination of the scrotum is done not only visually but through palpation. This is normally done without sedation. Any lesions or suspicious areas on the scrotum can be further investigated by ultrasonography or infrared thermography. These diagnostic procedures will provide the examiner with a thorough evaluation of these lesions, the degree of involvement, and the extent to which these lesions affect adjacent tissues.

Infrared thermography, which measures the amount of infrared radiation being emitted from the surface of a particular tissue structure, can be utilized as a noninvasive diagnostic procedure. These dermatone patterns depict abnormal increases or decreases of the surface temperature of the scrotum. Any degree of asymmetry within the thermal gradients found on the scrotal surfaces indicates an underlying change. Since normal spermatogenesis and epididymal functions are dependent on scrotal temperatures, the technique of infrared thermography has an obvious prognostic value.

SCROTAL TRAUMA

Etiology

The most common cause of scrotal trauma in a stallion is the blunt trauma resulting from a kick during mating. This usually results in contusions, lacerations, edema, hemorrhage, inflammation, and secondary bacterial infections.

Diagnosis

In order to perform a thorough examination of the tissues, the animal should first be tranquilized. The extent of injury can then be evaluated with comfort to the patient and less risk to the examiner. The examination begins on the scrotal surface where abrasions, lacerations, and puncture wounds would occur. Palpation of the deep tissues should then be performed to further evaluate the extent of the trauma.

It is often difficult to diagnose the difference between scrotal edema and scrotal hemorrhage. Aspiration with a needle will allow this differentiation. Thorough examination of the inguinal rings should be accomplished prior to needle aspiration in the event of the possibility that the scrotal swelling is due to a scrotal hernia. Scrotal hemorrhage becomes organized into a clot and forms fibrous tissues. These fibrous tissues eventually develop into adhesions which could possibly immobilize the testicle within the scrotum and interfere with the scrotum's ability to conduct thermoregulation. Changes in the circulatory pattern within these tissues could also lead to tissue degeneration, atrophy, and further decrease in thermal regulatory ability.

Treatment

Treatment of acute scrotal trauma is aimed at controlling the inflammatory reaction and reducing edema and hematoma formation. Systemic administration of nonsteroidal antiinflammatory medications and diuretics are useful in the treatment of scrotal trauma. Systemic administration of antibiotics should also be considered as a prophylactic measure. These modalities of treatment are certainly warranted, but the application of sound physical therapy techniques will also provide efficacious results. Basic cold therapy is not only the most inexpensive treatment that can be applied but is probably the most effective. Cold therapy can be applied every two to three hours throughout the day at twenty minute intervals. Cold packs can be applied to these tissues and held in place by a scrotal support. Massage of these tissues during the application of cold or immediately afterward mechanically reduces the edema. Topical applications of antibiotic cream and emollients help soothe the skin and provide antimicrobial activity.

Scrotal lacerations should be dealt with in a similar matter to any other laceration of the horse. The area should be thoroughly cleaned, debrided of any extraneous tissues, and closed surgically whenever possible. These lacerations usually result in a great deal of edema and inflammation and should be treated accordingly. Topical and systemic administrations of antimicrobial medications should be immediately initiated and a tetanus toxoid booster should be given.

CONTACT DERMATITIS OF THE SCROTUM

Contact dermastitis of the scrotal skin is the result of unsanitary conditions, the application of chemical irritants, fly bites, and *Onchocerca cervicalis*. Filthy conditions within the stall allow a build up of manure that can irritate and scald the delicate scrotal skin. This is easily remedied through a change in husbandry procedures. Fly sprays, disinfectants, various shampoos, and grooming products may also result in a localized

THE STALLION

Disorders: Testicular Habronemiasis, Testicular Trauma, 180 Degree Testicular Torsion

Artwork By S. Hakola / J. Dirig
Copyright Equistar Publications, Ltd.

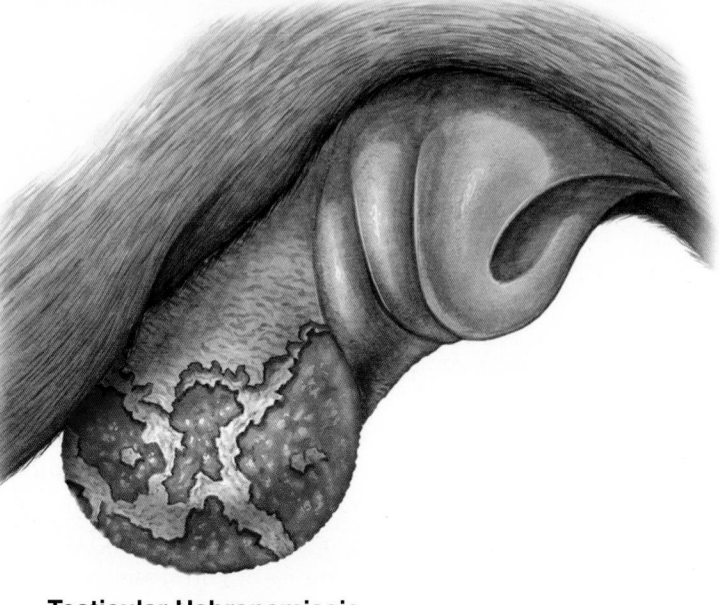

Testicular Habronemiasis

Normal testicular anatomy

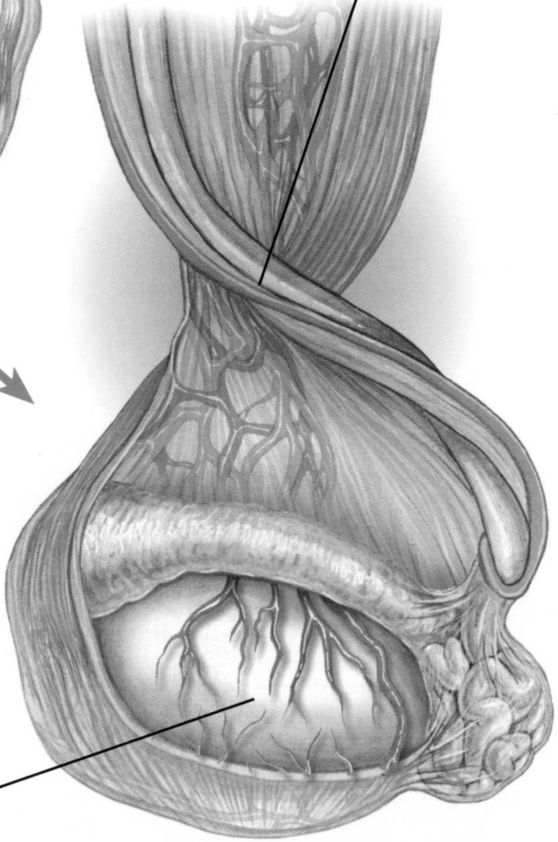

Area of inflammation without vascular compromise

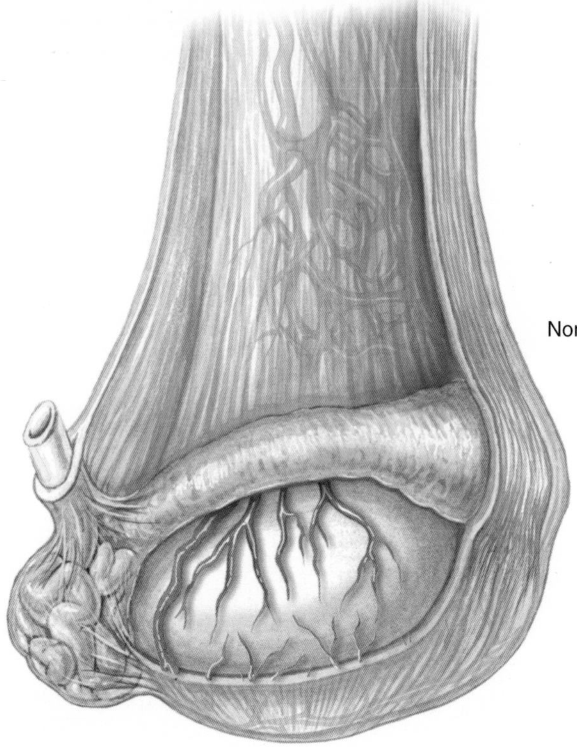

**180 Degree Testicular Torsion
(Torsion of the Spermatic Cord)**

Torsed testis

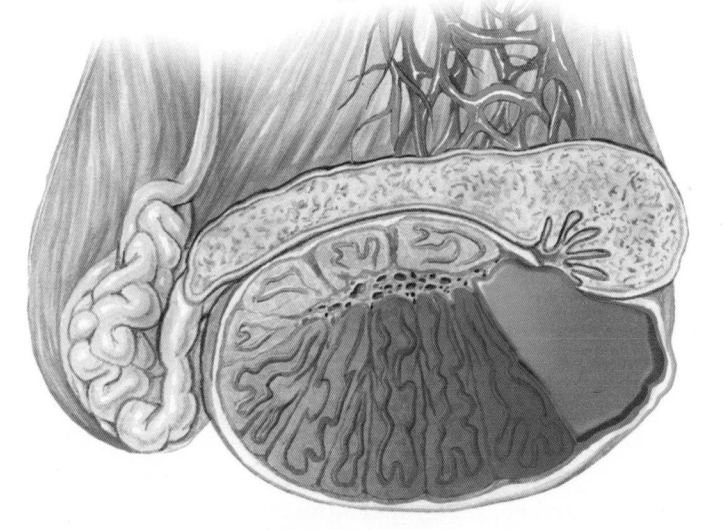

Testicular Trauma

inflammatory reaction of the scrotal skin. Eliminating further contact with the irritating substances prevents recurrences of dermatitis.

Onchocerca cervicalis is a parasite that localizes within the skin and can result in a mild scrotal dermatitis. It is actually the microfilariae of this parasite that produces these lessions. In most cases, it is not just the scrotum that is involved, but the entire ventral midline of the horse from the chest to the inguinal area. *Culicoides* is the vector of *Onchocerca* and the biting of this parasite will also cause a scrotal irritation. Ivermectin is the treatment of choice for this condition. When this medication is administered, it usually results in a local transient edematous swelling of the scrotal wall and ventral midline of the abdomen. Often times, these areas become infected and treatment to prevent these secondary infections is indicated.

CUTANEOUS HABRONEMIASIS (SUMMER SORES)

The common house fly and stable fly provides a vector for this parasitic skin disease. The house fly, *Musca domestica*, or stable fly, *Stomoxys calcitrans*, deposit larvae upon the moist body surfaces such as eyes, prepuce, penis, and scrotum. These infective larvae are the result of the following parasites: *Draschia megastoma*, *Habronema muscae,* and *Habronema microstoma*. Deposited larvae produce a pruritic granulomatous tissue reaction within the scrotum. A differential diagnosis must include cutaneous habronemiasis, neoplasms, and sarcoids.

NEOPLASIAS AND SARCOIDS OF THE SCROTUM

In older grey horses, it is not uncommon to find melanomas in the perianal and scrotal areas. These tumors arise from the skin and are potentially metastatic in nature. Sarcoids are nonmetastatic cutaneous tumors that are particular to the horse. They are commonly found on the head, limbs, and the ventral surface of abdomen, including the scrotum.

DISORDERS OF THE TESTES

TESTICULAR TRAUMA

There are two forms of trauma to the testes. Lacerations generally occur from a severe blow to the scrotum or direct blunt trauma. During the incidence of blunt trauma, a hematoma could result in an extravasation of blood into the testicular parenchyma.

When a laceration of the testis occurs, there is extensive hemorrhage within the tissues. When a testis is so affected, its sperm-producing potential is greatly reduced. Therefore, when the laceration is severe, unilateral castration is generally the treatment of choice. If this procedure is not acceptable, the animal should be placed under general anesthesia. The wound is cleansed, debrided, and closure of the tissues should be attempted surgically. Care must be taken with each layer of tissue to minimize the number of adhesions within these tissues that could interfere with thermal regulation of the testes.

When blunt trauma results in a hematoma within the testis, the integrity of the testicular capsule (the tunica albuginea) remains intact. Due to the vascularity of the testicular tissue, considerable hemorrhage will result within the testicular parenchyma. This can result in severe necrosis of these testicular tissues coupled with a complete loss of the testicular function.

Diagnosis

Ultrasonography is the most reliable noninvasive diagnostic method utilized in the diagnosis of testicular hematomas. Testicular tissue is homogenous; whenever an intratesticular hemorrhage or hemotoma occurs, a focal anechoic or hypoechogenic area will occur on the ultrasonogram.

Treatment

The treatments of choice for testicular hematoma are either hemicastration or systemic treatment with antiinflammatory and antimicrobial medications. If left untreated, the testis will undergo irreversable degeneration and become nonfunctional. The opposite testicle will undergo a compensatory hypertrophy. The determining factor indicating castration would be if the hemorrhage and consequent hematoma is contained within the tunica albuginea. If the hematoma occurs in the surrounding tissues, then castration could possibly help preserve the thermoregulatory mechanism.

TESTICULAR TORSION (TORSION OF THE SPERMATIC CORD)

Etiology

When there is rotation or twisting of the spermatic cord, there is an interference with the vascular supply to the testis. This results in an ischemic necrosis within the testis. It is actually not a disorder of the testis but is a torsion of the spermatic cord. Most spermatic cord torsions range from one hundred and eighty to three hundred and sixty degrees with the clinical signs exhibited by these dependent on the degree of torsion.

The etiology behind spermatic cord torsion is poorly understood. It is theorized that there is an elongation of the caudal ligament or the proper ligament of the testis which predisposes the animal to a spermatic cord torsion.

Clinical Signs

Clinical signs that occur with spermatic cord torsion vary depending on the degree of the torsion. In the case where the torsion is approximently one hundred and eighty degrees, the animal may not exhibit any clinical symptoms. There may be no pain or semen abnormalities present. It is possible that torsions of this degree

Artwork by S. Hakola / J. Dirig
Copyright Equistar Publications, Ltd.

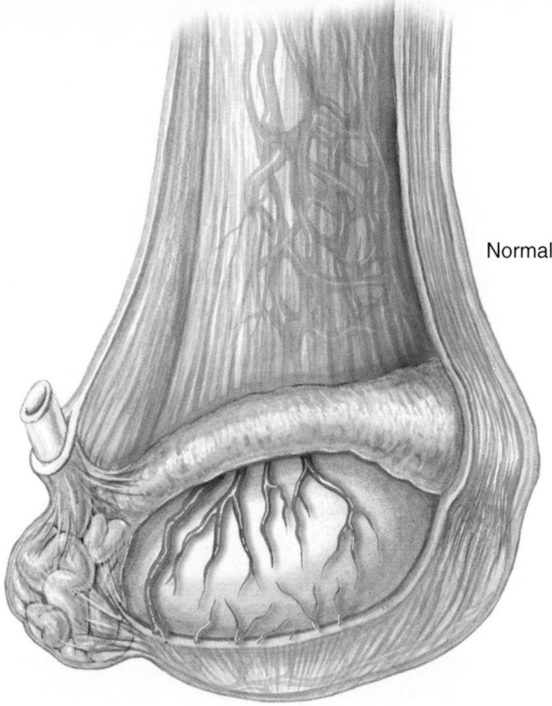

Normal testicular anatomy

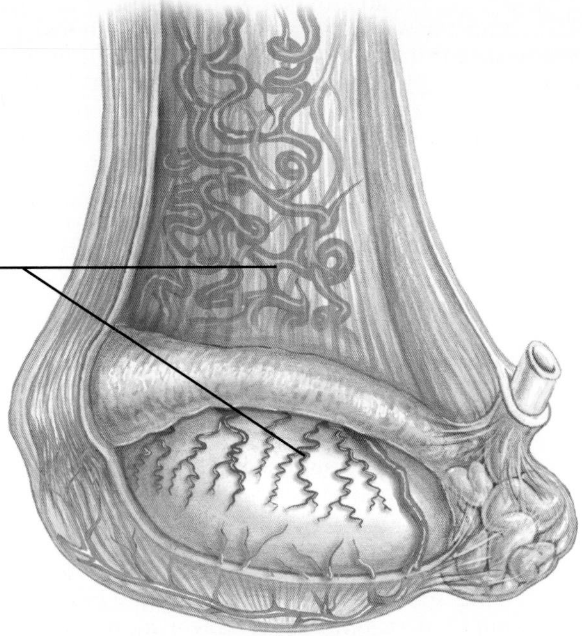

Tortuous venous structures

Varicocele

360 Degree Testicular Torsion (Torsion of the Spermatic Cord)

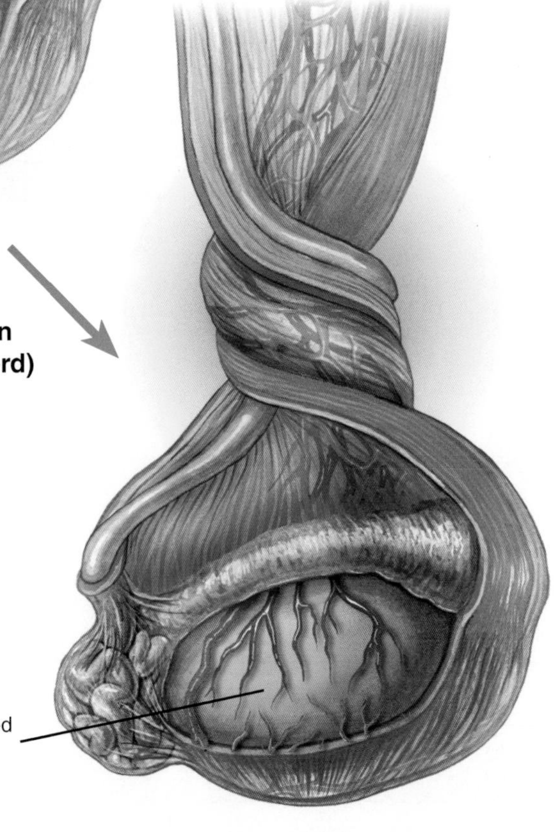

Torsed testicle with impaired vascular flow to structures distal to torsion.

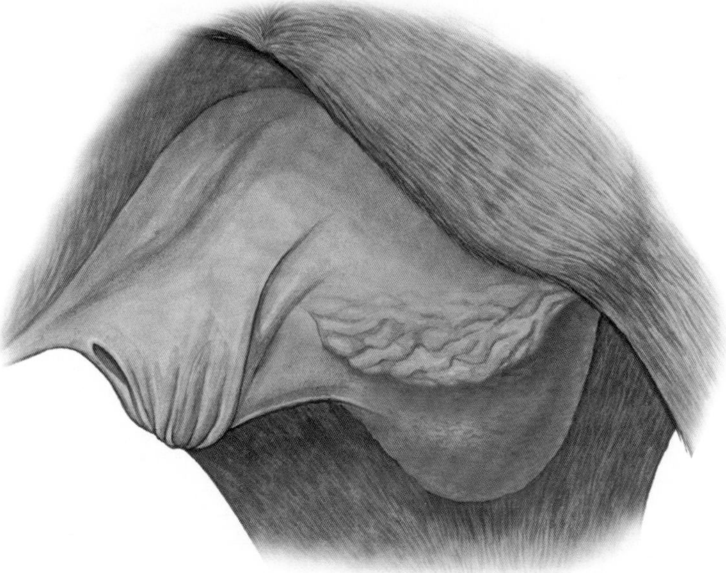

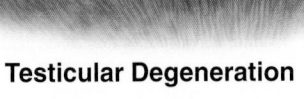

Testicular Degeneration

only exhibit intermittent scrotal pain that occurs for only short periods of time. It may be necessary to examine this animal on repeated occasions in order to diagnose this condition. Although the stallion may appear clinically normal and his semen sample appear within normal limits, it is often noted that these animals are reluctant to mount the mares or the collection dummy. It is possible that pain is only elicited during the mounting activity and therefore may be the only clinical sign evident.

Acute severe scrotal pain and localized edema and hemorrhage are present when there is a three hundred and sixty degree spermatic cord torsion. The animal exhibits symptoms of colic and lameness. This three hundred and sixty degree torsion results in a severe compensation of the circulation within the pampiniform plexus which results in possible hemorrhage and edema.

Diagnosis of Testicular Torsion

The diagnosis of one hundred and eighty degree torsion is relatively easy and can be accomplished through palpation on a normal genital exam. The caudal ligament of the epididymis and the cauda epididymis is normally located at the caudal pole of the testis. When these two structures are palpated within the cranial scrotum, there is a one hundred and eighty degree testicular torsion. These two structures are palpated in their proper scrotal positions with a three hundred and sixty degree torsion of the spermatic cord. However, other clinical signs such as pain, hemorrhage, and edema allow a diagnosis of the three hundred and sixty degree torsion. The testis itself will be painful and somewhat enlarged and the spermatic cord will be thick and edematous. Differential diagnosis for this condition should include an inguinal/or scrotal hernia.

Treatment

In most cases, it is not necessary to treat one hundred and eighty degree spermatic cord torsions. The testicle is manipulated back into its proper position manually. Mild tranquilization may be necessary in order to accomplish this procedure. In the animal that chronically torses, it

may be necessary to perform an orchiopexy. While the animal is under general anesthesia, a skin incision is made in the scrotum directly over the intended site of the epididymal tail. The torsion is then manually reduced and an incision is then made in the parietal tunic. The proper ligament of the testis is exposed through this tunic and then sutured to the adjacent tunica dartos. The vaginal tunic and scrotal skin are then sutured.

When there is a three hundred and sixty degree torsion, the recommended treatment is castration. The affected testes are usually damaged to such degree that their removal is the only feasible treatment. Because of the extreme pain and the edema within these tissues, it is imparative that surgery be completed as soon as possible after the diagnosis.

VARICOCELE

This condition depicts the distended and tortuous veins of the pampiniform plexus. Clinically, this appears as an abnormal thickening around the scrotal neck on the affected side. Varicocele is diagnosed upon digital palpation of the neck of the scrotum during the genital exam. The dilated tortuous vessels can be palpated and may extend several inches on the affected side. Varicocele is usually not painful and typically does not interfere with breeding performance. In severe cases, thrombosis has been reported. Varicocele with thrombosis can have an affect on the breeding performance and pain can often be elicited.

The only treatment available for this condition, especially when a thrombosis is present, is castration. A unilateral castration can be attempted when only one side is affected, thus preserving the fertility of the stallion.

TESTES DEGENERATION

Degeneration of the testes has numerous etiologies. When any of these causes occurs, there is damage to the germinal epithelium, allowing a testicular degeneration, which results in infertility or a subfertile state within the stallion. The most common causes of this testicular degeneration are

thermal injury, systemic or local infection, injury to the testicular vasculature, testicular tumors, age, and various drugs such as anabolic steroids.

Testicular degeneration can affect one or both testes. It can be temporary or permanent, depending on the severity and other etiological factors.

Diagnosis

Diagnosis begins with a good history so that one may differentiate testicular degeneration from testicular hypoplasia. In a case of testicular degeneration, there is a marked reduction in testicular size and consistency. The tunica albuginea becomes wrinkled and feels thickened as the testicle reduces in size. Testicular hypoplasia results in a slightly small testicle with normal turgidity and consistency. In the case of testicular degeneration, the epididymis will feel large when compared with the testicle. Testicular hypoplasia can be congenital or aquired since hypoplastic testes have an increased suseptibility to degenerative changes. They are hard to differentiate on physical exam and even upon examination of the semen. Testicular degeneration, however, may be reversible.

Treatment

The treatment of testicular degeneration is directed at removing the etiology causing the degenerative changes. Examples of this would include curing the systemic or local infection, discontinuing exogenous anabolic steroid administration, and simply lowering the fever that may be responsible for this condition. Treatment with gonadotropin-releasing hormone (GnRH) has been shown to be efficacious in improving semen quality in aged stallions.

Testicular size and consistency should be evaluated along with semen quality on a monthly basis to determine continued testicular improvement or degeneration. It will take several months before a normal spermatogenic function will be restored after removal of the causative degenerative factor.

Embryonal Carcinoma

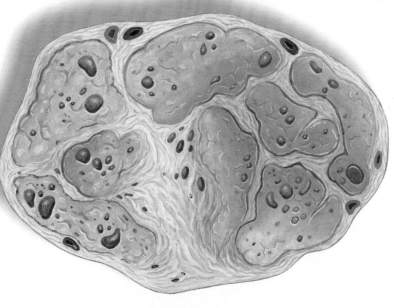

Leydig-cell Tumor

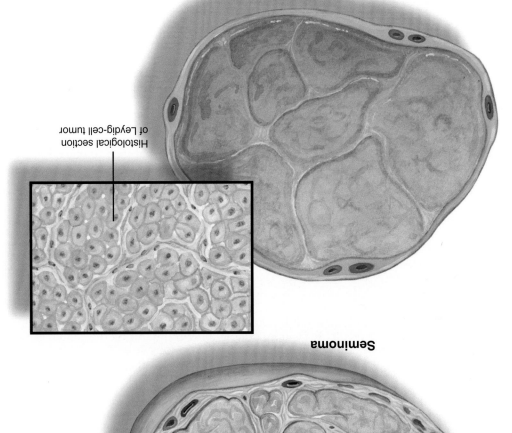

Histological section
of Leydig-cell tumor

Teratoma

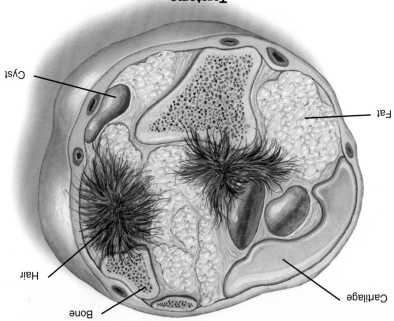
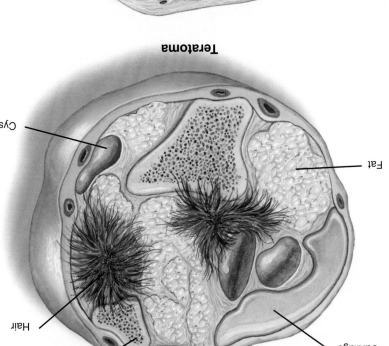

Cyst

Fat

Hair

Bone

Cartilage

Seminoma

Testicular Tumors

THE STALLION

TESTICULAR NEOPLASIA

The incidence of testicular neoplasia in a stallion is very rare, yet it cannot be statistically measured because most male horses are castrated when they are very young. Testicular neoplasms can be classified as either germinal or somatic depending on their cells of origin. Those neoplasms that originate from germ cells include seminomas, teratomas, and embryonal carcinomas. Those neoplasms that originate from nongerminal or somatic cell origin include Leydig-cell tumors, Sertoli-cell tumors, lipomas, and fibromas. Although the predisposing factors have not been established, cryptorchid testes have a much higher incidence of neoplasia in the stallion. Testicular tumors are usually unilateral in nature and should always be regarded as potentially malignant.

Diagnosis of testicular neoplasms should start with a thorough physical examination of the scrotum and its testicular contents. Since most tumors are unilateral, the normal testis should be palpated first through its entire length as well as its accompanied epididymis. The suspected enlarged testis should then be palpated for dimensions, consistency, and sensitivity to pain. The affected testis is usually heavier and harder in nature and remains freely movable within the scrotum. Ultrasonography will reveal the extent and dimension of testicular masses that may be undetectable through palpation. In the case of a cryptorchid, transrectal ultrasonography should also be utilized if a tumor is suspected or merely for evaluation of the undescended testis. Rectal palpation should also include all of the pelvic and abdominal organs and lymph nodes that can be evaluated.

If further diagnosis is required, the animal should be placed under general anesthesia and a biopsy performed of the affected testis. Care must be taken to avoid intratesticular hemorrhage. One should also be aware of the fact that in conducting this procedure, there is an increased potential for dissemination of the testicular tumor.

Castration is the treatment of choice for all testicular neoplasms regardless of their type. Since most tumors are unilateral in nature, unilateral castration is recommended so that the stallion can remain a viable breeding animal. This procedure should be done after the breeding season has been completed since the remaining testis will undergo a compensatory hypertrophy following the unilateral castration. Care must be taken during this procedure to handle the affected testes as little as possible to avoid iatrogenic metastasis.

SEMINOMA

Seminomas are the most commonly reported testicular tumor in the stallion. They arise from the germinal cells of the seminiferous tubules. Even though they are the most common tumor reported in the stallion, fortunately they are relatively benign. They invade the local tissue by spreading through intratubular and extratubular pathways. However, the tunica albuginea restricts this tumor's expansion. In most cases, the metastasis of seminomas to the thoracic and abdominal cavities can be traced to an iatrogenic cause. Large multiple lobules are seen on gross visual inspection of seminomas. They are grey-white in color, and are divided into smaller lobules by thick fibrous trabeculae. Diagnosis of seminomas are based on histological findings.

TERATOMAS

Teratomas are germinal cell in origin as they are derived from pluripotential germ cells. These complex tumors will be composed of all sorts of recognizable tissues that are not native to the testes. These tissues will include bone, cartilage, and even skin. They can be identified upon gross examination since they are multilocular structures found within the testes that contain a variety of tissues not normally found there.

EMBRYONAL CARCINOMAS

This tumor is rare in the horse and is also derived from pluripotential germ cells. This tumor is usually malignant. It differs from the teratomas in that these tumors have poorly differentiated germ cells, whereas teratomas contain only mature germ cell tissue.

LEYDIG-CELL TUMORS

This is an interstitial cell tumor as this tumor gains origin from the androgen-producing Leydig cells of the testicular interstitium. Diagnosis of these rare tumors is usually accomplished through the use of ultrasonography. These tumors are typically soft, oval, homogenous, and surrounded by a thin capsule. Definitive diagnosis of this tumor is based solely on a histological exam.

SERTOLI-CELL TUMORS

These are rare tumors in the horse. They arise from the somatic elements of the seminiferous epithelium. It has been reported in man that Sertoli-cell tumors usually secrete estrogen resulting in feminization. There is very little data available on the stallion and this feminizing tendency has not been reported. This tumor is locally expansive, grey to white in color, and is usually very firm. When they are large enough, their presence can be palpated digitally upon examination of the testis. A diagnosis of this tumor is made possible through histopathological examination.

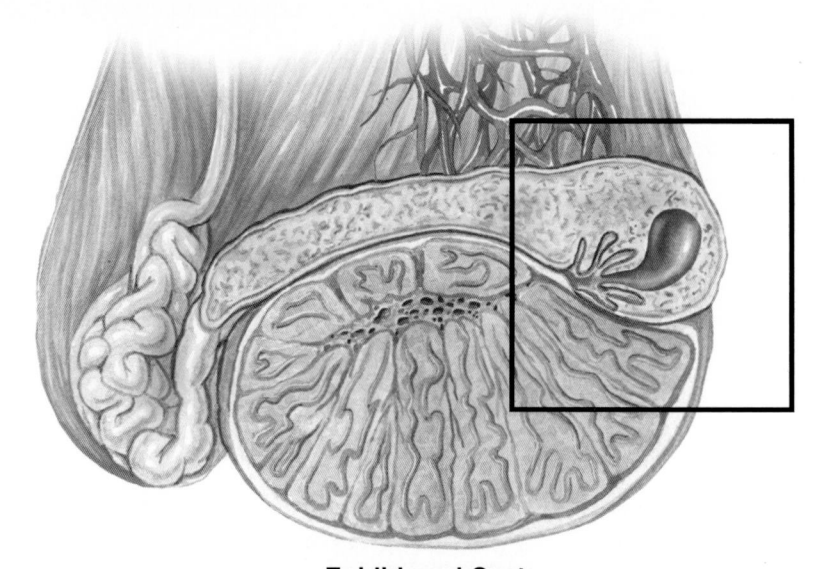

Epididymal Cyst

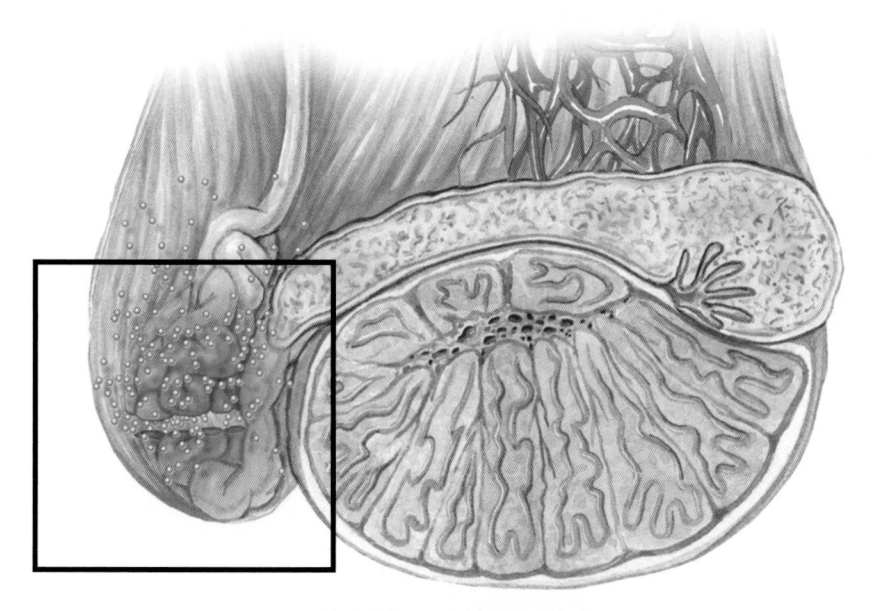

Epididymal Laceration

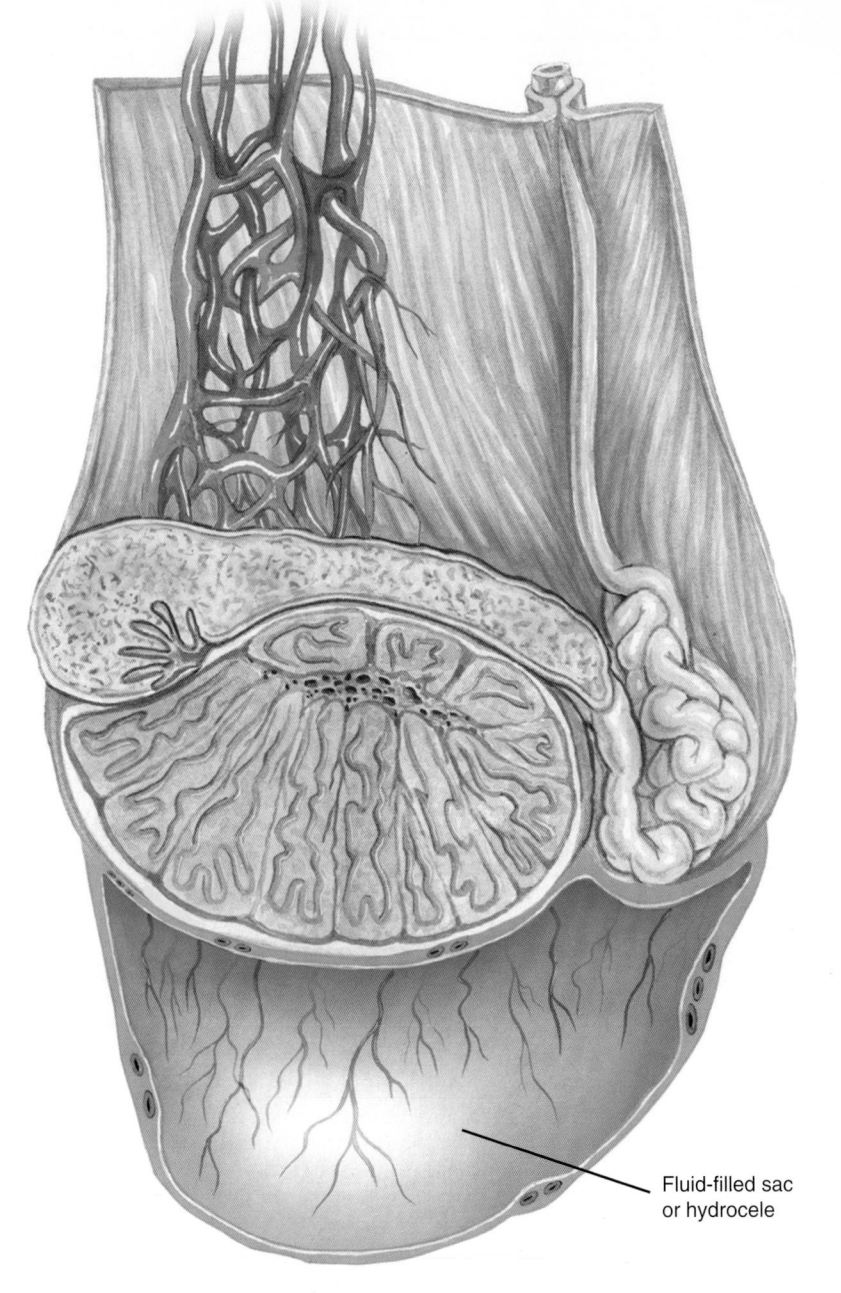

Fluid-filled sac
or hydrocele

Hydrocele

DISORDERS OF THE EPIDIDYMIS

All disorders of the epididymis are rare in the stallion. These disorders can be divided into three categories: congenital, physical, and infectious. The epididymis can usually be palpated digitally in the tranquilized stallion. In some cases, ultrasonography will reveal a definitive diagnosis.

EPIDIDYMAL CYSTS

This is a congenital disorder that develops in the blind vestiges of the extratesticular rete tubules (or mesonephric tubules), the blind cranial portion of each mesonephric duct, or detached segments of the mesonephric tubules. The lumina of all these tubules and ducts are lined with secretory epithelium, therefore allowing cystic dilation to occur. These circumscribed masses are usually palpable near the head of the epididymis at the craniodorsal aspect of the testicle. The significance of these cysts is that they usually do not interfere with the epididymal transit of spermatozoa. However, these blind tubules and ducts can become impacted with spermatozoa leading to local sperm granuloma formation.

PHYSICAL DISORDERS OF THE EPIDIDYMIS

There are three physical disorders that affect the epididymis: lacerations or trauma, thermal injury, and torsion of the spermatic cord.

Trauma to the scrotum can cause small lacerations within the epididymal tissue even when the trauma was nonpenetrating through the scrotal tissue. Laceration of the epididymis results in extravasated spermatozoa that will produce a granulomatous reaction. These are very difficult to diagnose and are usually only diagnosed through the use of ultrasonography. The first clinical sign is a swelling within the scrotum. It is very difficult to determine the cause of this swelling after traumatic insult. Unfortunately, the only treatment for this is

unilateral castration, including the removal of the lacerated epididymis.

Any etiological factor responsible for the increase in the local temperature of the epididymal tissue will interfere with spermatogenesis and impair the transit of epididymal spermatozoa. The mechanism behind this phenomenom is not clear, but it is similar to thermal insult to the testis.

Whenever there is a torsion of the spermatic cord, there is an interference within the vascular supply to the tissues distal to the torsion. This decreased vascularization results in ischemic necrosis. Therefore, any torsion of the spermatic cord will automatically result in a pathological change within the epididymal tissue.

EPIDIDYMIS INFECTIONS

Infections within the epididymal tissues usually occur secondarily to systemic infections within the horse. This can be secondary to a urinary tract or associated genital gland infection or even be the sequelae to a more generalized infectious disorder. Epididymitis is clinically manifested by a localized edema, pain, and a fever. Systemic treatment should be initiated immediately utilizing both antiinflammatory and sensitive-specific antimicrobial agents.

DISORDERS OF THE TUNICA VAGINALIS

There are two multifactorial disorders associated with the tunica vaginalis. The condition referred to as hydrocele and herniation of the bowel through the inguinal rings are both conditions involving the tunica vaginalis.

HYDROCELE

The term hydrocele simply refers to an abnormal collection of fluid between the visceral and parietal layers of the tunica vaginalis. This condition can be a sequelae from an inflammatory reaction

causing scrotal edema or it can occur without concurrent scrotal edema.

Etiology

The etiology of this fluid collection can be understood when one realizes that the vaginal cavity communicates directly with the peritoneal cavity. Therefore, any condition resulting in ascites within the abdomen could result in a transfer of this abdominal fluid into the vaginal cavity resulting in a hydrocele.

When aspirated, this fluid is usually serous in nature. This can be logically deducted then as a response to trauma to the visceral or parietal vaginal tunics. In almost all cases, these tunics are affected bilaterally. Unilateral hydroceles have been observed, however.

Diagnosis

Digital palpation of the scrotal contents can lead to an initial diagnosis of hydrocele. It will feel like a small fluid-filled sack, and it is generally not painful unless it is distended in size. Ultrasonography will evaluate the extent and dimensions of this fluid-filled area. A definitive diagnosis can be reached with needle aspiration of fluid from the vaginal cavity.

Treatment

Removal of the underlying cause of the hydrocele is the preferred treatment of choice. If the fluid is drained from the vaginal cavity, through the use of needle aspiration, it usually reaccumulates within a short period of time unless the etiology for the hydrocele is corrected.

Mild cases of hydrocele usually do not affect fertility within the stallion. However, accumulation of a significant amount of fluid greatly affects the thermal regulatory capabilities of these structures which ultimately results in a decline of semen quantity and quality. If the hydrocele is unilateral in nature and persists despite conservative treatment attempts, unilateral castration is indicated.

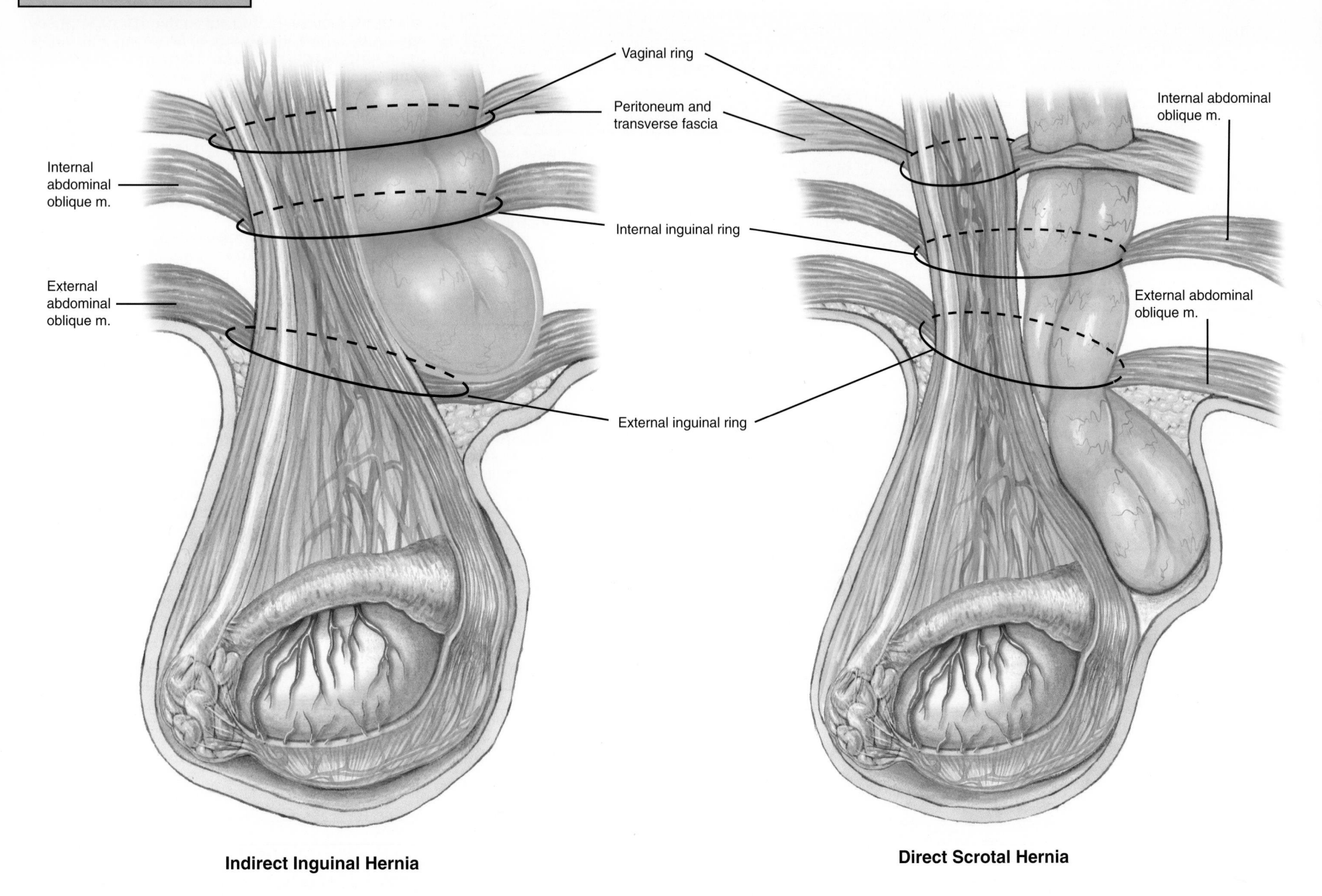

Vaginal ring

Peritoneum and transverse fascia

Internal abdominal oblique m.

Internal inguinal ring

Internal abdominal oblique m.

External abdominal oblique m.

External abdominal oblique m.

External inguinal ring

Indirect Inguinal Hernia

Direct Scrotal Hernia

INGUINAL HERNIATION

The terms inguinal or scrotal hernia are used to describe a protrusion of any portion of the abdominal viscera into the inguinal canal or scrotum. It is termed "inguinal" only if the viscera extends into the inguinal canal between the vaginal and external inguinal rings and "scrotal" if the viscera extends beyond the external inguinal ring and actually enters the scrotum. The portion of bowel that is usually herniated is the small intestinal tract. This condition can occur in either sex but is most commonly seen congenitally in colts and as an acquired condition in the adult stallion. There is a specific breed precedent for this condition. Arabians, Tennessee Walkers, Standardbreds, and American Saddlebreds seem to have a higher incidence than other breeds. Logic indicates that this congenital condition may be genetically inherited.

Etiology

The etiologies of herniation in the horse are congenital and acquired. Congenitally, the hernia will be present at birth or develop soon afterwards as a result of large vaginal rings. This could be caused by an excessive outgrowth of the extra-abdominal portion of the gubernaculum which results in a vaginal process with an unusually wide neck. Acquired herniation may develop following trauma such as a fall or result after breeding or exercise. Congenital hernias can be unilateral or bilateral and usually appear as a scrotal type. Clinically, they appear soon after birth as a viscera-filled scrotum. Manual reduction for these hernias can be accomplished and often times these do not recur. In some cases, these hernias reduce spontaneously over the first twelve weeks of life.

Treatment

Treatment of congenital hernias rarely requires surgery. Conditionally, a conservative form of therapy consists of manually reducing the herniated viscera several times daily. If the hernia persists after a few days of this treatment, a bandage can be applied after the hernia is reduced to apply pressure over both inguinal rings. Care must be taken not to provide pressure on the penis or to cover the anus. This bandage should be checked at least twice daily to ensure that herniation has not recurred. Acquired hernias occur in the adult usually in response to an incident of trauma. Clinically, these animals exhibit acute abdominal pain which can often be mistaken as a colic. Care must be taken in the diagnosis of inguinal hernias since palpation of viscera in the scrotum is not possible. A rectal examination will reveal viscera entering the vaginal ring. In most cases, strangulation of the visera results from the contraction of the muscles surrounding this anatomical area.

These acquired hernias require immediate treatment. It is possible, under heavy sedation, to reduce this hernia by externally massaging the entrapped viscera to gain reduction back into the abdominal cavity. Visceral retraction can be attempted per rectum while the horse is under general anesthesia while a second assistant performs external massage. The disadvantage to these nonsurgical reduction procedures is that it does not permit any evaluation of the herniated contents.

The ideal way to reduce the hernia is through surgery. In this case, the horse is placed under general anesthesia in a dorsal recumbency. The inguinal area and ventral midline are aseptically prepped. The incision is made over the external inguinal ring on the affected side and extended through the subcutaneous fascia to isolate the vaginal sack. An incision is performed longitudinally along the parietal tunic with care being taken not to incise the underlying viscera. The incision is then extended proximally to the external inguinal ring exposing the spermatic cord and the hernia. Upon examination of the viscera, if it is determined that these tissues are viable, they are immediately returned to the abdomen through the vaginal ring. Any portion of the bowel that has suffered irreversible vascular damage needs to be resected. Exteriorization of this portion of the bowel can be done through the superficial inguinal ring or through the ventral midline incision. An anastomosis of the remaining bowel should be performed and the viscera returned to the abdomen.

In most cases, the testis is removed from the affected side. If one tries to salvage the testis, there is a risk of reherniation. During this castration procedure, the vaginal sack is ligated and transfixed to the external inguinal ring. After this transfixion, the spermatic cord is then transected with an emasculator distal to the ligature. The external inguinal ring is then sutured as a guard against reherniation.

The inguinal fascia and skin should be left open to heal or it can be sutured if the incision is not long. If a midline incision was necessary, it should be closed in routine fashion. The remaining testis should still be fertile, and the stallion can still be used for breeding. There is an argument present discussing the heritability of inguinal herniation. Therefore, caution should be used in using these animals for breeding purposes.

DISORDERS OF THE ACCESSORY GLANDS

There are four accessory genital glands found in the stallion: the paired seminal vesicles, the paired ampullae, the bilobed prostate gland, and the paired bulbourethral glands. These accessory genital glands secrete substances which not only act as a vehicle for spermatozoal transport to the uterus, but also have a number of physiological functions.

BACTERIAL INFECTIONS

Etiology

The etiology of bacterial infections within the accessory genital glands include an ascending infectious urethritis, infectious cystitis, an expansion of an infectious epididymitis or orchitis, and the systemic spread of a generalized infection. The bacteria that are usually involved include *Pseudomonas aeruginosa*, *Klebsiella pneumoniae*, *Streptococcus* spp., *Staphylococcus* spp., and *Brucella abortus*. Bacterial infections can involve all four accessory genital glands; however, the vesicular glands are the most frequently affected.

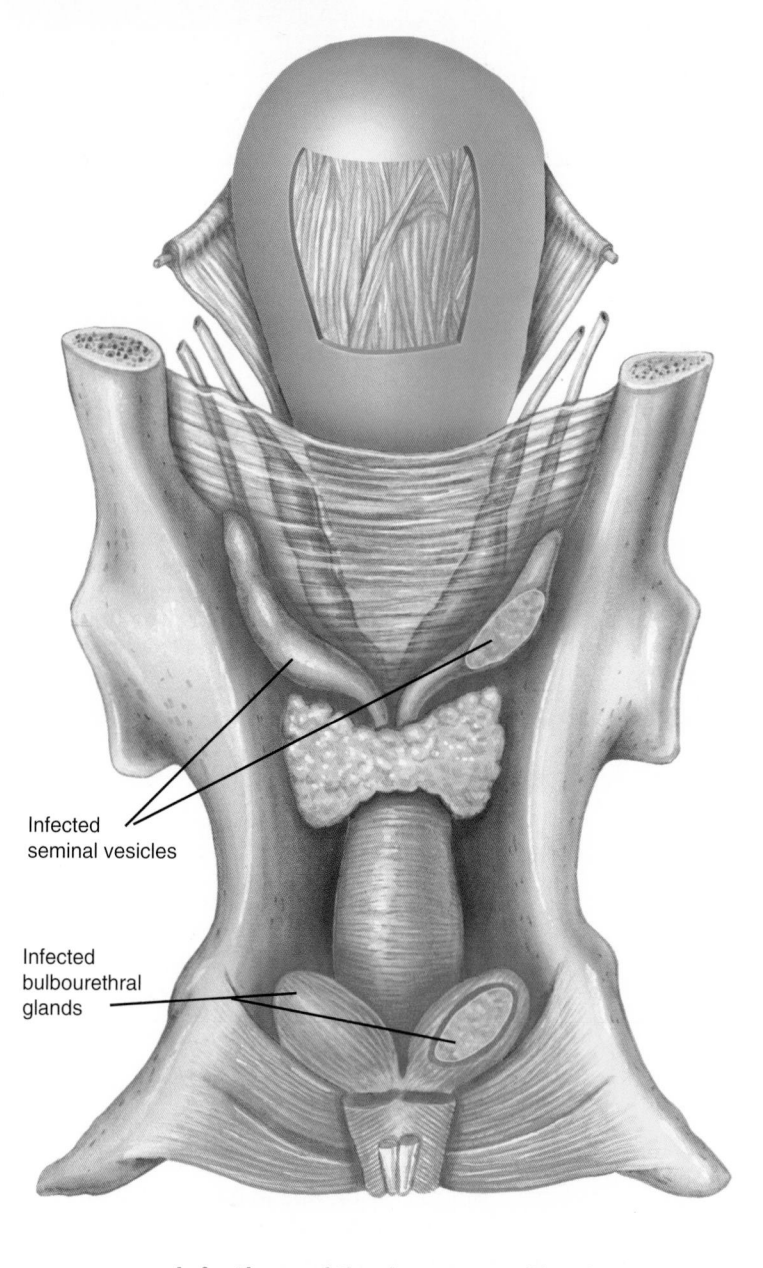

Infected seminal vesicles

Infected bulbourethral glands

Infections of the Accessory Glands

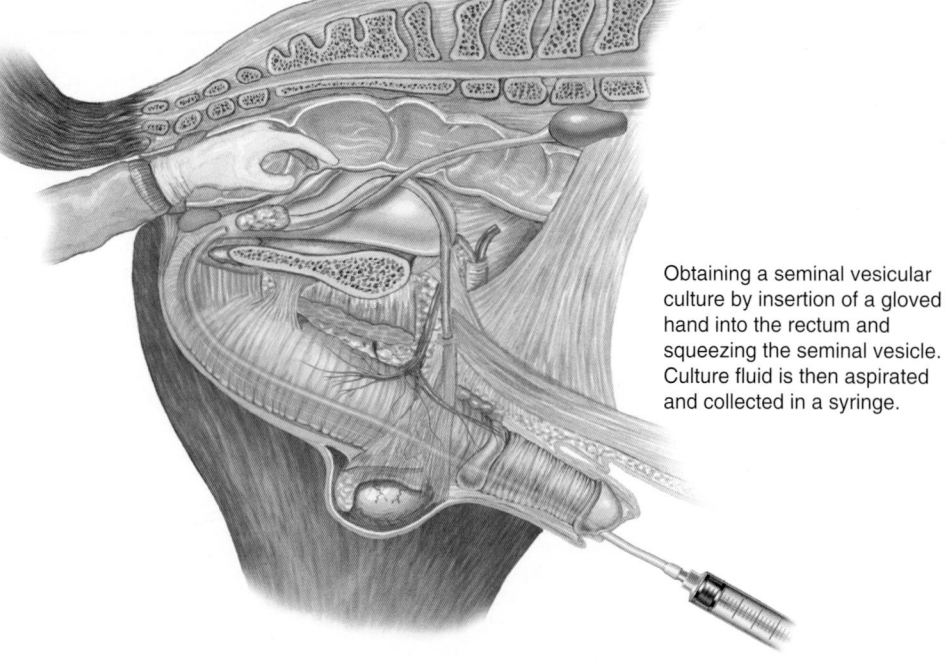

Obtaining a seminal vesicular culture by insertion of a gloved hand into the rectum and squeezing the seminal vesicle. Culture fluid is then aspirated and collected in a syringe.

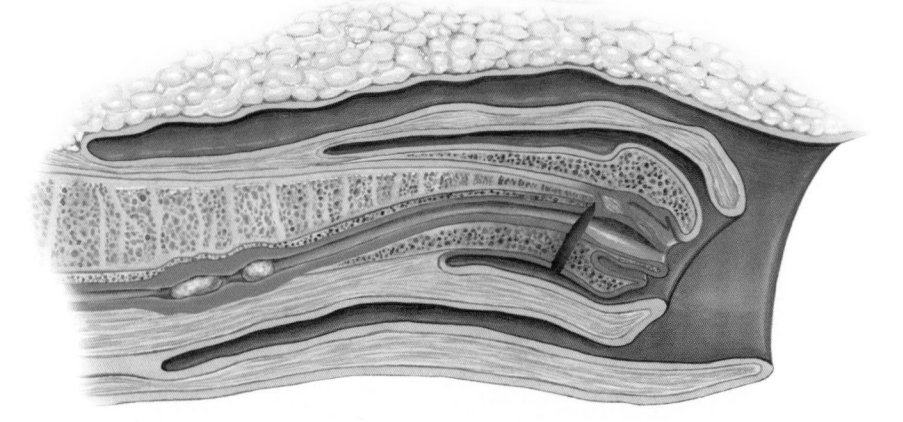

Urethral Calculi and Laceration of Urethra and Glans Penis

Clinical Signs

Clinically, these bacterial infections exhibit very few overt signs. The affected stallions are afebrile and usually exhibit no symptoms of pain through urination, defecation, or breeding. During systemic bacterial infections that are affecting the accessory genital glands; however, these animals are febrile and are usually reluctant to breed or ejaculate.

Diagnosis

The diagnosis of a bacterial infection within the accessory genital glands is made through gross and microscopic analysis of the semen which may appear blood-tinged and contain a high level of neutrophils and other purulent material. Bacterial cells may also be visualized microscopically.

Whenever an abnormal semen sample is discovered, a thorough genital exam is warranted. Examination of the accessory genital glands is usually done via rectal palpation which may reveal enlarged, firm, and lobulated vesicular glands. It is possible for this to be either unilateral or bilateral in nature. The vesicular glands can be further evaluated using ultrasonography and fiberoptic examination. All of the other accessory genital glands are difficult to evaluate by any diagnostic technique including rectal palpation.

Culture and cytological examination of the vesicular gland fluid is possible, whereas fluid collection from the prostate or ampullae is difficult to obtain. In order to get a good culture from the vesicular glands, the stallion should be teased for approximately fifteen minutes in order to fill the vesicular gland lumina with secretions. The distal end of the penis is then washed with surgical scrub, rinsed, and dried. A sterile one hundred centimeter catheter with an inflatable cuff is then passed into the urethra until its tip is immediately caudal to the seminal colliculus. The proper placement of this catheter is aided via rectal palpation. The cuff of the catheter is then inflated, and the fluid within the suspected vesicular gland is expressed by manual compression of the gland via the rectum. This fluid is then collected in a sterile container from the catheter opening at the urethral orifice. Using this technique, sterile samples can be submitted for culture and antimicrobial sensitivity.

The fluid from the bulbourethral glands can also be collected for evaluation. The stallion is teased until he gains an erection. The distal end of the penis is again washed, rinsed, and dried. While the stallion is still sexually excited, the glans penis is rubbed briskly in order to stimulate the release of clear preejaculatory fluid from the bulbourethral glands. Using this technique, it is difficult to distinguish a bacterial urethritis from an infection of the bulbourethral glands.

Treatment

Bacterial infections of the accessory genital glands have two consequences. There is a high degree of transmission of these bacteria to the mare during natural mating. This will lead to a myriad of problems involving infertility within the mare. Secondly, bacterial infections within the accessory genital glands can result in infertility within the stallion. Systemic antimicrobial treatment, even based on accurate culture results, is usually ineffective in resolving bacterial infections within the accessory genital glands. This is due to the inability of most antibiotics to diffuse into the lumen of the accessory genital glands. It is possible to instill antibacterial drugs into the lumina of the vesicular glands using a small diameter catheter passed through the urethra to the opening of the vesicular gland at the seminal colliculus. This catheter can be placed through the utilization of the biopsy channel of an endoscope. The catheter will allow lavage techniques and then infusion of specific antibacterial drugs into the lumen of each gland.

If infections within the accessory genital glands cannot be corrected, the stallion's breeding life may be extended through the use of minimal contamination breeding techniques. Artificial insemination programs allow the semen to be placed in seminal extenders containing antibiotics. Natural service programs require that the uterus be infused immediately before and four hours post-breeding with an antimicrobial solution. Antibacterial drugs can also be infused for one to three consecutive days postovulation.

DISORDERS OF THE URETHRA

There are three disorders that affect the urethra. They are physical damage to the urethra caused by trauma, infectious disorders, and a toxic disease that could irritate the urethra.

URETHRAL TRAUMA

Etiology

Trauma or physical damage to the urethra can occur many different ways. The urethra can be traumatized bluntly or with a penetrating wound such as a laceration or a bruise from a kick to the penis during breeding. Ischial damages can occur when any physical constriction is applied to the shaft of the penis. Iatrogenic injury to the urethra may occur during urethral catheterization or improper endoscopic passage. Cicatrization is the healing process that leaves a scar which is referred to as a cicatrix. Any indirect damage to the urethra may result in a focal cicatrization which is inelastic scar tissue that will tear repeatedly at the time of breeding because it can no longer dilate in response to engorgement of the corpus spongiosum penis. The resulting hemorrhage is then allowed to be mixed with the ejaculate.

Trauma to the urethra lumen can also be caused by calculi that are large enough to become lodged during transit. These calculi will result in a pressure necrosis to the tissues and a subsequent scarring of the mucosa. During the condition of cutaneous habronemiasis, there is cause for the surgical removal of the distal portion of the urethral process during treatment. This surgical removal will also result in a proliferation of scar tissue at the excision site.

Artwork by S. Hakola / J. Dirig
Copyright Equistar Publications, Ltd.

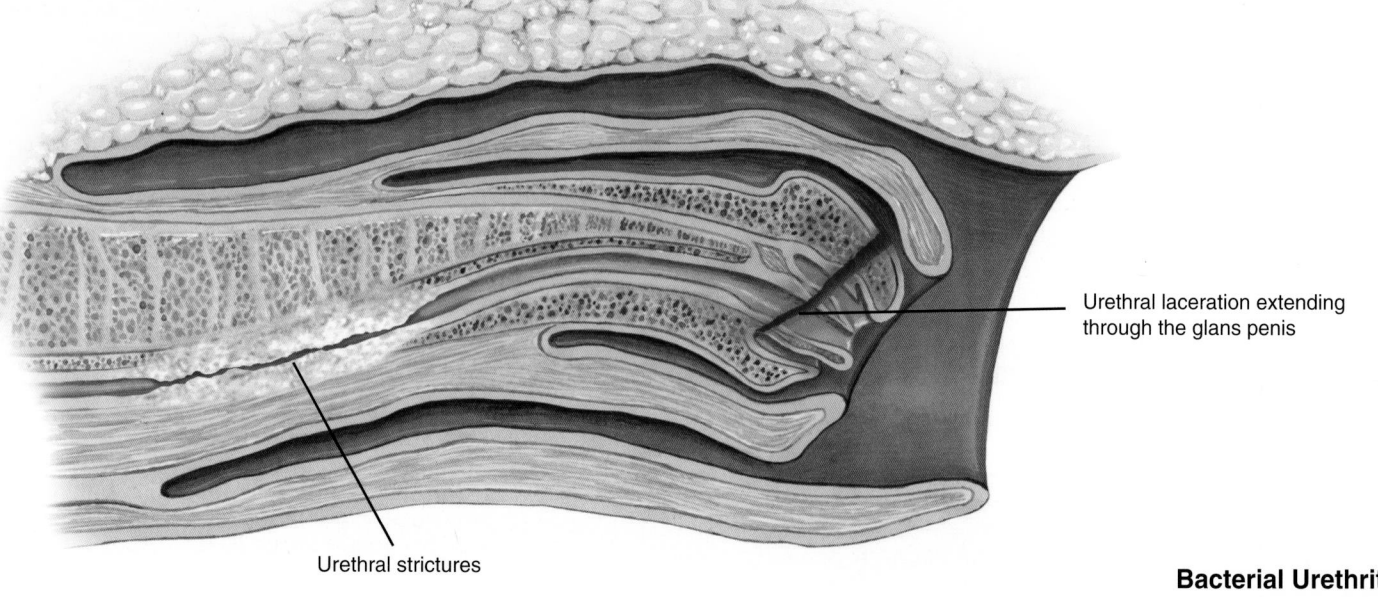

Urethral laceration extending through the glans penis

Urethral strictures

Urethral Strictures and Laceration

Bacterial Urethritis

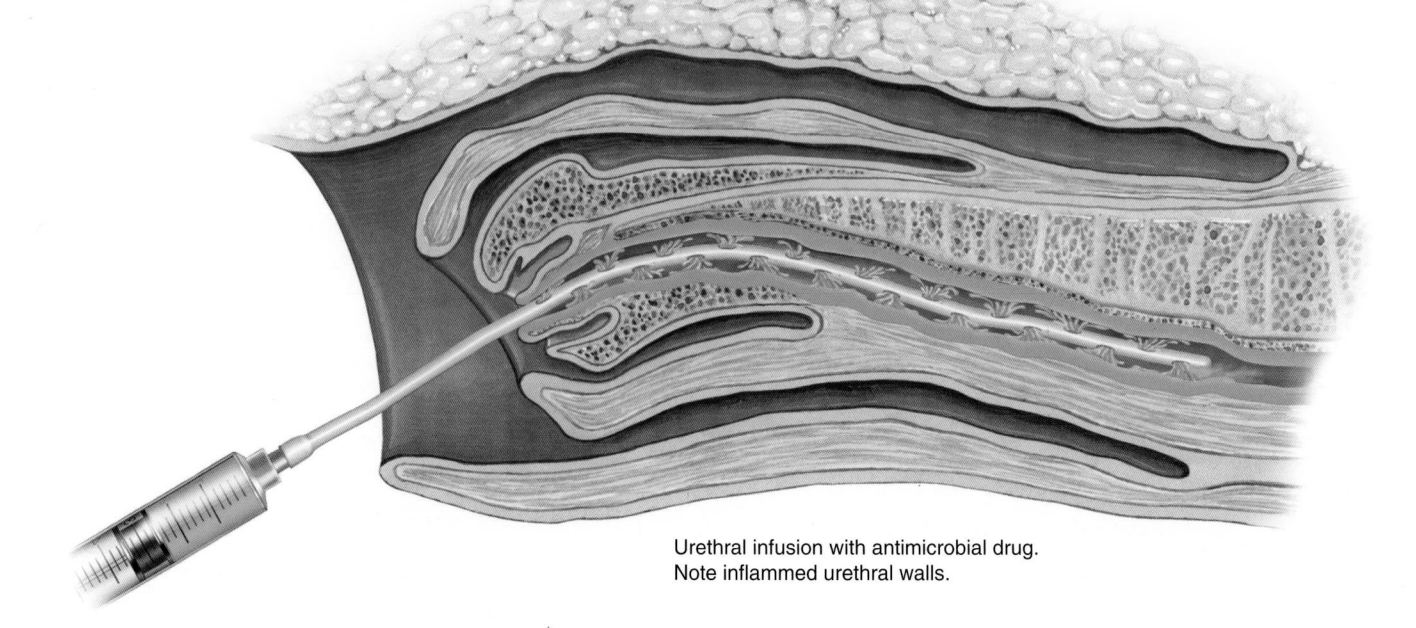

Urethral infusion with antimicrobial drug. Note inflamed urethral walls.

Diagnosis of Urethral Trauma

The stallion should be tranquilized to allow an exteriorizition of the penis to permit examination of the urethra. The entire length of the penis should be examined for the presence of any contusions, lacerations, or penetrating wounds. Circumferential depression resulting from improperly placed stallion rings should also warrant thorough examination.

Through the use of an endoscope, a definitive diagnosis of urethral lesions can be accomplished. This will reveal any ulcerations, lacerations, cicatrices, lodged calculi, and inflammation.

Contrast radiographic studies can be performed to detect space occupying lesions such as urethral strictures, pseudomembranes, lacerations, ulcerations, and fistulas within the urethra. Ultrasonography used in conjunction with endoscopy and radiography is useful for locating lodged urethral calculi.

Treatment

Treatment of these trauma-induced lesions varies depending on the type of injury present. Strictures and proliferative granulation tissue can be removed with curettage and local urethral dilation. Circumferential cicatrices of the urethral orifice can be treated with a gradual stretching of these tissues with urethral dilators, topical treatments, and sexual rest.

Iatrogenic injury to the urethra will usually resolve itself without complication with sexual rest for approximately two months. Calculi that are lodged within the urethral lumen need to be removed immediately through a urethrotomy. The stallion is usually heavily sedated and allowed to stand during this procedure. Epidural anesthesia and the application of local anesthetics allow a vertical skin incision to be made on the perineal midline. This incision is usually six to eight centimeters long and begins two to three centimeters ventral to the external anal sphincter muscle. The urethra is reached after dissection through the retractor penis muscles and through the bulbospongiosus muscles. It is helpful to catheterize the urethra to allow easier identification throughout this surgery. The corpus spongiosum penis is then incised longitudinally along with the urethral wall. Most calculi must be crushed before the forceps are introduced for retrieval of these small pieces. After the calculus is removed, the urethrotomy site is generally allowed to heal as an open wound. Systemic antiinflammatory and antimicrobial medications are administered as necessary.

Any lacerations of the urethral wall that communicate with the adjacent corpus spongiosum penis are usually refractive to healing. This is due to the increased blood pressure and movement of tissues within the corpus spongiosum penis during erection and micturition. During ejaculation or urination, bleeding into the urethral lumen is noted. Treatment for this condition consists of an ischial urethrotomy in conjunction with enforced sexual rest of at least two months. The incising of the corpus spongiosum penis converts this semiclosed cavernous space into an open one and encourages the blood to drain through the urethrotomy site rather than through the original laceration. Therefore, the intraurethral bleeding is prevented long enough to permit adequate healing time to the urethral wound.

BACTERIAL URETHRITIS

Bacterial infection within the urethra of horses is relatively uncommon. It can occur as a primary entity or as a sequel to infectious cystitis or infection from a local injury. Research has not yet determined the relationship of urethritis within the pelvic urethra to infections within the internal accessory genital glands.

Diagnosis

Diagnosis is based on bacterial cultures isolated from urethral swabs. Endoscopy is a valuable diagnostic tool since it permits direct visual examination of the mucosal lining throughout the length of the urethra. Evidence of pseudo-membranes may be seen with endoscopy or contrast radiographic studies that develop as a result of bacterial urethritis.

Treatment

The treatment of bacterial urethritis involves systemic antimicrobial therapy in conjunction with irrigation and infusion of antimicrobial drugs directly into the urethral lumen. Care must be taken during this irrigation and infusion technique to use antibiotic solutions that are nonirritating to the urethral mucosa. Treatments should last a minimum of seven to ten days with an additional sexual rest of another four to six weeks. Cultures should be taken of the urethra, urine, and semen after this period of time to ensure the elimination of the bacterial infection.

TOXIC DISORDERS OF THE URETHRA

The blister beetle contains cantharidin which is a potent irritant that primarily infects the gastro-intestinal tract, the urinary tract, and sometimes the cardiac structures of the horse. These beetles are frequently consumed inadvertently through the consumption of hay. Cystitis and urethritis are common manifestations of this toxication in horses that survive the initial phase of this disease. Clinical signs include frequent urination, dysuria, and hematuria.

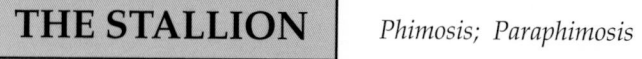

Phimosis

Paraphimosis

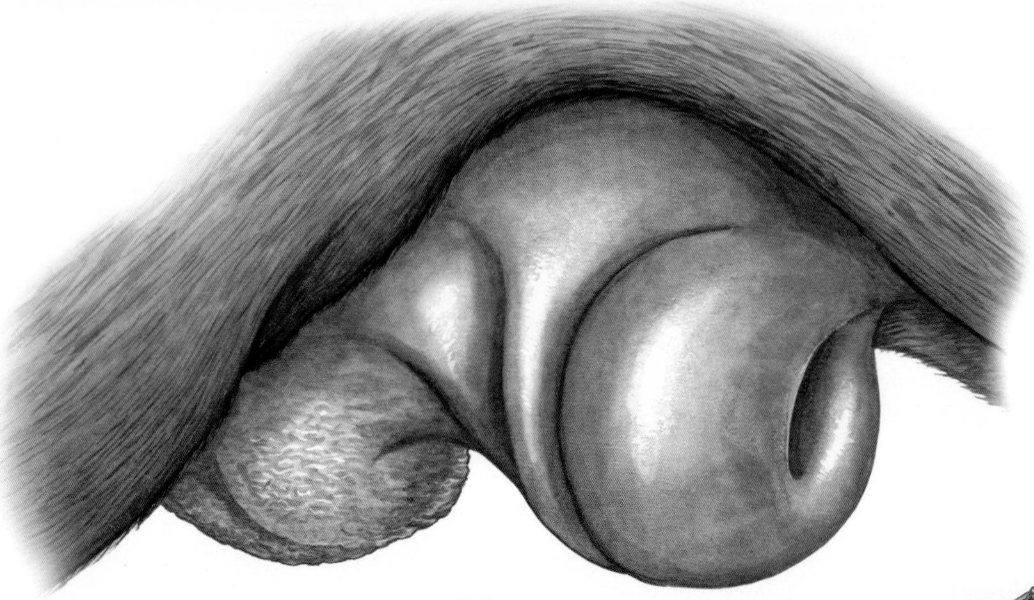

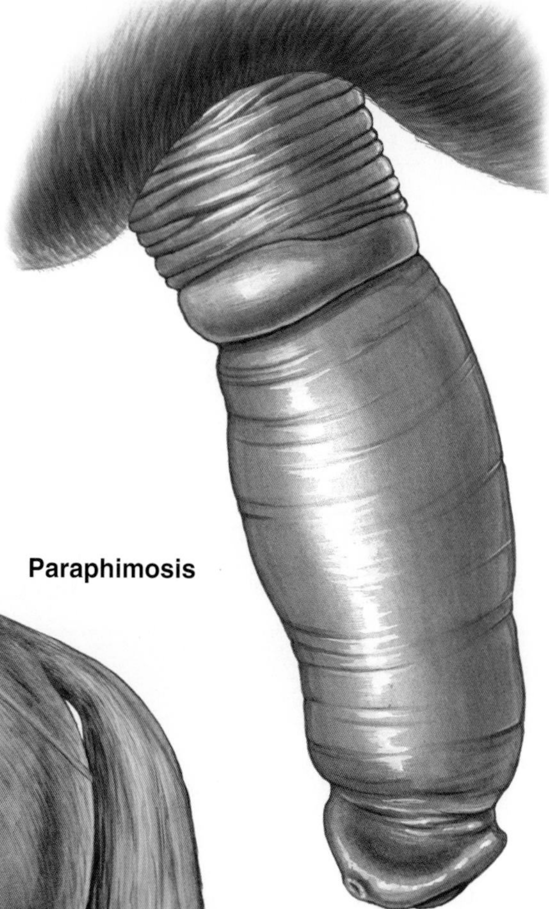

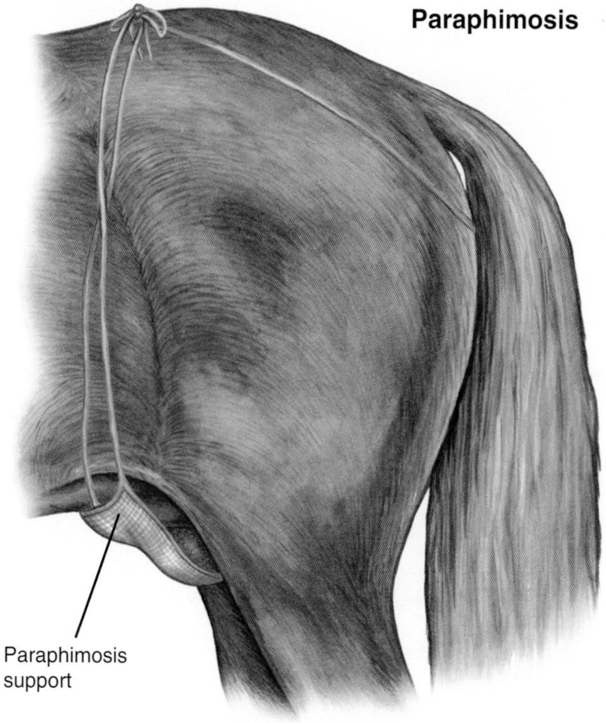

Paraphimosis
support

PHIMOSIS

The condition of phimosis is the inability of the penis to protrude from the prepuce. The etiologies behind this condition include preputial edema, chronic posthitis, and neoplastic or granulomatous lesions of the prepuce. Since the animal cannot exteriorize the penis to urinate, urine accumulates within the preputial tissues surrounding the penis which predisposes the penis to irritation and consequent inflammation. Due to the warm moist environment created within these tissues, bacterial infection is inevitable.

DISORDERS OF THE PENIS

Examination of the Penis

When the stallion is not sexually stimulated, the penis is detumescent and within the prepuce. Therefore, in order to perform a thorough examination of the penis, it is required that it be exteriorized from the prepuce.

There are two methods employed in obtaining penis exteriorization. In stallions that are familiar with being handled and washed for breeding, the penis can usually be extracted by passing a hand through the preputial orifice, grasping the penis from behind the glans, and manually removing it from behind the prepuce. The retractor penis muscles will contract and attempt to resist this technique. Tranquilization with intravenous xylazine or acepromazine usually produces a spontaneous exteriorzation of the penis. Utilizing tranquilizers usually allows a more thorough exam of the entire penis length without resistance from the stallion. Caution should be exercised, however, since phenothiazine tranquilizers such as acepromazine can lead to irreversible penile prolapse.

PARAPHIMOSIS

Etiology

This disorder is the exact opposite of phimosis in that it is the inability of the penis to be retracted back into the prepuce. In most cases, paraphimosis is the result of acute preputial trauma, but it may develop after penile paralysis or priapism following the use of some phenothiazine tranquilizers.

An inflammatory response resulting in edema within the prepuce is usually a consequence to direct preputial trauma. Following most castration techniques, preputial edema results simply from the forces of gravity. If the penis is exteriorized from the prepuce during this state of edema, the swelling within the prepuce mechanically prohibits penile retraction. After an occurrence of penile prolapse and the resulting edema within the tissues, penile retraction again becomes mechanically impaired.

Pathological Process

Edematous swelling of both the penis and prepuce occurs during penile prolapse. This is due to the impaired venous and lymphatic drainage within these tissues following the prolapse. The edema tends to localize near the preputial ring. Constriction caused by this localized edema often enhances the penile swelling. A vicious cycle occurs in that the more localized the edema which results in a constriction of the penis, the worse the vascular condition of the penis, which in turn creates more swelling within the penile organ. Unless treatment is initiated quickly, cellulitis develops. The integument becomes thickened, inelastic, desiccated, and finally necrotic. Gangrenous changes of both penile and preputial tissues can occur unless treatment is timely.

Treatment

The goal of treatment of paraphimosis is to replace the penis within the prepuce and reduce the edema. The penis should be immediately replaced within the preputial cavity and secured there with towel clamps or a pursestring retention suture placed around the preputial orifice. A simple penile retention device can be constructed from a half liter narrow-neck plastic bottle. After removing the base of the bottle and padding the edges with tape or gauze, two links of rubber tubing are secured to the neck of the bottle at their midpoints. The penis is placed within the plastic body until the urethral process opposes the opening at the bottle neck. The penis is then positioned normally within the preputial cavity along with its overlying plastic bottle. The bottle is held in position with tubing secured to the neck of the bottle. One length of the tubing is then passed laterally and dorsally around both flanks and tied over the horse's back. The other length of tubing passes caudally along each side of the scrotum between the hind legs and is fastened to the tubing over the horse's back. Urine can escape through the opening in the bottle neck. In addition, if further support is needed, a stud support can be applied exteriorly over the top of the prepuce. Twice daily, the penis should be exteriorized within the plastic body and treated topically with antibiotic ointments. This prevents irritation from collected urine and also drying and cracking of the integument due to the exteriorization.

Physical therapy techniques can play a vital role in the reduction of swelling in both the penis and prepuce. Gentle massage of these tissues will increase circulation and therefore, reduce the edema within the tissues. In an acute case, application of cold packs would also be of benefit. These techniques may have to be used in order to reduce the swelling within the penis to allow initial replacement of the penis within the preputial cavity.

Systemic antibiotics should be initiated as well as nonsteroidal antiinflammatory medication. Medications used in conjunction with aggressive physical therapy techniques yield more favorable prognoses toward recovery. If the penile paralysis or priapism associated with the paraphimosis is nonresponsive to treatment, surgical retraction of the penis or amputation of the penis may be required.

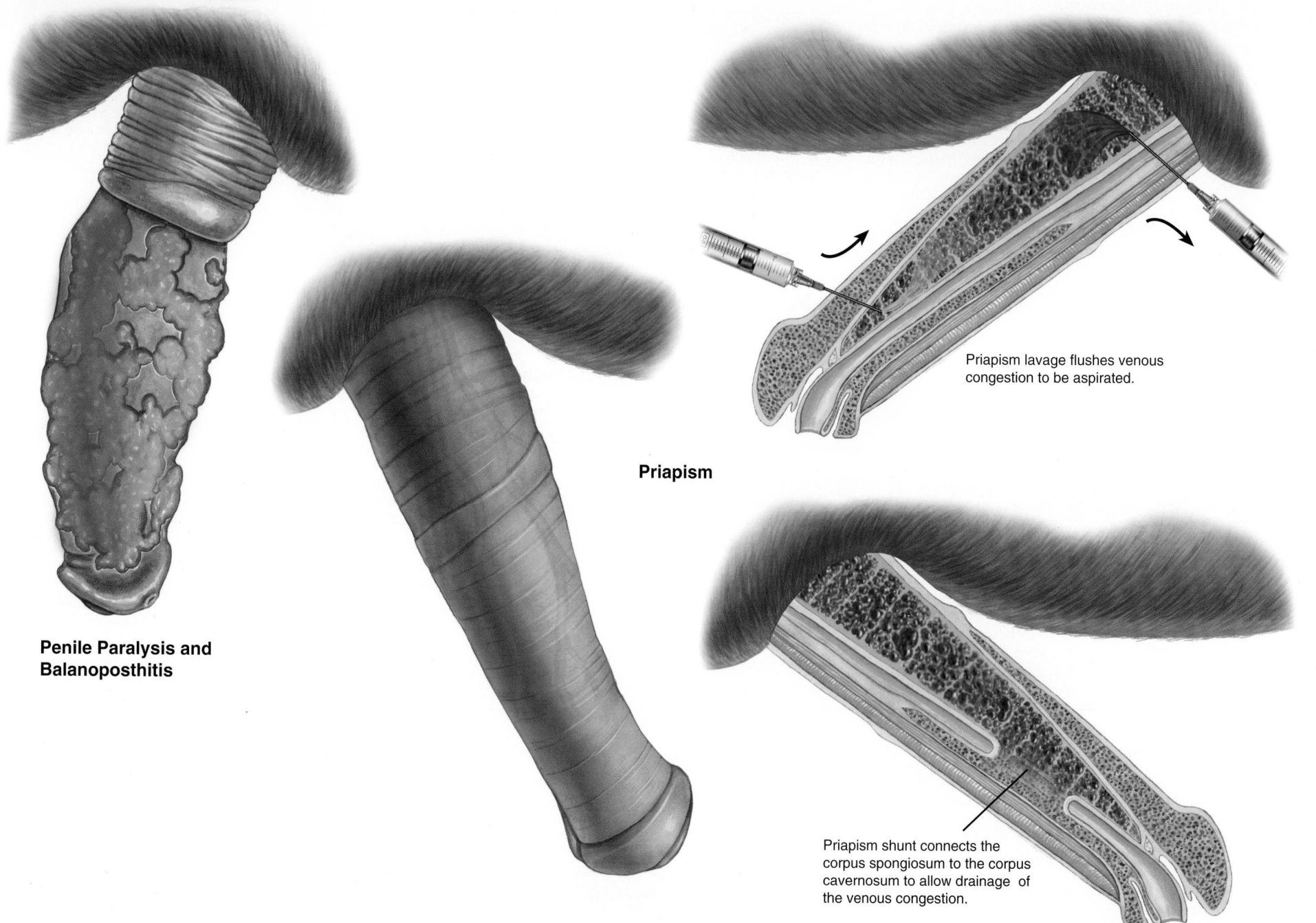

Priapism lavage flushes venous
congestion to be aspirated.

Priapism

**Penile Paralysis and
Balanoposthitis**

Priapism shunt connects the
corpus spongiosum to the corpus
cavernosum to allow drainage of
the venous congestion.

PENILE PARALYSIS AND PRIAPISM

Etiology of Penile Paralysis

When there is a reduction in the contractor penis muscle tone, penile paralysis occurs. This condition is seen in exhausted or debilitated horses, animals with myelitis or spinal disorders, and as a result of the use of phenothiazine-derivative drugs.

Pathological Process

This prolapsed penis is flaccid and due to compensated retractor penis muscles, it cannot be retracted back within the preputial cavity. Since venous and lymphatic drainage are impaired, fluid accumulates within the penile tissues producing an edematous condition. As this disorder progresses into a chronic ulcerated balanoposthitis, the epithelial surfaces of the exposed penis become dried, thickened, and inelastic. The pudendal nerves and smooth muscle cells of the erectile tissues as well as the retractor penis muscles are under constant gravitational pull, therefore resulting in damage to these delicate tissues. The sensory and motor innervation to the muscles and skin of the stallion's genitalia arise from the third and fourth sacral nerves. As this prolapsed condition continues, damage also occurs to these nerves which results in a long term penile paralysis and loss of cutaneous sensation within the penis epithelium.

Etiology of Priapism

The prolapsed paralyzed penis is flaccid, whereas a constant erection of the penis without sexual arousal is termed priapism. The etiology of this condition arises from a prolonged engorgement of the corpus cavernosum penis with blood. The precise cause of this change in blood flow, either arterial or venous, has not been determined. It has been theorized that it is basically a retardation of venous outflow.

Phenothiazine tranquilizers are the primary cause of priapism in horses. During tranquilization, the corpus cavernosum penis is filled with blood. Phenothiazine tranquilizers block the alpha sympathetic impulses that initiate detumesence. Therefore, there is a failure of the detumesence mechanism which would allow the blood within the corpus cavernosum penis to escape.

After a period of time, if the erection does not subside, penile and preputial edema occurs. This edema results in more edema and finally necrotic changes within these tissues. Penile paralysis in a state of priapism is differentiated from paraphimosis since in the case of paraphimosis, the penis cannot be retracted as a result of preputial injury or disease.

Treatment

Aggressive physical therapy techniques, mechanical slings, systemic administrations of medications (diuretics), and replacement of the penis within the preputial cavity constitute treatment of penile paralysis. Treatment of horses with the condition of priapism has generally been unsuccessful from a medical standpoint. Surgical treatment of priapism is indicated when physical therapy techniques and systemic medical treatments fail to restore venous outflow.

There are two surgical procedures utilized in the treatment of priapism. The first technique has a goal of removal of the congealed acidotic blood from the corpus cavernosum penis. After this is accomplished, shunts are created to establish venous drainage from the corpus cavernosum penis into the corpus spongiosum penis.

In order to remove the congealed acidotic blood, the animal is anesthetized and positioned in dorsal recumbency. A twelve gauge needle is inserted into the cavernosal tissue proximal to the glans penis and a heparinized saline solution is flushed under pressure into the corpus cavernosum penis. The congealed blood and saline solution are drained through one or two twelve gauge needles inserted into the corpus cavernosum penis ten to fifteen centimeters caudal to the base of the scrotum. This

flushing is continued until fresh blood is seen in the efflux. If fresh arterial blood is not seen in the efflux, this indicates that arterial damage has already occurred and evacuation of the cavernosal blood will be of no benefit.

In order to create a shunt from the corpus cavernosum penis to the corpus spongiosum penis, the corpus cavernosum penis is exposed caudal to the scrotum. A side to side anastomosis is created between these two cavernosum structures. Because the corpus spongiosum penis is not involved in the initial development of an erection, the penis drainage from these cavernous spaces should provide an exit route for the blood within the corpus cavernosum penis. The consequence of this surgery is that postoperatively, the stallion usually has an inability to develop an erection due to the shunt itself.

Both of these surgical procedures are salvage operations to try to save a stallion for breeding purposes. Some stallions can still impregnate mares even though the penis does not become rigid when fully engorged. In extreme cases of penile paralysis or priapism, surgical amputation of the penis or phallopexy may be indicated. In all cases, humane and economic considerations should be taken into account before these surgical decisions are made.

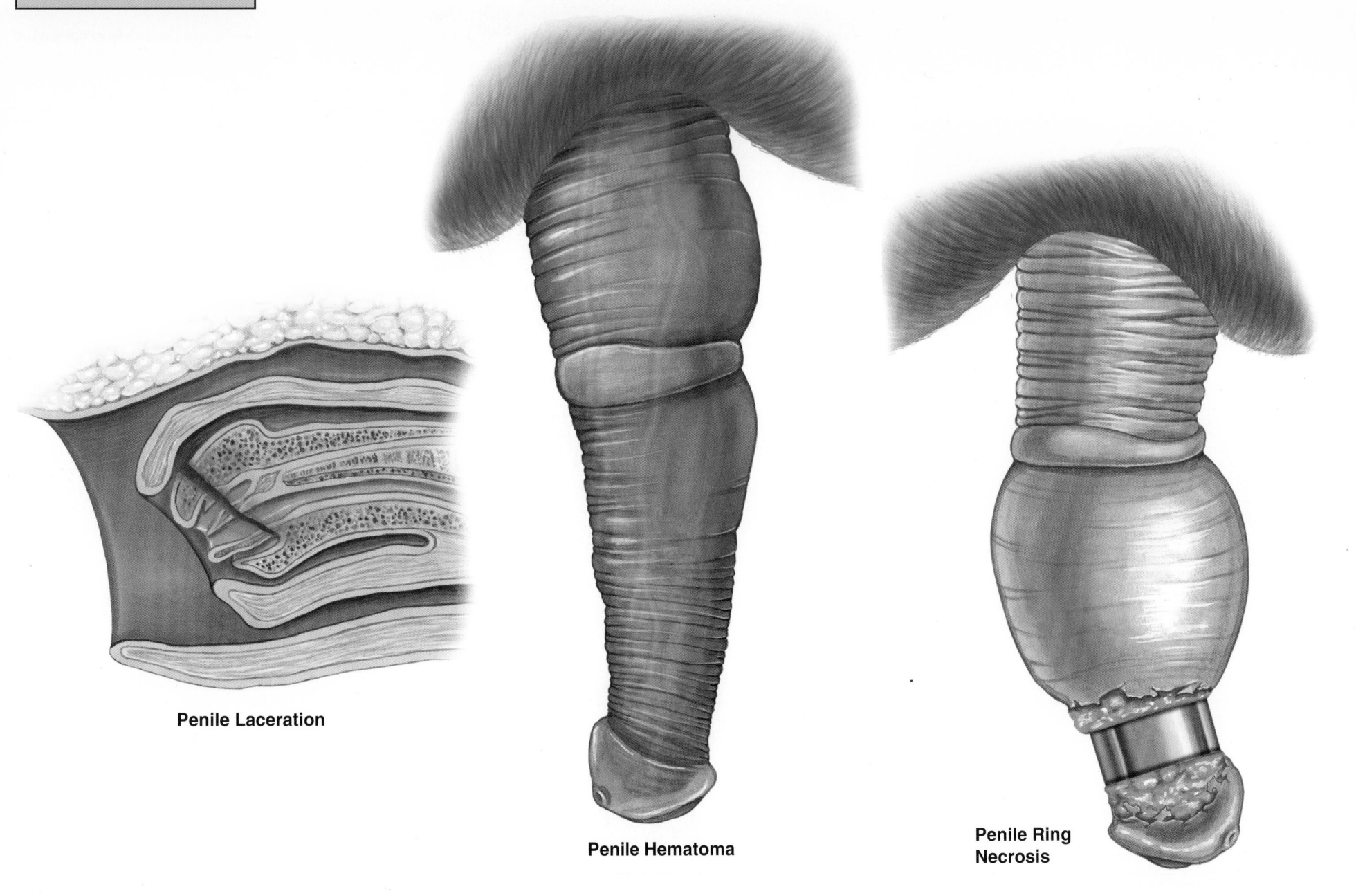

Penile Laceration

Penile Hematoma

Penile Ring Necrosis

PENILE LACERATIONS AND ABRASIONS

Etiology

Trauma to the penis occurs when the penis is erect. Sexual activity allows the penis a degree of vulnerability to trauma from kicks, sutures in the mare's vulva, improperly prepared artificial vaginas, breeding phantoms, and even the tail hairs of the mare. The conditions of penile paralysis, priapism, and paraphimosis also allow exposure to the penis for long periods of time. This predisposes the penis to trauma.

Treatment

Lacerations of the penis may be treated as open wounds or may require surgery when the cavernous spaces are involved. Superficial abrasions and lacerations heal well with a minimum amount of medical attention. One of the most critical aspects that needs attention is the controlling of the edema caused by these wounds. Sexual rest is essential to allow complete healing. Any penetration of the tunica albuginea that also results in hemorrhage or penetration of the cavernous spaces should be sutured. Surgical repair of these tissues will prevent infection and speed the healing process.

The key to treatment of a traumatized penis is the initial control of the inflammatory reaction and edema. Systemic antiinflammatory treatment should be initiated immediately along with physical therapy techniques to prevent and reduce edema. These techniques should consist of penile massage as well as cold therapy to the tissues. Antimicrobial therapy should be initiated as a prophylactic measure. A tetanus toxoid booster should always be considered.

PENILE HEMATOMA

Etiology

Hematomas result from blunt trauma to the erect penis. This occurs as a kick from the mare or a delayed deflection of the penis from a breeding phantom during semen collection.

The source of the hemorrhage is usually ruptured vessels on the dorsal surface of the penis superficial to the cavernous tissue. These hematomas can be numerous and at different locations along the length of the penis depending on the type of trauma imposed. On rare occasions, a hematoma can result from a rupture of the tunica albuginea and the underlying corpus cavernosum penis. Following the initial trauma, there is localized inflammation and edema. This edema may spread to both the scrotal and preputial tissues as well. When these hematomas go untreated, paraphimosis could result.

Treatment

Treatment of penile hematomas should occur in three stages: initial, systemic, and physical therapy. The initial goal is to stop the hemorrhage and reduce the swelling. Pressure bandages can be applied to the penis to reduce the hemorrhage. Cold packs should immediately be initiated to reduce the swelling and hemorrhage. If the hematoma continues to expand during these initial treatment attempts, surgery should be performed immediately to repair the tissues and accomplish hemostasis.

Systemic treatments involve antiinflammatory, diuretic, and antimicrobial medications. The goal of the antiinflammatory and diuretic medications is to reduce or prevent the swelling within the penile tissues. Antibiotic therapy is usually prophylactic in nature.

Physical therapy techniques are aimed at minimizing the formation of subcutaneous fibrous tissue. This tissue results after the hematoma is resorbed by the body. Fibrous tissues will often create adhesions which result in a directional deviation of the penis during erection. Penile massage along with topical medications are recommended on a daily basis to prevent this fibrous tissue formation. It is often necessary to continue this therapy for several weeks.

PENILE NECROSIS FROM STALLION RINGS

Pathological Process

Breeding stallions sometimes adapt the habit of masturbation. A nonexpansive band is usually placed immediately proximal to the glans penis to discourage this behavior. The theory behind these devices is that there will be a restriction in penile tumescence by causing pain to the penis when it becomes erect.

If this is a breeding management tool that is used, it must be properly fitted, cleaned, and changed at least every several days to insure that there are no pathological consequences in its use. When these appliances become too tight, they result in a compression of the underlying penile and urethral tissues. This then leads to ischemic necrosis and a constricting fibrosis. In severe cases, urethral strictures, failure of erection, and nerve damage may also develop. If damage from these stallion rings is suspected, endoscopic examination of the urethral lumen and possibly contrast radiography provide an evaluation of these tissues.

Treatment

Treatment of stallion ring-induced trauma revolves around correction of any urethral strictures and repair of the damaged erectile tissue. Urethral tissue regenerates fairly well and often times systemic treatment coupled with removal of the ring allows healing. Severe strictures can be treated with local curettage combined with luminal dilation. Erection dysfunction is usually the result of the inability of the corpus spongiosum glandis to fill properly with blood during sexual stimulation. If the nerves to these tissues are damaged, the prognosis is grave.

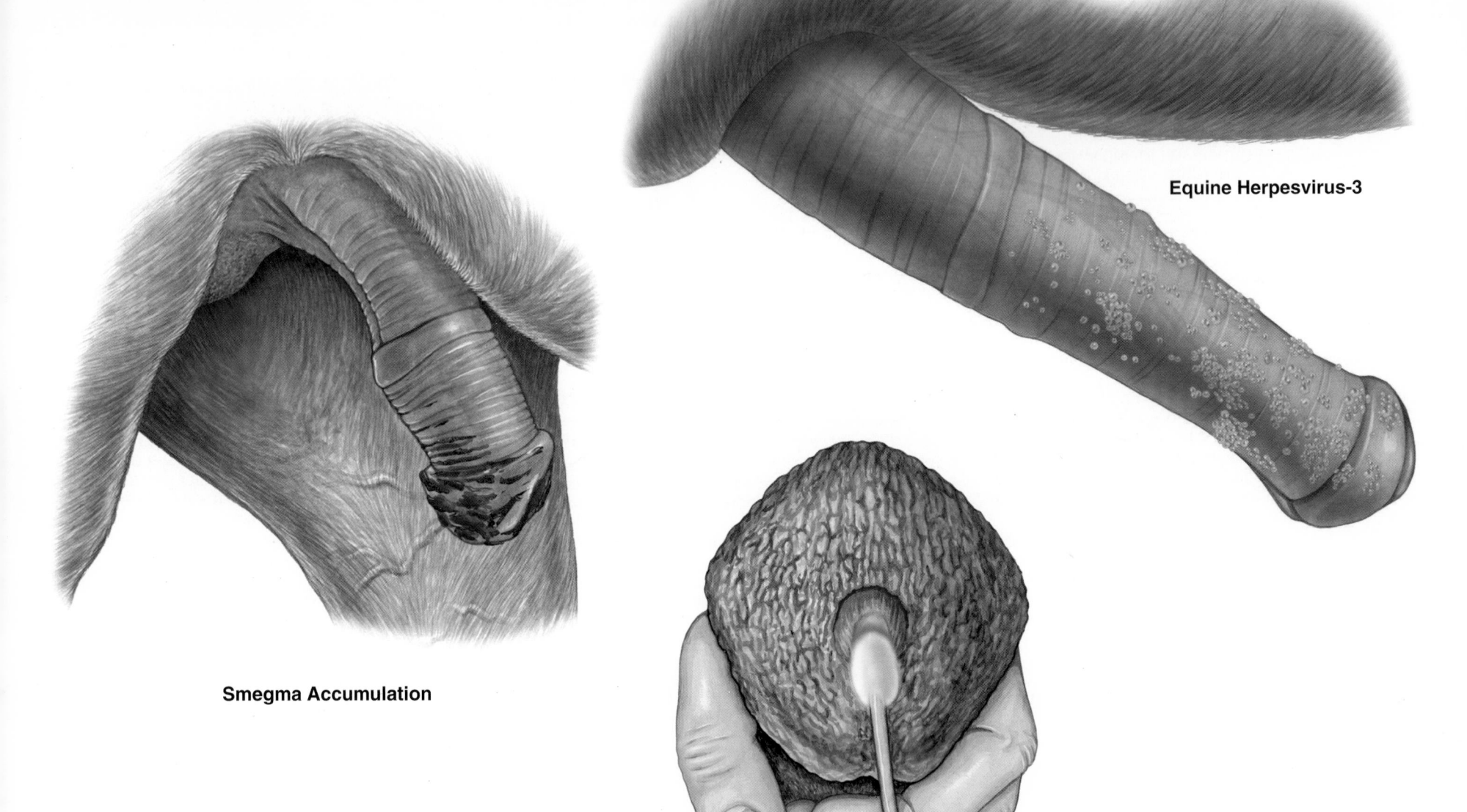

Equine Herpesvirus-3

Smegma Accumulation

Obtaining penile culture

PENILE SMEGMA

Smegma is the grey to black caseous, foul-smelling sticky substance formed from the secretions of sebaceous and sweat glands combined with dirt and dead epithelial cells. On the distal end of the penis, there are three recesses of the fossa glandis that become impacted with this material. This impacted material or smegma is often referred to as a "bean." Smegma may also collect on the outside of the penis and around the preputial folds.

There are two complications with this smegma compaction. When there is poor penile hygiene, this smegma can produce a low grade balanoposthitis. If the fossa glandis becomes completely filled with smegma, its physical pressure upon the urethra can cause pain during urination and ejaculation.

Penile hygiene should be a routine procedure performed at regular intervals. The penis and prepuce of geldings and stallions should be cleansed with plain warm water. Although soap will aid in the removal of smegma and make the job much more desirable, it also destroys the normal bacterial flora of the penis. When this bacterial flora is compromised, it allows for a possible overgrowth of potentially pathogenic organisms. Soap also leads to a drying and cracking of the penile skin and prepuce which leads to other complications.

EQUINE HERPESVIRUS-3

Etiology and Clinical Signs

Equine herpesvirus-3 (EHV-3) is the causative agent of a viral venereal disease in horses. It is referred to as coital exanthema. Clinically, this disorder is observed during the breeding season and appears as lesions on the external genitalia of stallions and mares. In the stallion, both the penis and prepuce will exhibit small white circumscribed vesicles or pustules that often become confluent. It is not uncommon for the genitalia of the stallion to exhibit some edema as a result of this disorder. Usually within forty-eight hours, these vesicles and pustules rupture to form superficial ulcers on the surface of the penis.

Treatment

Sexual rest allows resolution of this disorder within four to six weeks. This disorder is typically self-limiting as a virus and secondary bacterial infections are rare. Topical treatment with daily applications of ointments is usually of some benefit in the painful acute phase of this disorder. When breed regulations allow, it is possible to collect semen from the stallion using a phantom after the acute phase of the disease has subsided.

CONTAGIOUS EQUINE METRITIS (CEM)

Etiology

Contagious equine metritis is caused by the bacterium *Taylorella equigenitalis*. This is a very contagious venereal disease in horses and if untreated, can exist on the surface of the penis and prepuce indefinitely. It has not been reported that a migration of this organism occurs to the internal genitalia in the stallion.

Diagnosis

Diagnosis of contagious equine metritis is done through cultures obtained from the urethral sinus, urethra, penile skin, and preputial folds. It is often difficult to isolate this bacteria due to the normal bacteria flora that flourish on the external genitalia of stallions. These normal bacteria inhibit the growth of *Taylorella equigenitalis* on the culture plates or overgrow the cultures, making isolation difficult. If a stallion is suspected as being a carrier of contagious equine metritis, it is bred to properly screened test mares which are then checked bacteriologically and serologically to detect the presence of the disease. However, some positive stallions do not transmit the disease to all test mares since the site of bacterial seclusion may be in the deep recesses of the fossa glandis.

Treatment

Treatment of contagious equine metritis is quite successful. Daily washings of the penis, prepuce, and urethral fossa are done using a chlorhexidine solution for five consecutive days. Immediately following each cleansing, the prepuce and penis are dried and nitrofurazone ointment is applied topically.

Disease identification of CEM is of vital importance. Identification, isolation, and treatment of infected horses are mandatory to contain this disease. If this disease is even suspected, federal veterinarians should be contacted immediately.

BACTERIAL INFECTION

Etiology

The penis and prepuce of the stallion contains a normal population of microflora that rarely produces a genital infection within the mare. In certain instances, this normal bacterial flora is disrupted and a pathogenic strain of bacteria may colonize on the penis and prepuce. These pathogenic bacteria can then be trasmitted into the mare's genital tract at the time of breeding which results in an endometritis and consequential infertility. The two most common bacterial pathogens are: *Pseudomonas aeruginosa* and *Klebsiella pneumoniae*. Both of these organisms occur within the environment and are opportunistic when they florish on the external genitalia of the stallion.

The most common etiology of a pathogenic bacterial infection is the constant washing of the penis with soap. This frequent cleansing removes all of the nonpathogenic resident organisms and also dries the skin allowing cracks to occur where these pathogenic organisms can proliferate. The second most common cause of this pathogenic colonization of bacteria is the acquisition of these organisms during coitus with a mare that is already carrying this infection.

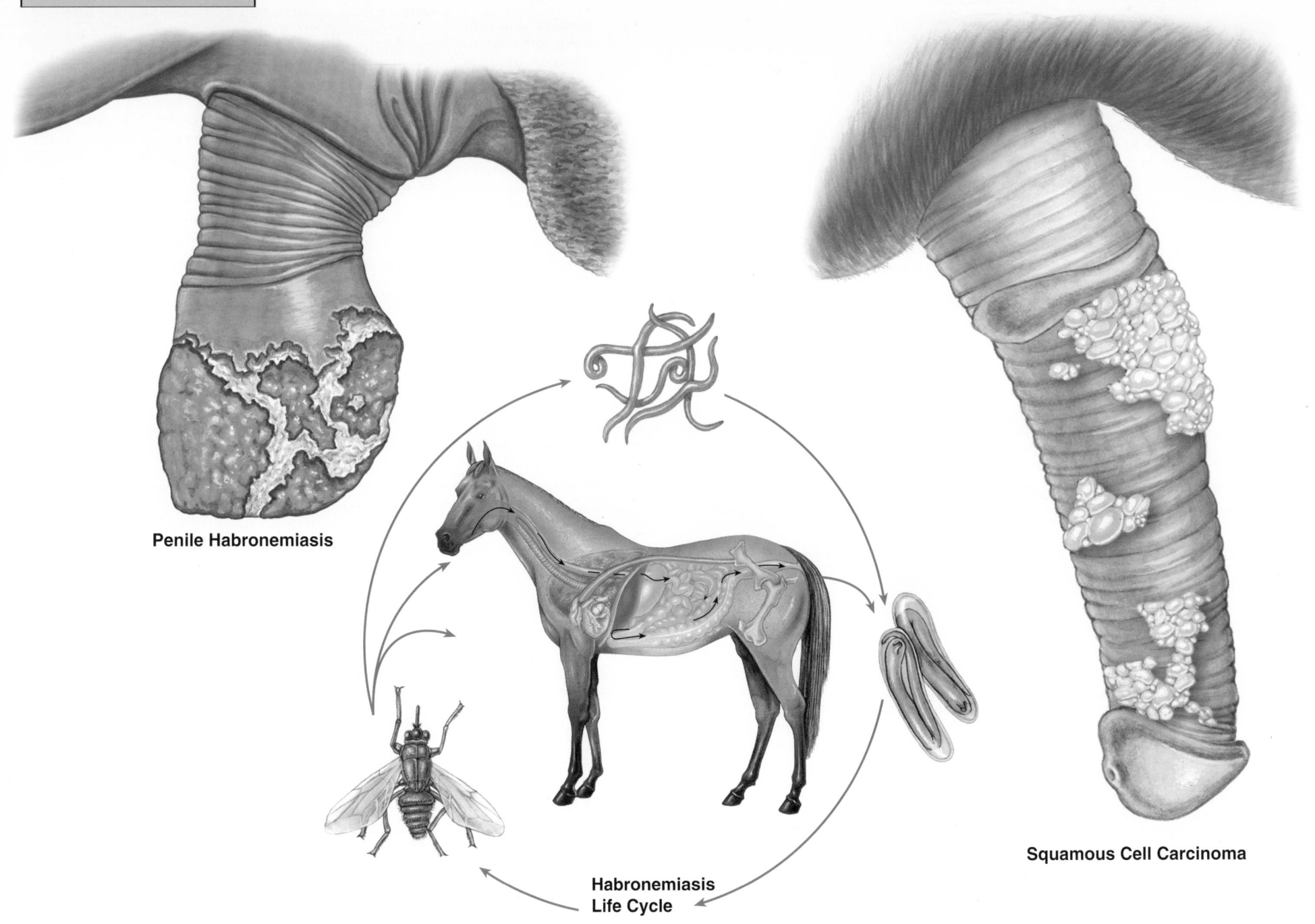

Artwork by S. Hakola / J. Dirig
Copyright Equistar Publications, Ltd.

Penile Habronemiasis

**Habronemiasis
Life Cycle**

Squamous Cell Carcinoma

Diagnosis of Penile Infections

Diagnosis is made via culture of these pathogenic organisms from culture swabs. The cultures are obtained from the preputial folds, the surface of the penis at several different locations, and the fossa glandis.

Treatment

Treatment of the penis for these pathogenic bacteria is very difficult. Treatment includes daily cleansing of the penis and prepuce with dilute hydrochloric acid solution or a weak solution of bleach. This is followed by applications of silver sulfadiazine cream or other emollients that protect the skin against chafing and cracking. This treatment regime is continued until culture swabs no longer reveal the pathogenic organisms.

CUTANEOUS HABRONEMIASIS

This condition is commonly called a summer sore. It is granulomatous in nature and caused by the infective larvae of the stomach worms: *Draschia megastoma*, *Habronema muscae*, and *Habronema microstema*. This condition usually involves the skin of the penis, but it also may affect the scrotum and the prepuce.

Parasitic Life Cycle

The life cycle involved with cutaneous habronemiasis is as follows: the adult worms live in the stomach wall of the horse and deposit eggs into the gastric lumen. These eggs are then passed in the feces, hatch, and are ingested by fly larva. When the adult flies land on the skin of the penis, or other warm moist areas, then the nematode larvae move down into the fly's labellum and are transferred onto the skin. Loss of skin integrity allows the larvae to gain entry to the skin. These developing larvae stimulate rapid production of granulation tissue within the skin. The larvae themselves may live for several weeks or months before they die. Fortunately, these parasitic larvae will never reach maturity within the skin lesions.

Diagnosis

The differential diagnosis for these granulomatous skin lesions should include squamous cell carcinoma, sarcoids, and exuberant granulomas. Diagnosis is based on the identification of the larvae within the lesions. The larvae are difficult to identify, and a biopsy is required to confirm the diagnosis. These biopsies are helpful and allow the differentiation of cutaneous habronemiasis from sarcoids and squamous cell carcinomas.

Treatment

Fortunately, there is one preferred treatment for cutaneous habronemiasis. Ivermectin, due to its larvicidal activity, is very effective in resolving cutaneous habronemiasis. Proper dosages should be administered every ten days to two weeks for three to five treatments. The lesions themselves will start to show clinical improvement within the first week of treatment. Antiinflammatory medications that are nonsteroidal in nature would also be of benefit to reduce any edema within the affected tissues. Sexual rest is essential until the lesions have healed sufficiently to avoid interference of breeding or infertility.

NEOPLASIAS OF THE PENIS

There are three types of neoplasic conditions that affect the external genitalia of the stallion. These are squamous cell carcinomas, squamous papillomas (warts), and fibrosarcomas. Squamous cell carcinomas are the most common neoplasm of the stallion followed by squamous papillomas and on rare occasions, fibrosarcomas.

SQUAMOUS CELL CARCINOMA

Etiology

Squamous cell carcinomas are seen mostly in the American Paint horses and Appaloosas. It is believed that the lack of pigmentation may predispose these breeds to this neoplastic condition. It is derived from the stratified squamous epithelium that originates primarily on the glans penis or internal lamina of the prepuce. It has also been theorized that constant irritation from smegma may also predispose the animal to this condition.

Clinical Signs

Squamous cell carcinoma appear clinically as small keratinized plaques on the genitalia. These plaques further develop as invasive papillary growths that have cauliflower-like appearances. These carcinomas usually grow very slowly and remain localized until later in the course of the disease. Metastasis can occur into the superficial and deep inguinal lymph nodes, but it rarely metastasizes to the liver or lung.

Diagnosis

Diagnosis of squamous cell cacinoma is based on a biopsy and histological exam of the lesion. These lesions may become secondarily infected by Habronema larvae and care must be taken to not overlook the primary carcinoma.

Treatment

Treatment of squamous cell carcinomas can include cryosurgery, hyperthermia, local incision, and phallectomy. When the lesions are in their early stages, and a definitive diagnosis has been obtained, cryotherapy with liquid nitrogen is sometimes effective. Several freezing cycles are recommended during this procedure. Following cryotherapy, care of the tissues is important since secondary damage to normal tissues cannot be

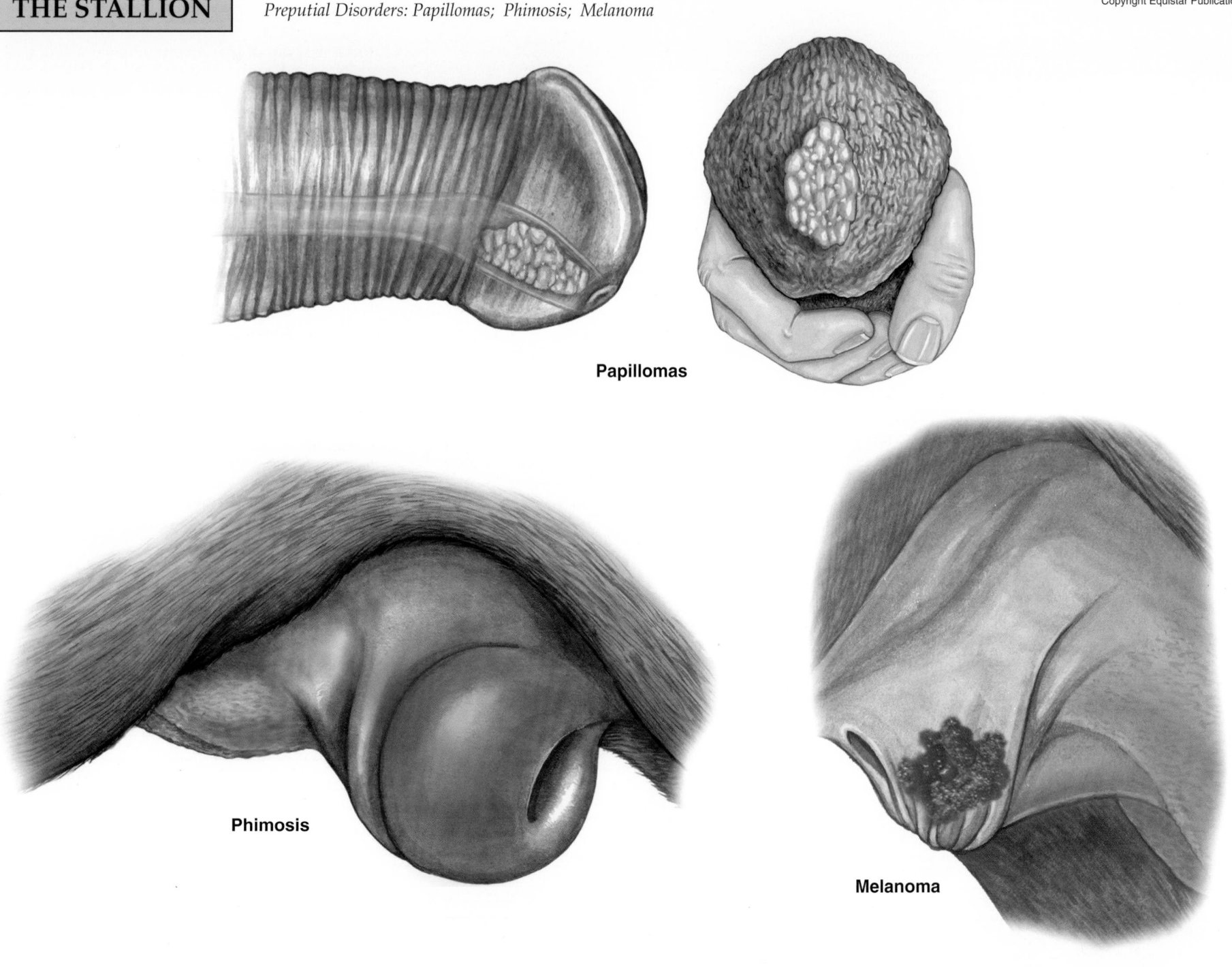

Papillomas

Phimosis

Melanoma

avoided. Phallectomy is a last resort in stallions and geldings where lesions are present that are too large or numerous to treat using other modalities. This is strictly a salvage operation for a horse to be used for purposes other than breeding. Both the quality of life and economics should be considered before this procedure is done.

PAPILLOMAS

Warts or squamous papillomas are common in horses but only rarely develop on the penis and prepuce. These are usually multiple cutaneous growths that are benign in nature. Diagnosis of this condition usually can be made strictly on clinical examination of the patient.

Treatment consists of creating an active acquired immunity to these squamous papillomas. Simply removing several of these growths surgically exposes this tissue to the blood stream and results in a spontaneous regression of the remaining papillomas. Genital squamous papillomas are usually quite refractive to treatment by topical means. Cryosurgery is successful when the papilloma is isolated.

FIBROSARCOMA

Fibrosarcomas are rarely found on the genitalia of the horse. If this condition is diagnosed on the penis and prepuce, it almost certainly involves other tissues in the horse. Therefore, further diagnostic techniques should be considered to gain an appreciation for its occurrence within the animal.

DISORDERS OF THE PREPUCE

PHIMOSIS

Etiology and Symptoms

Any condition that results in the inability to exteriorize the penis is referred to as phimosis. This condition may be congenital or acquired in nature. Congenital phimosis occurs normally in the free portion of a penis of a newborn colt. This free portion can be adhered in the internal lamina of the internal prepuce during the first few weeks of postnatal life. Separation of the epithelia of the apposed penis and prepuce integuments usually occurs four to six weeks after birth.

Acquired phimosis occurs secondarily to an acute or chronic posthitis or space occupying lesion of the prepuce. Posthitis, or preputial inflammation, accompanies any physical injury to the prepuce or an infectious process. Any episode of trauma will result in edema within these tissues. This edema will produce a prolapse of the external prepuce, therefore trapping the penis and the swollen internal prepuce with a constricting preputial ring. Paraphimosis results if the penis extrudes from the prepuce during this edematous episode.

Any neoplastic or granulomatous lesion of the prepuce may contain the penis within the preputial cavity. These lesions may involve the preputial orifice sufficiently that it becomes a form of physical blockage for the extrusion of the penis.

Treatment

Treatment of this acquired phimosis involves systemic antiinflammatories and aggresive physical therapy. Massage of the tissues as well as cold pack applications should be included in any physical therapy regime to reduce the edema within the preputial tissues. These techniques should be initiated immediately so that the pliability of these tissues would not be impaired by the formation of adhesions or fibrous scar tissue.

In the case of neoplastic granulomatous lesions, surgical correction is often required.

PREPUTIAL TRAUMA

Any trauma to the preputial tissues usually results in an acute posthitis. After injury to the preputial tissue, it is severely susceptible to edema formation due to its dependent position. Phimosis or paraphimosis may develop if this trauma is not attended to immediately.

Treatment will be determined by the type of trauma that occurs. Any open lesions may require sutures and in all cases, aggressive physical therapy techniques should be initiated to reduce any possible edema. Systemic antiinflammatory and antimicrobial treatment should be considered in all instances.

PREPUTIAL NEOPLASIA

The preputial tissues, as those of the penis, can be afflicted with squamous cell carcinomas, squamous papillomas, melanomas, and sarcoids. The squamous cell carcinomas and squamous papillomas are handled in the same manner as that when they are found on the tissues of the penis. Sarcoids are nonmetastatic locally-proliferated cutaneous tumors found in horses. These can appear anywhere on the body and are occasionally found on the prepuce or scrotum. A discussion of this neoplastic condition will be found in a section on disorders of the skin.

Melanomas are commonly found in grey horses. These are highly metastatic tumors that arise from melanocytes. These tumors are occasionally found on the prepuce and scrotum of geldings and stallions. A further discussion of this neoplastic condition will occur in the chapter on the skin.

Artwork by S. Hakola / J. Dirig
Copyright Equistar Publications, Ltd.

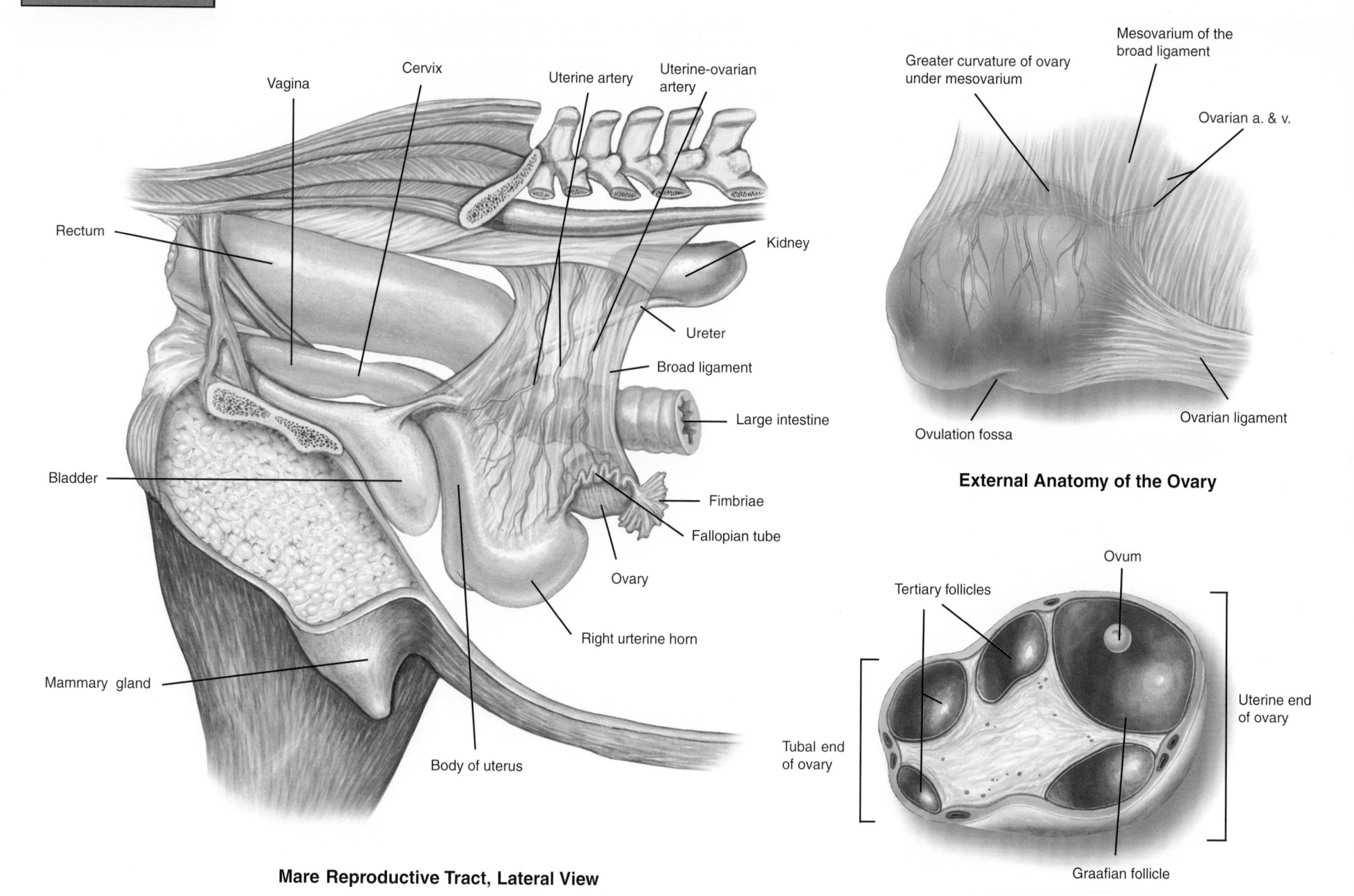

Mare Reproductive Tract, Lateral View

External Anatomy of the Ovary

Longitudinal Section of Ovary

2 The Mare

REPRODUCTIVE ANATOMY AND PHYSIOLOGY

Some consider anatomy a dead subject. When dealing with the reproductive system of the mare, the dynamics of living anatomy and the relationships of these structures allow for the biological and physiological functions that are performed within the reproductive system.

There are five primary structures within the reproductive tract of the mare. These are the ovaries, the oviducts or uterine tubules, the uterus, the vagina, and the vulva. The reproductive tract of the mare is located ventral to the fourth or fifth lumbar vertebrae, and travels caudally through the pelvic cavity to the structure of the vulva. The ovaries, oviducts, and uterine horns lie on either side of the descending colon and its mesocolon. The uterine body and cervix are ventral to the terminal portion of the descending colon and the rectum. Ventral to the uterine body and cervix is the bladder with its corresponding urethra coursing caudally and ventrally to the vagina. The urethra terminates into the vestibule at the urethral orifice. The vagina relates dorsally to the rectum, ventrally to the bladder and urethra, and laterally to the pelvic wall.

The actual position of the internal reproductive genitalia of the mare is dependent upon the movement of the intestines, the distention within the bladder, and the condition of pregnancy. When the bladder is distended and the descending colon is full, the uterine body can be displaced to one side. In the nonpregnant mare, the position of the ovaries, uterine tubules, and uterine horns can vary from contact with the dorsal abdominal wall to a location among the intestinal coils. Various ligamentous structures on the ovaries, oviducts, and uterine horns allow for this mobility.

The Ovaries

The ovaries of the mare are kidney-bean shaped with a prominent depression on the free or ventral border. Different mares have different sized ovaries. The rule is that they are usually larger in the younger animals than in the older mares. It is not unusual to find one ovary larger than the other. The average length of the equine ovary is approximately seven to eight centimeters, and it is usually three to four centimeters thick. A convex dorsal border is often called the greater curvature of the ovary. Each ovary can be described as having two surfaces, (lateral and medial), two borders, (dorsal or attached and ventral or free), and two poles (cranial or tubule and caudal or uterine). The poles are rounded in shape with the cranial pole attached to a portion of the fimbriae of the oviduct. The caudal pole is attached to a point just caudal to the end of a uterine horn by the proper ligament of the ovary. The dorsal or attached border is enclosed by part of the broad ligament which is termed the mesovarium.

The ovary in a nonpregnant mare may ride on the intestines, and the mesovarium may be loose. The right ovary is often approximately fifteen centimeters behind the corresponding kidney. The left ovary is usually more caudal than the right. The ovary may vary in distance from the uterine horn by as much as five centimeters. The average distance from the ovaries to the vulvar orifice is approximately fifty to fifty-five centimeters in a mare of average size. The convex surface of the ovary is referred to as the hilus. The term hilus is defined as that part of an organ where nerves and vessels enter and leave. Most of the surface of the ovary is covered by peritoneum, but the peritoneal tissues are absent at the attached border of the hilus. The medial and lateral surfaces are covered by the mesovarium. The visceral layer of the peritoneum is connected to more than half of the total surface of the ovary where it is loosely attached. It is within these loose connective tissues between the visceral layer and the ovary itself where the arteries, veins, and stored fat are contained.

In the ovary of the adult mare, the structure is such that the medullary or vascular zone is superficial, and the cortical zone, which contains the oocytes and follicles, is partly in the interior of the structure. The cortical zone only reaches the

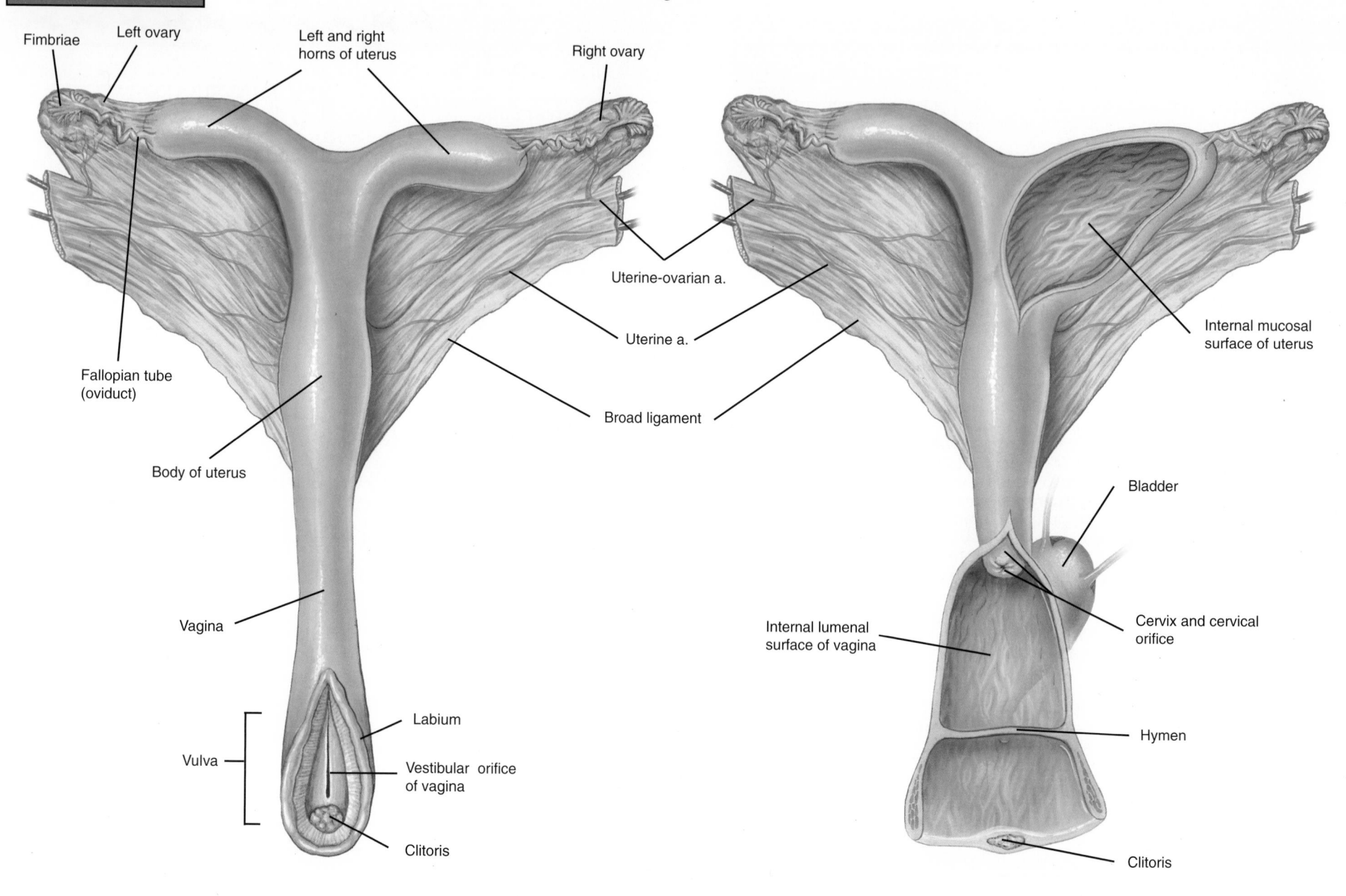

THE MARE *Anatomy of the Fallopian Tubes, Uterus, Cervix, and Vagina*

Fimbriae

Left ovary

Left and right horns of uterus

Right ovary

Uterine-ovarian a.

Uterine a.

Internal mucosal surface of uterus

Fallopian tube (oviduct)

Broad ligament

Body of uterus

Bladder

Vagina

Internal lumenal surface of vagina

Cervix and cervical orifice

Labium

Vulva

Vestibular orifice of vagina

Hymen

Clitoris

Clitoris

Dorsal View of the Mare's Reproductive System

surface at the ovulation fossa on the free border. This is the only area on the ovary where normal ovulation can occur. The corpus luteum is also seen within the ovulation fossa. During folliculogenesis, maturing follicles move toward the fossa and enlarge in diameter. These follicles can enlarge to four and a half to six centimeters in diameter just before ovulation. These mature ovarian follicles become less turgid. Following ovulation, a corpus hemorrhagicum forms. The corpus luteum does not bulge from the ovary, as in other species, but projects slightly into the ovulation fossa. This structure then becomes yellow. Secondary corpora lutea form at forty days of gestation from other rapidly growing follicles.

Oviducts (Uterine or Fallopian Tubes)

The cranial end of the oviduct is the beginning of the continuous lumen of tubular genitalia which begins with this structure and ends at the labia. The oviducts function to convey the ova from the ovary to the uterus. The oviducts in the mare can be divided into an infundibulum, ampulla, and isthmus. Cumulatively, they are twenty to thirty centimeters long in structure.

The most cranial portion of the oviduct is the infundibulum. Its cranial margin contains an irregular process called the fimbriae. This structure is attached to the cranial pole of the ovary to form the cranial margin of the ovulation fossa. When ovulation occurs, the infundibulum covers the ovulation fossa to facilitate the entry of the ova into the oviduct. The ampulla of the oviduct is that portion which extends from the abdominal opening to where it gradually narrows into the isthmus at the lateral surface of the ovary's caudal pole. The isthmus comprises the remainder of the oviduct and opens into the uterine horn slightly caudal to the blunt end of the horn.

Externally, the oviduct is covered by a serous coat formed by the mesosalpinx. On the fimbriae, the serous membrane meets with the mucous lining that occurs internally. Circular muscle fibers, along with some longitudinal fibers, occur as a derivative of the broad ligament. The lumen of the oviduct is lined by a mucous coat that is thin and very placated.

These folds are longitudinal in structure and are continuous onto the fimbriae. The lumen is lined with an epithelium containing a single layer of columnar ciliated cells. These cilia produce a current directed toward the uterus that aids in the transport of the recovered ova.

The Uterus

The uterus of the mare consists of two horns and a body. The horns of the uterus are located entirely within the abdominal cavity lying on or within the intestinal coils. The body of the uterus is situated partially in the abdominal cavity and partially in the pelvic cavity where it is continuous caudally with the cervix. The walls of an estrus or anestrus uterus are quite flaccid and appear like part of the bowel. During diestrus, the tone of the uterus increases as it does during early pregnancy. The uterine horns range in length from twenty to twenty-five centimeters. The diameter of the horns increases from the point of their attachment to the oviducts to their junction with the body of the uterus. The body of the uterus averages eighteen to twenty centimeters in length.

The broad ligaments of the uterus attach the body and uterine horns to the abdominal and pelvic walls. These broad ligaments extend on either side of the sublumbar region and the lateral pelvic wall to the dorsal border of the cornua and the lateral margins of the body of the uterus. Dispersed through these ligaments are the vessels and nerves of the uterus and ovaries, connective tissue, and a large amount of unstriped muscle fibers which are continuous with those of the uterus. Along the parietal margins are the ureters. The lateral layer of each gives off a fold (the round ligament of the uterus) which blends with the parietal peritoneum over the abdominal inguinal ring.

The lumen of the uterus contains numerous prominent endometrial folds. These folds are arranged longitudinally and average between five and ten in number.

Histologically, the uterine wall contains three layers: the perimetrium, the myometrium, and the endometrium. The perimetrium is the serosa layer

of the uterus and is continuous with the broad ligaments. The myometrium consists of a thick inner circular layer of smooth muscle and a thin outer longitudinal layer. Between these two layers of muscle is a vascular layer which supplies blood to these tissues. The endometrium consists of an epithelial lining and a lamina propria which is composed of two layers: the stratum compactum and the stratum spongiosum. The lamina propria of the uterus contains glands opening on the surface of the endometrium and extending down into the depth of the stratum spongiosum. The epithelial lining of the endometrium is secretory in nature and consists of high columnar epithelial cells that may be ciliated.

The Cervix

The cervix is often times considered a portion of the uterus. It is a thick walled firm structure that is five to seven and a half centimeters in length and three and a half to four centimeters in diameter. A portion of it projects into the cavity of the vagina. During estrus, the structure becomes flaccid and relaxed in nature. Within the lumen of the cervix are numerous folds arranged longitudinally. These are continuous with the endometrial folds of the uterine body. A distinct feature of the equine cervix is the dilatability of the lumen and the lack of any noticeable cervical rings.

The cervix has three functions. It produces a large amount of mucus that may act as a lubricant or a sealant. The lumen can be occluded so that it is impermeable to foreign material and bacteria. Lastly, it can expand in size to a point where it will allow the passage of the foal during parturition.

The Vagina

The vagina of the mare extends from the cervix to the labia of the vulva. It is tubular in structure and approximately fifteen to twenty centimeters in length. When slightly dilated, the vagina is about ten to twelve centimeters in diameter. It is situated within the pelvic cavity ventral to the rectum, dorsal to the bladder and urethra, and lateral to the pelvic wall. The lumen of the vagina is extremely dilatable and is limited only by the pelvic wall.

Anatomy of the Vulva and Mammary Gland; Perineal Conformation

Artwork by S. Hakola / J. Dirig
Copyright Equistar Publications, Ltd.

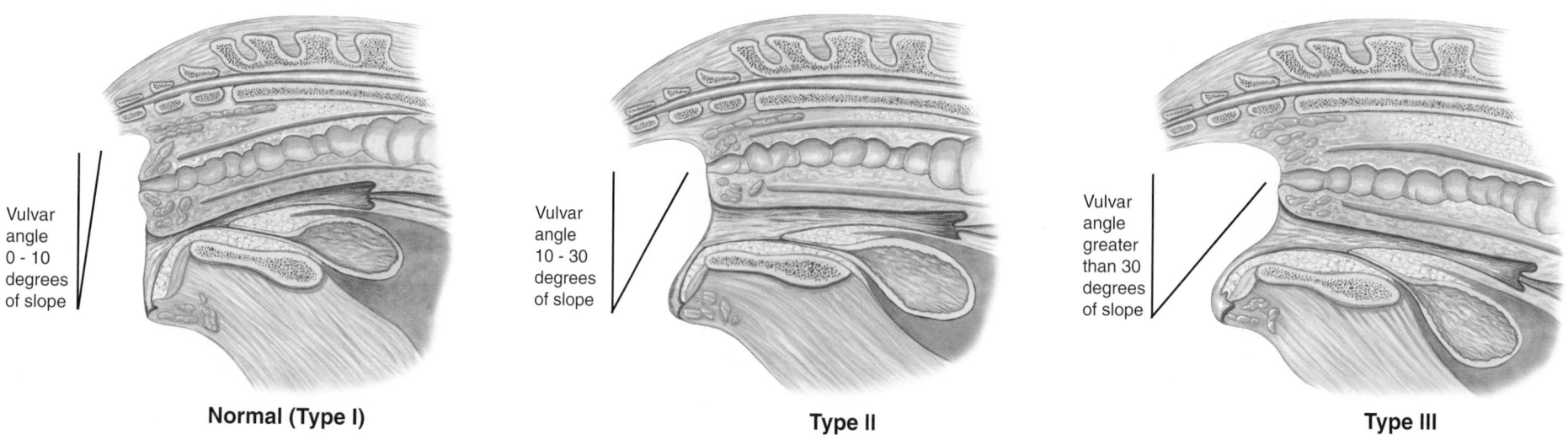

Ilium

Anus

Ischial
tuber

Vaginal
orifice

Labium of
vulva

Relationship of Perineum and Pelvis

Subcutaneous fat

Lactiferous
ducts

Cranial lactiferous
sinus

Caudal lactiferous sinus

Caudal papillary duct

Cranial papillary duct

Mammary Gland

Vulvar
angle
0 - 10
degrees
of slope

Normal (Type I)

Vulvar
angle
10 - 30
degrees
of slope

Type II

Vulvar
angle
greater
than 30
degrees
of slope

Type III

Perineal Conformation

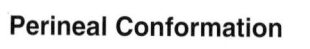

Caudally, the vagina and all of the vulva are covered by a fibrous tissue and a large amount of intermuscular connective tissue. This muscular layer is composed of a thin layer of longitudinal fibers and a thicker layer of circular fibers. The mucous layer is highly elastic and is covered by a stratified epithelium which has no glandular structures. The fornix is an annular cavity around the projecting caudal portion of the cervix. Therefore, an annular recess is formed around the cervix.

The Vulva

The vulva consists of two labia and the clitoris. It is the terminal portion of the genital tract and is continuous in front with the vagina and opens externally at the vulvar cleft five to seven centimeters below the anus. There is no distinct line of demarcation between the vagina and vulvar structures. The structure of the vulva is related dorsally by the rectum and anus, ventrally by the pelvic floor, and laterally to the sacrosciatic ligament and semimembranosus muscle. The external orifice consists of a vertical slit twelve to fifteen centimeters long which is sometimes referred to as the vulvar cleft. This cleft is bound by two prominent labia which form an acute angle above and a rounded junction below. The acute angle of the labia is termed the dorsal commissure whereas the rounded junction below is termed the ventral commissure. The ventral commissure is situated approximately five centimeters below the arch of the pelvis. Any instrumentation, such as a speculum, should enter the vulva at an upward angle.

The clitoris is the female homologue of the penis and consists of very similar structures. The corpus clitoridis is about five centimeters long, and its diameter is about that of one's small finger. It is attached to the ischial arch by two crura. The glands clitoridis is the rounded and enlarged free end of the organ and occupies the fossa clitoridis in the ventral commissure of the vulva.

The Mammary Glands

The udder of the virgin mare is very small and inconspicuous. Each gland is placed on either side of the median plane in the prepubic region. It consists of a glandular mass or body and the papilla or teat. The base is attached to the abdominal wall by areolar tissue which contains a venous plexus, the superficial inguinal lymph gland, and a variable amount of fat. The teat is flat transversely and varies in length from two and a half to five centimeters.

The skin covering the mammary gland in the mare is thin, pigmented, and chiefly hairless. The skin contains numerous large sebaceous and sweat glands. Beneath the skin are two layers of fascia except on the teat. On either side of the median plane, two lamina from the abdominal tunic descend and form a septum between the two glands constituting a suspensory ligament. The parenchyma or glandular substance is pinkish gray in color and of a somewhat firm consistency. It is enclosed by a fibroelastic capsule which sends numerous trabeculae inward. These trabeculae form an interstitial tissue and divide the gland into lobes and lobules. Secretory tubules and alveoli unite to form larger ducts. Each lobe has a duct which opens at the base of the teat at a space called the lactiferous sinus and from this, two lactiferous ducts pass through the extremity of the teat. The lining of these ducts consists of a nonglandular mucous membrane which is covered by a stratified squamous epithelium. A sphincter is formed by a circular arrangement of unstriped muscle tissue.

An average sized lactating mare produces around ten liters of milk daily. The fat content of equine milk is quite low, approximately one point six percent. The lactose content is extremely high, approximately six point one percent.

External Perineal Conformation

The conformation of the external genitalia of the mare is important since abnormal perineal conformation will lead to pneumovagina, cervicitis, endometritis and/or a state of subfertility. The mare's vulvar and perineal structures have a great influence on the animal's reproductive health.

Anatomically, the perineum is the body wall encompassing the outlet of the pelvis and surrounding urogenital passage and anal canal. The structure is bounded dorsally by the base of the tail and coccygeal muscles, laterally by the sacrosciatic ligaments and the semimembranous muscles, and ventrally by the ischial arch and the udder.

The vulva includes the clitoris and labia. The labia consists of the mucocutaneous vulvar lips and constrictor muscles. An acute angle, referred to as the dorsal commissure, is formed approximately five centimeters below the anus. The ventral commissure is thick and rounded and lies approximately five centimeters behind and below the ischial arch. The opening of the vulvar cleft between the dorsal and ventral commissures is approximately twelve to fifteen centimeters long. This vulvar length is actually under hormonal influence. Progesterone, which causes an increase in vulvar muscle tone, shortens the vulvar length. Estrogen relaxes and lengthens the vulva. "Winking" is the inversion of the clitoris when the mare exhibits a sign of estrus. It is a function of the contraction of the vulvar constrictor, the constrictor vestibuli, and the retractor clitoridis muscles.

Normal perineal conformation is the first barrier between the external environment and the uterus. The other anatomical barriers that are present in the mare's reproductive tract are the transverse fold and the cervix. In the case of optimal conformation, the right and left vulvar lips should be apposed evenly and appear full and firm. The dorsal commissure of the vulva should be no more than four centimeters above the pelvic floor. The vulvar lips should be in a vertical position with a cranial-to-caudal slope of no more than ten degrees from vertical.

Artwork by S. Hakola / J. Dirig
Copyright Equistar Publications, Ltd.

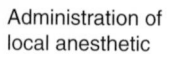

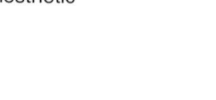

Administration of
local anesthetic

Removal of mucosa to reveal
submucosal gap of 8-10 mm.

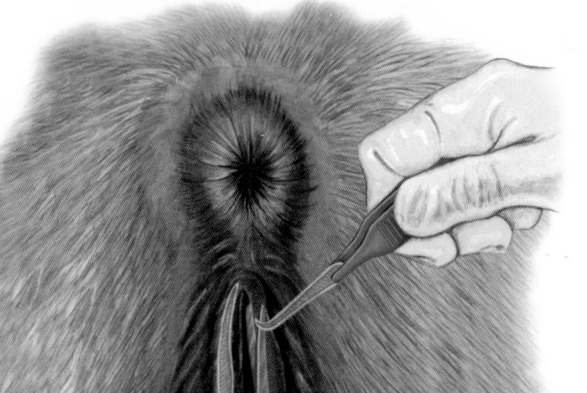

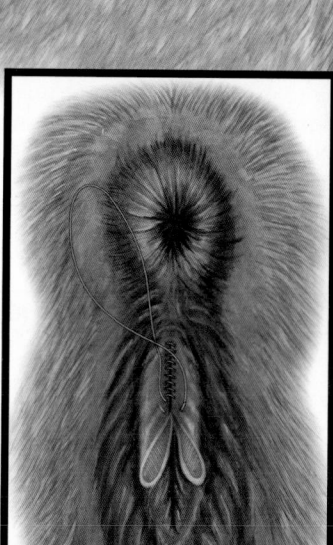

Continuous
suture
pattern

Caslick's Vulvoplasty Surgery

- Triggered by daylight or photosensitization
- Follicular development leads to secretion
  of **ESTROGEN**
  - increased sexual receptivity
  - relaxation of cervix & vagina
  - stimulation of secretions within
    uterus, cervix, and vagina
- Ovulation occurs 24 - 48 hours prior to the
  end of estrus

ESTRUS (FOLLICULAR) PHASE
5 -7 Days

19 - 22 Days
(Average of
21 Days)

14 - 15 Days
DIESTRUS (LUTEAL) PHASE

- Formation of corpus luteum following ovulation
  produces **PROGESTERONE**
  - prohibits sexual behavior
  - aids in closure of cervix
  - prepares entire reproductive
    tract for pregnancy

The Estrous Cycle

When the conformation of the vulvoperineum is varied, the mare is predisposed to reproductive problems. There are three distinct vulvoperineal conformational types:

Type I mares: Anatomically, these animals have less than two to three centimeters of vulva dorsal to the pelvic brim. In most cases these are young animals and rarely require a Caslick operation.

Type II mares: These mares have a length of six to seven centimeters between the dorsal commissure and the pelvic floor. These mares will usually need a Caslick operation at the point of their life when the angle of declination of the vulva increases because of the general relaxation of the organs and muscles in the pelvic region.

Type III mares: These mares anatomically measure five to nine centimeters between the dorsal commissure and the pelvic floor. There is a definite angle of declination within the conformation of the vulvar structures. These mares require a Caslick operation at an early age.

There are many causes to these variations in perineal conformation. Genetic heritability is probably the most common etiology of poor perineal conformation. Debilitation of the animal's general physical condition can predispose the mare to abnormal conformation even though the mare may have normal conformation when not debilitated. As the mare gets older, the effective length of the vulva will increase. Trauma during foaling or an external trauma can also result in perineal abnormalities.

Any abnormal perineal conformation results in a compromised vulvar seal and predisposes the animal to pneumovaginitis, cervicitis, vaginitis, or endometritis. Urine pooling or urovagina can occur if the urethral orifice is pulled cranial to the ischium. When the urine is voided, it cannot pass completely through the caudal vagina and vulvar lips. This results in a retention of urine in the interior portion of the vaginal canal which causes chronic irritation of the tissues and predisposes the reproductive tract to subfertility. Any chronic irritation from urine, air, or fecal material will decrease the mare's ability to conceive. Contamination of the vagina can even cause early embryonic death and abortion since the aspiration of air can lead to a placentitis resulting in fetal septicemia.

Perineal Surgery

Surgery is performed on the perineum of the mare to correct abnormal perineal conformation or to repair damage from breeding or foaling. Care must be taken to try to surgically correct any of the protective barriers of the vagina. Predisposition to pneumovagina, urovagina, or urine pooling can be corrected through a combination of medical and surgical procedures.

Surgery is performed on the perineum, vestibule, or vagina while the mare is in a standing position. Tranquilization is often helpful as a form of restraint for this procedure. Xylazine, butorphanol, or detomidine hydrochloride may be utilized to achieve tranquilization.

The infiltration of a local anesthetic or epidural anesthesia should be performed in conjunction with tranquilization. Epidural anesthesia can be accomplished with a two percent lidocaine solution injected into the first intercoccygeal space at a dose of one ml/one hundred lb. body weight. The needle is directed at right angles to the skin and guided into the first intercoccygeal space. Local anesthesia is performed with infiltration of a two percent lidocaine solution along the margins of the vulvar labia. Local anesthetics are administered until the vulvar margins are distended from the dorsal commissure to a point just below the level of the ischial arch.

After appropriate tranquilization and local perineal anesthesia has been performed, a Caslick vulvoplasty is performed on the standing mare. An eight to ten millimeter strip of vulvar mucosa is removed from the level of the mucocutaneous margin cranially from a point just below a level of the ischial arch to and including the dorsal commissure. This is completed on both vulvar labia. The vulvar cleft is then closed using a continuous suture pattern so that the tissue apposes along the denuded tissue surfaces. A nonabsorbable suture is commonly used and removed ten to twelve days after the procedure.

A common measuring device is used to determine the proper amount of closure to the vulvar cleft. A tube speculum is inserted through the vulvar cleft into the vagina and the sutures are placed in a fashion to easily permit passage of this speculum. Excessive closure of this vulvar cleft will predispose the animal to splashback of urine producing a urovagina.

The Estrous Cycle

Sexual activity in the mare is influenced by the season of the year, nutrition, and climate. These characteristics allow classification of the mare as a seasonal polyestrous animal. In the northern hemisphere, the majority of the mares will undergo cyclic sexual activity during the breeding season which consists of the spring and summer months. There are exceptions to the rule and the odd mare will stay reproductively active during the late fall and winter. The reproductive activity in the mare is primarily regulated by the photoperiod. Therefore, when the day length increases in the early spring, ovarian activity is gradually stimulated. The increased day length creates a transition from an anestrous state to a breeding state. Follicular development progresses from irregularity to the first ovulation of the season. After the first ovulation, the mares will generally continue to have regular ovulatory cycles.

The estrous cycle is that sequence of events that prepares the mare for conception. This estrous cycle can be divided into a follicular phase, known as estrus, and a luteal phase, known as diestrus. When the mare is sexually receptive to the stallion, a follicle develops which secretes estrogen. This is termed estrus. During the last twenty-four to forty-eight hours before the end of this estrus period, ovulation occurs. When the mare is not receptive to the stallion, and the genital tract is prepared to accept a conceptus, the period is termed diestrus. Upon ovulation, the ruptured follicle develops into a corpus luteum which secretes progesterone. This increased progesterone secretion causes the mare to reject any sexual advances from a stallion. Therefore, the term luteal phase of the cycle is derived from that period of time when the corpus luteum secretes progesterone.

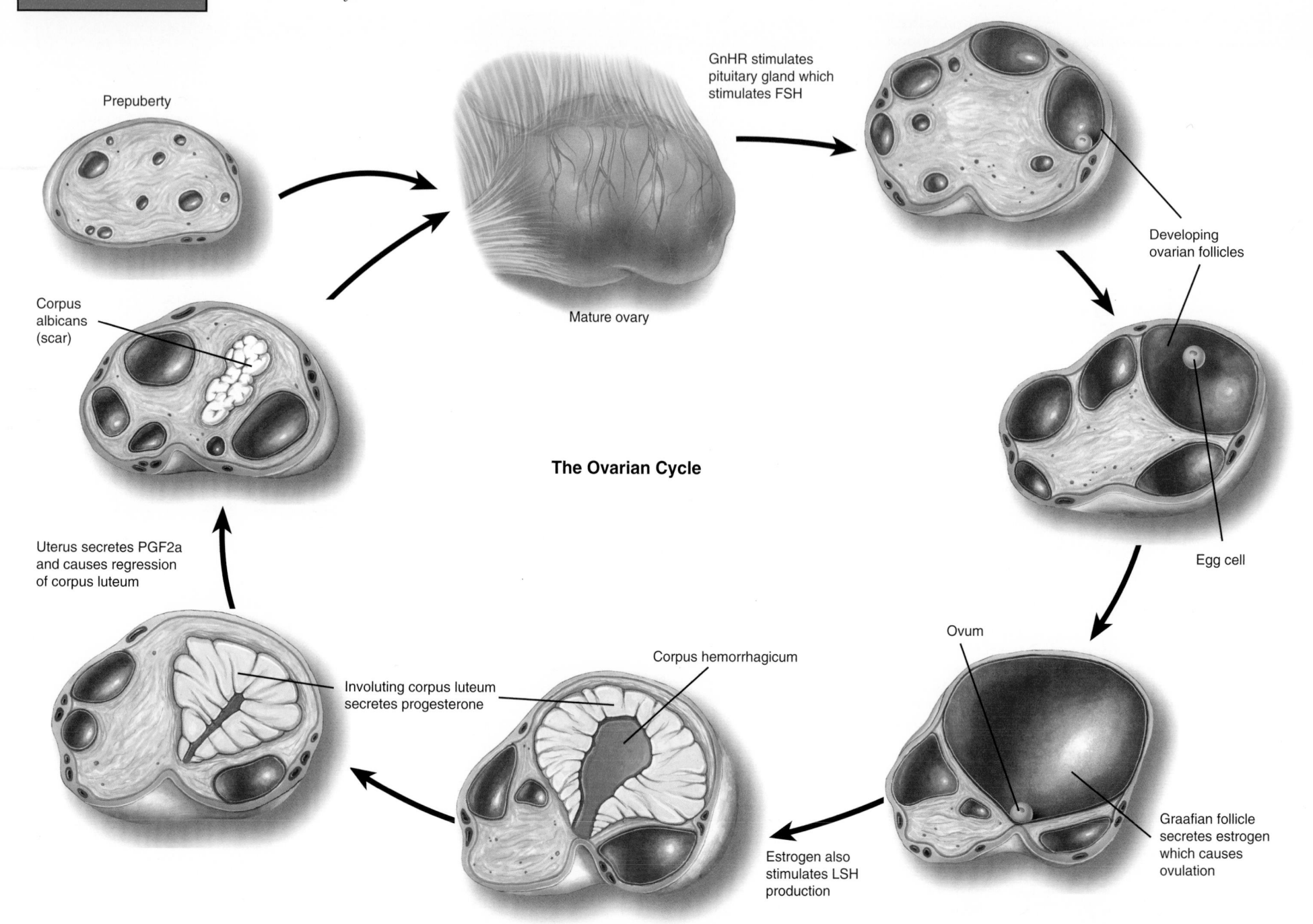

THE MARE

The Ovarian Cycle

Prepuberty

GnHR stimulates pituitary gland which stimulates FSH

Mature ovary

Developing ovarian follicles

Corpus albicans (scar)

Egg cell

The Ovarian Cycle

Uterus secretes PGF2a and causes regression of corpus luteum

Ovum

Corpus hemorrhagicum

Involuting corpus luteum secretes progesterone

Graafian follicle secretes estrogen which causes ovulation

Estrogen also stimulates LSH production

The average estrous cycle is twenty-one days in the mare. Diestrus averages fourteen to fifteen days and estrus averages five to seven days. An estrous cycle is that cyclic interval from the beginning of one estrus to the beginning of the next. Simply, it can be defined as the period between two ovulations.

Using the technique of ultrasonography, it has been found that follicles within the ovary tend to grow in waves. In most cases, there are one to two waves per cycle. At approximately the time of ovulation, the follicles that are two to five millimeters in size become identifiable within the ovaries. These small follicles grow at a rate of two and a half to three millimeters per day during the luteal phase of the cycle. At the time of luteolysis, these follicles have reached a diameter of approximately twenty-five to thirty millimeters. One or two of the follicles then become dominant and continue to grow while the remaining follicles regress. In some instances, a second follicular wave appears in the midluteal phase after regression or a diestrous ovulation of the follicle which developed during the first wave.

Luteolysis occurs and the largest follicle usually becomes the primary ovulatory follicle. This primary ovulatory follicle increases from its size of thirty millimeters to greater than forty-five millimeters less than twenty-four hours before ovulation. The diameter of these primary ovulatory follicles is greater during the breeding season than those diameters seen during the rest of the year.

Ovulation is a specific event that takes very little time. The follicle has ripened over many days, yet when ovulation occurs, the follicular fluid disappears in less than two minutes. After ovulation, the follicular cavity fills with blood and is termed the corpus hemorrhagicum. It is a soft mushy structure that usually reaches its maximum size in two to two and a half days. Ultrasonography can be used to differentiate a follicle from the corpus hemorrhagicum. This corpus hemorrhagicum develops into a corpora lutea. During pregnancy, accessory corpora lutea develop from unruptured follicles.

On the average, sixteen percent of the mares have two ovulations. These multiple ovulations are influenced by breed, genetic disposition, and the time of the year. These double ovulations do not appear to affect the duration of the estrous cycle, estrus or diestrus. The progesterone concentrations are very similar in mares with either one or two corpora lutea.

Progesterone and estrogen have a dramatic effect on the oviducts, uterus, cervix, vagina, and vulva. The effect of higher concentrations of estrogen upon the uterine tissue results in a state of edema within these tissues. The uterus feels heavier upon palpation and has only slight tone and tubularity. After ovulation, the edema begins to disappear and the tone and tubularity increase. When the uterus is under the influence of progesterone, secretions within the uterus can be scanned using ultrasonography. There is little or no edema present within the tissues. During anestrus, the uterus loses its muscular tone and becomes flaccid.

Through the use of a vaginal speculum, the changes within the cervix can be visualized during the estrous cycle. Just prior to the onset of estrus, the cervix softens and relaxes. The vaginal mucosa around the cervix becomes more engorged with blood and edema. Secretions through the cervix become more abundant in the amount of fluid and consistency. Therefore, as estrus progresses, there is a change in color, hyperemia, edema, secretions, and relaxation. When progesterone levels are elevated during diestrus, the cervix is closed tightly, and there is only a scant amount of viscous mucus.

The changes in the vagina and vulva during estrus are the same as those seen in the cervix and uterus. The vagina becomes more relaxed, and secretions within the structure are increased. The vulva relaxes somewhat and becomes visually more edematous. During the period of diestrus, the vagina and vulva are dry, small in structure, and tightly closed.

Endocrinology of Reproduction

The photoperiod of the day increases and produces a stimulation to the pineal gland within the brain. This stimulation results in a decrease in the production of melatonin which allows the hypothalamus to increase the secretion of gonadotropin releaseing hormone (GnRH.). GnRH stimulates the secretion of two gonadotropins: luteinizing hormone (LH) and follicle-stimulating hormone (FSH). These hormones then reach the ovarian tissues through the systemic circulation.

Using day zero of the estrous cycle as the day of ovulation, the levels of luteinizing hormone are at their lowest level from day five to day sixteen of the cycle. Approximately two days after ovulation, the levels of luteinizing hormone are at their highest. These levels progressively decrease over the next four or five days. After luteolysis, the level of progesterone within the systemic circulation creates a negative feedback upon the pituitary production of luteinizing hormone. When this negative feedback is removed, the estrogen that is secreted by the follicles stimulates the production and secretion of the luteinizing hormone.

One of the functions of luteinizing hormone is the stimulation of the primary follicle through development and maturation. This results in an increase in the estrogen production which sequentially produces a closed positive-feedback loop.

The mare is unique in the fact that there is not any preovulatory peak in luteinizing hormone that is commonly found within other species. Therefore, the precise role of luteinizing hormone during ovulation in the mare is unknown. The equine species has a relatively high rate of double ovulations, and this could be the result of the high levels of luteinizing hormone present for a long time during the postovulatory period.

The secretions of follicle-stimulating hormone in the mare are biphasic in nature. There is a relatively smaller peak at the end of estrus and a larger peak approximately ten days before the next

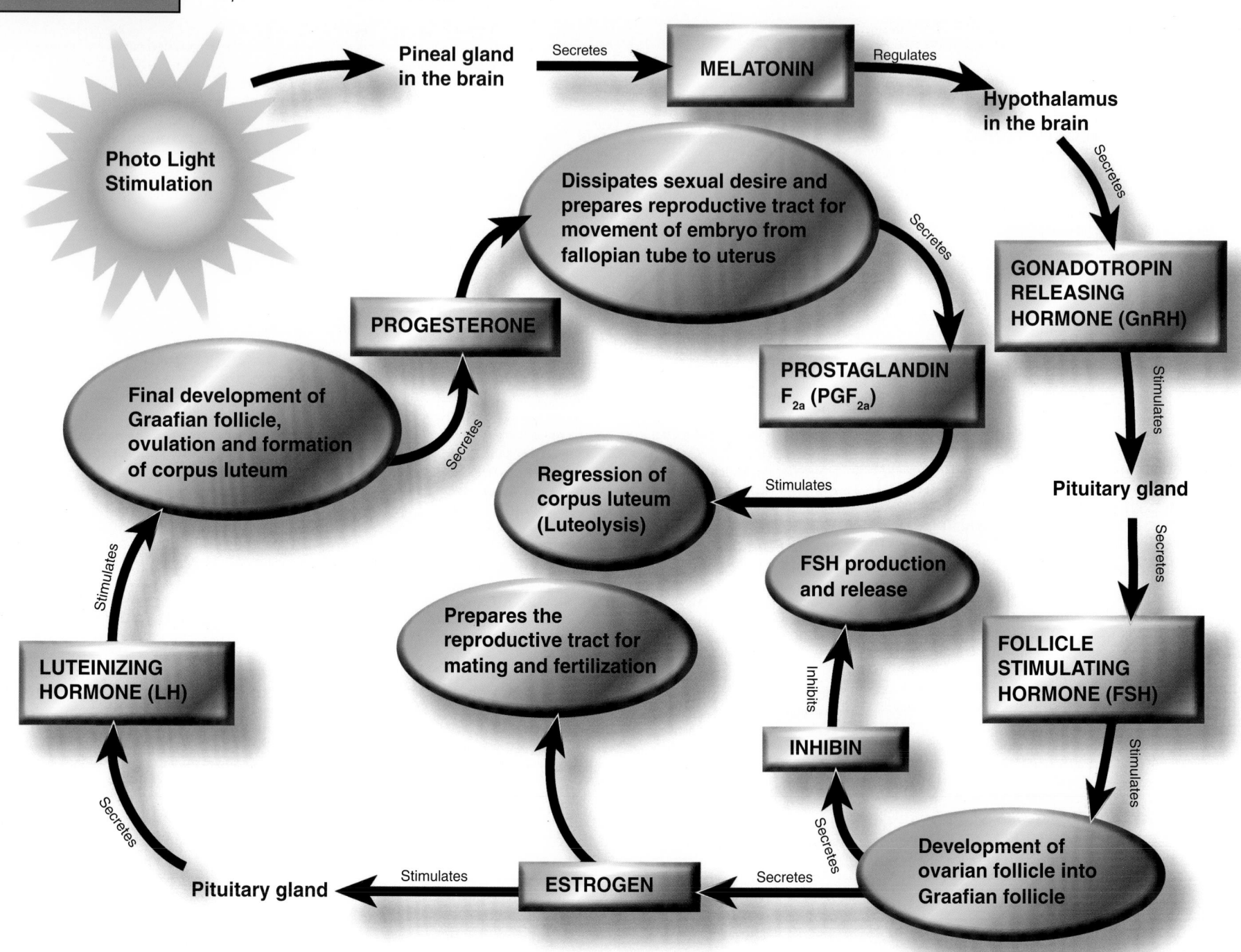

THE MARE

Reproductive Hormonal Flow Chart

Photo Light Stimulation

Pineal gland in the brain — Secretes → **MELATONIN** — Regulates → **Hypothalamus in the brain**

Hypothalamus in the brain — Secretes → **GONADOTROPIN RELEASING HORMONE (GnRH)**

GONADOTROPIN RELEASING HORMONE (GnRH) — Stimulates → **Pituitary gland**

Pituitary gland — Secretes → **FOLLICLE STIMULATING HORMONE (FSH)**

FOLLICLE STIMULATING HORMONE (FSH) — Stimulates → **Development of ovarian follicle into Graafian follicle**

Development of ovarian follicle into Graafian follicle — Secretes → **ESTROGEN**

Development of ovarian follicle into Graafian follicle — Secretes → **INHIBIN**

INHIBIN — Inhibits → **FSH production and release**

ESTROGEN — Stimulates → **Pituitary gland**

ESTROGEN → **Prepares the reproductive tract for mating and fertilization**

Pituitary gland — Secretes → **LUTEINIZING HORMONE (LH)**

LUTEINIZING HORMONE (LH) — Stimulates → **Final development of Graafian follicle, ovulation and formation of corpus luteum**

Final development of Graafian follicle, ovulation and formation of corpus luteum — Secretes → **PROGESTERONE**

PROGESTERONE → **Dissipates sexual desire and prepares reproductive tract for movement of embryo from fallopian tube to uterus**

Dissipates sexual desire and prepares reproductive tract for movement of embryo from fallopian tube to uterus — Secretes → **PROSTAGLANDIN F_{2a} (PGF_{2a})**

PROSTAGLANDIN F_{2a} (PGF_{2a}) — Stimulates → **Regression of corpus luteum (Luteolysis)**

ovulation. The primary role of follicle-stimulating hormone is to stimulate the growth of small follicles. Graafian follicles produce a protein substance which inhibits the secretion of follicle-stimulating hormone. During the late diestrus phase, increased levels of follicle-stimulating hormone are responsible for follicular development. When these follicles reach the preovulatory stage, inhibin is produced which then inhibits follicle-stimulating hormone secretions. In sequential events follicle-stimulating hormone is inhibited, estrogen and luteinizing hormone are secreted in increased levels, and further development of immature follicles is halted.

There are many functions of the estrogen hormone within the mare. Estrogen is responsible for an increased sexual receptivity, a relaxation of the cervix and vagina, and a stimulation of secretions within the uterus, cervix, and vagina. The main source of estrogen is the follicle. The level of estrogen within the systemic circulation peaks one to two days before ovulation. These levels decrease to their baseline levels within two days after ovulation.

Progesterone levels are at their lowest during the estrus phase of the estrous cycle. Circulating progesterone prohibits estrus behavior, aids in the closure of the cervix, and prepares the entire genital tract for the maintenance of pregnancy. The luteal phase begins after ovulation which results in rapid increases in the levels of circulating progesterone. The level of progesterone falls around day fifteen when the corpora lutea begin to regress.

The uterine endometrium releases prostaglandin approximately thirteen to fifteen days after ovulation. This is the agent responsible for luteolysis. The regression of the corpora lutea parallels the decline in the levels of circulating progesterone.

In pregnant mares, the primary corpus luteum begins to regress at a point approximately forty days after conception. The primitive placenta forms endometrial cups which secrete equine chorionic gonadotropins. These chorionic gonadotrophins have historically been referred to as pregnant mare serum (PMS) or pregnant mare serum gonadotropin (PMSG). Equine chorionic gonadotrophins appear around day forty of gestation, reach a maximum circulating level around day sixty of gestation, and start to decline at day one hundred and twenty of gestation. The function of these gonadotropins is to stimulate the maternal ovary to produce more ovarian follicles. These follicles ovulate and form accessory corpora lutea while some of these developing follicles luteinize without ovulation. At approximately day one hundred eighty of gestation, these accessory corpora lutea begin to degenerate. In addition, the equine chorionic gonadotropins also stimulate the fetal gonads of both sexes to increase in size.

The Initial Onset of the Estrous Cycle

Throughout the months of November to Janurary in the Northern Hemisphere, the period of sexual incompetence called anestrus occurs. During this period, the mare may develop some follicles, but they are not ovulated and the ovaries actually go through a palpable reduction in size. Any sexual behavior toward the stallion has ceased to exist. Most mares will act very negatively towards the stallion if presented.

Since the mare is a polyestrous seasonal breeder, the transition from the anestrus state to that of the breeding season is a vague and misleading time of the year. There is a traditional pressure upon veterinarians and breeding farms to have mares conceive in the early part of the year during this transitional phase. This is not only very frustrating in most cases but also reproductively inefficient. During this transitional phase, the mare may exhibit sexual behavior coinciding with renewed secretions of pituitary and ovarian hormones. Rectal examination may reveal a large preovulatory follicle that never ovulates and merely regresses after a week of instigating strong sexual behavior in the mare. It is important to guide the mare through this transitional phase as quickly and efficiently as possible in order to achieve reproductive efficiency with the next cycle.

Artificial light is the most consistent method utilized to accelerate the breeding season in the mare. The key to this system is to trick the mare's endocrine (hormonal) system into the transitional phase earlier in the year. In this way, the mare will be through all of the transitional events earlier in the year allowing for an efficient reproductive cycle to occur in Janurary and February instead of April.

The initiation of the artificial lighting system utilized in altering the onset of the estrous cycle should be done in a rhythmic manner which mimics the naturally occurring photoperiod that is normally found within that geographical area. Stimulation by artificial light should be gradually increased with corresponding periods of darkness that creates a natural photosensitive period.

Equine breeding farm managers often will question as to how much light intensity is enough. Studies have revealed that if a mare is kept in a twelve foot by twelve foot stall, the intensity of light emmitted from a 100-watt incandescent bulb is sufficient for photosensitization. This can be measured with the photometer present within most single-lens reflex cameras. A diffuser is made out of a simple styrofoam cup placed over the lens of the camera so that light is not measured on a particular focal point. The ASA is set at 400 and the shutter speed is placed at 1/4 second. The camera is then placed so that the lens is at the eye level of the horse. The aperature is set for proper exposure and the light intensity can then be measured. A light intensity of ten footcandles (107 lux) is sufficient to result in photostimulation. This method of measurement will also take into account any light being received by the animal's eye from other sources such as the security light on the outside of the barn.

Since the transitional phase may last forty to sixty days, it is important to initiate an artificial lighting program at the appropriate time. If the breeder wanted to begin breeding in February, the artificial lighting program should begin around the first of December and not in Janurary. In most cases, it is important to have the mares pass through several estrous cycles before breeding. This allows an opportunity to obtain cultures and treat infectious fertility problems. Therefore, it may be advantageous to start the photostimulation regime even as early as November to accomplish these goals.

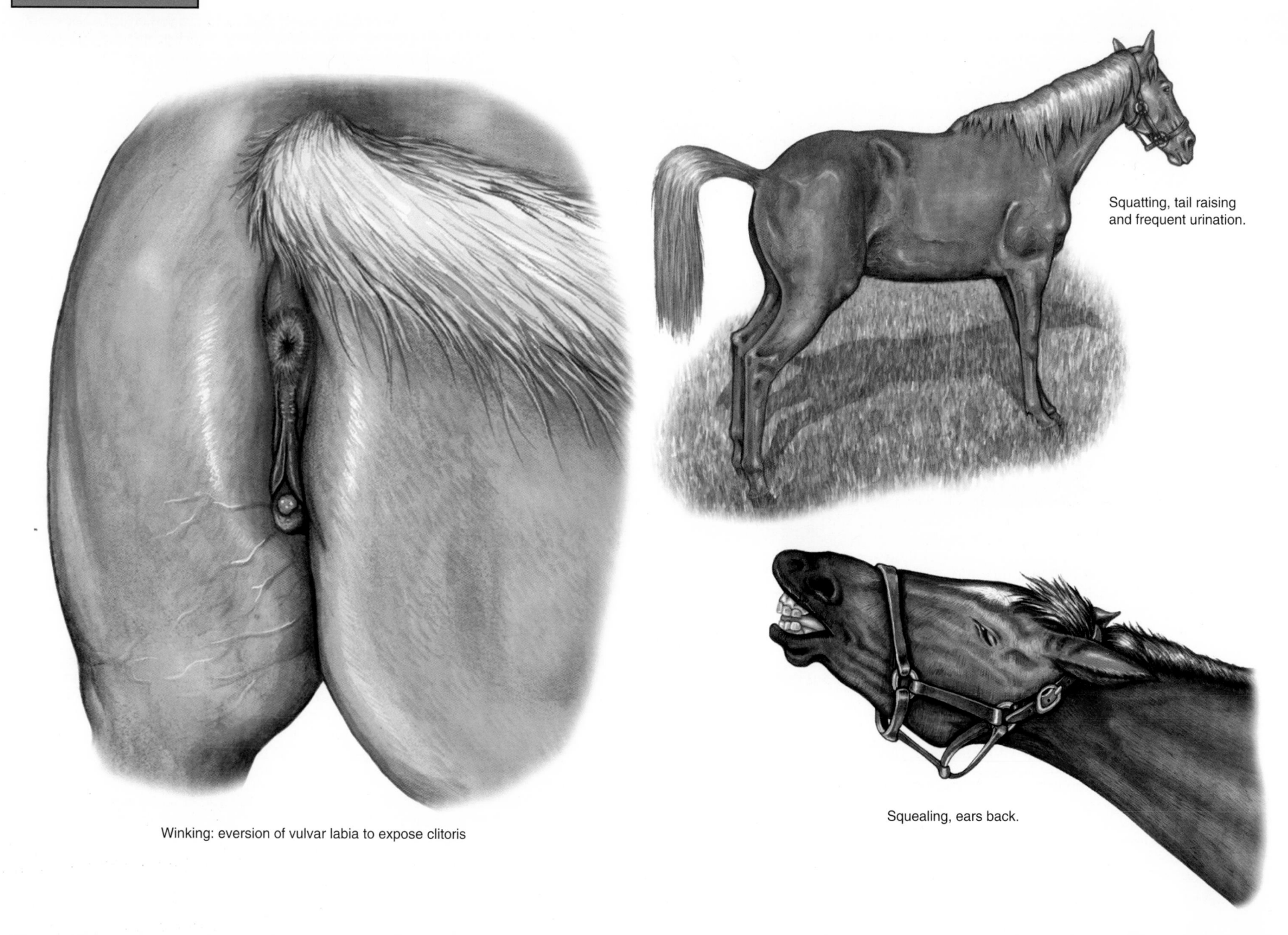

Winking: eversion of vulvar labia to expose clitoris

Squatting, tail raising and frequent urination.

Squealing, ears back.

The management system of the farm may have to be changed to accomodate an artificial lighting regime. The barren mares may have to be kept in a box stall at night whereas they are normally turned out on pasture during this time. A large paddock may have to be constructed outside with sufficient light to cause photostimulation. This can be an expensive proposition and may require a construction consultation.

It has been proven that the anestrous mare requires 14.5 hours of photostimulation to elicit a reproductive response. This is not a figure that is chiseled into concrete and varies dependent upon the geographical location. The easiest way to accomplish this task is to increase the day length through artificial means with each day beginning at dusk. The artificial light should be initiated when the intensity of light from natural sources falls below the level of 107 lux. This artificial means could then merely be supplied through the use of a timer on the lights that was adjusted each week to accommodate the natural timing of sunset. In this manner each anestrous mare is exposed to 10 - 12 footcandles of light for an additional two to two and one-half hours per day.

The Signs of Estrus

A successful breeding program relies upon the detection of estrus in order to inseminate or breed mares at the time of ovulation. The ability of the staff on the breeding farm to detect the signs of estrus often determines the success of the reproductive rates for that farm. In most cases, the lowest paid and least experienced employee of the farm is tasked to the laborious and boring task of estrus detection. This is a huge mistake and should be the task of the most skilled employee that the breeding farm has to offer. Classically, the best technique for estrus detection is the exposure of each individual mare to the stallion approximately fourteen to fifteen days after the completion of the last estrus. It is also important to tease all of the mares individually that are already exhibiting signs of estrus to determine receptivity to the stallion.

The most common behavioral signs of estrus include the following: "winking"(eversion of the vulvar labia), squatting (as if urinating), tail raising, urinating excessively, ears back, kicking, squealing, striking with the front limbs, and fence pushing. On mares where estrus detection is difficult, it is often advantageous to tease them to two stallions instead of one. There are occasions where a mare is disinterested in one and exhibits behavioral signs to the second.

It is a common practice to use pony teaser stallions on small breeding farms where a breeding stallion is not available. The cost involved in the maintenance of this animal is nominal compared to that of a breeding stallion. Historically, the effectiveness of the pony stallion in the stimulation of mares is not that of a horse stallion; therefore, use of pony stallions facilitates estrus detection.

When a stallion is not available, it is possible to treat a mare with androgens so that she exhibits stallion behavior characteristics. Testosterone propionate and boldenone undecylenate are commonly administered to mares for several weeks at a dosage needed to exhibit male sexual behavior.

The role of the stallion in the stimulation of estrus in the mare is often overlooked. Mares that have actual physical contact with the stallion readily exhibit detectable estrus more than those mares that do not have contact. The ideal teaser stallion should be controllable yet aggressive towards the mares. The stallion should not be rough but have a degree of libido that will not allow him to give up on a mare that does not immediately exhibit behavioral signs of estrus.

The flehmen response or stance is the most common characteristic of the male sexual behavior when the stallion is exposed to an estrus mare. This consists of a curling of the upper lip as if an olfactory response is made to urine or vaginal secretions. Stallions have the ability to sniff the urine or even feces and detect the odors of estrus on those animals in that stage of the cycle.

Reproductive Examination of the Mare

The first step in the reproductive evaluation of the mare is to assess the general condition of the mare and compile a medical history that is as thorough as possible. A physical exam should determine the age of the animal and the general body condition of the mare. The mare should be positively identified through the use of registration papers, tattoos, markings, brands, and photographs. The weight of the mare should be recorded with an evaluation of her underweight or overweight status. The status of her current immunizations and parasite control should be questioned. The status of her teeth and feet should be noted, and any deficiencies in these areas should be corrected. A superficial lameness exam should reveal any musculoskeletal disorders present and determine if the animal is in any state of discomfort. An evaluation should be made of the mare's attitude and behavior since this often has a significant effect on the animal's reproductive performance.

The medical and reproductive history should be recorded. This information may be essential in the final evaluation and possible selection of therapy regimes. Any medical problems should be immediately evaluated to determine their effect on the reproductive status of the mare. Reproductive records should be as accurate as possible and include any previous foaling data, estrous cycle patterns, previous uterine infections and therapy, abortions, and any previous medications that may effect reproduction. "Is the mare in foal now?" should be the first question of the reproductive history. This should be followed by: "How many foals has she had in her lifetime? How many have survived? How often has she been diagnosed pregnant and then found open at a later date? What has been the length of her gestations?" If information of the previous season's estrous cycles is available, these records should be added to the information collected from this season's cycling patterns. The question regarding the performance of any reproductive surgery on the mare should be asked and evaluated as to the significance to this breeding season. All of this information is important and should be collected and evaluated before the first physical examination of the mare is conducted.

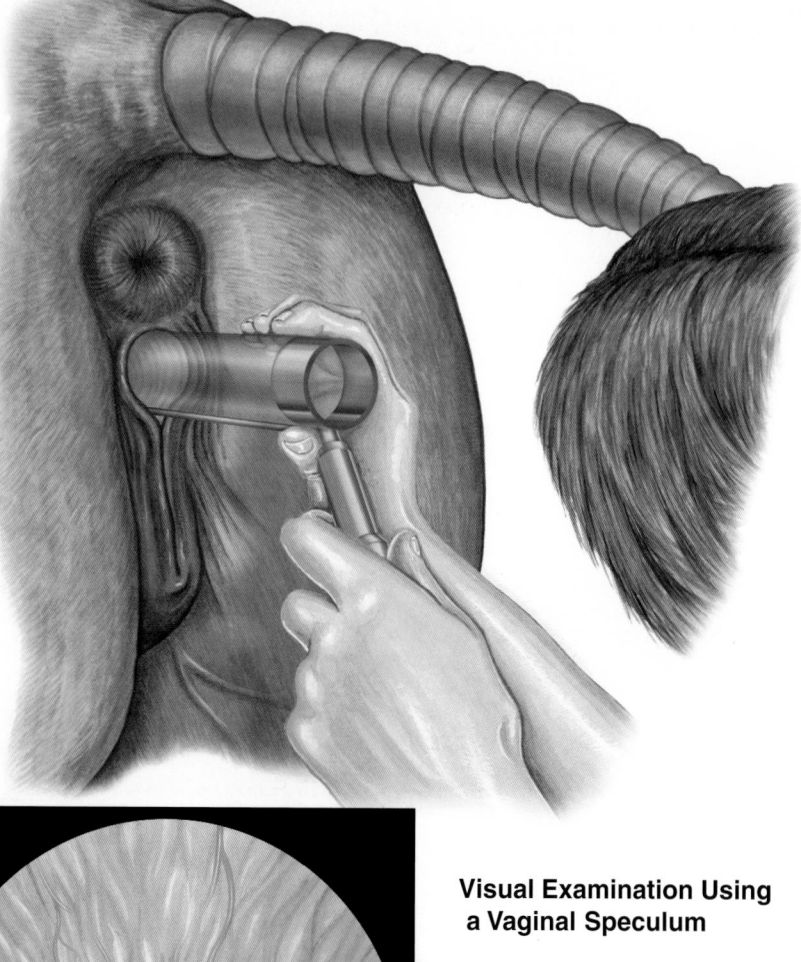

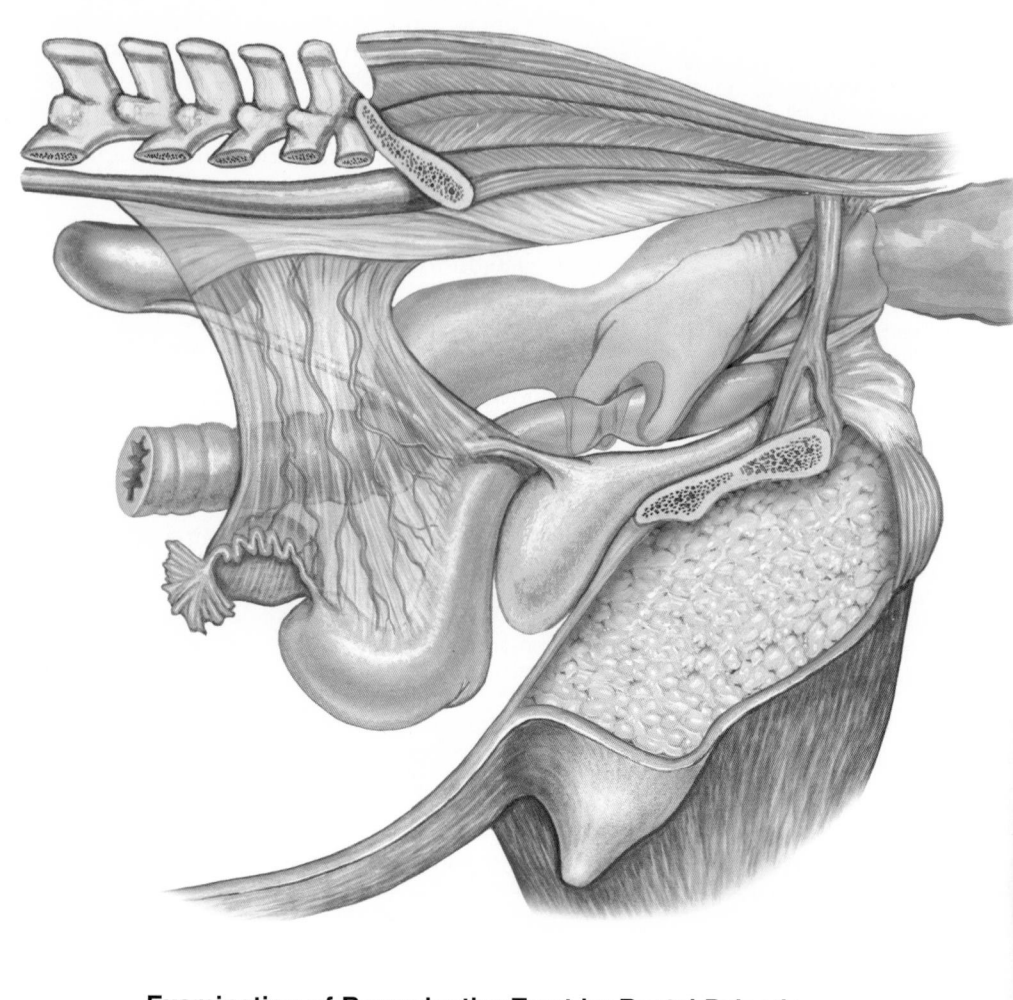

Examination of Reproductive Tract by Rectal Palpation

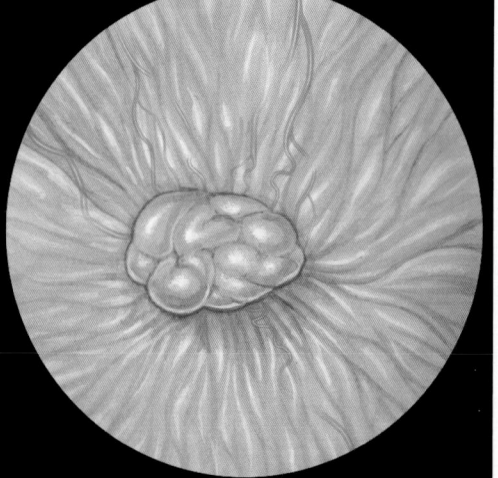

Visual Examination Using a Vaginal Speculum

Visual field of proximal vagina and cervix seen through a vaginal speculum.

Perineal conformation should be evaluated to determine its effect upon the reproductive tract of the mare. Any faults should be noted and addressed as required for correction. Evidence of previous Caslick operations, episioplasty, or laceration repair should be noted as part of the reproductive history.

The Internal Reproductive Examination

Rectal examination or palpation is the technique employed to permit direct examination of the genitalia of the mare. This method of examination will provide all of the information required to perform a fertility and pregnancy examination. Other ancillary techniques of examination are now available such as ultrasonography. Their efficacy usually depends upon a sound rectal examination. A thorough rectal examination can only be accomplished if the conditions are safe for both the mare and the examiner. Ideally, a set of stocks is available to provide restraint and safety for this procedure. If these facilities are not available, suitable restraint should be utilzed such as a twitch, lip chain, or chemical sedation. In extreme cases, a set of hobbles can be applied to the mare, but this technique is very time consuming. Copious amounts of lubrication and a rubber or plastic sleeve are the two essential materials required for rectal examination. When a large number of palpations are required, such as on a large stud farm, additional protective clothing should be worn to protect against soiling from fecal material. If a mare insists on excessive straining during the palpation procedure, a small amount of topical anesthetic such as lidocaine can be added to the lubricant to anesthetize the rectal mucosa.

There are three major objectives for the rectal examination which include the following: 1) determining the presence of physical abnormalities within the reproductive tract, 2) manually examining the ovaries, 3) determining the endocrine function stage of the cycle, and 4) diagnosing pregnancy. The presence of normal ovaries, oviducts, uterus, and cervix are fundamental for the mare to be fertile. Any abnormalities such as a change in size, location, tone, and engorgement should be noted as significant. The types of structures that are found upon the examination of the ovaries will determine the stage of the cycle and the endocrine functions currently present. The absence or presence of follicles will determine if the mare is influenced by estrogen or progesterone. This hormonal influence can also be evaluated upon uterine and cervical palpation as they are also responsive to the hormonal influences of estrogen and progesterone. A determination of pregnancy is made upon rectal palpation about 17 to 22 days after ovulation with a closed cervix and excellent uterine tone being noted. During the later stages of pregnancy, rectal palpation provides a very accurate pregnancy diagnosis.

The first obstacle of the rectal examination is the anal sphincter. A cone-shaped, well lubricated hand should be carefully inserted into the rectum using patience and responsibility. All fecal material should be removed with repeated applications of lubrication to the examining hand. After this is accomplished, most mares will relax to some degree to allow the completion of the examination. Orientation is provided through identification of the pelvic brim and the cervical structure.

The examination continues to the body of the uterus which is usually very soft, pliable, flat, and even flaccid. The size and tone of the uterine body and horns are noted and recorded. The uterus should be followed laterally and cranially to the ovary which will be attached to the uterine horn by the utero-ovarian artery and the oviduct. Suspension is provided by the broad ligament of the uterus. The greater curvature should be palpated, and this will allow orientation to the convex surface which contains the ovulation fossa. The surface of the ovary should be evaluated for smooth fluctuant areas that are the follicles. These should be evaluated for size, tone, and the degree of maturation. Any change in size or texture of the ovary should be noted and correlated with the season and cycle of the mare. The opposite uterine horn and contralateral ovary should be examined in the same manner. Before the examination is complete, an evaluation should be made of the cervix to determine its size and texture. Hormonal influence will have a positive correlation with these findings.

Visual examination of the vagina will aid in the identification of the stage of the estrous cycle, allow the diagnosis of any pathological process within the vaginal cavity, and identify any anatomical variations or problems present. Due to the hormonal influence upon this structure, visual examination of the cervix will help in the estimation of the stage of the estrous cycle. When this structure is relaxed and opened, then it can be surmised that it is under the influence of estrogen. It is not unusual to discover purulent exudates originating from the cervix in addition to inflammed tissues from urine pooling. Genetic remnants and a persistent hymen can often be visualized during this procedure.

To allow a visual examination of the mare, she is restrained and the tail wrapped or tied out of the way. The entire perineal area should be cleansed with special attention given to the clitoral fossa and the folded edges of the labia. A speculum should then be inserted into the vaginal vestibule craniodorsally at a 45 degree angle. The speculum should be sterile and be either disposable or glass. A focused bright direct beam of light allows visualization of the structures within the vagina. The source of this light is usually a halogen or a simple penlight.

The hormonal influences upon the cervix are unique in the characteristics that can be visualized during a vaginoscopic examination. During diestrus approximately ten days after ovulation, the cervix appears hard and the folds are well defined. On the first day of estrus, the cervix is slightly swollen with the folds being shallow and less defined. The orifice of the cervix is open. At the end of estrus, around the sixth day, the cervix is markedly swollen and relaxed with the folds hanging down over the orifice in a membranous fashion. The orifice appears as a horizontal slit. During pregnancy, the cervix is hard and budlike in appearance with the orifice tightly closed and covered by a pasty mucus. During the winter, most mares are anestral with no hormonal influence upon the cervical structure. In these cases the cervix appears almost white in color and flaccid. It is not unusual for the orifice to gape open during this stage.

Artwork by S. Hakola / J. Dirig
Copyright Equistar Publications, Ltd.

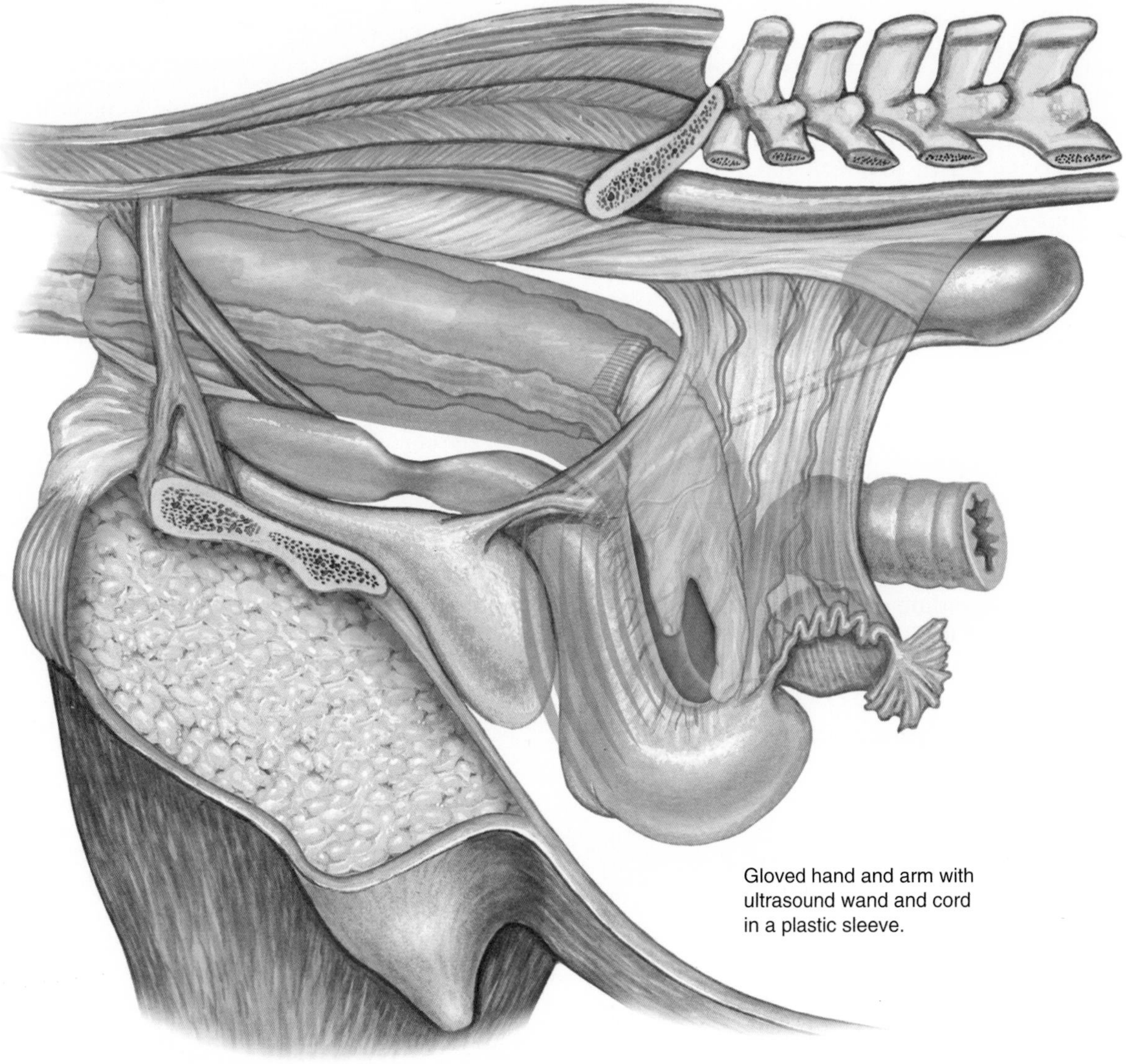

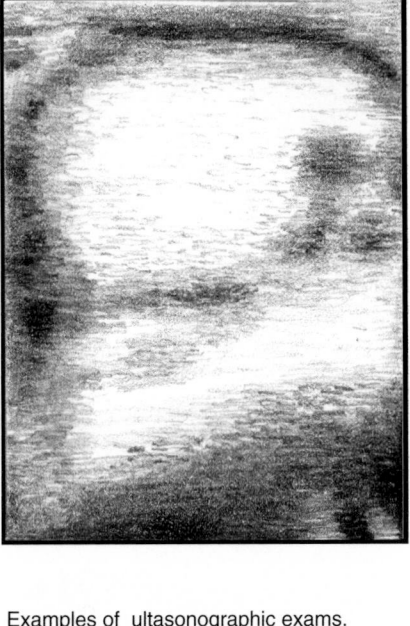

Examples of ultasonographic exams.

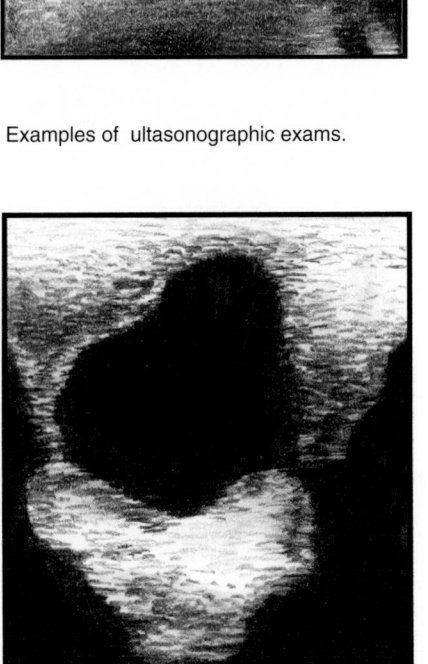

Gloved hand and arm with
ultrasound wand and cord
in a plastic sleeve.

Ultrasonographic Examination of the Mare's Reproductive Tract

When exudates are discovered during the vaginal examination, their source can be easily determined. On the first day of estrus, the mare may appear clean upon examination; yet on the third or fourth day, the examination reveals a grayish to white purulent discharge on the vaginal floor. Due to the increased level of secretions at this stage, this discharge may actually be visualized passing out of the cervical orifice. The source of the exudate can then be concluded as that from an endometritis and not from a case of pneumovagina.

Urine pooling can easily be determined upon vaginal examination. This is usually seen in older, multiparous mares that suffer from pneumovagina. In certain instances, this diagnosis can only be made during estrus when the estrogen levels are high and the perineal region is relaxed. One must be sure that the visualization is indeed urine and not an abundant level of normal secretions.

Endometrial cultures can be obtained through a vaginal speculum utilizing a guarded uterine culture swab. The possibility of any contamination from the vaginal walls is minimized. Using this technique, the culture should be taken while the mare is in heat if possible. This allows for a more representative culture that is not confused with nonpathogenic contaminants. The swab should then be submitted to a lab for the identification of the organisms and antibiotic sensitivity testing.

Ultrasonographic Examination of the Reproductive Tract

Historically, ultrasonography was merely utilized for the diagnosis of pregnancy. With the new versatile equipment that is now available, ultrasonography should be utilized as a routine part of the reproductive examination of the mare.

Ultrasonography utilizes sound waves that are produced by a transducer, transmitted through the tissues, and reflected back to the transducer. These reflected sound waves are then converted to an electrical impulse and displayed upon a screen. This is analogous to radar where energy is emitted out into the air and bounces back to a receiver when a dense object is encountered. These sound waves are reflected back in a direct proportion to

the density of the tissue that they encounter. Ultrasonic sound waves travel easily through fluid but have a more difficult time through tissues. The surface between these two mediums can then be easily determined on the ultrasound since the fluid-filled structures will appear black, or anechoic, upon the ultrasound screen.

The type of equipment that is utilized for an ultrasonic evaluation will determine the detail in the picture on the screen. Ultrasound frequencies are measured in megahertz units (Mhz; 1 hertz (Hz) = 1 sound wave). The higher the frequencies of the sound waves produced, the greater the detail of the structures that are under study. However, these high frequencies do not penetrate the tissues as well as the lower frequencies. Therefore, the lower frequencies are utilized in the study of larger structures that are further away from the transducer. An example of this concept is as follows:

    1.) A 3.0 - 3.5 MHz transducer will detect follicles when they reach about 6 - 8 mm in diameter and can detect a pregnancy around day 13 of gestation.

    2.) A 5.0 MHz transducer will be able to detect follicles when they are 3 mm in diameter and can detect a pregnancy at day 10 of gestation.

The technique for intrarectal ultrasonic examination is very similar to that of rectal palpation. It is important to understand that the transducer emits a linear sound beam that reflects all of the structures with which it comes in contact. This appears as a cross-sectional image on the screen. It is necessary to keep the probe in direct contact with the tissues to avoid scanning errors and omissions. The examination should be done in the same manner each time in a systematic fashion. The routine technique for a right handed palpator would be as follows: uterine body, right uterine horn, right ovary, uterine body, left uterine horn, left ovary, uterine body, and cervix.

One can determine the size and shape of the equine uterus through rectal palpation but a thorough evaluation of the uterine structures can be accomplished through ultrasonography. The ultrasound probe is usually held in a sagittal plane in relation to the uterus. The structures therein are

usually seen in cross-section. During anestrus, the uterus appears flat, irregular, and remains in contact with the surrounding abdominal organs. It is during this stage that no endometrial folds are present using ultrasonography. When the mare is in estrus, the uterine horns are round and easily distinguished. The endometrial folds are quite prominent, and edema is noted within the structures. These characteristics have the appearance as that of a sliced orange. During diestrus, the uterus is not as flaccid, but there are usually no endometrial folds present.

Ultrasonographic evaluation of the uterus and its corresponding endometrial folds becomes really significant when scanning for embryos in the early stages. It could be concluded that if an early embryonic vesicle is identified in a uterus with prominent endometrial folds, this pregnancy will most likely be aborted.

Uterine fluid accumulations and cysts can be evaluated utilizing ultrasonography. Rectal palpation can detect fluid accumulations within the uterus only when these accumulations are large. Intraluminal fluid during estrus in cycling mares is not that uncommon and does not appear to affect the fertility rate among these mares. However, intraluminal fluid accumulations during the diestrus phase of the cycle, resulting in a significantly lower fertility rate, is a good indication that endometritis is present. Endometrial cysts usually arise from endometrial glands or are lymphatic in origin. These cysts can be mistaken for early embryonic vesicles but can be differentiated from these vesicles by their lack of mobility, their spherical appearance, and their growth rate. In some cases, the presence of these cysts is the cause of early embryonic death. Other uterine lesions can be identified using ultrasonography. Air within the uterine lumen can be distinguished and is usually found normally after artificial insemination. Tumors, abscesses, and hematomas can be recognized and evaluated for further therapy.

Utilizing ultrasonography, an examination of the ovaries will result in an estimation of the stage of the estrous cycle, an assessment of the preovulatory follicles, the time of ovulation, an

Artwork by S. Hakola / J. Dirig
Copyright Equistar Publications, Ltd.

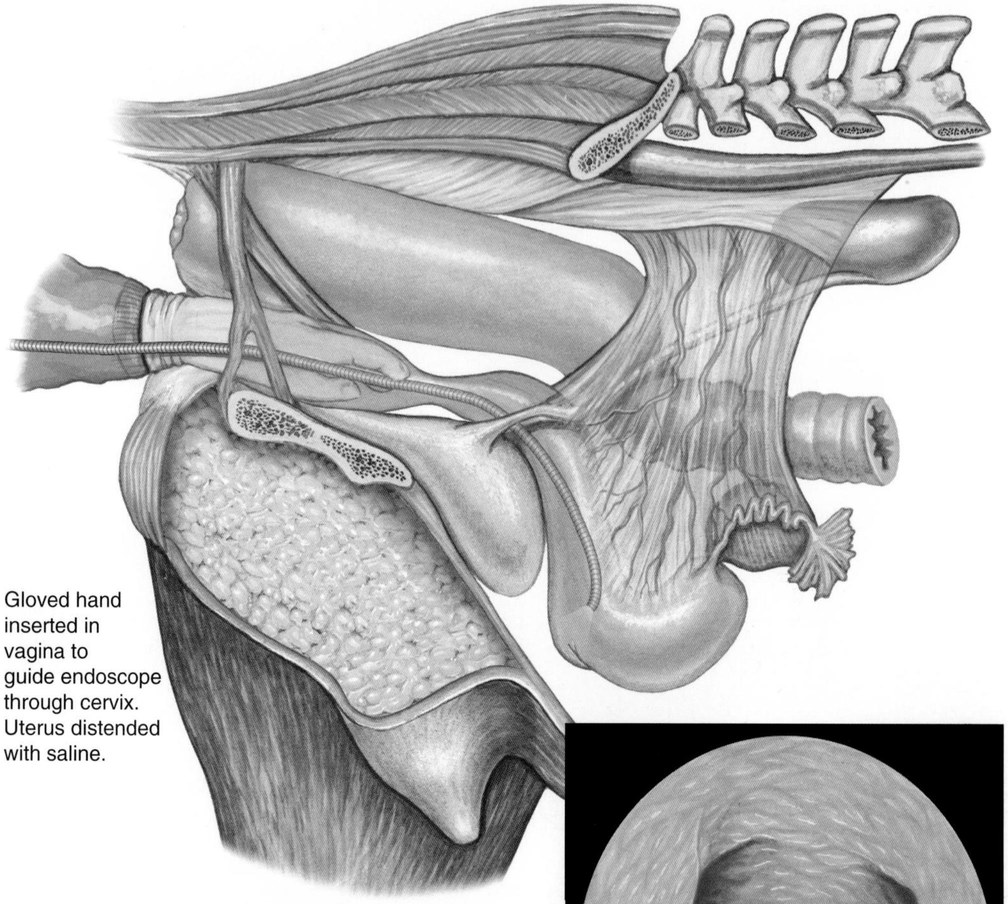

Gloved hand
inserted in
vagina to
guide endoscope
through cervix.
Uterus distended
with saline.

Fiberoptic Examination

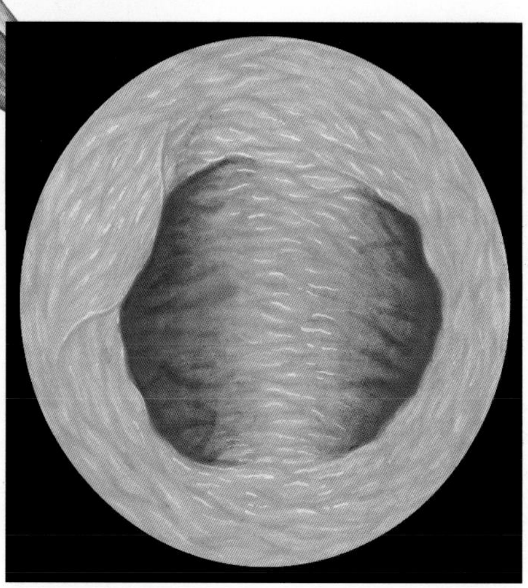

Visual field of uterine
horn bifurcation.

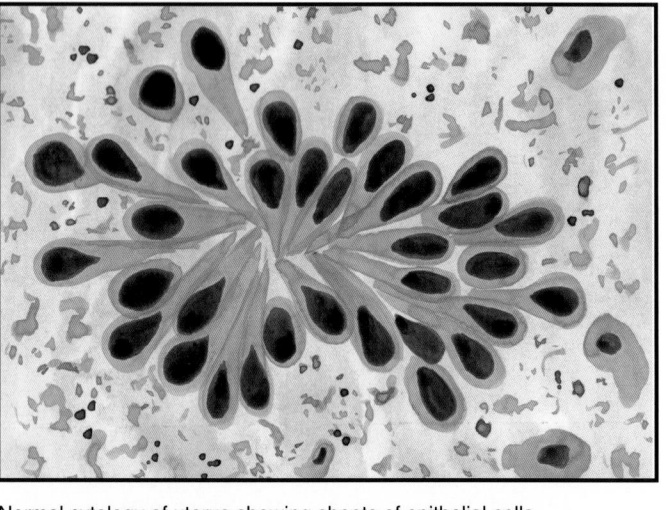

Normal cytology of uterus showing sheets of epithelial cells.
(Diff-Quick stain)

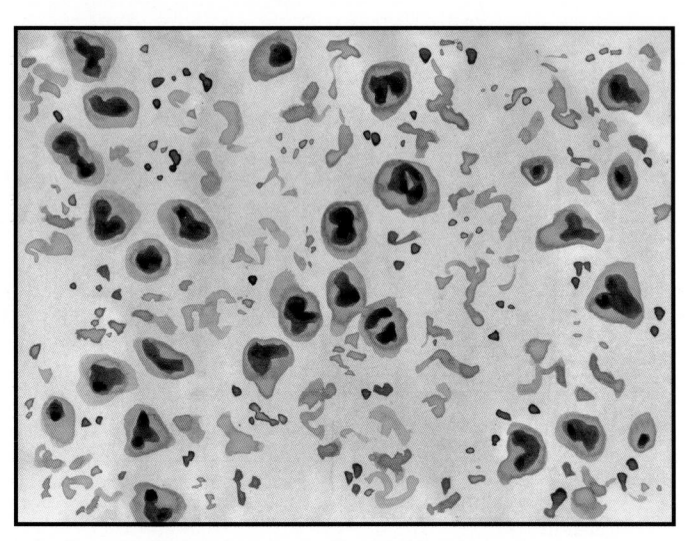

Endometritis cytology with hematoxylin-eosin stain. Many neutrophils,
some of which have degenerated, phagocytosed bacteria, and
degenerated epithelial cells.

examination of the corpus luteum, and the diagnosis of ovarian pathologies and lesions.

The stage of the estrous cycle can be determined through an evaluation of the ovarian stroma by ultrasonography. When the mare is in the anestrus state, the ovaries are inactive with no visible corpus luteum or follicles. During the transitional phase of the cycle, numerous large follicles are seen until one becomes dominant and ovulates, which allows a visualization of the corpus luteum. After the ovulatory season is established, multiple small follicles ranging in size from 2 - 5 mm in diameter occur during early diestrus. These mature at an accelerated growth rate and then begin final maturation approximately 6 days before ovulation. The remaining nonovulated follicles then regress just a few days before ovulation.

Preovulatory follicles can be assessed to determine an accurate time of ovulation. As the follicle matures preceeding ovulation, it undergoes a softening and an obvious change of shape. Normally the follicle is very spherical in shape but becomes visibly irregular just prior to ovulation. Ovulations can also be accurately detected using ultrasonography. The fluid-filled area disappears and is replaced by a definitive corpora lutea. Multiple ovulations can also be visualized for the prevention of twin pregnancies or the scheduling of two recipients in an embryo transfer program.

Numerous other ovarian abnormalities can be visualized using ultrasonography. Unruptured or hemorrhagic follicles, persistent corpora lutea, neoplastic conditions, and ovarian cysts can all be diagnosed with a higher degree of accuracy utilizing ultrasonography.

Uterine Fiberoptic Examination

Uterine abnormalities can be visualized using a flexible fiberoptic instrument. This procedure should be considered when all other noninvasive diagnostic techniques have failed to provide an answer to the cause of infertility. It is extremely important to observe sterile technique when employing this procedure. The endoscope should be gas sterilized or repeatedly washed with a surgical scrub. The perineal area should be thoroughly cleansed, and surgical gloves should be worn when handling the endoscope.

In order to visualize the uterus, it must be distended with either fluid or air. Distention with a sterile saline solution causes less straining in the mare than distention with air. A small Foley catheter is placed through the cervix before the introduction of the endoscope. The endoscope is then passed laterally to the catheter. One to two liters of warm sterile saline solution is then infused into the uterus to obtain distention. It is often necessary to also insert a gloved finger to help seal the cervix against leakage. Diestrus mares are more suitable for this procedure since the tight cervix facilites sealing which allows for distention of the uterus.

After the distention is completed to the satisfaction of the examiner, the uterine body, bifurcation, and uterine horns can be visualized. Cystic structures, endometrial changes, and adhesions can be detected and proper therapeutic regimes can be initiated.

Cytological Examination of the Endometrium

A normal uterine lumen contains a resident population of bacteria. Any bacteria that are pathogenic in nature have the ability to cause a disease and initiate an inflammatory response within the uterus. This inflammatory response is characterized by the migration of neutrophils from the circulatory system. These neutrophils have the ability to destroy any pathogenic bacteria that initiated their response. Examination of a normal lumen of the uterus will reveal zero neutrophils present within the cytological sample. Bacterial cultures will often reveal findings of a positive nature. However, these findings could be the result of contamination and should be correlated with cytologic findings before a treatment regime is initiated.

Several techniques are available which allow the collection of a uterine cytological sample. The easiest and most convenient to use is that which employs a guarded culture swab. These sterile swabs are guarded by a plastic tube which has a cap that is popped off when the swab is advanced to obtain a culture. When this is done within the lumen of the uterus, the cap is attached to the end of the rod but is very mobile in nature. After the swab has been saturated for the microbial culture, it is withdrawn back within the tube. The tube should then be positioned where the cytological sample is to be taken and then given several rotations. This allows the cap to collect a sample of endometrium and uterine fluid. The instrument is then withdrawn, the cap removed, and a slide prepared from the cells and fluids that it contains. The slide is then allowed to air dry and then stained in order to visualize the cells.

The chief disadvantage to this method is that there is collection of material from only one site and using this technique, there may be a distortion of cells within this sample. If this is a concern, uterine lavage will provide a more suitable cytologic sample for examination. During lavage, a guarded instrument is placed within the uterine lumen and a ballooned-tipped catheter is passed through this instrument to allow placement for collection. By inflating the balloon on the catheter, the uterine lumen is sealed, and the distal portion of the uterine horn can be flushed and collected.

If staining of this sample reveals epithelial cells, then the sample had to be collected properly from the uterus. The epithelial cells from normally cycling mares are tall and columnar in shape. When the mare is in the anestrus state, these cells are cuboidal in shape and are usually nonciliated, although some ciliated cells may be found in the diestrus stage. These cells exhibit basophilic staining nuclei and a cytoplasm which contains vacuoles that stain light blue in color. Maiden mares and younger mares will exhibit smears that contain a large number of epithelial cells with overlapping cytoplasm and mucus. Anestrus mares have cuboidal or low columnar epithelial cells with little cytoplasmic vacuolation.

Whenever there is a bacterial infection within the uterus, the neutrophils are the most predominant cells found. When a mare is not infected, neutrophils are rarely present within the

Artwork by S. Hakola / J. Dirig
Copyright Equistar Publications, Ltd.

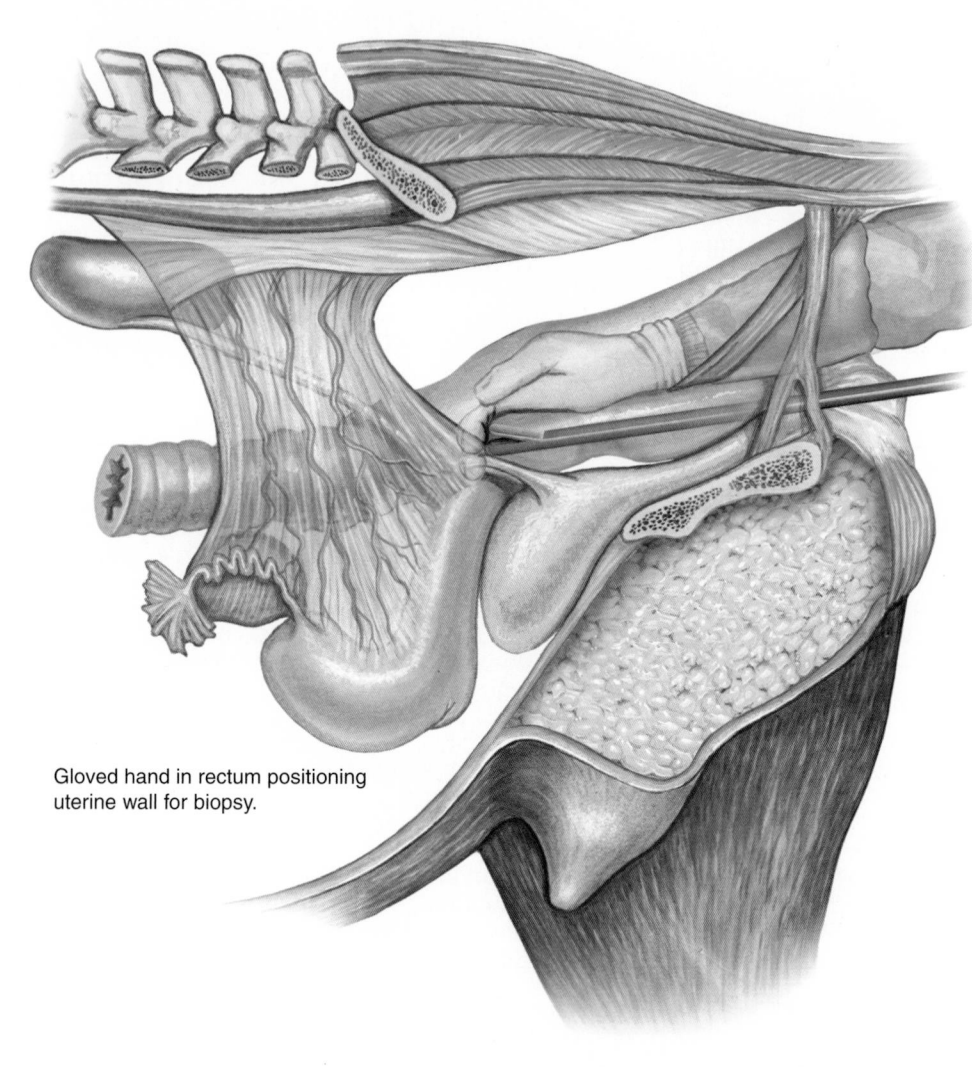

Gloved hand in rectum positioning
uterine wall for biopsy.

Endometrial Biopsy

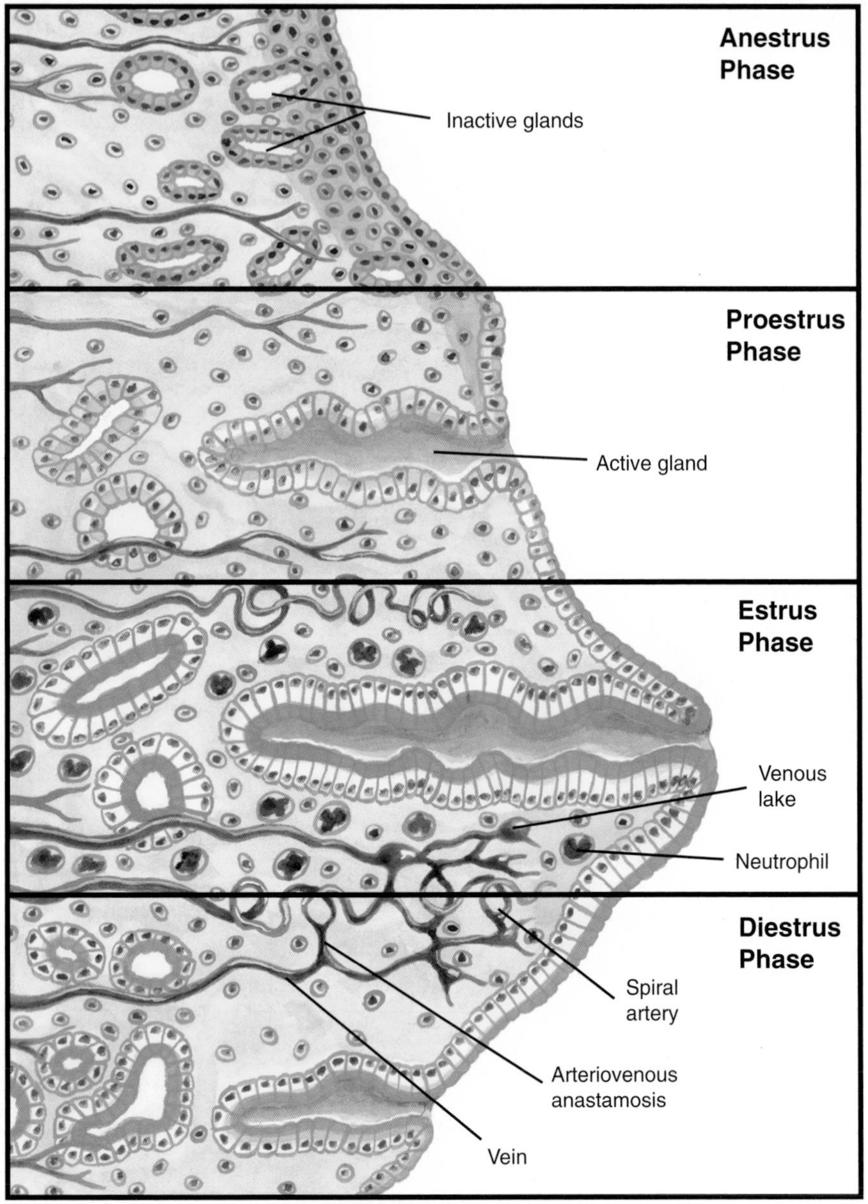

Anestrus Phase

Inactive glands

Proestrus Phase

Active gland

Estrus Phase

Venous lake

Neutrophil

Diestrus Phase

Spiral artery

Arteriovenous anastamosis

Vein

Endometrial Changes During the Estrus Cycle

cytological sample. Neutrophils will, however, appear after breeding, foaling, or immediately following a uterine lavage. Neutrophils are a type of leukocyte or a white blood cell with a primary function to fight off infection. Large macrophages and lymphocytes are also seen within the uterine cytology. Macrophages are usually found along with red blood cells and neutrophils immediately after the mare has foaled. In the case of a chronic infection or chronic endometritis, lymphocytes can sometimes be found. These are white blood cells that help fight infection.

In cases of severe acute endometritis, or immediately after foaling, one may see red blood cells (RBCs) within the uterine cytology. If a cytological sample is obtained right after an endometrial biopsy, it is not unusual to find red blood cells present. The trauma to the tissues that is associated with foaling can easily explain the presence of RBCs within the cytological samples collected at this time.

By using special staining techniques, bacteria, yeast, and fungi can be seen under the microscope. Just the mere presence of bacteria on the cytological sample does not mean that treatment is necessary, but yeast and fungal infections seen on these samples may hasten an initiation of therapy while culture results are pending.

It is possible to rapidly diagnose a condition within the uterus by utilizing uterine cytology through the examination of endometrial smears. This is important when one must decide whether or not to cover a mare for breeding during that cycle.

Endometrial Biopsy

Endometrial histological findings are an integral part of a complete reproductive examination. This procedure is an additional tool that can be utilized to assess a mare's reproductive viability. This procedure should never be undertaken without a complete physical exam, a thorough rectal palpation, and ultrasonography of the reproductive tract. A determination of pregnancy must be made before a uterine biopsy is attempted since the biopsy procedure on a pregnant mare would almost invariably result in an abortion.

Candidates for an endometrial biopsy include: barren mares, repeat breeders, mares with a history of early embryonic death or abortion, and in all nonpregnant mares presented for fertility evaluation even as part of a prepurchase examination. This procedure should be accomplished as early as possible in the breeding season. The mares will need a period of time for recovery from the procedure and may require additional treatment to correct any disorders discovered through the biopsy. Ideally, biopsy samples should be collected during the transition phase from winter anestrus to the first cycle.

Numerous instruments can be utilized in obtaining endometrial biopsies. The most important consideration is that the specimen collected should be of sufficient size to provide at least one to two centimeters of the endometrium for histological examination. In most cases, one sample will be representative of the entire endometrium. However, when rectal palpation reveals a uterine disorder present, endometrial biopsy samples should be collected in each of these specific areas in addition to a sample obtained that is representative of the rest of the uterine lumen.

The tail is wrapped and the perineal area is surgically prepped to be as aseptic as possible. Being careful not to expose the instrument to any outside contamination, the biopsy instrument is inserted through the cervix and placed inside the uterine lumen. The technician's hand is then removed from the vaginal area and inserted into the rectum. Palpating the uterus through the rectal wall allows the placement of the instrument to that area of the endometrium chosen for biopsy. The biopsy instrument is then turned on its side and a portion of the endometrium is placed between the side walls of the biopsy instrument with the index finger of the hand in the rectum. Patience and care must be exercised so that the biopsy instrument does not cut through the entire uterus resulting in a perforation into the abdominal cavity.

The biopsy specimen should be handled very gently so that the tissues are intact for histological examination. A small-gauge hypodermic needle can facilitate the removal of the specimen from the basket. This sample is then placed in a ten percent

formalin or Bouin's solution. If Bouin's solution is used, the specimen should be transferred to ten percent formalin after being immersed in Bouin's solution for two to four hours. This specimen is then sent to a pathology lab for a histopathological examination and diagnosis.

Normal Endometrial Anatomy

In order to interpret the pathological findings of the endometrial biopsy, normal endometrial anatomy should be taken into consideration. As the stage of the cycle varies, so do characteristics of the endometrium. The luminal epithelial cells, the configuration of the glands, and the amount of edema in the lamina propria will change. There may also be a variation within multiple samples collected from an individual mare.

During the anestrus phase of the estrus cycle, the endometrial glands undergo atrophy to an inactive stage. The glandular ducts are usually arranged in straight lines. The luminal epithelial cells during this phase are cuboidal and atrophic. It is rare to find any edema within the lamina propria. The glandular lumens may contain trapped secretions.

During the proestrus stage of the cycle, the luminal epithelium will reflect different degrees of activity. The epithelium is generally columnar in appearance, but the cells are very short. There is a slight increase in the edema within the lamina propria which may appear to push the glands into clumps. The glands themselves appear more active than the luminal epithelium.

The luminal and glandular epithelial cells are usually columnar in appearance during the estrus phase of the cycle. There is a considerable amount of edema in the lamina propria, and this results in the glands appearing less dense. There is usually a layer of neutrophils present around the capillaries beneath the epithelium. This is the only stage of the cycle which exhibits neutrophils.

The luminal epithelium varies during the diestrus stage of the cycle. The cells range from a low cuboidal shape early in diestrus to an increased height as estrus approaches. One sees glandular proliferation and a reduction of edema in diestrus.

Artwork by S. Hakola / J. Dirig
Copyright Equistar Publications, Ltd.

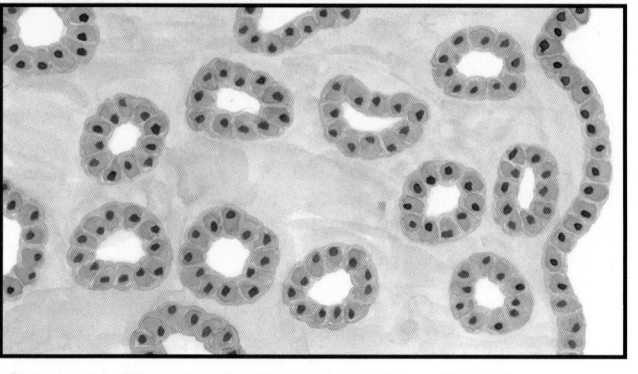

Category I: Normal and active endometrium with random active glands and infrequent inflammatory cells.

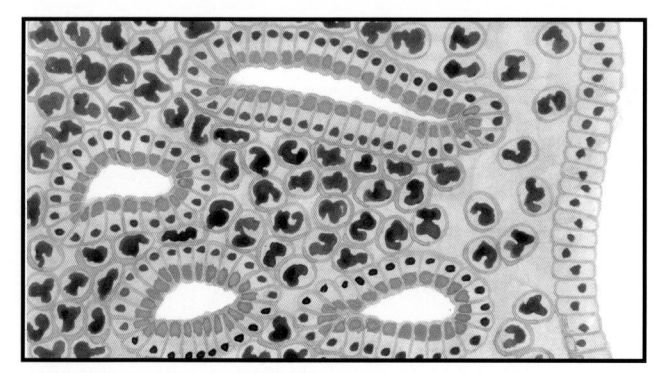

Category II: Chronic endometritis with widespread neutrophil infiltration.

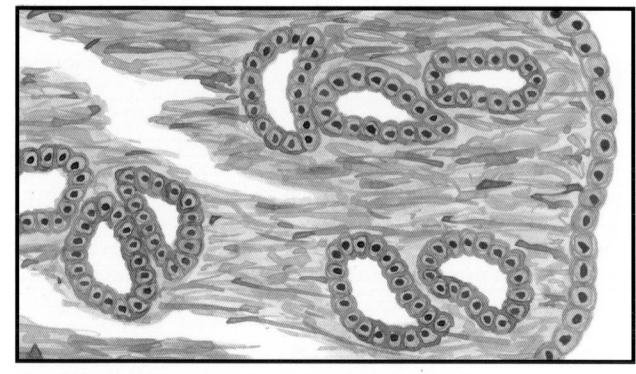

Category III: Clumping of glands caused by widespread periglandular fibrosis.

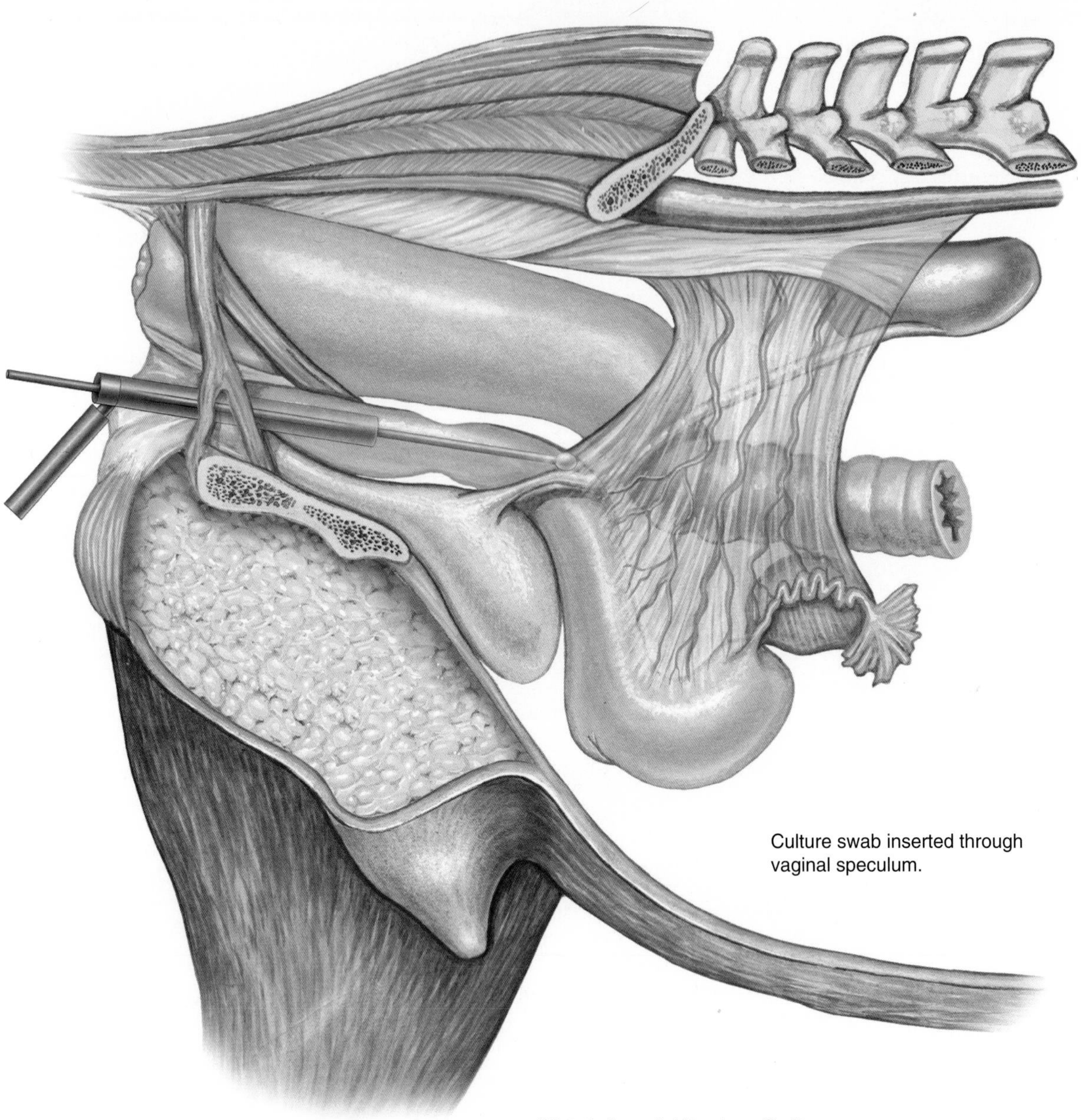

Culture swab inserted through vaginal speculum.

Obtaining A Uterine Culture

Categorization of the Endometrium

Inflammation, fibrosis, and lymphatic stasis are the usual pathologic changes found within endometrial biopsies. These changes within the endometrium allow a classification system to be utilized in rendering a diagnosis and prognosis regarding reproductive efficiency for the mare.

Inflammation within the endometrium results in an increase number of inflammatory cells within the lamina propria. When this inflammation is acute, the predominant cell type is the neutrophil. When a chronic endometritis is present, lymphocytes and macrophages are present along with the neutrophils.

When the inflammatory reaction has been long standing or there has been damage to the glandular cells, a fibrosis of the endometrium can occur. This fibrosis interferes with the functions of the glands within the endometrium and results in early embryonic death. These mares will usually fail to sustain a pregnancy beyond seventy days.

Lymphatic lacunae are formed from dilated lymphatics resulting in a fluid-filled space lined with endothelial cells. These lesions can be differentiated from an artificially induced edema because the edema lacks a regular margin with the tissues. The finding of this lesion correlates with a reduced state of fertility within the mare.

The evaluation of these pathological changes allows the mare to be categorized into three different diagnostic and prognostic groups. These are listed as follows:

Category I: which is a normal group.

Category II: which is a group that contains some endometrial changes that result in a lower level of fertility but that are perceived reversible with proper management and veterinary care.

Category III: which is the severely affected group.

Categorically, mares that are in Category I have a greater than seventy percent chance in producing a live foal. Mares that fall within the Category II

parameters have approximately a fifty to seventy percent chance of producing a live foal, whereas mares in Category III have less then a ten percent chance of being fertile.

When there is no evidence of hypoplasia within the glands of the uterus and there is no atrophy present, this mare is categorized as having a Category I uterus. There may be one or two slightly scattered areas of inflammation present, but this still allows inclusion within this Category I group.

Category II mares have mild or moderate endometrial changes. These changes can be reversed through proper management and result in conception and the maintenance of a normal pregnancy. Endometrial changes within this category include scattered areas of inflammation or fibrosis, periglandular fibrosis, neutrophilic cellular infiltration, and widespread lymphatic stasis.

Category III endometrial biopsies result when changes are found histologically that are essentially irreversible. There is usually wide spread periglandular fibrosis, severe cellular infiltration, lymphatic stasis, endometrial atrophy, and severe inflammation.

Other factors such as age, the number of years the mare is barren, and the breeding management techniques that are utilized also enter into the establishment of a prognosis concerning the fertility of the mare. Older mares will normally have an increased level of endometrial fibrosis. Therefore, the age factor should be considered when evaluating an endometrial biopsy from an older mare. Mares that have had numerous barren years may have difficulty in clearing the bacteria from the uterus following breeding. The age of the mare should also be considered when evaluating an endometrial biopsy from a mare that has been barren for several years. Special techniques utilized in breeding management may reduce the effects of fibrosis and the number of years the mare has been barren to increase the fertility prognosis.

Uterine Cultures

The value of the cultures taken from the mare's genital tract are controversial in nature. The question of when to take them, from where to take them, and the significance of their findings is debatable. These genital swabs should be cultured for microorganisms and be utilized in the screening for venereal disease, acute endometritis, and aid in the diagnosis of genital abnormalities. Swabs should be collected from the endometrium during early estrus and can also be collected from the vagina and clitoral fossa. Cultures will allow screening for numerous organisms including *Taylorella equigenitalis* which causes contagious equine metritis. Nonvenereal acute endometritis can also be identified through bacteriological cultures. Uterine bacteriological swabs should also be collected on any mares that have aborted or failed to conceive at the end of the breeding season.

These bacteriological uterine cultures serve numerous functions. Through identification of a venereal organism, contamination of the stallion's genitalia is prevented. Those mares with nonvenereal acute endometritis are identified before mating which allows for proper treatment resulting in an improved chance for successful conception and gestation.

In order to collect a meaningful uterine culture, the mare should be properly restrained, have her tail wrapped and tied off to the side, and the perineal area thoroughly washed with warm clean water. Care must be taken when using disinfectants in this area since they may favor the growth of pathogenic bacteria and may also irritate these delicate tissues.

There are numerous culture instruments available for the collection of the uterine swab. Remember that the laboratory results are only as good as the samples that are collected. The swab must be guarded and not exposed to the tissue to be cultured until it is immediately apposed to those tissues. Confusion occurs if one cultures the mare in the winter during anestrus before the mare starts to cycle regularly. It is possible at this time to culture bacteria that is not associated with the causative organism. During diestrus, bacterial

Ovarian Tumors: Granulosa-Theca Cell, Teratoma

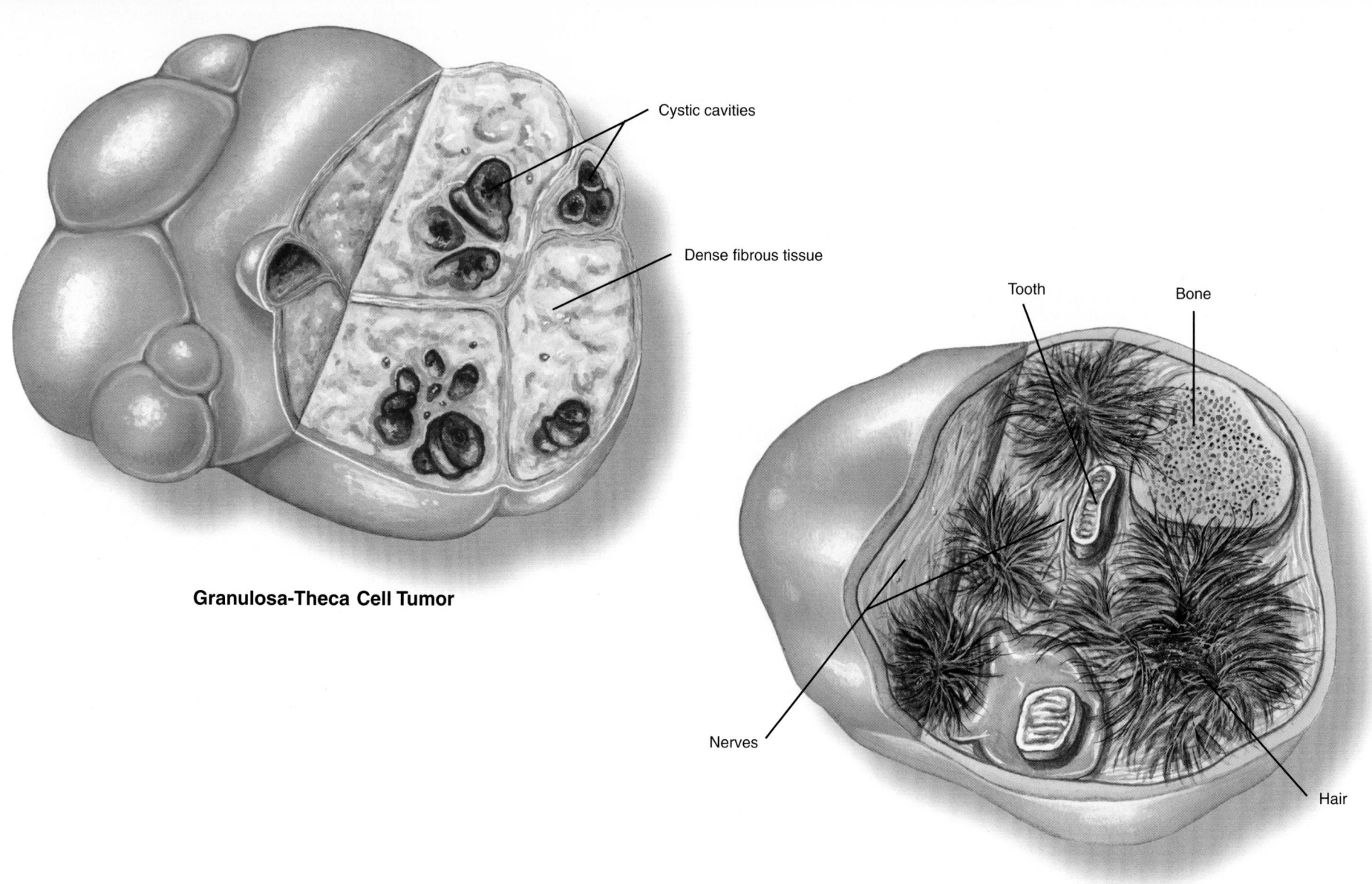

Cystic cavities

Dense fibrous tissue

Granulosa-Theca Cell Tumor

Tooth

Bone

Nerves

Hair

Teratoma

recovery is also difficult due to the dryness of the endometrium. The ideal time to obtain a uterine culture is the first day of standing estrus when the cervix is not fully relaxed and secretions from the endometrium allow a moist swab to be obtained. There is a high degree of correlation between cervical and uterine cultures. It is just as easy to obtain a uterine swab as it is to obtain a cervical culture.

It is important to exercise great care in the handling of the collected samples. If the sample is handled improperly, it could become contaminated or favor the growth of an organism that would lead to an error in diagnosis. As soon as the swab is collected, one must transfer this swab to a transport medium since bacteria are lost as the swab dries. Amies transport media is the standard all-purpose bacteriological media used in equine practice. Traditionally, nutrient broth was used for transportation or storage of swabs, but this broth proved to promote a proliferation of contaminating bacterial species.

It is important that swabs within the transport medium be sent to a laboratory and arrive there within twenty-four to thirty-six hours after collection. These samples should be protected against all extremes of temperature and should be kept out of direct sunlight. In most cases, when the swab arrives at the lab, it is fairly simple to grow and identify those organisms that cause endometritis. When a quick diagnostic decision needs to be rendered, it is the common practice to obtain two uterine swabs. Transport one to the commercial laboratory and grow one either in the laboratory at the breeding farm or at the local veterinarian's or human hospital laboratory. Cultures are started on blood agar and a Gram-negative selected medium. They are incubated at thirty-seven degrees Centigrade under microaerophilic conditions. The number of colonies are then counted and identified with antibiotic sensitivity tests being set up after isolation.

There are several pathogenic organisms that are significant: *Beta-hemolytic streptococci, hemolytic E. coli, Pseudomonas spp, Klebsiella spp.,* and *Candida spp.* Once these organisms are recovered and

correlated with physical and cytological evidence, a diagnosis can be rendered. The physical exam will usually reveal a high degree of inflammation within the tissues, and the cytological exam will exhibit the neutrophilia within the tissue sample. Any organism can be considered the cause of the endometritis when it is recovered in pure culture and in large numbers from the mare.

DISORDERS OF THE OVARY

There are three types of common disorders of the equine ovary: neoplastic, disorders of physical causes, and disorders that are self-originating. Neoplasic conditions include granulosa cell tumors, teratomas, adenomas, and adenocarcinomas. There are other neoplastic conditions; however, they are extremely rare. Those disorders of physical origin include hematomas, abscesses, and ovarian cysts. The self-originating disorders include instances when the mare has a particular abnormality within the estrous cycle. These include periods of prolonged diestrus, periods of anestrus, and ovulation failures.

GRANULOSA-THECA CELL TUMORS

Etiology

Granulosa-theca cell tumors are the most common neoplastic condition of the equine ovary. These tumors are benign in nature and cause abnormal behavior, masculinity, and irregular estrus cycles. The clinical signs that are seen with this neoplastic condition are dependent upon the hormone levels caused by this tumor. These tumors produce testosterone, the male hormone, at an abnormal level causing many of these masculine manifestations. High levels of progesterone and estrogen may also result in these abnormal clinical signs. They may be aggressive in behavior with a masculine demeanor. These mares may mount other mares that are in estrus.

Diagnosis

The diagnosis of these granulosa-theca cell tumors is based on the mare's history, behavior, rectal palpation, ultrasonographic scanning, and serum testosterone levels. Upon rectal examination, the ovary will be enlarged, firm, and feel multicystic. Ultrasonographic scanning will reveal a multilobular "honeycomb" ovary that contains numerous dense areas as well as fluid-filled cystic structures. Testosterone levels will be greater than fifty pg/ml which will be significant but not absolutely diagnostic. The differential diagnosis for this disorder should include teratomas, adenomas, adenocarcinomas, and numerous ovarian cysts.

Treatment

Treatment for any secreting ovarian tumor is excision or ovariectomy of the affected ovary. Following a successful removal of a granulosa-theca cell tumor, it is possible for the contralateral ovary to be fertile and the mare to remain fertile. Normal cyclic activity will resume and the prognosis for fertility is favorable.

TERATOMA

Etiology

The second most common ovarian tumor is the teratoma. The etiology of this tumor is the germ cell; therefore, these tumors are benign and nonsecretory in nature. Upon histological exam of these tumors, structures such as bone, skin, teeth, cartilage, nerves, and hair are found.

Diagnosis

Diagnosis of an ovarian teratoma is based on rectal and ultrasonographic examination. It is possible that the contralateral ovary is normal which would allow the mare to cycle and ovulate normally. Teratomas normally do not interfere with fertility unless they are large enough to cause a physical impediment upon the reproductive tract.

Ovarian Tumors: Adenocarcinoma; Ovarian Hematomas; Prolonged Diestrus

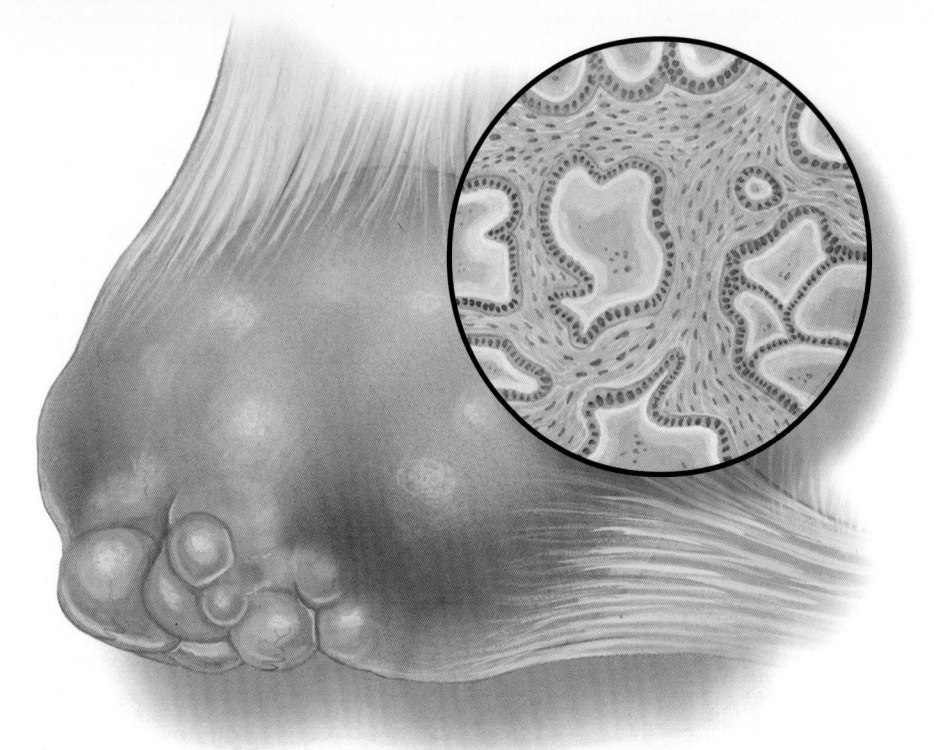

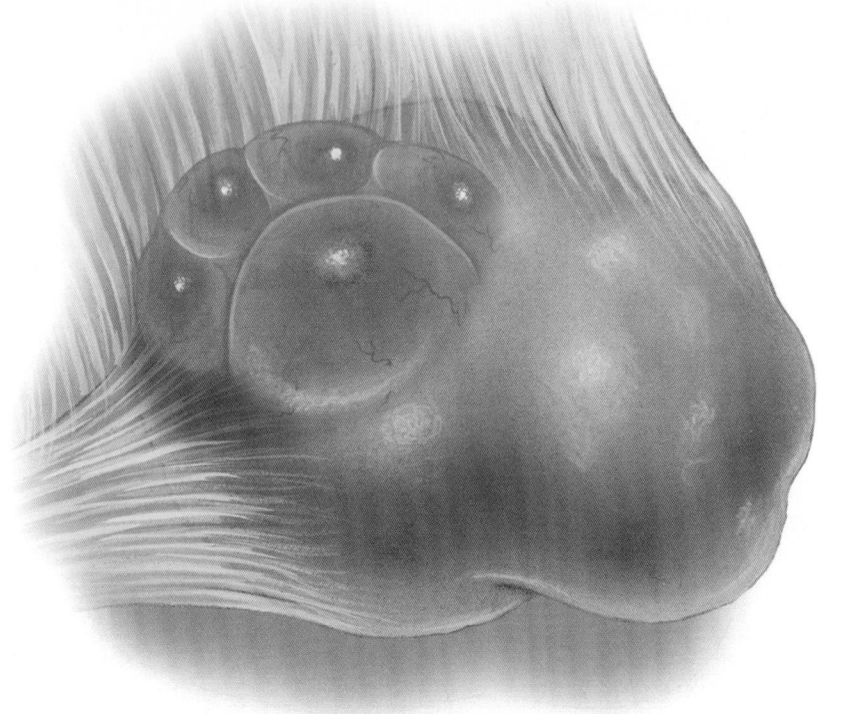

Adenocarcinoma of the Ovary

Ovarian Hematoma

Prolonged Diestrus

Ultrasound as seen
in prologed diestrus.

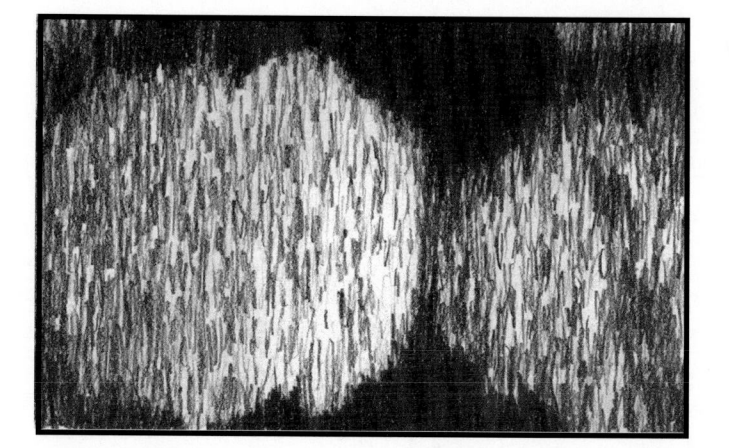

If it would be advantageous to remove the teratoma, an ovariectomy is performed. This surgical removal should be considered if the teratoma is large enough to impinge upon the other portions of the mare's reproductive tract.

ADENOCARCINOMS

Adenomas and adenocarcinomas are nonsecratory ovarian tumors. These originate from epithelial tissues and are usually located on the surface of the ovulatory fossa or oviductal fimbriae. These tumors are usually unilateral in nature, and if a cysts occurs with them, they are referred to as cystadenomas. If the adenoma is metastatic in nature, it is classified as an adenocarcinoma. Clinical signs of a mare with an adenocarcinoma include loss of weight, periodic bouts of colic, and recurring abdominal fluid. A definitive diagnosis can only be rendered when these tumors are excised and examined histologically.

OVARIAN HEMATOMAS, ABSCESSES, AND CYSTS

Hematomas of the ovary are relatively common and may be easily confused with ovarian tumors. This condition is rarely pathological since hemorrhage into the follicular lumen normally occurs during ovulation. Ovarian hemotomas occur when there is an excessive amount of hemorrhage following ovulation. This distends the former cavity of the follicle and can range in size from fifty millimeters to thirty or forty centimeters. Depending on size, hematomas can persist on the ovary for up to several months. In the meantime, normal ovarian cyclic activity continues even though the hematoma is present. These are differentiated from ovarian neoplastic conditions by their occurrence or formation following estrus. Hematomas usually shrink in size over a period of time, whereas a tumor will not.

Treatment of ovarian hematomas is rare. They usually regress on their own over a period of time with the only consequence being a partial destruction of ovarian germinal tissue. Areas that contain an ovarian hematoma are usually very firm and almost never contain any follicular activity.

Ovarian abscesses are usually the sequelae following needle aspiration of an ovarian cyst. These abscesses typically do not effect the normal ovarian cyclic activity. Ultrasonographic examination will differentiate an ovarian abscess from other ovarian conditions such as a tumor. Treatment of these ovarian abscesses include surgical drainage, systemic antimicrobial medications, and in severe cases, ovariectomy.

One of the most common misdiagnoses made upon rectal palpation of the mare is that of "cystic ovaries." Follicular and luteal cysts that are normally found in the bovine do not exist in the equine. Mares can have multiple preovulatory follicles, ovarian hematomas, or prolonged estrus cycles during the breeding season, but these are not true "cystic" conditions.

Under normal conditions, the mare ovulates only one follicle during each estrous cycle. There are certain breeds such as thoroughbreds, warm bloods, and draft breeds that have a higher incidence of multiple ovulations. Rectal palpation in conjunction with an ultrasonographic examination can be used to determine when to breed mares with multiple ovulations. These mares should be bred twelve to twenty-four hours before ovulation of the most promising follicle.

SELF-ORIGINATING OVARIAN DISORDERS

There are four main self-originating or idiopathic disorders of ovarian origin that occur in the mare causing abnormalities within the estrus cycle. Theses include a prolonged state of diestrus, periods of anestrus during the breeding season, diestrual ovulation, and failure to ovulate.

PROLONGED DIESTRUS

Etiology

There are two main etiologies for a prolonged diestrus period. If a normal pregnancy occurred that resulted in early embryonic death, the mare may not return to a normal estrus cycle. This early embryonic death may be a sequel to an endometritis or may result in a case of pyometra. The second most common cause for the failure of the mare to return to an ovulatory cycle is the presence of a persistent corpora lutea on the ovary. This prolonged luteal phase of the cycle can last thirty to ninety days and is due to a failure of normal luteolysis. This failed luteolysis is from inadequate levels of or the nonrelease of prostaglandins by the endometrium.

Diagnosis

Diagnosis of these two conditions consists of an ultrasonic examination for pregnancy and a thorough rectal palpation. If ultrasonography fails to detect a pregnancy when one was detected earlier in the history of the mare, then it can be assumed that this prolonged diestrus was a result of an early embryonic death. A persistent corpora lutea can be diagnosed when a mare has a history of failure to return to estrus for long periods of time and typical diestrus characteristics are present when the mare is palpated. In this case, there would be a firm, elongated cervix and an excellent tone to the uterus.

Treatment

Treatment of a prolonged diestrus period involves luteolysis. The most efficient and cost effective treatment is the administration of prostaglandins. Care must be taken to thoroughly examine the mare for other problems such as endometritis since this may have caused early embryonic death.

Anestrus; Contagious Equine Metritis

Anestrus

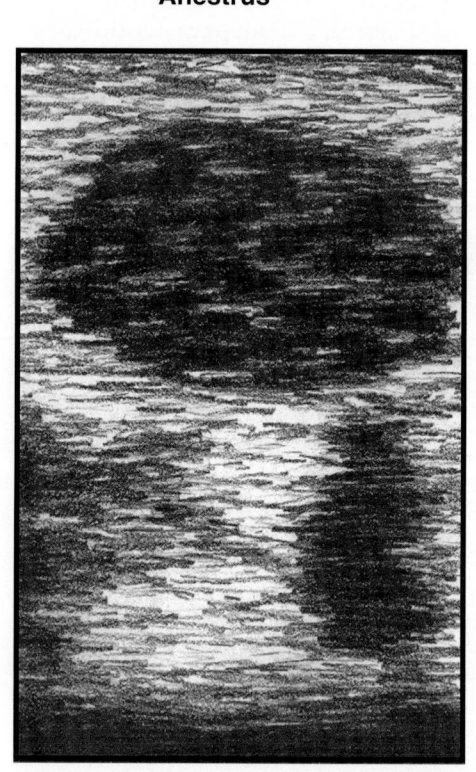

Ultrasound during anestrus

Contagious Equine Metritis (CEM)

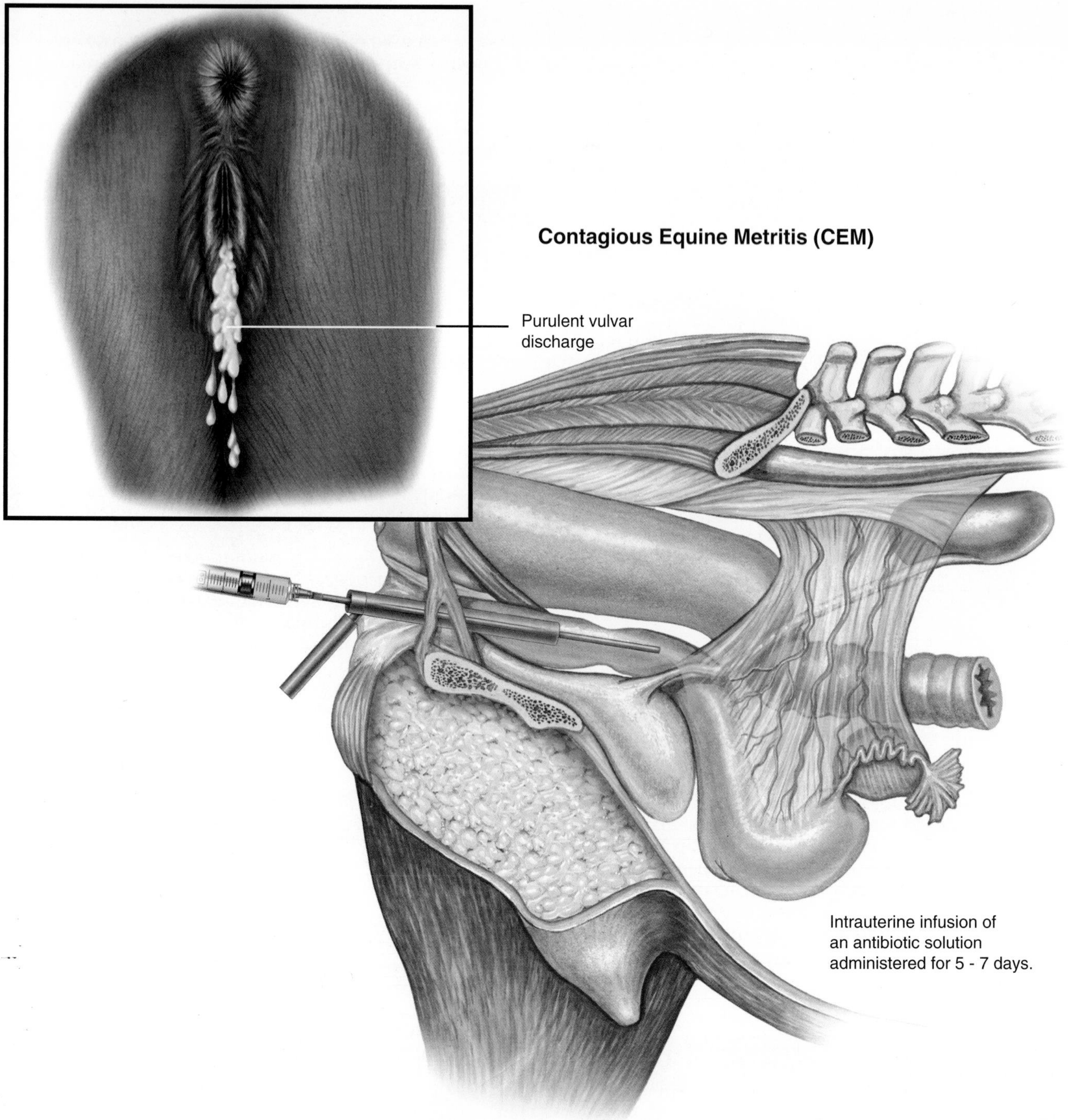

Purulent vulvar discharge
Intrauterine infusion of an antibiotic solution administered for 5 - 7 days.

ANESTRUS

Etiology

Mares that develop an anestrus period during the breeding season are very frustrating to all those involved in the breeding operation. There are two possible causes for this ovarian atrophy and loss of uterine tone: stress (from poor nutrition or environmental factors) and a state of lactational anestrus. A mare that is overprotective of her foal and lacking behavioral signs of estrus should not be mistaken as anestrus. These mares, although not showing behavioral estrus, when checked rectally will have follicular activity on their ovaries and ovulate normally.

Diagnosis

The diagnosis of this anestrus period is based upon the physical exam of the mare and periodic assays for circulating progesterone. When rectally palpated, mares that are exhibiting lactational anestrus, will have small, firm, inactive ovaries, an open cervix, and a uterus that lacks tone. These mares may have come into a normal postpartum estrus at eight to fourteen days after foaling and then not show signs of estrus again for three to four months. If a serum progesterone test is taken, the levels will consistently be less than one mg/ml.

Treatment

Treatments for these anestrus periods are mostly unsuccessful. Administrations of prostaglandin usually show little effect in returning this mare to a normal estrus cycle. Oral progesterone administration for a ten day period of time has only been effective in some of the cases. Unfortunately, treatment usually consists of waiting for the mare to return to a normal cycle.

DIESTRUS OVULATION

Mares that ovulate in the presence of a functional corpora lutea usually do not show any signs of estrus. This is referred to as a diestrus ovulation. The etiology behind this condition is unclear, but if mares are examined regularly during the diestrus phase of the cycle, ovulations can be detected. In rare instances, these ovulations can even be normal. The mare can conceive, carry, and deliver a foal after breeding in conjunction with this diestrual ovulation.

During the breeding season, mares do not fail to ovulate. During the autumn and transitional period early in the spring, follicles can be produced that do not ovulate. These are commonly called autumn follicles or persistent follicles. These persistent follicles can exist for up to sixty days during the transitional phase of the mare. Upon rectal palpation, these persistent follicles are large, tense, and fluid-filled structures on the ovary. The ovaries may contain multiple developing and regressing follicles at this time. However, these are not cystic by definition. Ultrasonic examination of these follicles will render an evaluation of their size, structure, and the tissues surrounding them. Treatment of these autumn follicles usually consists of the administration of chorionic gonadotropin coupled with the administration of prostaglandins.

UTERINE DISORDERS

CONTAGIOUS EQUINE METRITIS (CEM)

Etiology

The first outbreak of contagious equine metritis occurred during the 1977 breeding season in the New Market area in England and was later identified in parts of Ireland. It is a highly contagious venereal infection that was first found in thoroughbreds. It is caused by a Gram-negative coccobacillus identified as *Taylorella equigenitalis*. The original outbreak spread to several countries including the United States where it affected several breeding farms in Kentucky in 1978.

Taylorella equigenitalis requires microaerophilic culture conditions. This organism can not be grown on conventional culture media but grows on Eugon agar in five to ten percent carbon dioxide at thirty-seven degrees centigrade. It is often helpful to run these cultures on a medium containing streptomycin and also without streptomycin. The antibiotic streptomycin will inhibit growth of contaminating organisms that are present on the culture swabs. This organism can survive for a long period of time on the external genitalia of stallions, the caudal vagina, and clitoral areas of the mare.

Clinical Signs

The most common clinical sign of contagious equine metritis is that of acute endometritis which results in a copious, grayish vulvar discharge that can be seen visually. This discharge usually appears approximately eight to ten days after the mare has been covered by a carrier stallion. Care must be taken not to confuse mares that do not show outward signs of this disease since thirty percent of the mares exposed may not exhibit this discharge. Uterine cytology will reveal the presence of neutrophils within the sample. This may be the definitive reason to specifically include contagious equine metritis in the differential diagnosis.

Diagnosis

There are two important differential diagnoses that should be considered when contagious equine metritis is suspected: any bacterial endometritis and injuries to the vaginal tissues that result in a discharge.

A diagnosis of contagious equine metritis can be rendered simply through a positive culture of *Taylorella equigenitalis* or through serological testing. Bacteriological samples for culture should be collected using sterile swabs from the endometrium, cervix, clitoral fossa, and the vagina.

Artwork by S. Hakola / J. Dirig
Copyright Equistar Publications, Ltd.

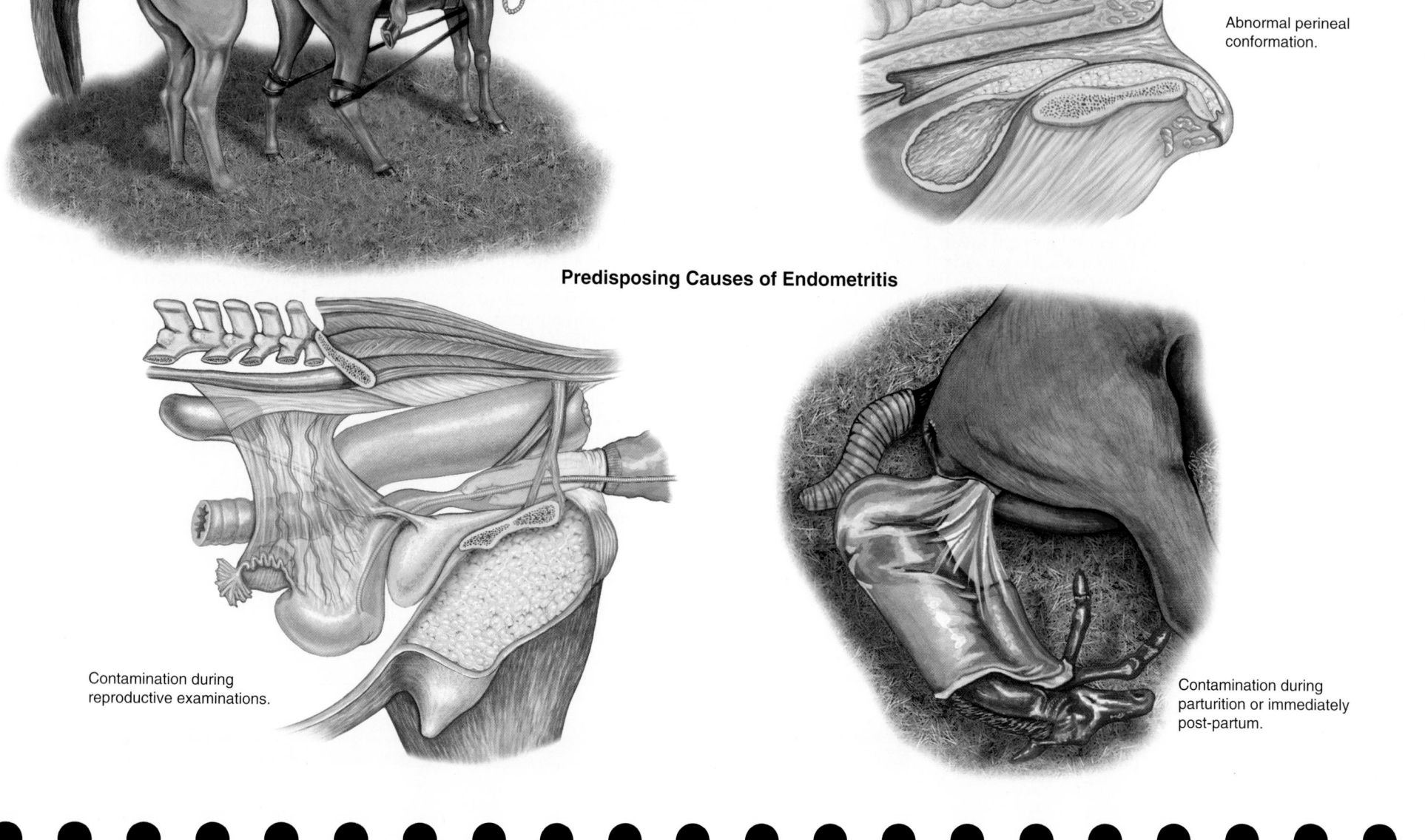

Contamination of uterine lumen via live cover breeding.

Abnormal perineal conformation.

Predisposing Causes of Endometritis

Contamination during reproductive examinations.

Contamination during parturition or immediately post-partum.

These culture samples should be transported to the laboratory in a liquid transport medium such as Amies with charcoal. Cultures should be prepared using chocolate agar and ten percent horse blood plates. Remember that the plates should be incubated at thirty-seven degrees centigrade in a five to ten percent carbon dioxide atmosphere.

Serological testing for the presence of *Taylorella equigenitalis* is based on testing that can detect the animal's antibodies against this organism present in the serum. Numerous serological tests can be utilized. The two most common tests are the complement fixation test and the serum agglutination test. The complement fixation test is useful in the diagnosis of chronically infected mares and is usually valid about ten days after the initial infection. The serum agglutination test has an advantage because there are no false positives or false negatives associated with this test. This assay is used to confirm the results of complement fixation tests. An enzyme-linked immunosorbent assay is very reliable and economic to use. This is commonly referred to as an ELISA test.

Treatment

Treatment of mares that are affected with CEM usually consists of intrauterine infusions of an antibiotic solution. It should be noted that the acute endometritis that results from this organism seems to resolve itself with or without antimicrobial therapy. Asymptomatic carriers result in about twenty percent of the infected mares regardless of treatment with antibiotics or sexual rest. In most cases, antimicrobial therapy consists of a suitable antibiotic solution that is infused for a period of five to seven days. This administration of antibiotics is done in conjunction with a thorough cleaning of the clitoral fossa and vaginal areas.

The spread of contagious equine metritis is prevented through the utilization of quarantine measures and breeding restrictions. In the United States, this is a reportable disease and the appropriate state agencies must be notified with any suspicious cases. Unfortunately, immunizations of mares against CEM have proven unsuccessful.

ENDOMETRITIS

Endometritis simply refers to an acute or chronic inflammatory reaction within the endometrium. Endometritis is the most significant cause of reduced reproductive efficiency in the mare. The organisms that cause this inflammatory reaction are no more than common opportunistic skin, soil, and fecal organisms that become established within the uterine tissues when the mare's natural defenses fail. Despite the availability of sophisticated antimicrobial drugs, the incidence of endometrial infections is the same as before the day that penicillin was discovered. Unfortunately, the economic relevance within the horse breeding industry due to endometritis, is actually increasing as the value of our average horse increases.

Etiology

Contamination of the uterine lumen results as a sequel to breeding, parturition, defective perineal conformation, and reproductive examinations. The uterine lumen must have a healthy environment in order to sustain embryonic and fetal life. Any contamination of the uterine lumen that is not handled by the normal defense mechanisms of the uterine tissue will result in a reduction of reproductive efficiency.

Under normal circumstances, within the normal fertile mare, there is a great deal of contamination of the uterine lumen following breeding and foaling. These contaminating microorganisms and the resulting inflammatory byproducts are cleared from the uterus within days after contamination. During estrus, there is increased mucus, exudates, and transudates flowing from the uterine lumen to the outside of the mare. Physically protecting the uterine lumen is the valve-like action of the cervix, the vestibular sphincter, and the vulva. These structures serve to keep foreign contamination out and allow a flow of fluid from the uterine lumen to the external environment.

The mare's natural defense mechanism occurs histologically within the uterine tissues. Neutrophils migrate rapidly from the circulation to

the uterine lumen. The cells then ingest and kill any contaminating microorganisms. These cells, and their cellular debris, are then eliminated mechanically by the flow of fluids from within the uterine lumen to the outside environment. Timing is critical for this process to occur since the embryo descends from the uterine tube into the uterine lumen at approximately five and one half days after ovulation. Therefore, in order for the embryo to survive, the transient endometritis has to be removed from the uterine lumen by day four following ovulation to allow a pregnancy to become established.

Following parturition, the demands on this natural defense mechanism within the mare are even greater. The uterus is involuting, or decreasing in size, and all of the contamination that was induced within these tissues must be removed within a short period of time. Therefore, it is easy to understand that even on the best managed mares, a fifty percent conception rate following natural service on foal heat is acceptable.

Reproductive efficiency is determined not only by the ability of the natural immune defense mechanisms, but also the age of the mare, the number of times she has foaled, and any anatomical abnormalities within the reproductive tract. Treatment of these mares will be nonrewarding unless the underlying etiology that resulted in the infection is corrected. Changes in perineal conformation, integrity of the vulva and cervical structures, and repeated parturition tends to stretch and remold the reproductive anatomy in such a way that an increased amount of contamination will occur.

Endometritis can be caused by numerous common surface, fecal, and soil organisms. Natural service usually results in the normal contamination of the reproductive tract with billions of organisms from the penis, prepuce, and urethra. Vulvar contamination is also a factor during natural service since these organisms are added to the ejaculate and usually are deposited directly into the uterine lumen. The most common bacteria that result in endometritis are *Streptococci spp.*, *Pseudomomas spp.*, *Klebsiella spp.*, *E. coli*, and even yeasts such as Candida. Yeasts and fungi can

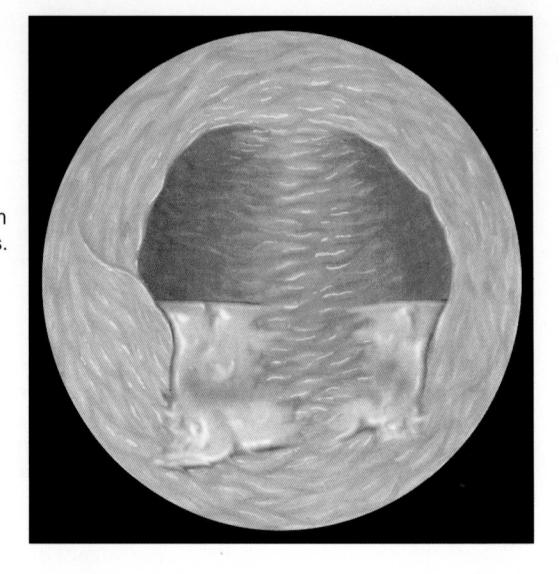

Inflammed uterine tissue with mucopurulent accumulations.

Treatment of Endometritis

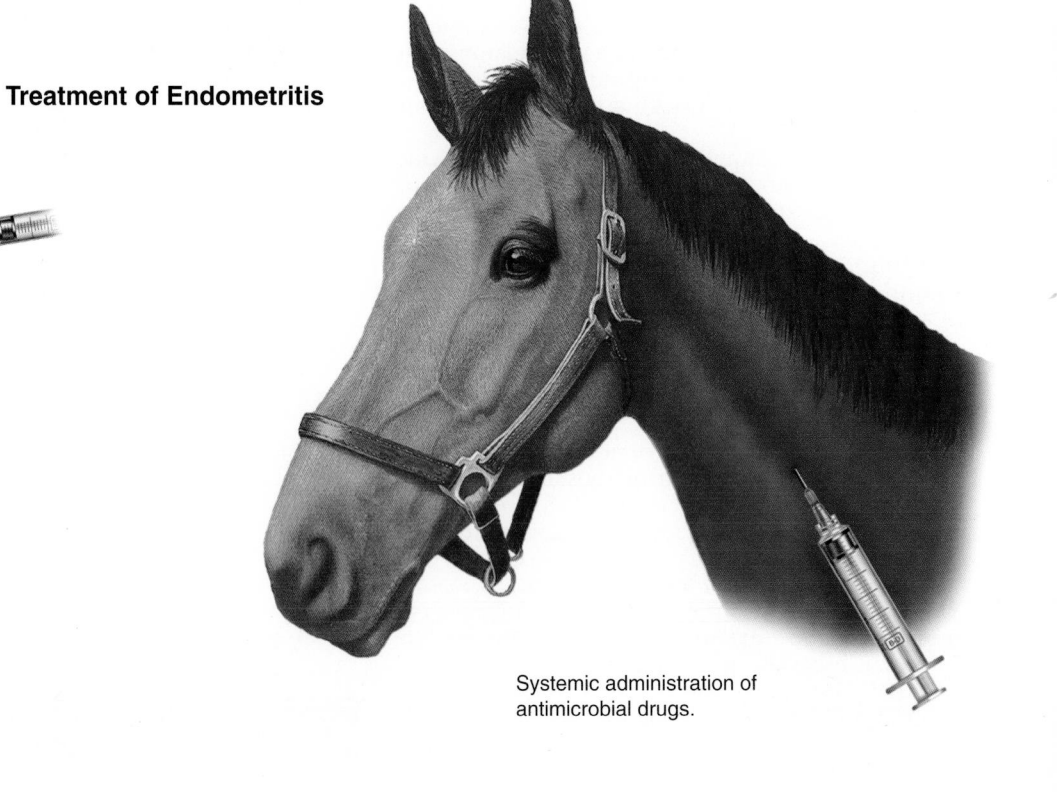

Treatment of endometritis using administration of antibiotics via intrauterine infusions.

Systemic administration of antimicrobial drugs.

become established within the uterine lumen as a result of the resistance of these tissues being lowered when there is constant antimicrobial therapy.

Clinical Signs

The most obvious clinical sign of endometritis is a mucopurulent discharge from the vulva. Unfortunately, this clinical sign is not always present. A thorough reproductive examination will reveal numerous other clinical signs. Rectal palpation will reveal uterine fluid present within the uterine lumen, a swelling within the cervix, and a generalized thickening of the uterine tissue. Examination with a speculum will reveal inflammatory changes within the mucosa and may reveal the presence of a purulent exudate that is not seen externally.

Diagnosis

Confirmation of uterine inflammation is the key to the diagnosis of endometritis when a mucopurulent discharge is seen upon physical examination. The diagnosis is obvious and the need for ancilliary diagnostic techniques is not necessary. However, in most cases, other diagnostic aids are helpful in obtaining an accurate diagnosis of endometritis. Uterine cytology will reveal more then one neutrophil per ten endometrial epithelial cells. It is important to note that the mere presence of bacteria within the cytological sample is not enough to diagnose endometritis since these bacteria may be part of the normal flora found within these tissues. A uterine flush should be clear in appearance when the uterine tissue is not inflammed. This becomes cloudy and upon microscopic examination, will contain neutrophils when there is inflammation present within the endometrium. The endometrial biopsy is diagnostic when a neutrophilic migration occurs throughout the tissues. The degree of histological change within this biopsy will be valuable in assessing future breeding prognosis. An ultrasonographic examination will reveal a fluid layer within the uterine lumen.

To make a diagnostic decision between normal, chronic, and acute endometritis, evidence of inflammation within the reproductive tract should be corrolated with cultural findings. It is important to completely evaluate the entire reproductive situation and to have an accurate diagnosis before treatment is initiated. This will allow complete communication between the breeding manager, the owner of the horse, and the veterinarian so that the reproductive process can be as efficient as possible.

Treatment of Endometritis

Treatment of mares with endometritis should involve three steps. Initially, there should be a correction of any anatomical defects that predispose the mare to endometritis. Treatment should then be initiated so that the end result is a reduction in the inflammatory reaction and the bacterial numbers within the uterine lumen. Lastly, measures should be taken to prevent a recurrence of the disorder. Chemotherapeutic agents can be administered either locally, through intrauterine infusion, or systemically to reduce the number of offending organisms within the uterine lumen. Efforts should be made to also enhance the natural defense mechanisms within the uterine tissue. This is accomplished through a uterine lavage. Unfortunately, there are no specific guidelines that can be applied to each mare. The selection of the chemotherapeutic agent, the routes of administration, the dosage, and the treatment schedule are usually based on experience, anecdotal information, and the innate creativity of the practicing veterinarian or breeding farm manager.

Uterine Infusion

Traditionally, the infusion of various chemotherapeutic agents, dissolved or suspended in water or saline directly into the uterine lumen during estrus, have been used in the treatment of endometritis. This is a type of local antimicrobial therapy since the goal of this therapy is to achieve a high concentration of the therapeutic agent at the specific site of inflammation within the endometrium. Efficacy of this intrauterine local antimicrobial therapy relies on the sensitivity of the

organisms to the chemotherapeutic agents used. This is easily accomplished through accurate culture results before treatment is initiated. Intra-uterine infusion should be administered during the estrus part of the cycle when the cervix is relaxed and the natural defenses are at their highest level. This therapy should be done on a daily basis and end when ovulation is detected.

There are several problems associated with direct intrauterine infusion of chemotherapeutic agents. There may be an irritation of the endometrium by the drug itself. The organisms within the uterine lumen may develop a resistance or be resistant to the chemotherapeutic agents utilized, which results in an ineffective treatment. The worst problem associated with this however, is the possibility of predisposing the uterine lumen to a superinfection by other organisms such as yeast or fungi. When this localized intrauterine therapy is accomplished, all of the pathogenic as well as the normal bacteria are killed. This allows an overgrowth of yeast and fungi.

Irritation of the endometrium is a consequence of several therapeutic agents used in intrauterine infusion. The most common of these irritating substances is a Lugol's solution (ten percent solution) and chlorhexidine. Both of these substances along with other irritating antiseptic agents should be used with great care. These will cause a chemical curettage within the uterine tissue. Further damage may result within these tissues when these antiseptic agents are utilized. Ulceration, fibrin formation, and fresh blood may appear in the uterus after an irritating solution is utilized.

The most effective antibiotic, determined through uterine culture, should be utilized in the treatment of endometritis through the route of intrauterine infusion. The most commonly used antibiotics for the treatment of endometritis through the use of intrauterine infusion are penicillin, tetracycline, gentamicin, ampicillin, streptomycin, amikacin, chloramphenicol, nitrofurazone, ticarcillin, polymyxin B, and neomycin. Care should be taken to follow adequate dilution or buffering when using any antibiotic solution. Gentamicin and amikacin are acidic in nature and should be

Artwork by S. Hakola / J. Dirig
Copyright Equistar Publications, Ltd.

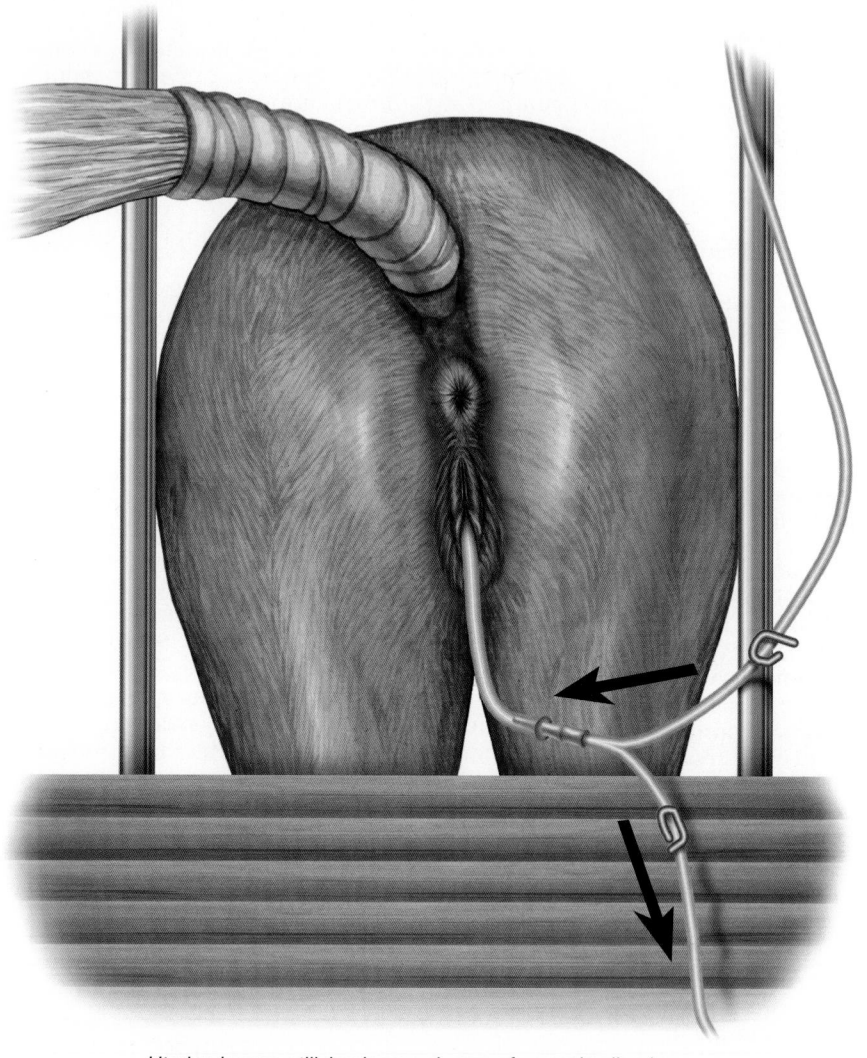

Uterine lavage utilizing large volumes of normal saline is
a very effective treatment modality for endometritis.

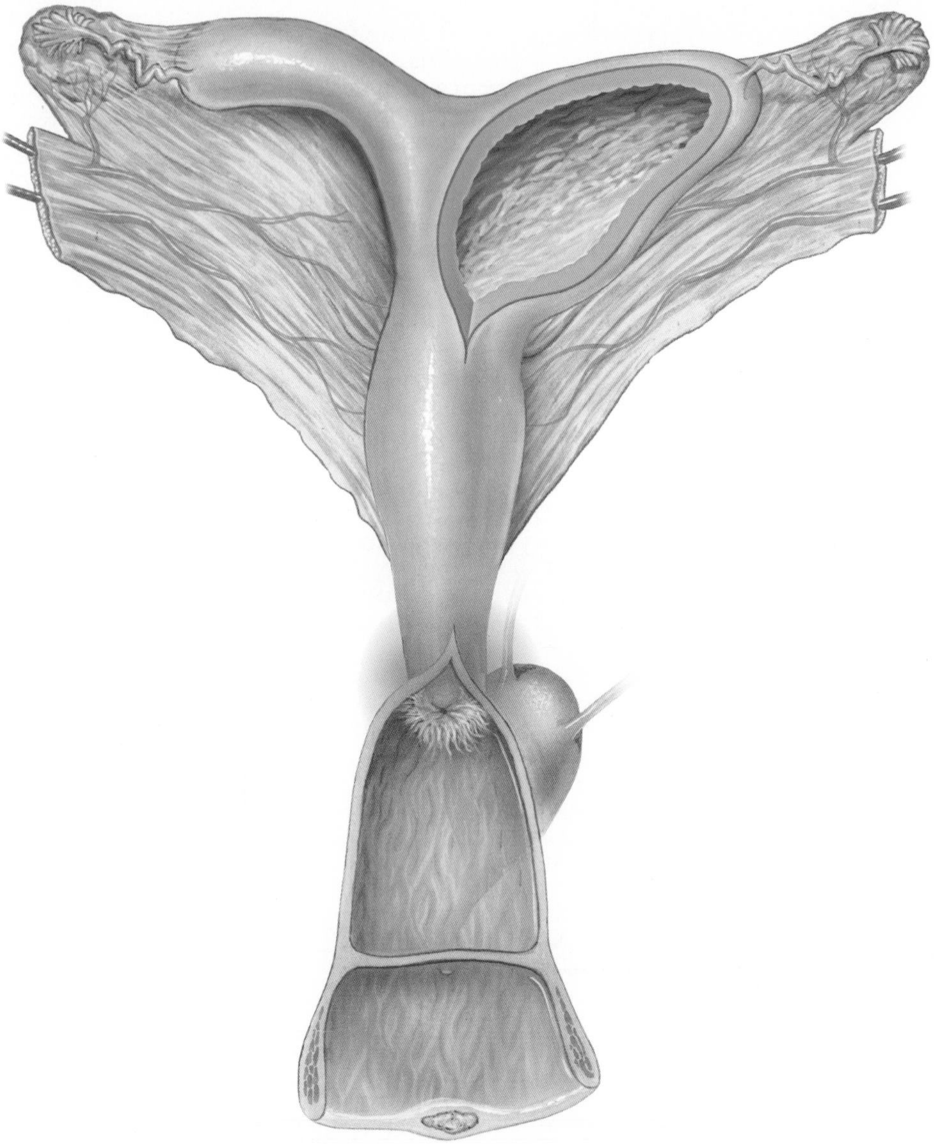

Pyometra with large accumulations of pus and inflammatory
exudates within the uterus. Note the cervical adhesions.

neutralized before infusion. The tetracycline drugs are also irritating and need to be diluted and buffered properly before infusion. Unfortunately, one of the more common risks associated with direct intrauterine infusion is the change of the pathogenic bacteria into resistance strains. For example, if not treated properly, a mare that has cultured positively for a streptococcal infection may reculture a growth of resistant *Pseudomonas spp.* after treatment.

The treatment regime that is utilized with intrauterine infusion of various antibiotics is usually based on convenience rather than the length of time the antibiotic is active in the uterus. Traditionally, intrauterine infusions are done daily for three to five days. In some instances every other day infusions are utilized for three to five treatments. Unfortunately, it is usually not practical to infuse mares more than once per day. The correct dosage and usage of antibiotics is essential if treatment is to be successful and resistance is to be avoided.

In most cases, approximately sixty milliliters of fluid is needed to cover the endometrial surface of the normal mare's uterus and one hundred to five hundred milliliters is required to cover the entire endometrial surface of an abnormal uterus. The goal of treatment is to infuse a sufficient volume of fluid so that the substance that is infused comes in contact with the entire endometrial surface.

Systemic Antibiotic Therapy

There are several advantages in the utilization of systemic antibiotic therapy for the treatment of endometritis. This allows for a significant tissue concentration of the antibiotic within the endometrium. There is a lesser degree of contamination of the uterine lumen utilizing this technique verses localized intrauterine infusion. The therapy can be administered systematically during diestrus with little risk to the tissues. The chief disadvantage to this approach is strictly economics since a six to ten day regimen of properly administered antibiotics is going to be more expensive than intrauterine infusion. The same dosages of any particular antibiotic are used for treating endometritis as for any systemic

infection. In numerous cases, it is often advantageous to administer systemic antibiotics in conjunction with intrauterine infusion of the same drug.

Uterine Lavage

Uterine lavage is a very effective treatment for endometritis. The advantages in utilizing this technique include the following: the mechanical removal of accumulated uterine fluid and other uterine contents, the stimulation of uterine contractility, and the recruitment of neutrophils and serum proteins to the site of phagocytic activity. Therefore, this technique actually enhances natural uterine defense mechanisms. Also, the fluid can be inspected which will render immediate information concerning the nature of the uterine contents.

Large volume uterine lavage requires the placement of a catheter that can be kept within the cervix to allow copious fluid to pass into and out of the uterine lumen. The external genitalia of the mare is prepped aseptically; the tail is wrapped and tied to the side. Proper restraint is used so that safety of the mare and the technician is observed.

Normal saline is utilized as a preferred fluid for lavage. This is due to its mildly irritating activity within the endometrium. It is clear, which allows easy inspection of recovered materials. This fluid should be warmed to forty-five to fifty degrees centigrade because warm fluid enhances uterine contraction. A thirty French catheter eighty centimeters long is introduced manually through the cervix. The cuff is inflated which seals the cervix off and allows administration of fluid within the uterine lumen without leakage. Care must be taken to clamp the end of the catheter that is outside the mare to prevent aspiration of air into the uterus. Utilizing gravity flow, one to two liters of fluid is infused into the uterus. Manipulation of the uterus per the rectum may facilitate exposure of the entire endometrium to this fluid. The fluid is then recovered in a separate container and measured to monitor the amount that is siphoned off. The mare's uterus may be large enough to require up to ten liters of fluid to completely fill it. Repeated filling and emptying of the uterus will

allow complete evacuation and removal of any accumulated uterine fluid and inflammatory debris. In most cases, uterine contraction is evident upon rectal palpation during the lavage.

PYOMETRA

Pyometra differs significantly from endometritis in that pyometra is a large accumulation of pus or inflammatory exudate within the distended uterus. The etiology behind the occurrence of pyometra is some form of interference with the natural fluid drainage from the uterus. In most cases, this is due to cervical adhesions or an abnormally constricted, tortuous, or irregular cervix. The second most common etiology is that of a chronic infection with *Pseudomonas spp.* or fungi. In most cases of pyometra, the corpus luteum persists beyond its normal life span.

Clinical Signs and Diagnosis

In most cases, there is a lack of any outward clinical sign of this disorder. The cycle length is varied but rarely are there any signs of weight loss, depression, septicemia, or anorexia.

Rectal palpation and ultrasonic examination are necessary in the diagnosis of pyometra. Care must be taken to rule out the possibility of pregnancy. Palpation per rectum will reveal a uterine wall that is thicker and more edematous than found in the normal pregnancy. Ultrasonography will confirm the fluid-filled uterine lumen.

Treatment

The most important consideration in the treatment of pyometra is the re-establishment of drainage through the cervix. Once this drainage is established, repeated treatment of uterine lavage with large volumes of warm saline should be initiated. Luteolysis of the corpus luteum can be accomplished with systemic administration of prostaglandin. In severe cases, hysterectomy should be considered if the mare is to be kept for purposes other than breeding. Care should be taken during the surgical hysterectomy to not contaminate the peritoneal cavity.

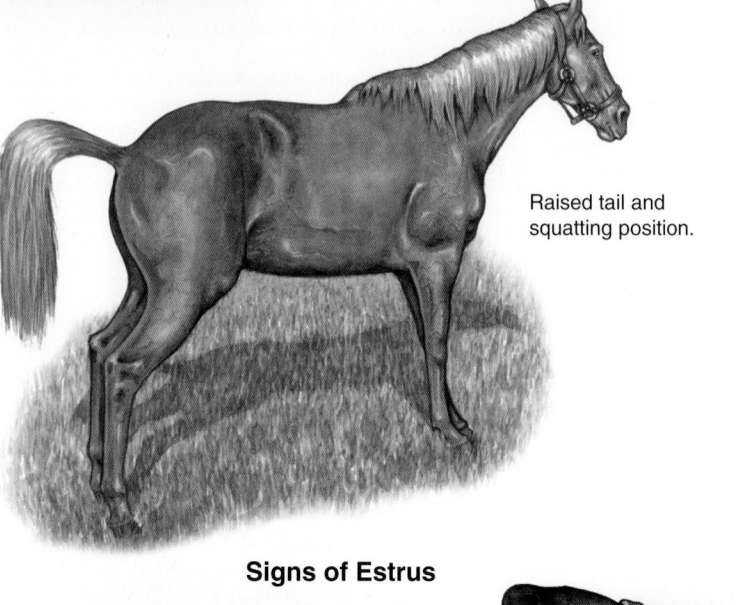

Raised tail and squatting position.

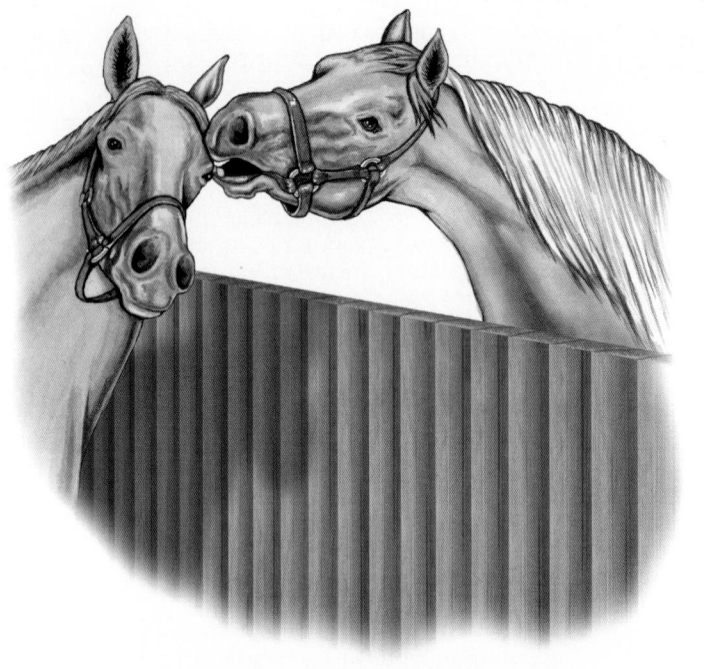

Mare exposed to a breeding stallion in adjacent stall with teasing wall to detect the beginning of estrus.

Signs of Estrus

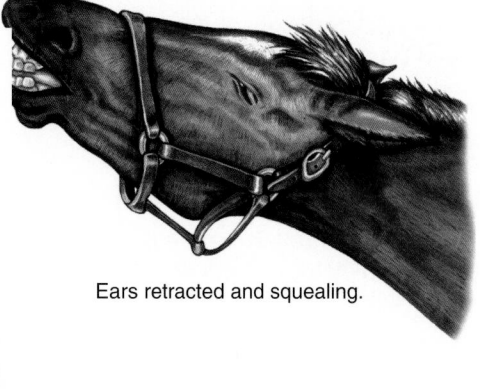

Ears retracted and squealing.

Determination of Proper Breeding Time

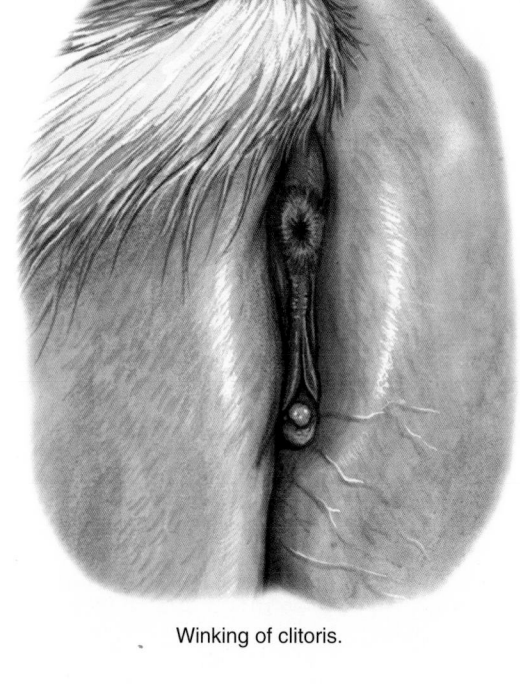

Winking of clitoris.

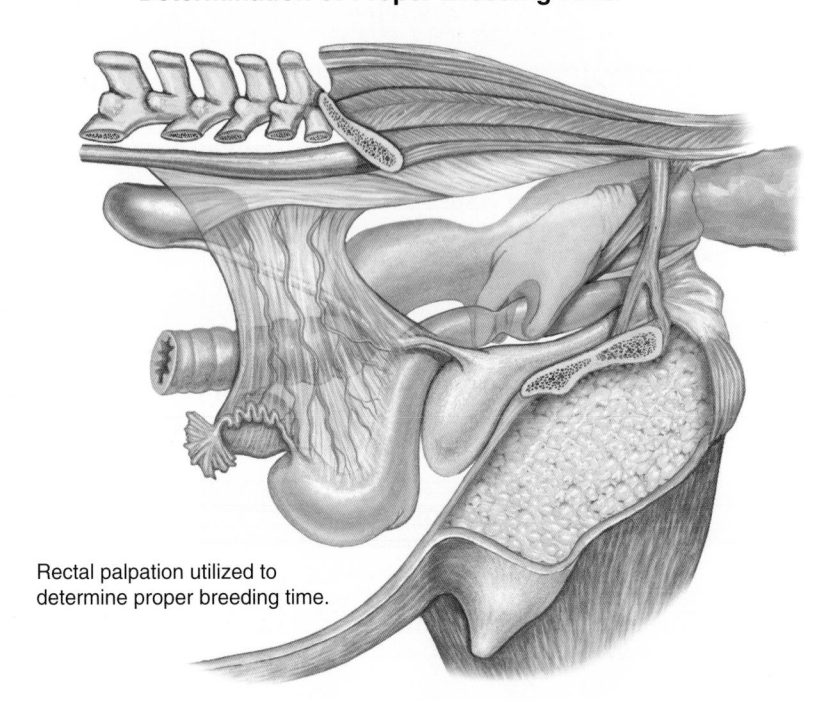

Rectal palpation utilized to determine proper breeding time.

BREEDING MANAGEMENT OF THE MARE

Heat (Estrus) Detection

The two most common man-made causes of infertility in the equine are the lack of detection of estrus and the improper selection of a breeding time. All of the managerial and scientific advantages in breeding programs are insignificant without the ability to recognize the stage of the estrous cycle that signals estrus, along with the failure to breed the mare at a time that is conducive to conception.

Estrus detection within the brood mare band should be the responsibility of an employee or breeder that has an understanding of the estrous cycle and knows the importance of his or her task. An effective heat (estrus) detection program should be designed with a designated individual for each particular farm. That individual should also have the knowledge of each individual mare's estrous cycle and unique behavioral characteristics.

Recognizing the Signs of Estrus

Internally, increased levels of estrogen stimulate the development of the uterine endometrium. The entire reproductive tract begins to prepare for estrus. Characteristic behavioral patterns depict a receptive attitude toward the stallion. The most common of these include frequent urination, a squatting posture, a raised tail, and spasmatic "winking" of the labia. Mares that are presented with a foal at their side or overly shy mares will exhibit extremely passive and sometimes protective behavioral characteristics during estrus. Skillful observation by the breeding management will be invaluable in the detection of estrus within these animals.

Teasing the Mare

Proper teasing of mares is an important key to any successful equine breeding program. Mares will exhibit estrus in different individualistic manners. It is important to tease each mare an adequate amount of time and under comfortable environmental conditions in order to detect the beginning of estrus. Trained observations and patience are essential qualities in the person handling this task. During the early part of the breeding season, abnormal estrous behavior and variable estrus durations are to be expected. If these mares are teased carefully during the early breeding season, it allows the breeding manager to follow the mare from a transitional anovulatory state to that of a receptive ovulatory state. This is one of the most important aspects of the breeding program. Even with diligent teasing, some mares will just not show estrus after extensive teasing with an intact stallion. Mares that displayed behavioral signs of estrus at the home farm may be intimidated by new surroundings at the breeding farm and may not show heat. There are those mares that have already ovulated and quickly gone out of heat before they reached the breeding farm. Maiden mares that have never been to a breeding farm or around a stallion are particularly hard to tease.

The ideal teaser is a well-mannered and vocal breeding stallion, whereas an ill-mannered stallion requires constant restraint and is more likely to injure a mare or her handlers. In rare instances, he may even intimidate the mare into not responding to the teasing process. This stallion should also be aggressive enough to continue to tease mares day in and day out.

One must be careful when using the actual breeding stallion to serve as a teaser. When the stallion is used as a teaser, it may discourage his normal libido or sexual drive. Pony stallions, vasectomized horses, or other stallions could be used instead of the breeding stallion. Just like any other animal on the farm, it is important to keep the teaser stallion in good physical and mental condition by providing him a balanced ration, adequate shelter, exercise, and routine health care.

The methodology of teasing horses allows a close association between the teaser stallion and the mare for several minutes in order to detect estrus. It is important to consider safety, the size of the brood mare band, and the availability of farm labor when developing a teasing facility. One of the most common methods of teasing mares is to turn the mare loose in a stall adjacent to the stallion in which a sliding partition between the two stalls allows the stallion access to the mare. The teaser can get his head and neck into the stall with the mare when this partition or sliding door is lifted. In other instances, a padded teasing wall which is about four feet high and ten feet long allows the teaser stallion and mare to be in close proximity to each other and prevents injuries to both animals. In large breeding operations when labor and time are limited, a teaser stallion is sometimes penned in the center of a small pasture or paddock where a small brood mare band is enclosed. Lastly, it is not uncommon in small operations with limited labor to have a pony or vasectomized stallion running directly with the brood mares even though this procedure has numerous disadvantages.

Rectal Palpation for the Detection of the Proper Breeding Time

Traditionally, rectal palpation has been utilized to predict the time of ovulation in mares. Rectal examination should be done very carefully and judicially to allow safety to the mare as well as the palpator. A shoulder length obstetrical glove coated with adequate amounts of lubrication should be utilized in performing rectal palpations of the reproductive tract. The lubricated and gloved hand should be gently inserted through the anus into the rectum. All manure within this region should be carefully and slowly evacuated. Once this is accomplished, orientation within the bony pelvis and identification of the pelvic brim will aid the palpator in finding the cervix and corresponding uterine horns for palpation.

During the stages of diestrus and pregnancy, the uterine wall palpates as a firm tubular structure. The cervix feels like a hard dense tube at the bottom of the pelvis or just over the pelvic brim.

Artwork by S. Hakola / J. Dirig
Copyright Equistar Publications, Ltd.

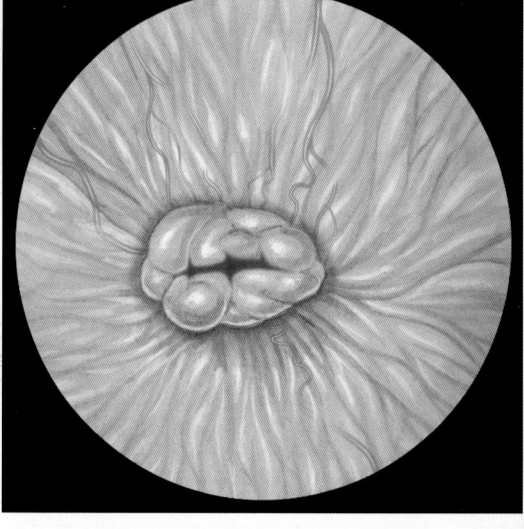

Cervix during estrus prior to ovulation.

Examination of Cervix to Determine Ovarian Cycle and the Optimum Breeding Time

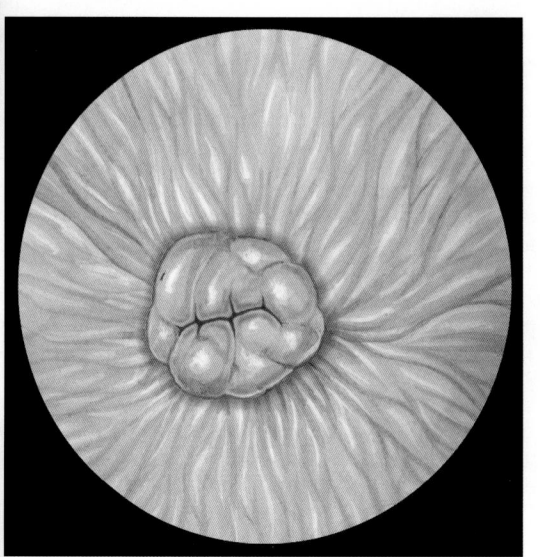

Diestrus cervix

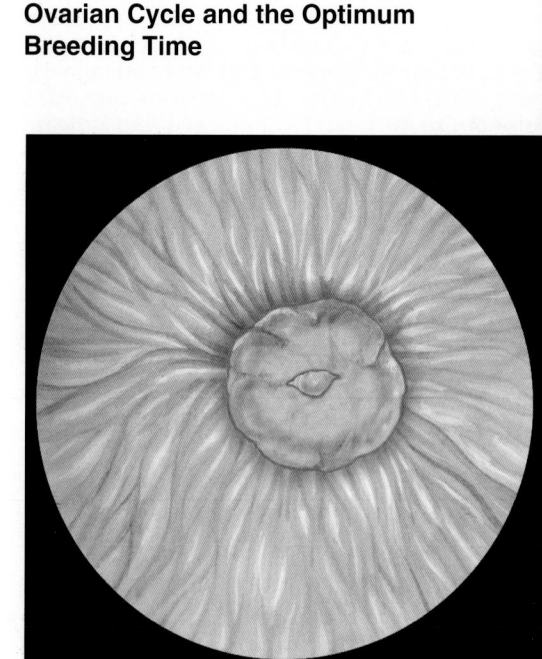

Cervix during pregnancy.
Note mucous plug sealing
cervical oriface.

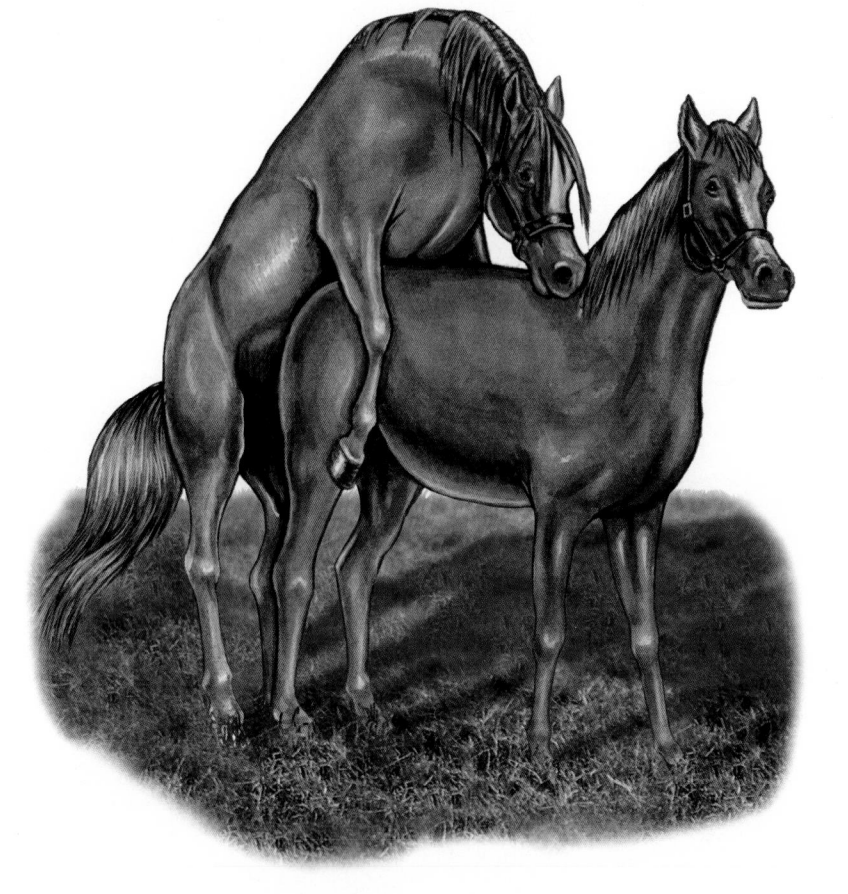

Pasture Breeding

During estrus, the uterine wall has a flaccid tone and palpates as if swollen. Cervical folds relax and the cervix becomes easily palpated during estrus. Careful evaluation of the cervix is usually a significant aid in breeding at the optimum time.

In the first stages of estrus, the maturing follicle on the ovary is a dense structure approximately one centimeter in diameter. Numerous follicles can be palpated, but one is usually larger than the others. This primary follicle typically increases in size by 10 centimeters. Ovulation will probably occur within the next three days. An experienced palpator will note that this primary follicle softens within twenty-four hours prior to ovulation. This change in consistency is a far better predictor of ovulation than that of follicular size.

In summary, the cervix should be relaxed and open, the uterine wall should be flaccid and swollen, and the primary follicle should soften when the optimum time for breeding exists. Ideally, all three of these criteria are met when a recommendation for breeding is made. However, most animals will exhibit only two of these three criteria and sometimes only one when their optimum breeding time occurs.

Utilization of a Vaginal Speculum to Determine Optimum Breeding Time

Through the use of a vaginal speculum and a good light source, a trained breeding technician can detect the estrous-related changes upon the cervix. When the animal is in heat, or estrus, the cervix softens and drops towards the floor of the vagina. Approximately twenty-four hours before ovulation, the cervix of the mare will actually flatten on the vaginal floor. The opening of the os will appear horizontal. The change in appearance of the cervix is due to the increased amount of estrogen secretion from the developing follicle. The tissues around the cervix are usually edematous and mucus secretions can be noted. Estrogen also has an effect on the blood supply to the cervix at this stage. This results in a state of hyperemia which literally means that it is more pink in color and the vasculature can be easily visible.

When the mare is in the diestrus stage, the cervical and vaginal surfaces become pale and dry when visualized with a vaginal speculum. The tissues within this region appear gray or even pale white in color. The external cervical os projects into the cranial vagina from high on the wall and is tightly contracted.

During pregnancy, the cervix usually is intensely white and appears tightly closed. During late pregnancy, the cervix is covered by a thick, sticky exudate. It is sometimes difficult to examine the cervical os because of this exudate and its position within the vagina.

Breeding the Mare at the Optimum Time

Traditionally, it has been recommended that the mare should be bred on her third day of estrus and then every other day thereafter until she is no longer receptive to the stallion. In most mares, ovulation will occur approximately twenty-four hours prior to the end of estrus or heat. However, this ovulation may take place anywhere from forty-eight hours before to twenty-four hours after this point. The ovulated ovum begins to disintegrate within the oviduct twelve to twenty-four hours postovulation. Sperm retain their motility for at least twenty-four to forty-eight hours. Therefore, it is important that a viable ovum and motile sperm are present in the oviduct for conception at the right time. Optimum conception rates are achieved at the breeding farm when breeding takes place within the time period of twenty-four hours prior to ovulation and no later than two hours post-ovulation. This well-timed mating is a product of careful observation, judicious use of the stallion, and an accurate assessment of each mare's reproductive status.

BREEDING METHODS AND PROCEDURES

There are four basic methods for breeding horses: pasture breeding, hand breeding, artificial insemination, and embryo transfer. Each of these breeding methods have distinct advantages and

disadvantages. Each farm has its own unique management and physical structures available for the breeding program. To summarize an efficient breeding procedure for that particular operation, one should consider the number of mares that are bred yearly, facilities and space available for the breeding activities to occur, and the breed restrictions that are applicable to that program.

Pasture Breeding

The basic methodology of pasture breeding involves simply placing a stallion with a group of mares in an area that is large enough to imitate natural breeding behavior. The disadvantages of this breeding method usually outweigh the advantages even when simple economics requires the breeding management to maximize production and minimize cost. However, there are certain instances where this is an ideal breeding method for a particular farm.

Caution should be utilized when using a pasture breeding program. Most importantly, steps should be taken to ensure that the stallions and mares are healthy and free of any infectious organisms. Having just one mare carrying an infection would allow the possibility of this organism to be transmitted throughout the entire herd via the stallion, which could result in infertility of the entire group. Care should also be taken in introducing the stallion to a mare or group of mares since an inexperienced or overanxious stallion could result in injuries to either the mares or himself. Routine observation should be conducted on more than a daily basis for injury, illness, and to ensure that the stallion is servicing the mares. In addition to these visual observations, several of the mares should be checked for pregnancy as soon as possible to determine whether or not the stallion is settling this group of mares.

Pasture breeding allows a herd to revert back to natural breeding patterns. Since the species has survived for thousands of years, this in itself is not detrimental to fertility. However, there are many disadvantages and actual limitations with a pasture breeding program.

Artwork by S. Hakola / J. Dirig
Copyright Equistar Publications, Ltd.

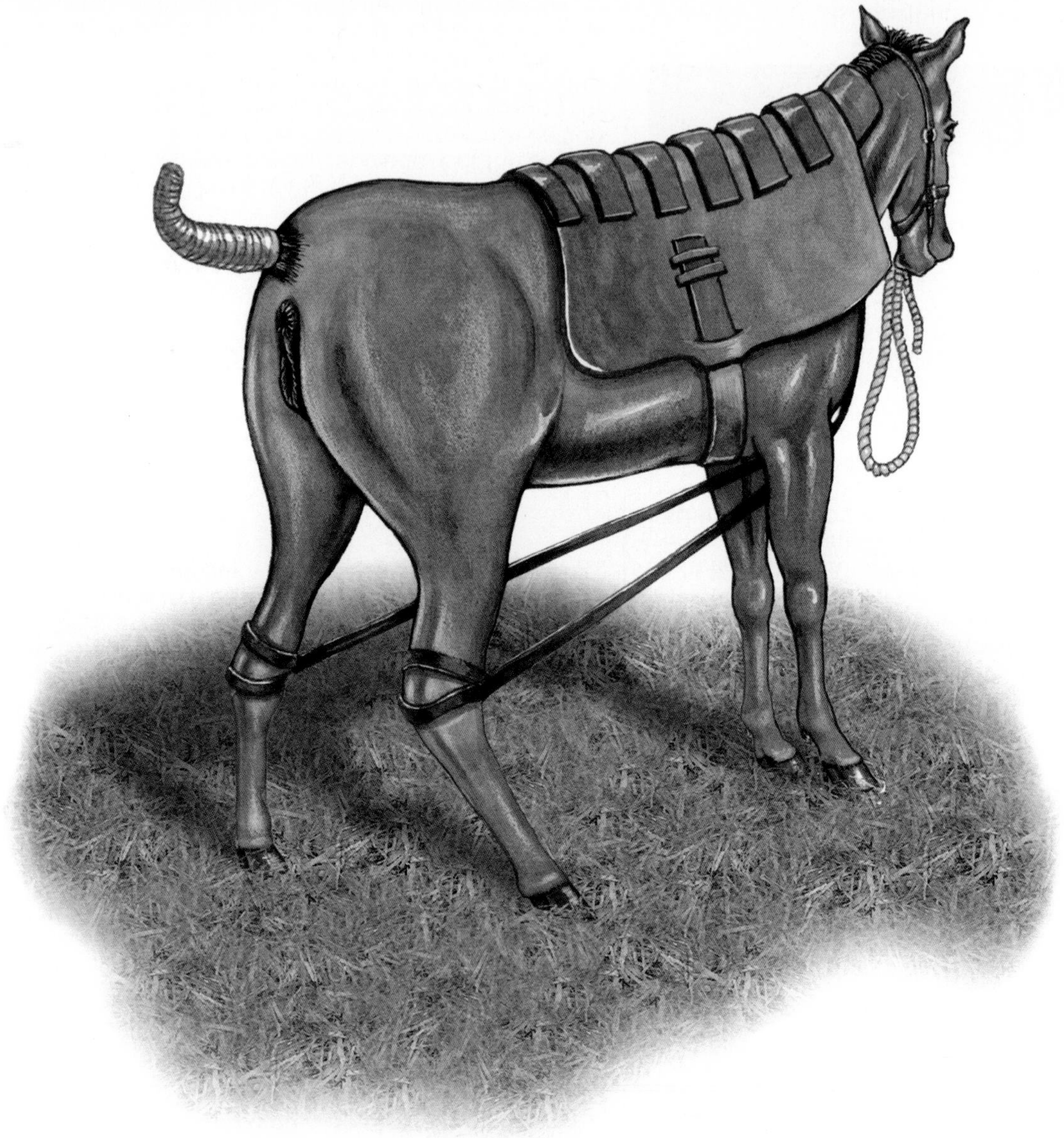

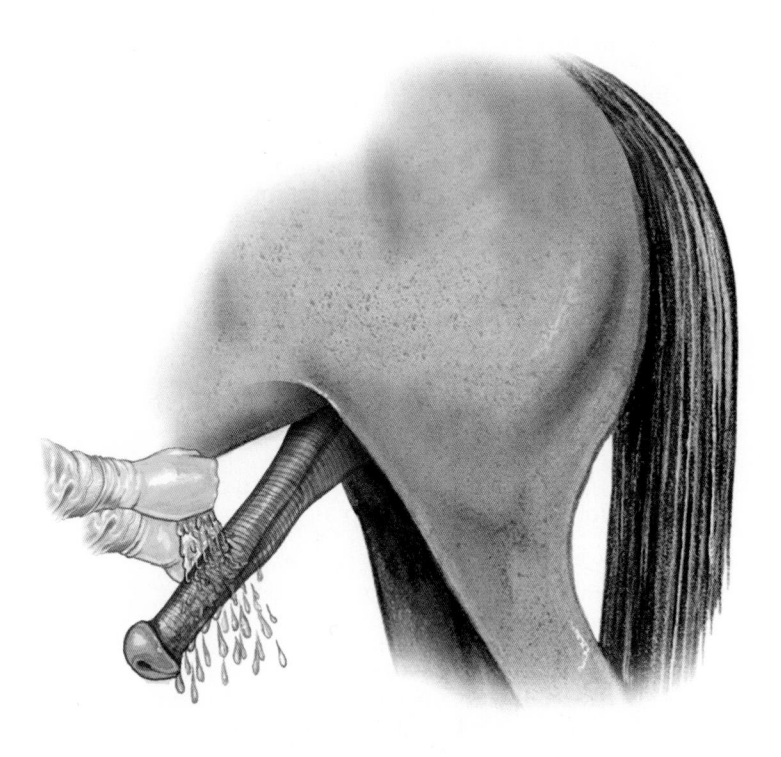

Cleansing of the Stallion's Genitalia.

Mare Prepared for Live Cover: Proper Restraints, Hobbles, Protective Neck Mat, Wrapped Tail.

The following are disadvantages to a pasture breeding program:

1. A pasture bred stallion can only settle a limited number of mares when compared to what a stallion can settle in other breeding programs.

2. It is difficult to observe the mares in a pasture bred program. Any management technique such as palpation of the mares becomes time consuming and impractical when a pasture breeding program is utilized.

3. It only takes one infected mare to contaminate the stallion who will then expose all the other mares to the pathogen.

4. Valuable breeding stock can be easily injured in a pasture breeding program due to an overanxious stallion or a mare protective of her foal.

5. Record keeping of exact breeding dates becomes difficult, which results in mares that foal without the benefit of human supervision.

There are certain instances where pasture breeding will work very effectively with a small number of healthy farmed-owned mares bred to a fertile, aggressive stallion. Certain mares will conceive only when there is an absence of management-related stresses that effect the estrus cycle of these mares. A pasture breeding program is also economical in the sense that stalls, paddocks, shutes, and labor costs are usually eliminated.

Hand Breeding

In the hand breeding program, mares and stallions are both handled as individuals. This allows for close examination by the management personnel of idiosyncrasies and individual fertility problems. Hand breeding programs will be unique to each farm with the equipment, the facilities, and even the breeding procedure itself reflecting that farm and the management personnel of that farm.

Physical facilities utilized in the hand breeding program are unique to each farm yet should have

the following common characteristics:

1. The entire area should be as clean as possible to minimize any contamination of the male and female genitalia.

2. The stallions and mares should have good footing at all times (even in the wash areas) to reduce the chances of a horse slipping and falling, which could result in an injury.

3. The area should be enclosed and protected from the elements. This also minimizes distractions for the personnel, the stallion, and the mares.

4. Wash areas and holding pens should be designed into the facilities to allow cleanliness and less stress to the mares.

5. There are times when a mare is much taller than the stallion and an elevated or recessed area should be available to allow the stallion to cover this animal.

6. Accurate and up-to-date records should be kept on each day's activity which allows proper management and identification of any potential fertility problems.

Preparing the Mare for Breeding

When the ideal time to breed the mare has been determined, there is a standard procedure in preparing this mare for breeding. The mare's tail is wrapped in some fashion and the external genitalia and perineum are washed before breeding. This should be done in a wash area that has adequate flooring and drainage. Plain warm water should be utilized for the cleansing of mares and stallions. Excessive scrubbing or washing with antimicrobial compounds alters the normal bacterial flora of these anatomical areas which encourages the growth of opportunistic pathogens. The mare should be inspected to see if she has had a recent Caslick operation. If this is the case, extra care should be taken to clean this area. It may be necessary to remove the sutures and open her up to allow entry of the stallion's penis.

Although most mares in estrus usually stand quietly to be bred, care must be taken to properly restrain specific mares in order to prevent injury to themselves as well as the breeding stallion. Protection of a mare's neck from an overly aggressive stallion is accomplished through the use of a leather protective mat that attaches to the halter and extends from just behind the head down to the middle of the back. The most common restraint used, beside the twitch, is a set of breeding hobbles. These hobbles prevent the mare from kicking the stallion during breeding. Quite simply, hobbles are leather straps that buckle around the mare's neck just in front of her shoulder which are attached to ropes or other strips of leather that are attached to leather straps that buckle around the mare's hocks or pastern. Using this equipment, the mare can walk but not kick. Care should be taken so that a stallion and a mare should not become entangled. In certain instances, sometimes all that is necessary is a one-legged hobble on the front leg to prevent the mare from kicking.

Preparing the Stallion

The stallion should be allowed to tease the mare briefly to encourage him to extend his penis. After the penis is extended, the stallion should be moved to the wash area where his genitalia is cleaned with luke warm water and rinsed prior to breeding. It is normal for the stallion to move his feet repeatedly or kick at this time. Therefore, it is important to be patient with the young stallion and train him to be well-mannered during the wash process. Most stallions do not object to the washing before breeding after this procedure has been repeated for several days. In many instances, stallions will become accustomed to extending their penis as soon as they sense that they are in the wash area.

Overzealous washing of the stallion's penis can sometimes do more harm than good. Luke warm water should be the only thing that is utilized in the cleansing process of the penis. Soaps and antimicrobial sanitizing solutions may irritate the stallion's penis and may disrupt the normal bacterial flora that occur on the surface of these

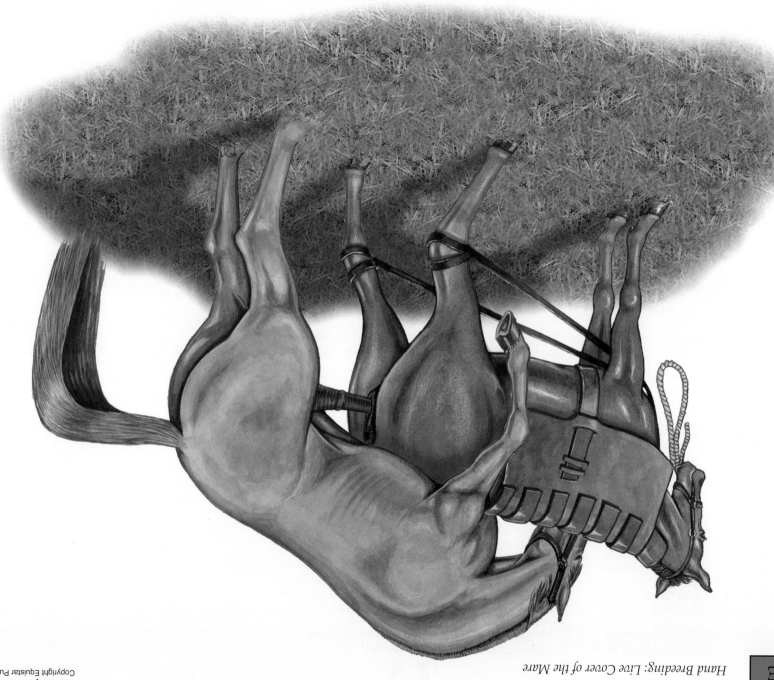

Hand Breeding: Live Cover of the Mare

THE MARE

tissues. This may predispose the growth of disease-causing organisms which could result in future breeding problems. Some stallions will even become overstimulated by the prebreeding wash which will effect the concentration and amount of ejaculate during that service. Stallions who are bred on a regular basis and who are kept clean sometimes are not washed before breeding but washed only after they have covered a mare.

Covering the Mare

Each stallion will exhibit individual sexual behavior. Some mature stallions may take as little as 15 seconds of sexual stimulation to achieve an erection to breed a mare. Younger stallions, however, may need as long as 20 - 25 minutes before an erection is achieved to allow a successful mount. This stimulation period is very important because if an erection is not achieved, the stallion cannot penetrate the mare. If the stimulation is too long, the stallion may actually lose interest in the mare. In all cases the knowledge and skill of the individual person that handles the stallion is invaluable.

It is important that the stallion approach the mare slowly and at a slight angle to avoid contact if the mare decides to kick the stallion. The handler should maintain control over the stallion from a short distance. The stallion should be discouraged from mounting until he obtains a full erection. He should not be allowed to charge the mare and startle her. The stallion should be reprimanded during breeding for any objectionable vices such as severe biting or ravaging the mare. Care must be taken during this behavior modification because excessive correction during the breeding process may have psychological effects on the stallion that result in a reduced libido or even a refusal to mount that particular mare.

After the stallion has obtained an erection, it may be necessary for the handler to guide the stallion's penis for proper intromission. Handling should be kept at a minimum and exam gloves utilized so that any dirt cannot be deposited on the penis. An assistant should be available to hold the mare's tail to one side and possibly offer guidance to the penis.

In most cases, hand breeding requires an intensive amount of labor. An individual is required to hold the mare and restrain her, one is required to hold the stallion, and a third individual may be required to hold the mare's tail to the side, direct the stallion's penis, and possibly maneuver the breeding rod into position if this is needed.

A breeding rod is utilized when it is desirable to prevent complete entry of the entire length of the stallion's penis into the mare. It is usually comprised of a long, padded cylinder, 5 inches in diameter and approximately 18 inches long. It is placed inside a plastic disposable sleeve or glove that is changed after each use. It is positioned between the pair just above the stallion's penis. This prevents the stallion from penetrating the mare too deeply. This is helpful when breeding maiden and anatomically smaller mares.

Each individual stallion will breed mares in his own unique fashion. Some stallions may require only a few thrusts before ejaculation occurs. Other stallions may thrust anywhere from thirty seconds to two minutes before ejaculation. There are two ways to note whether or not the stallion has ejaculated. Most stallions will flag their tails during ejaculation. If the base of the penis is held gently, pulsations will be felt along the urethra on the ventral surface of the penis.

After ejaculation, the stallion should be allowed to rest for a short period of time. He should dismount at his own pace dependent upon which side he mounted. The mare should be turned away from him to prevent possible kicking. The stallion should be backed away from the mare and at the same time, the mare should be turned away from the stallion to prevent contact. Most stallions will then allow their penis to be washed again without any obvious objections.

It is important to be aware of the safety of both the mare and the stallion during the entire hand breeding process. Aggressive stallions may injure the mare. It is up to the handler to prevent a rapid dismount after ejaculation that may cause injury to the mare's vagina or vulva which could result in a pneumovagina. Any experienced breeding farm manager will remember an instance where the

stallion has lost consciousness after ejaculation. In some cases, the stallion may actually fall off the mare but since his body is typically relaxed, he is usually unharmed by the landing. If the horse is injured by the fall or remains unconscious for an extended period of time, veterinary care may be required.

Traditionally, mares have been walked quietly for approximately 15 minutes after breeding. However, there is no proof that this procedure affects conception rates. Walking the mare after a poor cover does not improve conception rates.

Hand breeding is one of the most commonly used breeding techniques within the horse industry. Care must be taken that it does not result in overuse of the stallion. During the height of the breeding season, scheduling problems will arise since several mares must be breed to the same stallion on the same day. Careful management and scheduling can overcome some of this problem; however, the biggest disadvantage to hand breeding is that it limits the number of offspring a stallion can sire within a particular breeding season.

ARTIFICIAL INSEMINATION

There are numerous advantages in utilizing artificial insemination within the breeding program. They are as follows:

1. Utilizing artificial insemination prevents overuse of the stallion in that an ejaculate can be divided into several insemination doses permitting a more efficient use of the stallion's semen. Therefore, the number of mares that can be booked to a stallion within a particular breeding season can be increased exponentially.

2. There is a great reduction in venereal transmission of bacterial diseases. The addition of antibiotics and seminal extenders which contain protective and nutrient factors for the spermatozoa greatly reduce the chance of bacterial infection and enhance pregnancy rates.

Artwork by S. Hakola / J. Dirig
Copyright Equistar Publications, Ltd.

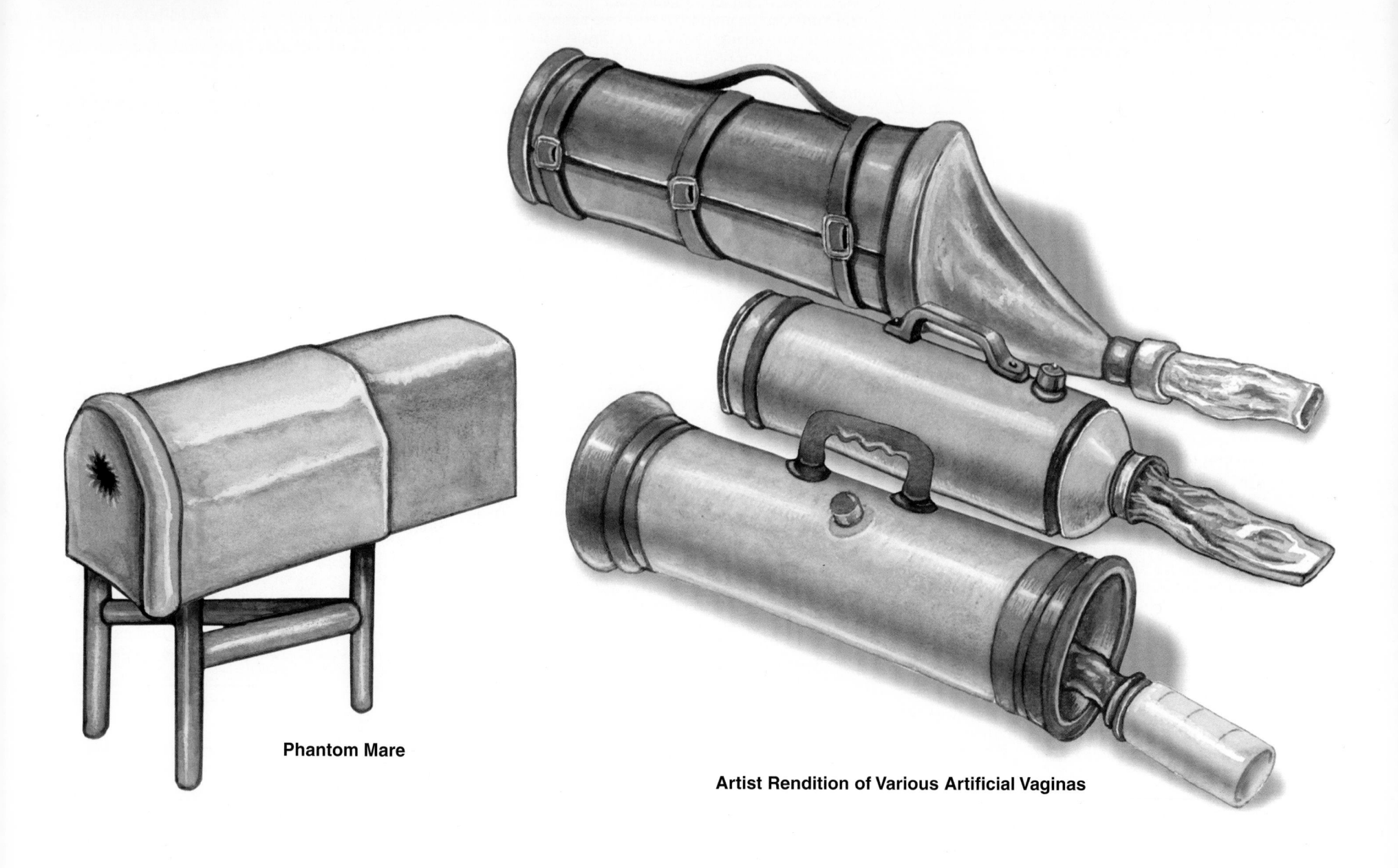

Phantom Mare

Artist Rendition of Various Artificial Vaginas

3. Artificial insemination, through the use of a phantom mare, will greatly reduce the chances of injury to the mare or the stallion.

4. There is a close evaluation of seminal quality throughout the breeding season. Changes in the number of spermatozoa per ejaculate, sperm motility, and sperm maturity can be detected immediately and corrective measures be implemented.

5. Conception rates are usually improved through the use of artificial insemination. Physical stress that is associated with live cover is eliminated through the use of artificial insemination. In addition, the use of an infusion or insemination pipette allows the semen to be deposited directly into the mare's uterus so that the spermatozoa have easier access to the egg.

6. Some stallions have lost the ability to live cover a mare through arthritis, injury, or old age. Artificial insemination techniques have allowed the continued use of these stallions.

Facilities and Equipment

The physical layout of the artificial insemination facility for the collection of semen will improve the efficiency and safety of the entire breeding program. The actual semen collection area should be a well lighted indoor area with good footing and adequate space to provide optimum efficiency. The facility should be constructed so that semen collection can be done during inclimate weather and during periods of the day when there is no sunlight. When constructing this facility, distraction for the stallion should be kept at a minimum. The facility should provide an environment in which the stallion consistently associates this space with breeding.

The phantom or dummy mare should be the same size or slightly smaller than the anticipated stallions who will utilize it. This phantom should be padded and covered with a material that is durable and yet easy to clean. Consideration should also be given to cover the "phantom mare's neck" with a material that the stallion can grip with his teeth to maintain balance.

Adjacent to the breeding area should be a environmentally controlled laboratory. This laboratory should be properly equipped for both the evaluation of semen and the preparation of the artificial vaginas.

An artificial vagina is an essential piece of equipment needed to collect high quality semen from the stallion. Several models are available commercially which include the Colorado State University model, the Missouri model, and a Japanese model. Most of these commercially available models should include an in-line filter which will yield an ejaculate of superior quality during seminal collection.

Because the stallions are sensitive to both temperature and pressure, there should be individual conditions within each artificial vagina in order to obtain a superior ejaculate. Each stallion will have a preference and the knowledge the breeding manager has of each stallion's preferences will enhance the quality of the semen collected. The preparation of the artificial vagina should therefore be timed to coincide with the washing of the stallion. This will allow an optimum temperature and pressure to be present within the artificial vagina during the collection process.

Artificial vaginas should be cleaned and disinfected after each use. The utilization of hot water is usually all that is needed to clean most artificial vagina liners. Care must be taken not to use any soaps or disinfectants that would leave a residue that could be damaging to the sperm or be spermicidal. These include any concentrations of iodine since concentrations as low as .05% have been shown to render spermatozoa completely immotile within one minute of contact. In certain instances, gas sterilization can be utilized, but it is necessary that the equipment be allowed to air out for at least 48 - 72 hours before it is reused.

There are certain stallions that will resist the use of an artificial vagina. Stallions that have been used in the past for natural live cover and some young stallions are usually in this category. In these cases, a condom is used for seminal collection. Sometimes a condom will be just as objectionable

to the stallion as will an artificial vagina. Ejaculate collected in a condom is usually of an inferior quality due to contamination. There is also an increased risk for human injury while applying the condom to a stallion's erect penis and its retrieval after use.

Semen Collection

The actual collection of semen can be accomplished with a live jump mare or a breeding phantom. Live jump mares can be normal mares exhibiting behavioral estrus or be mares that have had their ovaries removed. Ovariectomized mares are more predictable with regards to their sexual receptivity than those mares that are showing imbehavioral estrus. These mares require exogenous estrogen therapy to mimic signs of behavioral estrus. They then exhibit behavioral estrus on a continual basis to allow a constant stimulation source for semen collection. In any case the jump mare should still be restrained in order to maximize safety for both the handlers and the stallion.

The use of a breeding phantom to collect semen from stallions is much easier than the maintenance of ovariectomized mares. Most stallions will require only a minimum amount of training to treat the breeding phantom as a sexual object and readily mount it. On numerous instances, experienced stallions will prefer to mount a breeding phantom without an estrous mare anywhere in the vicinity. However, some breeding stallions will still require a live estrous mare in the area to obtain an erection.

As a stallion mounts the phantom or live jump mare, the collector usually maneuvers along the stallion's left side and deflects the stallion's penis gently into the artificial vagina. Care must be taken not to force the artificial vagina on to the stallion since most stallions will recognize this movement as abnormal and become discouraged. Once the stallion has entered the artificial vagina, support against the stallion's thrust can be gained by steadying the artificial vagina against a mares thigh or buttock. If the stallion decides to dismount, the artificial vagina should not follow the stallion's penis since this again would be interpreted as abnormal to the stallion.

**Perineal Prep Necessary Prior to
Artificial Insemination**

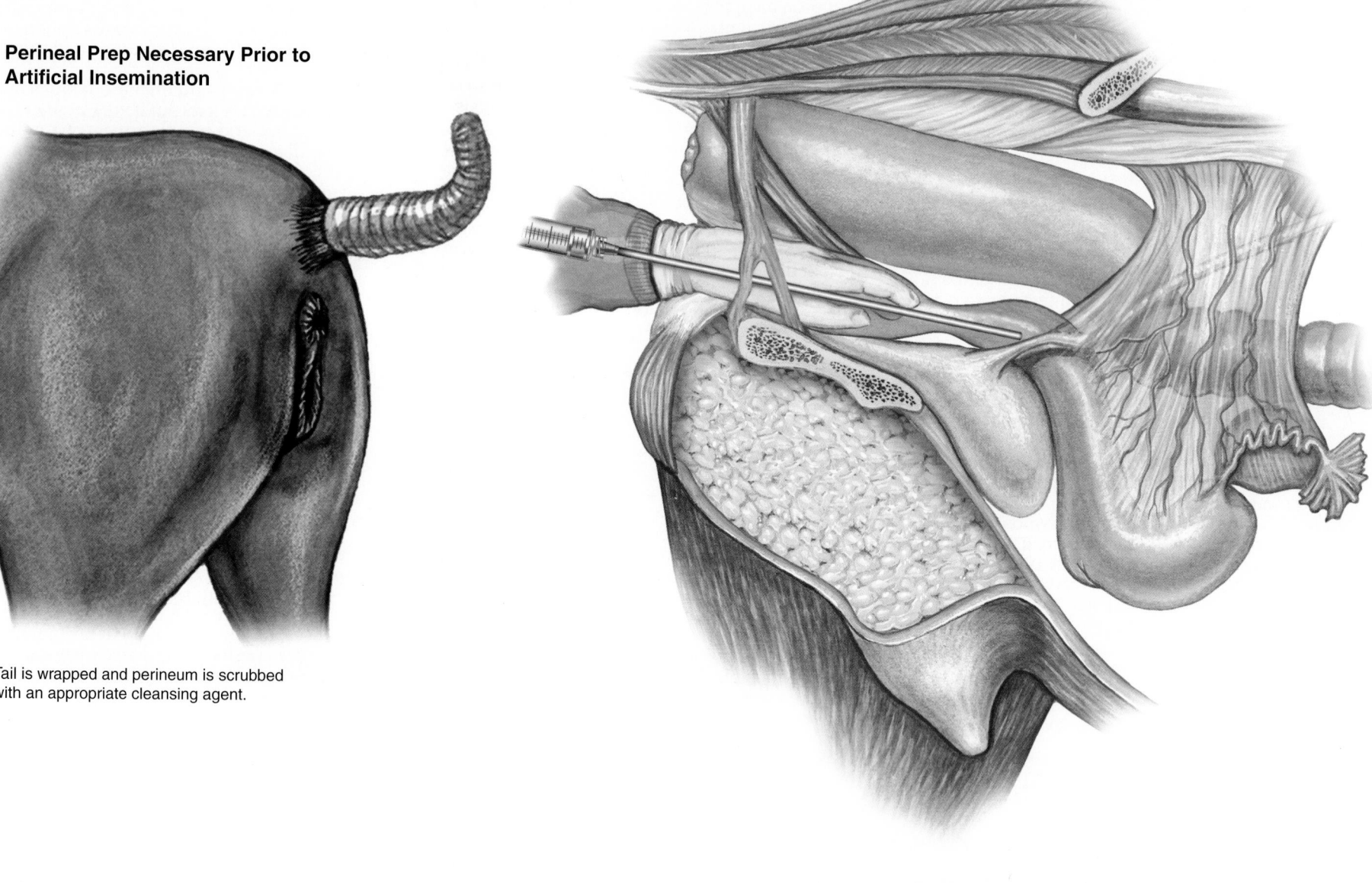

Tail is wrapped and perineum is scrubbed
with an appropriate cleansing agent.

Artificial Insemination Using an Infusion Pipette

Ejaculation can be detected through the palpation of pulsations along the base of the stallion's penis. Ejaculation will usually last at least 10 seconds. Approximately 75% of the sperm are present within the first 7 - 8 seconds of ejaculation. The end of the artificial vagina into which the collection bottle is attached should be lowered as the stallion ejaculates to facilitate the collection of the sperm rich fraction of the ejaculate.

Once the stallion ejaculates, he should be allowed to rest on the jump mare or phantom mare until he is ready to dismount. When the stallion dismounts, water is released from the pressure jacket so that the semen descends into the collection bottle. Care should be taken not to expose the collection bottle to the environmental factors of cold and sunlight. The collection bottle should be taken immediately to the laboratory for processing.

Care and Processing of Collected Semen

Immediately after collection of the semen sample, it should be transported to the laboratory with minimal agitation, exposure to light, or temperature changes. Care must be taken to prevent the gel fraction from contaminating the sperm rich fraction. Most artificial vaginas have a filtering device built into the collection apparatus. If not, the sample should be immediately filtered after collection through sterile gauze or a milk line filter to separate these fractions.

A measurement should be taken of the gel free volume in a prewarmed measuring device such as a graduated cylinder. Again, minimal agitation of the sample should be maintained. The cylinder should be tilted and the sample poured slowly to avoid damage to the sperm cells. Motility and concentration should also be determined before the insemination dose can be calculated. The semen should also be evaluated for morphology, white blood cell counts, and all other tests that are relevant at this time.

The standard goal for the utilization of an artificial insemination program is that each mare be

inseminated with 500 million progressively motile sperm cells at each insemination. Research has shown that inseminating mares with dosages exceeding 500 million sperm do not enhance conception rates. Regardless of whether the semen is to be used immediately or preserved, an appropriate extender should be added. This protects the spermatozoa and provides a supportive medium immediately after ejaculation. Even if the raw semen is to be divided into several doses and inseminated into several mares immediately after collection, there are several advantages to adding an extender to this sample. The greatest advantage lies in the addition of antibiotics within the extender to the semen sample that allows control of any undesirable organisms within the sample.

The most common equine semen extenders are as follows:

1. Cream-Gel Extender
Knox gelatin (unflavored)	1.3g
Distilled water (sterile)	10 ml
Half-and-half cream	1 pint (475 ml)
Penicillin, crystalline	100,000 units
Streptomycin, crystalline	100,000 ug
Polymyxin B sulfate	20,000 units

2. Heated Skim Milk Extender
Skim Milk	100 ml
Polymyxin B	100,000 units

(Heat skim milk to 92 - 95 degrees Celsius in a double boiler for 10 minutes; cool and add polymyxin B.)

3. Nonfat Dry Milk Solids Glucose Extender I
Nonfat Dry milk solids	2.4 g
Glucose	4.9 g
Penicillin, crystalline	150,000 units
Streptomycin, crystalline	150,000ug
Sterile deionized water	q.s. 100 ml

4. Nonfat Dry Milk Solids Glucose Extender II
Nonfat dry milk solids	2.4 g
Glucose	4.9 g
Gentamicin Sulfate (reagent grade)	150,000 units
8.4% $NaHCO_3$ (Sodium bicarbonate)	2 ml
Deionized water (sterile)	92 ml

(Mix liquids before adding nonfat dry milk solids or gentamicin will curdle the milk.)

Insemination Procedure

The goal of insemination should be to deposit 500 million progressively motile sperm cells within the mare's reproductive tract within 48 - 72 hours before ovulation. Traditionally, mares are inseminated every other day beginning the second or third day of estrous until ovulation is detected or until the mare no longer exhibits behavioral signs of estrus. The introduction of the semen into the mare's reproductive tract cannot be a completely sterile procedure, but techniques can be utilized to minimize any contamination. Therefore, all equipment utilized in this technique should be as clean as possible and sterilized whenever practical. If possible, a sterile pathway from the exterior of the mare through the mare's vagina and into the cervix and uterus should be established for the introduction of the semen. This can be accomplished through the use of sterile plastic tubing, a sterile insemination pipette, and a sterile syringe with a plastic plunger.

The mare requiring insemination should be adequately restrained, in stocks if possible, and her tail wrapped and diverted either off to one side or up over her rump. The entire perineal area is then scrubbed and rinsed repeatedly until clean. All fecal contamination around the vulva should be removed. Rinsing should be thorough to eliminate any residual soap that is not only spermicidal but may possibly irritate the mare's genitalia.

The inseminator's arm that enters the mare's reproductive tract should be covered with a sterile lubricated sleeve and glove. The tip of the insemination pipette is usually covered in the gloved hand. Care should be taken when this hand

Artwork by S. Hakola / J. Dirig
Copyright Equistar Publications, Ltd.

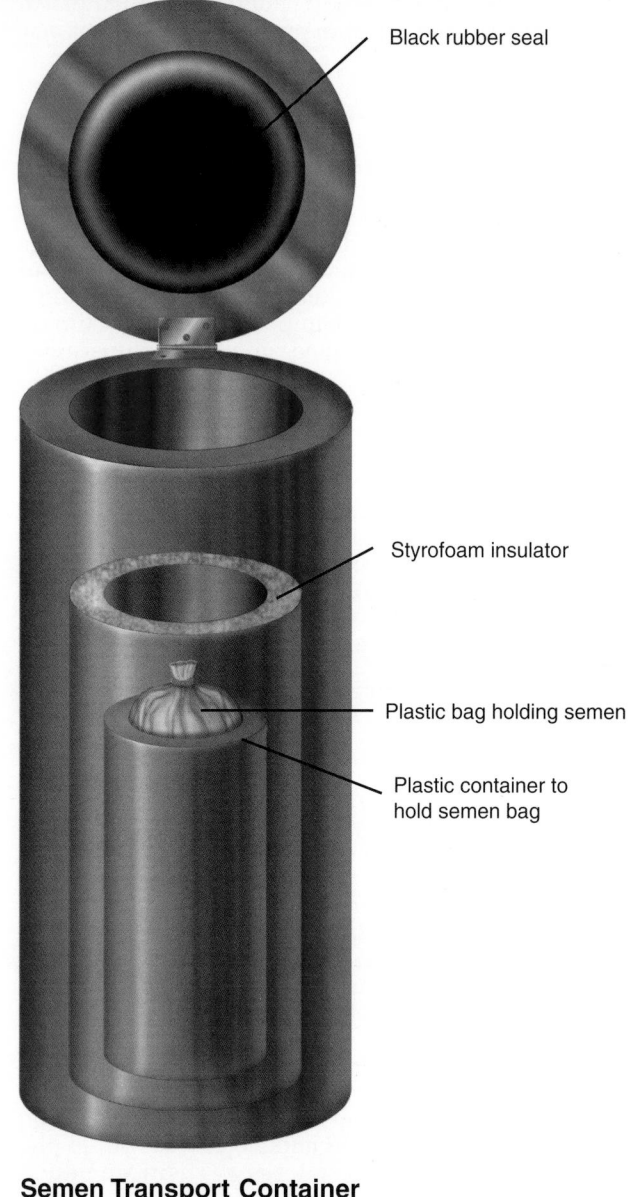

Black rubber seal

Styrofoam insulator

Plastic bag holding semen

Plastic container to
hold semen bag

**Semen Transport Container
With Transparent Schematic
Representation to Show
Interior Components**

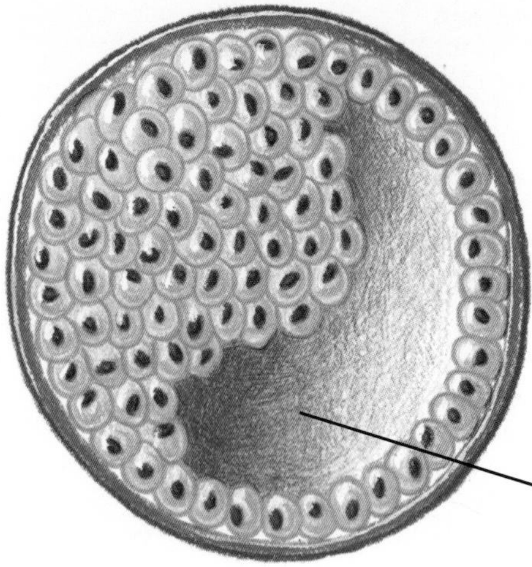

**Cross-Section of a
7 Day Old Blastocyst.**

Interior cavity

Embryo Transfer

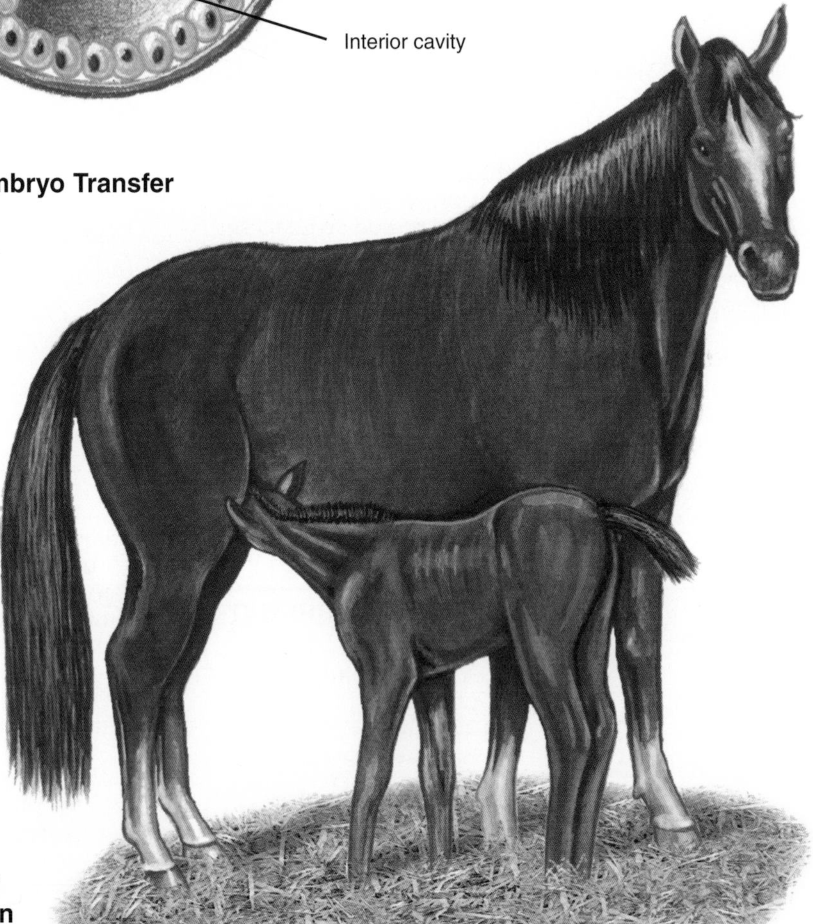

**Successful Embryo Transfer
Results in a Healthy Newborn
Foal Raised by a Surrogate Mare.**

is passed through the vulvar lips into the cranial vagina to avoid any contamination. The cervix is identified and penetrated with the index finger of the inseminator's hand. The insemination pipette is then advanced through the cervix to the uterine body where the semen is deposited. Semen should be injected slowly through the use of a syringe to avoid damage to the sperm. After the semen sample is deposited, the arm should be removed in a slow downward motion to prevent a sudden rush of air into the reproductive tract.

Preservation of Semen

Utilization of cooled, transported semen can achieve pregnancy rates equal to those obtained utilizing artificial insemination with fresh, extended semen. There are numerous advantages that can be obtained when one has the ability to transport stallion semen to the mares rather than having to transport the mares to the stallion. Economic advantages are obvious in that there is tremendous savings to the mare owners since they do not have to ship the mare, or the mare and her foal, and board her at the breeding facility. Health advantages are also obvious in that the mare, or the mare and her foal, can remain in her relatively stress-free home and not be exposed to the potential disease-causing organisms that occur when animals are transported to a central location from numerous geographical points. There is also an advantage to the stallion owner in that the stallion can be utilized between shows or performance events since a mare's estrous cycle can be manipulated and synchronized to coincide with the arrival of transported semen.

Insemination techniques for cooled, extended semen are the same as those for fresh, extended semen. It is not necessary to warm the cooled semen before insemination. However a small sample of the cooled extended semen should be placed on a warmed 37 degree Celcius microscope slide to evaluate spermatozoa motility following storage.

Communication between the veterinarian and other personnel involved with the reproductive management of both the mare and stallion is

essential when utilizing cool transported semen for breeding. Insemination timing is critical; therefore, an accurate prediction of ovulation is essential. The semen must be collected, packaged, and shipped. Time must be allotted for seminal transportation so that it arrives at the optimum time for breeding. Insemination of the cooled transported semen should be made within 24 hours of ovulation.

The use of cool transported semen has been made possible through the development of the Equitainer (TM) system. The unique design of this shipment container allows extended semen to be cooled slowly to 4 - 8 degrees Celsius. This container allows this temperature to be maintained for up to 72 hours while the semen is being transported to its destination for insemination. When semen from fertile stallions is processed and handled correctly, it can be transported and stored within this system and achieve the same pregnancy rates as that which are achieved utilizing artificial insemination with fresh extended semen.

Utilization of frozen semen within the equine industry is becoming more popular. Unfortunately, there is a huge variation among individual stallions in post-thaw spermatozoal viability. This lowered viability can be seen with pregnancy rates for frozen/thawed semen ranging anywhere from 6 to 70%. Consistent methods for freezing and thawing equine semen have yet to be determined because there is such an individual variation not only between stallions, but also between ejaculations of the same stallion.

EMBRYO TRANSFER

Embryo transfer is simply the process of removing a fertilized seven day ovum from a donor mare and introducing it into a recipient mare's uterus utilizing nonsurgical or surgical techniques. This assisted-reproductive technique is advantageous in that it obtains foals from older problem mares. Embryo transfer allows an increased number of foals from genetically superior mares. It also allows one to obtain offspring from mares that

would foal late in the season or even two year old mares that are in training. Donor mares have to meet certain criteria before they should be considered for an embryo transfer program. Since this is an assisted-reproductive technique, the ultimate value of the donor mare's offspring should be the primary consideration involved in the decision to perform an embryo transfer from this mare. Donor mares should have a normal reproductive cycle, be free of any uterine infection or endometritis, and be free of any evidence of adhesions, tears, or other physical injuries to the reproductive tract. Mares that have any evidence of endometritis are treated and usually allowed to cycle twice before any embryos are recovered.

Selection of recipient mares will usually determine the success of any equine embryo transfer program. These mares should be in good body condition, have an age of 3 - 10 years, and have a reproductive history of producing foals. These recipient mares should also be subjected to a thorough reproductive exam that identifies any evidence of physical injuries. In addition, uterine cultures and biopsies should be obtained to insure that this animal is free of any evidence of infection.

Embryo transfer can only be successful if both the donor and recipient mare have synchronized estrous cycles. Ideally the stallion, the donor mare, and recipient should all be at the same facility so that the donor mare's estrous cycle and recipient mare's cycle can be monitored and synchronized as closely as possible. In most instances, it is advantageous to synchronize two recipients for each donor mare. Since the time of ovulation is so variable in the equine, even though the recipient's and donor's estrous cycle have started on the same day, the odds are better with two recipients that one will ovulate on the same day as the donor.

Synchronization of the donor and recipient estrous cycles can be accomplished in several ways. The easiest program to follow is to provide increased artificial daylight early in the breeding season to both the donor and recipient. After 60 days of increased artificial light, both recipient and donor receive 2.2 milligrams of Altrenogest per hundred pounds of body weight orally for 15 days. When the Altrenogest is withdrawn, both the mare and

Embryo Transfer

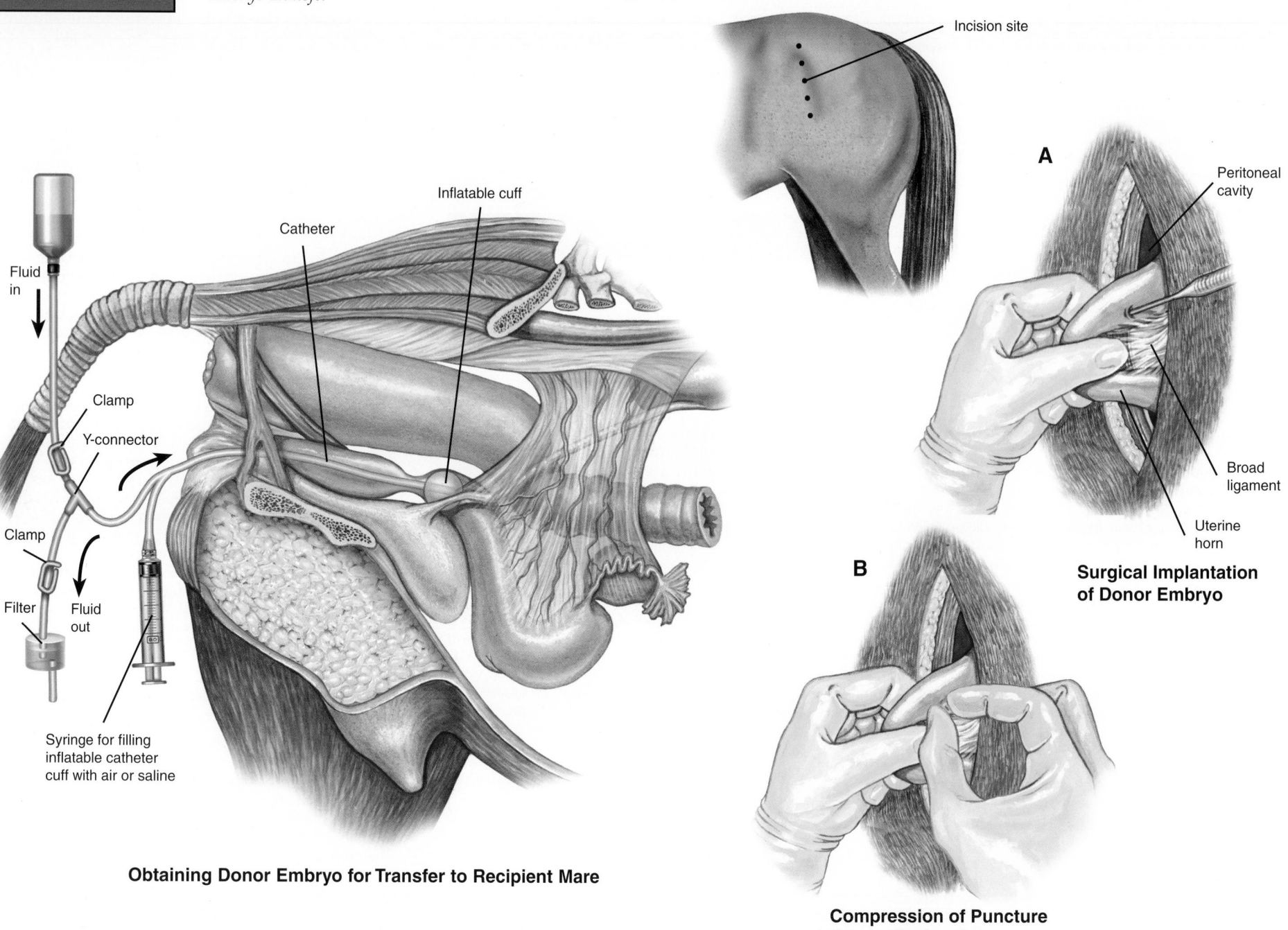

Incision site

Inflatable cuff

Catheter

Peritoneal cavity

A

Fluid in

Clamp

Y-connector

Clamp

Filter

Fluid out

Syringe for filling inflatable catheter cuff with air or saline

Broad ligament

Uterine horn

Surgical Implantation of Donor Embryo

B

Obtaining Donor Embryo for Transfer to Recipient Mare

Compression of Puncture Site in Uterine Horn

recipient should have synchronized estrous cycles. Prostaglandins can be administered twice, 14 days apart, with an injection given to the recipient mare one day after injection given to the donor mare as another means of synchronization. This product will induce luteolysis when a mature corpus luteum is present and results in a synchronized estrous cycle. There are also injectable progesterone pharmaceuticals available that can be systemically administered that will replace Altrenogest for the synchronization of the cycles. Ideally, the goal of this estrous synchronization is to have the recipient mare ovulate on the same day or within 24 hours of the donor mare.

Since the synchronization of ovulation is generally difficult to control between the donor and the recipient, it is possible to use ovariectomized mares as recipients. These mares are given 300 mg of progesterone IM daily for 5 days before the embryo transfer. The progesterone treatment in the ovariectomized mares should correspond to the day of donor ovulation. Recipient mares that remain pregnant after the embryo transfer are continued on progesterone treatment until day 150 of the pregnancy.

A nonsurgical transcervical recovery procedure is used to obtain the 7 day equine embryo from the uterine lumen of the donor mare. This mare is usually placed in stocks with her tail wrapped and pulled out of the way. Her genital area and buttocks are prepped with a dilute iodine scrub as if surgery would be performed. The technician will wear a sterile surgical glove over a palpation sleeve and introduce a French Foley catheter into the vagina and through the cervix approximately 4 - 5 centimeters into the uterine body. A cuff on the Foley catheter is then inflated with either air or sterile saline and drawn back against the internal opening of the cervix to ensure a seal.

Flushing is done through gravity flow using approximately 3 liters of prewarmed modified Dulbecco's phosphate-buffered saline solution combined with 1% fetal calf serum. The uterus is filled with these fluids and allowed to infuse by gravity into both the right and left uterine horns. The inlet tubing is then clamped, and the outlet tubing is connected to a specially designed embryo

filter positioned above the collection cylinder. The clamp is opened and the fluid is again allowed, through gravity flow, to drain out of the uterus, passing through the filter and into the collection cylinder. It is important to collect nearly all of the infusion media from the uterus. This fluid should be examined carefully to make sure that it is free of cellular debris or blood. After the medium is recovered, the cuff on the Foley catheter is deflated, and the catheter is withdrawn from the uterus. The medium is then searched through the use of a microscope to recover the seven day embryo. Once located, the embryo is then rinsed from one dish to another through fresh medium comprised of Dulbecco's phophate-buffered saline plus 10% fetal calf serum. This will dilute any possible contamination and keep the embryo in a viable environment. Ideally, the embryo should be transferred to the recipient as soon as possible, but the embryo can be maintained in a culture dish at room temperature for up to an hour after recovery.

Storage of fresh embryos for 24 hours has been accomplished without loss of quality. A solution known as Ham's F10 medium is used. The embryos are suspended in this solution during the cooling process down to 5 degrees centigrade. Pregnancy rates using this technique have proven to be the same as that rate obtained through immediate transfer.

Actual transfer of the embryo to the recipient can be accomplished by one of two methods: surgical or nonsurgical. The nonsurgical technique involves the embryo loaded into an insemination pipette or frozen semen straw which is then introduced transcervically into the uterine body. Care must be taken to gently dilate the cervical lumen of the recipient mare when this embryo is introduced. It is important to gently handle the embryo as well as the uterine tissue to guard against trauma to the uterine lumen and agitation of the embryo.

Surgical transfer of the embryo is done through a flank incision using a local block and a systemic tranquilizer for sedation. The flank of the recipient is surgically clipped and scrubbed from the last rib to the tuber coxae and from the transverse process of the lumbar vertebrae approximately 40

centimeters ventrally. A 15 - 20 centimeter vertical skin incision is made over a local line block of anesthetic beginning approximately 10 centimeters beneath the transverse process of the lumbar vertebrae. This incision should be made on the same side of the uterus where ovulation has occurred. A hand is introduced into the peritoneal cavity, and the uterine horn is located and then exteriorized. Using the blunt end of a large cutting needle, the uterine wall is punctured in an avascular location. The embryo is introduced through this puncture into the uterine lumen. The puncture site is then compressed for approximately 1 minute. The uterine horn is replaced in the peritoneal cavity. Closure of the incision is routine and systemic antibiotics are administered for at least 7 days.

Recipient mares are examined in 15 days for the pregnancy utilizing ultrasonography. Pregnancy examinations are again conducted at 25 days, 35 days, 60 days, and 90 days. At this point, the mare is returned to the farm for the completion of her gestation.

Collection and transfer of equine embryos has become a routine assisted-reproductive technique. A 65% pregnancy rate is considered normal after surgical embryo transfer. Expanded use of embryo transfer in the equine will depend somewhat on breed registry, regulations, and new technological advances. Cryopreservation of equine embryos has met with very little success. Different mediums and techniques are currently being explored since this would allow frozen embryos to be transported long distances and even internationally. Transportation of cooled embryos is possible through the use of the Equitainer (TM) system utilizing Ham's F10 medium and 10% fetal calf serum. This way, it is not always necessary to have the recipient at the same geographical location as the donor. Within the next few years, technological progress will be made in both embryo collection and in vivo and in vitro fertilization techniques.

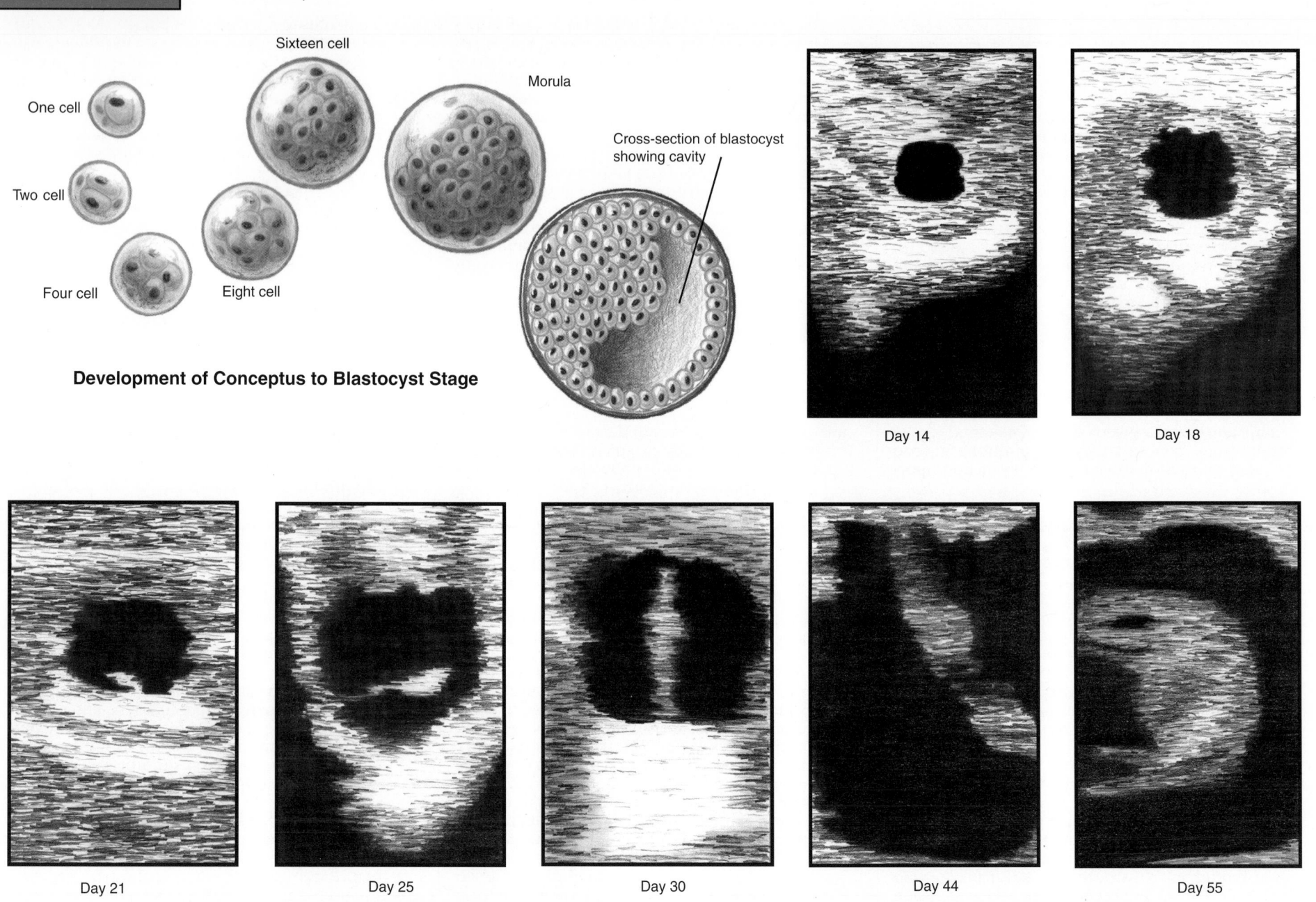

Artwork by S. Hakola
Copyright Equistar Publications, Ltd.

One cell

Two cell

Four cell

Sixteen cell

Eight cell

Morula

Cross-section of blastocyst showing cavity

Development of Conceptus to Blastocyst Stage

Day 14

Day 18

Day 21

Day 25

Day 30

Day 44

Day 55

Monitoring Early Fetal Development Utilizing Ultrasound Exams

CONCEPTION AND FETAL DEVELOPMENT

Fertilization of the equine ovum occurs at the ampullary and isthmus junction of the oviduct and is the culmination of months of planning and preparation during the first part of the equine reproductive year. If a viable oocyte and spermatozoa culminate in fertilization, the first phase of breeding management ends. The focus of attention is now spent on the care of the pregnant mare and the foal's various stages of development. When this fertilization occurs, the 32 chromosomes from the mare pair up with the 32 chromosomes from the stallion. At this point, the foal's inherited characteristics and genetic potential are determined.

The fertilized ovum is then transported down through the lumen of the oviduct and into the uterine lumen at approximately 5 - 6 days postovulation. If fertilization occurs on day zero, the initial cleavage of the cells occurs approximately every 24 hours. Therefore, the initial cell that occurred from the combination of the ovum and sperm divides into two cells, then four cells, then eight cells at approximately two days postovulation. Division of the embryo from eight to sixteen cells occurs on the third postovulation day. The thirty-two to sixty-four cell embryo, which is classified as a morula, occurs from day four through day six of development. When utilizing embryo transfer on day six or day seven postfertilization, a late morula or early blastocyst is what is usually recovered. This blastocyst is recognized as an embryo with a cavity or fluid-filled area within its structure. Embryos at day seven to eight postovulation are visible to the naked eye.

Between 12 - 16 days postovulation, the conceptus is extremely mobile within the uterine lumen. This movement occurs between the uterine horns and the uterine body. It is also during this time that the conceptus prevents the release of or inhibits the function of prostaglandins. Prostaglandins normally cause luteolysis of the corpus luteum, which would return the mare to estrus, which would in turn terminate the pregnancy.

Ultrasonographic examination of the uterus can be accomplished on days 12 - 15 postovulation. This early examination can detect the presence of twins at a very early stage which can then be monitored for future management. It is not unusual to find a transuterine migration of the embryo up until day seventeen. At that time, migration has usually ceased. Care must be taken when ultrasonically scanning these early vesicles. Scanning must be done slowly and systematically to avoid missing a portion of the reproductive tract. It should also be treated very gently to prevent trauma or agitation of the embryo. At day twelve to seventeen postovulation, the ultrasonographic image is going to be a very small, almost perfectly round vesicle.

By the seventeenth day postovulation, the embryonic vesicle has stopped moving within the uterine lumen and appears irregular in shape on the ultrasound scan. This embryonic vesicle usually becomes fixated on the caudal portion of the uterine horn near the bifurcation. The uterine wall begins to thicken, and when palpated, there is an increase in uterine tone. This can account for the irregularity of the vesicle on the ultrasound scan. At approximately day sixteen to seventeen postovulation, tiny blood vessels begin to develop within the embryo. These are very difficult to see on the ultrasound scan.

The embryo itself can usually be visualized ultrasonographically within the vesicle at approximately day twenty to twenty-five. Due to the thickening of the uterine wall and the massaging action of the uterine contractions, the vesicle rotates upon implantation. The embryo can be visualized in the most ventral position. The viability of this embryo can be determined around this time as this is when the heartbeat can usually be detected.

By day twenty-five, the yoke sac contracts and the allantois expands. This allantoic sac is vascularized and quite large compared to the embryo. Ultrasonography will reveal this developing allantois and the regression of the yoke sac. At approximately thirty days, the ultrasonic image will reveal the fetus in apposition of the yoke sac and allantois, which results in an image that appears as a vertical line.

At approximately day forty, the yoke sac has deteriorated, and the fetus has gravitated to the ventral floor. Usually the umbilical cord can be visualized as it elongates from the dorsal pole. The fetus assumes a position of dorsal recumbency from day fifty onward.

By day fifty-five of the pregnancy, the equine fetus has several unique characteristics. The hocks and fetlocks are evident on the legs of the fetus. There is no evidence of hair anywhere on the fetus, but reproductive organs such as the vulva and the penis can be visualized. The head depicts a prominent cranium, and the eyelids are closed except for a small slit indicating where they would part.

By day sixty of the equine pregnancy, the fetus now has a conformational characteristic that is unmistakably equine in nature. The soles of the feet are evident, and even the frogs can be visualized. If the uterus would be dissected at this stage, a ring of endometrial cups would be seen. There is still a remnant of the yoke sac in the amniotic cavity enclosing the umbilical cord for a considerable distance.

By day eighty, the pregnancy fills both uterine horns. The fetus has a head and neck that are in normal position. The points of the shoulders and hips can now be visualized. At approximately the one hundredth day of pregnancy, the first hair will appear on the lips, chin, muzzle, and eyelids of the fetus. The fetus will be approximately 25 - 28 centimeters in length and will weigh approximately 70 grams. It will be easy at this stage to start recognizing some of the muscle groups, and the coronary band on the hoof will be evident. On the cranium, the ears will be approximately one centimeter long and will probably curl forward and down. The fetus' eyes will appear to be slightly bulged.

At approximately 150 - 160 days, the ears will appear very developed. Eyelashes will appear around the eyes. Ergots of approximately five millimeters in size will appear on the legs.

THE MARE

Fetal Development; Twins; Early Embryonic Death

Stages of Fetal Development

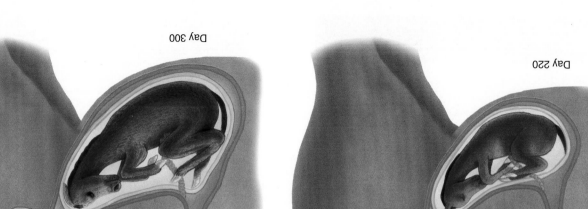
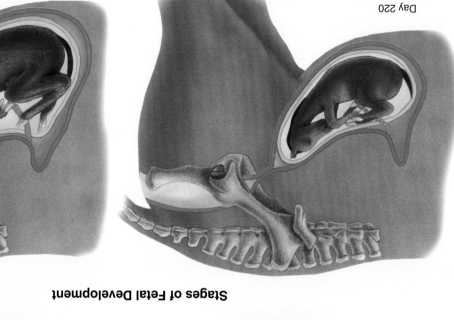
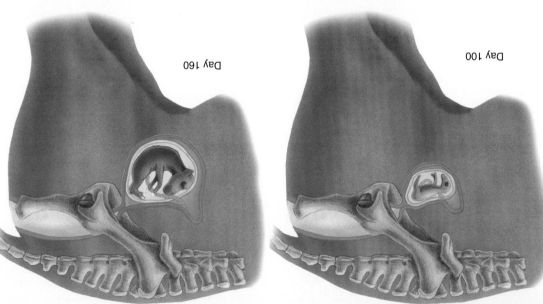

Day 100

Day 160

Day 220

Day 300

Twinning and Early Embryonic Death

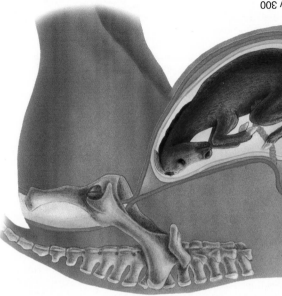

12 day old twins prior to splitting

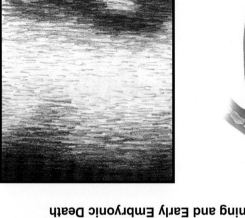

Twin conceptus after splitting

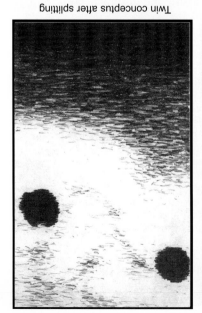

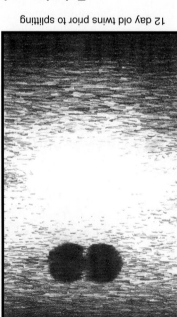

Early embryonic death as shown on ultrasound

At approximately 220 days from conception, the fetus will be between 55 - 60 centimeters in length and will weigh close to nine kilograms. Mammary glands can be noted on the females at this time. At this developmental stage, the most unique characteristic will be the development of mane and tail hair.

When the fetus is approximately 270 - 280 days into the pregnancy, it will be approximately 80 - 90 centimeters in length from head to tail and weigh between 18 - 20 kilograms. The entire body will be covered with fine hair, and the tail will actually appear as a switch. By day 300 the fetus will have a full hair coat. The average pregnancy in the equine is approximately 340 days gestation with 14 to 20 days above or below considered normal. At this time, the fetus will be approximately 90 - 100 centimeters in length from head to tail and weigh between 42 and 50 kilograms. The developmental phases of the fetus are considered complete. The fetus is now mature and the pregnancy is terminated by birth or parturition.

TWINNING

The equine species appears to be the only mammal that cannot successfully maintain two pregnancies at the same time. The reason being is there is simply not enough room for two different placentas. After a certain stage, there will be a competition between the placentas which results in either weaker and less desirable foals or abortion.

The second leading cause of abortion in mares is twin pregnancies. In almost every case, a mare that carries a twin pregnancy to term will require assistance with the birthing process. The resulting foals are usually weak, more susceptible to infections, and develop very slowly. When an abortion occurs in a mare during the late stages of pregnancy, the mare usually retains her fetal membranes. She will probably be very difficult to get to recycle. Therefore, there is a great reduction in the reproductive efficiency of this particular mare.

Twinning within a species occurs either by the division of a fertilized ovum or by multiple ovulations with multiple ovum becoming fertilized, the latter being the most common. Close monitoring of ovulation and timed breeding can prevent a good percentage of twinning which is most undesirable. When a twin conception occurs, there are two treatments available to manage these twin pregnancies. Early detection through ultrasonography is key to identifying the twin pregnancy between twelve and sixteen days postovulation. At this point, the smaller of the two vesicles can be manipulated to the tip of the uterine horn and crushed manually. After day seventeen when the vesicle becomes fixed within the uterine wall, a systemic administration of prostaglandins should terminate the pregnancy, recycle the mare, and allow rebreeding. The prostaglandins should not be administered after day forty since the endometrial cups have begun to form and efficacy in the termination of the pregnancy is not as high. In these extreme cases, when it is desirable to terminate these later pregnancies, an infusion of saline solution into the uterus should be considered.

Early detection using ultrasonography of the twin pregnancies is the key to its proper management. Even after one of the twins has been eliminated, it is important that the pregnancy be monitored every few days to ensure that the single fetus is still developing. After the administration of the prostaglandins, it is also important to monitor the result of this treatment through the use of an ultrasonic reproductive examination.

EARLY EMBRYONIC DEATH "EED"

Early embryonic death in the mare is regarded as the loss of viability to the embryo before forty days of gestation has passed. Through the use of ultrasonography, repeated reproductive exams can easily diagnose this condition. There are embryonic, maternal, and intentional causes which can result in this early pregnancy loss.

Early embryonic loss is easily diagnosed using ultrasonography. An ultrasound exam will reveal an abnormal appearance to the vesicle, a continued mobility of the vesicle, fluid surrounding the vesicle, an absence of a heartbeat within the vesicle, and disruption of the conceptus membranes. All of these signs indicate an impending early embryonic death. One of the first signs that can be noted on the ultrasound exam is a granular appearance of the conceptus and then a decrease in size coupled with a loss of definition of the vesicle. At this point the vesicle collapses, and the contents can be visualized via ultrasonography within the uterine lumen. Manual palpation will reveal a loss of uterine tone. A palpable bulge in the uterus can be present for up to one week after the embryonic death.

The cause of early embryonic death may be as simple as a chromosomal abnormality within the embryo leading to the loss of pregnancy. Certain family lines and stallions may have a higher incidence than others of early embryonic death due to genetic abnormalities.

A form of prostaglandin, designated E2, has been theorized to be secreted by the equine embryo and is responsible for transport of the embryo through the oviduct. If the embryo is unable to produce a sufficient quantity of E2 prostaglandin, transportation through the oviduct may not be possible; therefore, pregnancy may not be established.

The movement of the embryo throughout the uterine lumen is essential for the prevention of luteolysis. If the embryo fails to move throughout the uterus and inhibit luteolysis, early embryonic death will result. This is due to interaction between the mare's uterus and the embryo mechanisms itself. Without the inhibition of luteolysis, the embryo never becomes fixated; therefore, the pregnancy fails.

There are numerous factors originating from the mare that can result in early embryonic death: such as insufficient levels of progesterone, prostaglandin release, endometritis, other pathological agents such as venereal disease, and

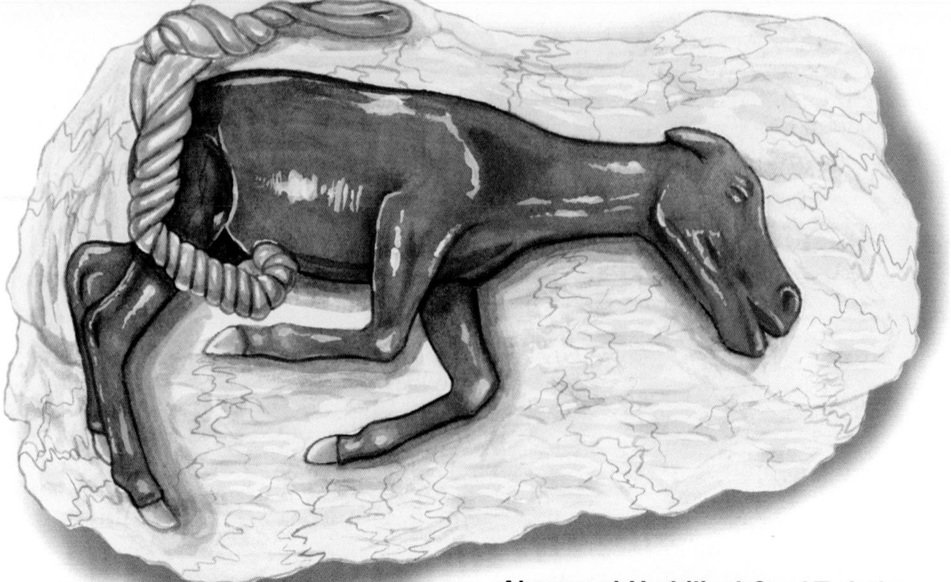

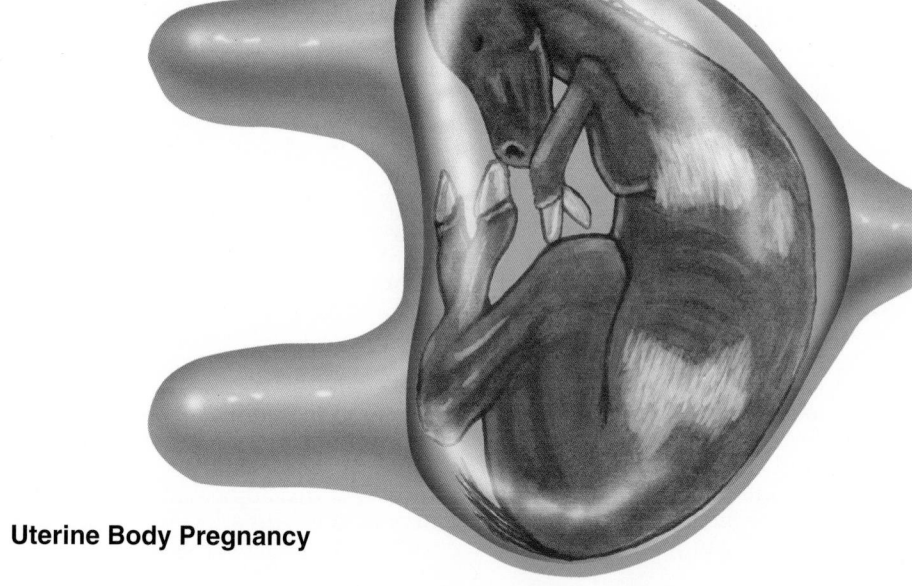

Abnormal Umbilical Cord Twisting

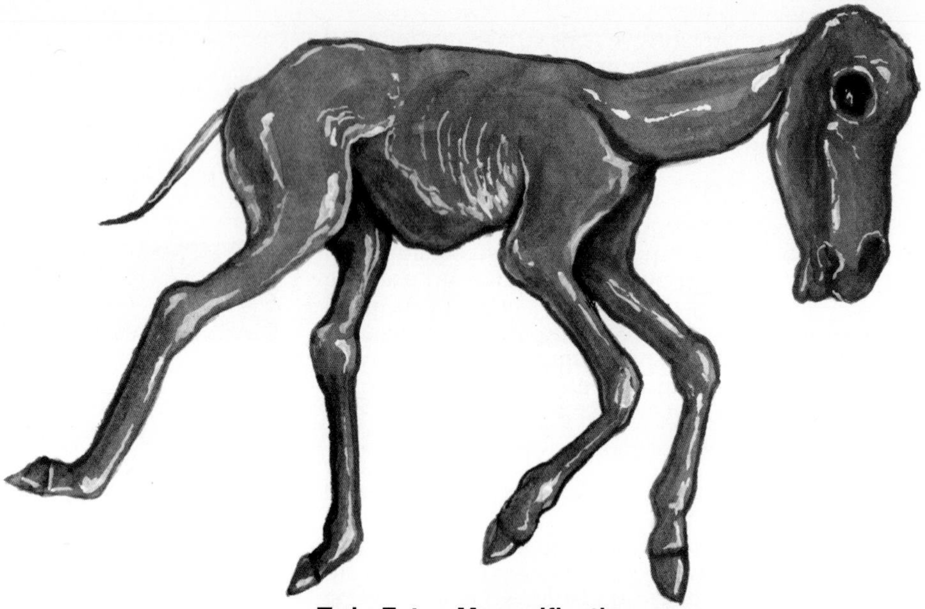

Twin Fetus Mummification

Uterine Body Pregnancy

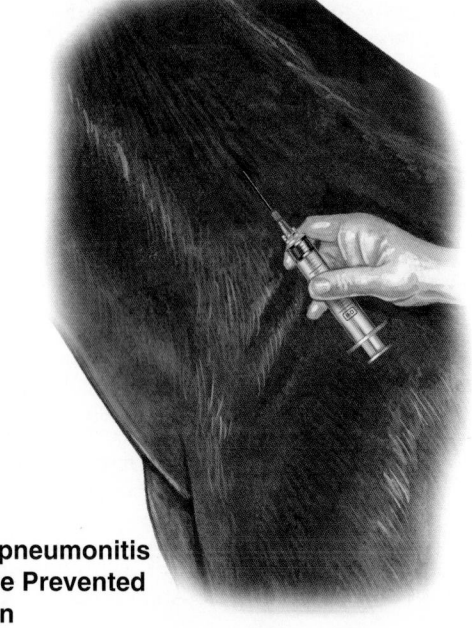

Equine Rhinopneumonitis Virus-1 Can Be Prevented By Vaccination

physical causes such as oviductal pathology. Prevention or treatment of early embryonic death revolves around diagnosis and treatment of endometritis prior to breeding and the administration of progesterone orally to help ensure the maintenance of the pregnancy.

Proper diagnosis and treatment of endometritis will allow a pregnancy to be established without the complications of early embryonic death. If a premature release of prostaglandins is thought to be the attributable factor in the very early stages of implantation, successful treatment has been accomplished through the use of flunixin-

meglumine systemically. The exogenous administration of a daily dose of 100 mg of progesterone in oil or 22 mg of altrenogest will help maintain the pregnancy. This should be continued for the first four months of gestation until the placenta can provide adequate progesterone for pregnancy support.

The normal gestation length for the mare is approximately 340 days and by definition, abortion means termination of this pregnancy before 300 - 320 days of gestation. There are a wide range of causes for abortion in the mare. In general, older mares have a higher incidence of abortion than do younger mares. Fetal loss after 300 - 320 days of gestation should be termed a still birth.

The causes of abortion can be noninfectious which include twinning, fetal trauma, abnormal umbilical cord twisting, and abnormalities within the reproductive tract such as a problem with the placenta or a body pregnancy. Infectious types of abortion include viral, bacterial, fungal, mycoplasmic, and protozoal agents.

COMMON CAUSES OF ABORTIONS IN MARES

Noninfectious causes of abortion:

CAUSE	ETIOLOGY	CLINICAL SIGNS	CHARACTERISTICS	DIAGNOSIS	PREVENTION
Twinning	Multiple ovulations, or division of a fertilized ovum, poorly timed breeding, placental insufficiency.	Abortion usually occurs between 8 - 11 months gestation.	Mummification of one of the twin fetuses; twin fetuses.	Twin fetuses usually including a mummy.	Early detection of the twin pregnancy using ultrasonography; termination of one of the embryos.
Uterine Body Pregnancy	The placenta fails to extend fully into the uterine horns.	Abortion can occur at any stage of the pregnancy but usually occurs at 8 - 11 months of gestation.	A visual examination of the expelled placenta depicts the portion that would project into the horns to be very small.	Visual exam of the placental membranes.	This noninfectious cause cannot be prevented.

Infectious causes of abortion:

Equine Rhino-pneumonitis Virus "EHV-1"	Equine herpes virus-1.	Initially depicts itself as a respiratory disease with abortion occuring 1 - 4 months after the respiratory outbreak. Can result in still births or weak foals.	Autopsy of the fetus usually reveals necrotic foci in the liver, a generalized mild icterus, pulmonary edema, and congestion.	Intranuclear inclusions found on histopathology. Viral isolation.	Vaccination will reduce the incidence. Isolation from the general population of all infected animals, especially from the brood mares.

Aspergillus Fungal Placental Infection

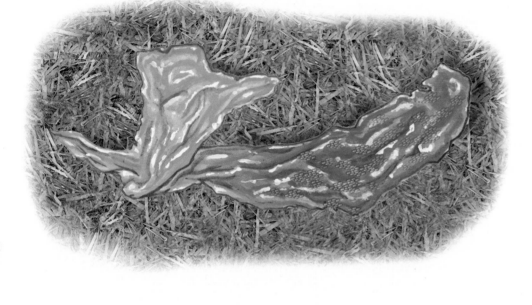

Leptospirosis
Moon Blindness

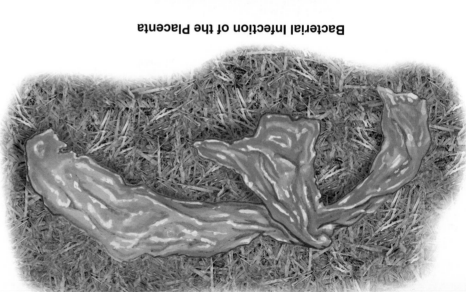

Leptospirosis Autolytic Fetus

Bacterial Infection of the Placenta

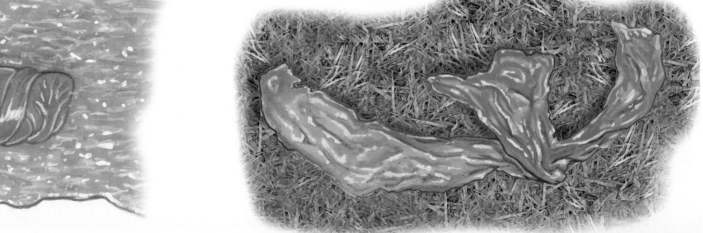

Infectious Causes of Abortions

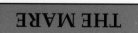

THE MARE

Infectious causes of abortion (Continued from page 104):

CAUSE	ETIOLOGY	CLINICAL SIGNS	CHARACTERISTICS	DIAGNOSIS	PREVENTION
Equine Virus Arteritis "EVA"	Togavirus	This is a rare systemic disease with abortion as a complication. Abortion occurs usually within two weeks after onset of the virus.	Both the fetus and the placenta are very necrotic.	Serology and viral isolation of fetal tissues.	Proper management of semen and vaccination with state or federal approval.
Equine Infectious Anemia	Retrovirus	Abortion occurs usually in the last half of the gestation period.	No specific placental or fetal lesions are present.	An AGID test 45 days later.	No vaccine or effective treatment is available.
Bacterial Abortion	E. coli, Pseudomonas spp., Klebsiella, Staphylococcus spp., Streptococcus spp., and Taylorella equigenitalis.	Abortion can occur at any stage of the pregnancy.	The fetus will be septic in appearance and the placenta will show placentitis and areas of necrosis.	Cultures from the placenta or fetus.	Complete treatment of endometritis before breeding; proper management of semen; sanitary techniques.
Lepto-spirosis	Leptospira interrogans-serotypes: canicola, pomona, autumnalis.	Moon blindness - periodic opthalmia abortion usually occurs in the last half of gestation.	The fetus is necrotic and autolytic.	Culture of lepto-spira; dark field or phase contrast microscopy; paired serum samples.	Vaccination within endemic areas.
Equine Mycotic Abortion	Aspergillus fumigatus, Allescheria boydii.	Abortion usually occurs between 5 - 11 months of gestation.	Placentitis, small fetuses that may contain lesions within the lungs.	Culture of the lungs, placenta, and liver; fungal organisms found within the placenta or fetal stomach contents.	Sanitation and proper diagnosis; treatment of the uterus before breeding.
Protozoal Abortion	Badesia caballi or equi	Mares are usually jaundiced and stressed.	The fetus usually appears icteric and has excessive fluid in the pleural cavity.	CS test of the sera.	There is no effective treatment.

Abortions

Artwork by S. Hakola / J. Dirig
Copyright Equistar Publications, Ltd.

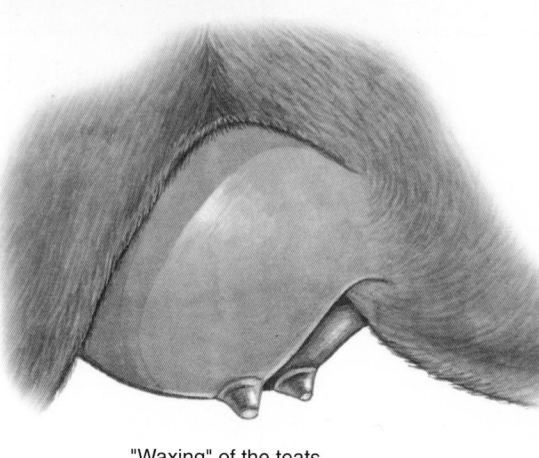

"Waxing" of the teats

Signs of Impending Delivery

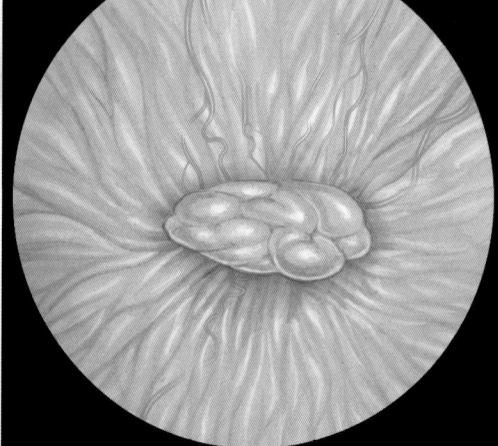

Softening of the cervix

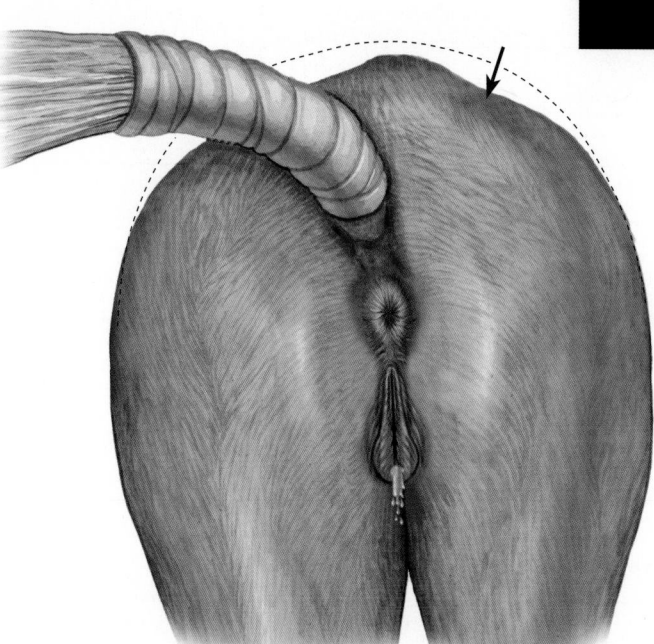

Relaxation of the sacrosciatic
ligaments and vaginal discharge.

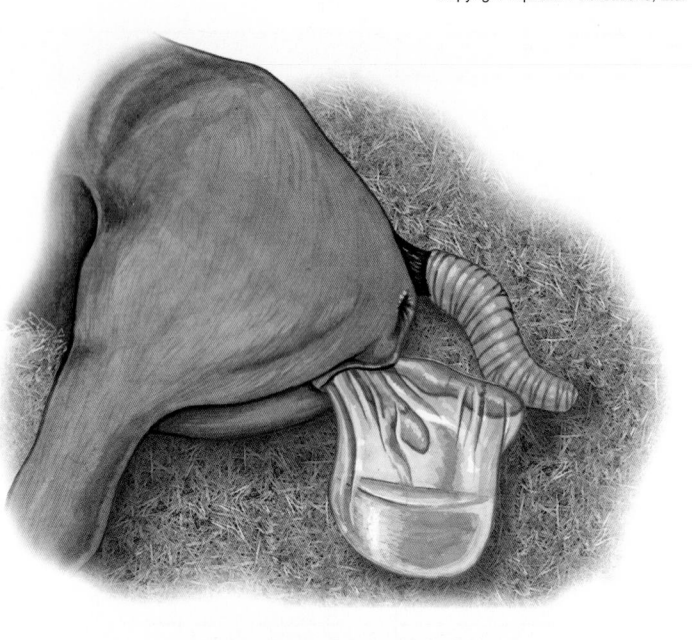

Progression of Parturition

PARTURITION

After the fetus has fully developed and reached maturity, parturition occurs which terminates the pregnancy. Parturition is synonymous with birth, and literally translated, the word parturition means "a bringing forth". The exact mechanisms which initiate birth or the birthing process are not clearly understood. It is a combination of the preparation of the foal for independent life, the mare for labor, the hormonal exchange between the mother and the foal, and the changes in the uterine tissue itself which activates the uterine musculature to initiate labor.

During the time of the last month of pregnancy, before foaling, the mare should be examined on a regular basis for clinical signs of the physiological changes that indicate the nearness of delivery. These changes include an increase in udder size and secretion, relaxation of the sacrosciatic ligaments, a development of vulvar laxity and edema, slight discharges from the vulva, and a softening of the cervix.

The most obvious physical indicator of impending birth is increase in udder size and secretion. During the last month of gestation, the mare's mammary glands will grow and become distended. Several days before foaling, the udder will become engorged with a mammary secretion termed colostrum. The term "waxing of the teats" is the accumulation of a waxy secretion on the teat ends from early colostrum formation. This usually occurs 24 - 96 hours before foaling. However, it is not unusual to see mares wax two weeks before parturition. If this precious colostrum should start to leak from the teats several days before foaling, it should be collected without stimulation to the mare for oral administration to the foal. In severe cases of leakage, it is possible to seal the ends of the teats with a latex teat dip that is used in cattle.

Even though the delivery of the foal is a continuous process, it can be divided into three different stages. The first stage is a preparatory stage. The second stage of parturition occurs after cervical dilation is complete and ends with the delivery of the foal. The third stage of parturition involves the passage of the placental membranes.

First Stage of Parturition

The initial onset of the first stage of parturition is difficult to determine. The mare may appear to have a mild bout of colic. This is caused by an increased level of uterine contraction and the rotation of the foal from a dorsopubic or dorsoilial to a dorsosacral position. The mare may appear restless, pace the stall, frequently get up and down, or merely just turn around and stare at her flanks. The mare may have patchy areas of sweating behind the ears, behind the elbows, along the neck, and even in the flanks. Other physical behavioral signs that can occur during this stage may include pawing, yawning, curling her lip, swishing her tail, biting her sides, or merely shifting her weight repeatedly from one hind leg to the other. All of these physical signs can occur as early as 4 - 8 hours before the actual birth of the foal. During this first stage of labor, the mare's tail should be wrapped, the vulva should be washed, and every effort should be made to attend to the comfort and privacy of the mare. Usually there is a level of excitement in the stable as the foaling time approaches. It is absolutely essential that everyone remain quiet and not disturb the mare in any fashion. The end result of the first stage of parturition is the dilation of the cervix and the passage of the chorioallantoic membrane through the cervix until her membrane ruptures.

Second Stage of Parturition

Rupture of the chorioallantoic membrane allows the release of the allantoic fluids through the vulva which has been given the common term "breaking water." This initiates the second stage of labor. The uterine contractions facilitate the movement of the fetus into the birth canal. This passage into the birth canal stimulates abdominal contractions which work in combination with existing uterine contractions in order to expel the foal. At this point the mare will usually lay on her side and periodically strain forcefully in active labor. Usually within a short period of time,

visualization can be made of the amniotic membrane (white glistening membrane surrounding the fetus) between the vulvar lips.

The first sign of the foal should be one forefoot with the soles of the hooves directed downward. Within one or two contractions, the second forefoot and possibly the nose of the foal should be noticed. At this point it is not uncommon for mares to stand and lie down repeatedly. When the foal,s head and shoulders are in the pelvic cavity, the most forceful contractions of labor usually occur. It is at this time that the amniotic membrane usually ruptures. Assistance should be offered only if it is absolutely necessary. Gentle traction on the foal's forelimbs in synchrony with the mare's uterine and abdominal contractions may facilitate the delivery. This stage of labor is usually completed in less than ten minutes, but it is not unusual for a mare to take 20 - 30 minutes to expel the foal. The only intervention that the foaling manager should render is a gentle traction in synchrony with the mare's contraction, breaking of the amniotic sac so the foal can breath, and clearing the fluid from the foal's nose. All managerial type procedures should be done as quietly and as carefully as possible so as not to disturb either the mare or the newborn foal.

After the foal's hips have exited the pelvis, the mare will usually rest for 15 or 20 minutes. Care must be taken not to disturb the mare and the foal because sudden movements may break the umbilical cord prematurely. It is important to allow the umbilical cord to be connected for at least several minutes following delivery to allow the completion of blood flow from the placenta to the foal's circulatory system. Under normal circumstances with the mare undisturbed, the umbilical cord will separate naturally when the mare stands or when the foal struggles in its first attempt to rise. The umbilical stump should be inspected for hemorrhage and disinfected with an appropriate chlorahexdine or iodine solution.

Artwork by S. Hakola / J. Dirig
Copyright Equistar Publications, Ltd.

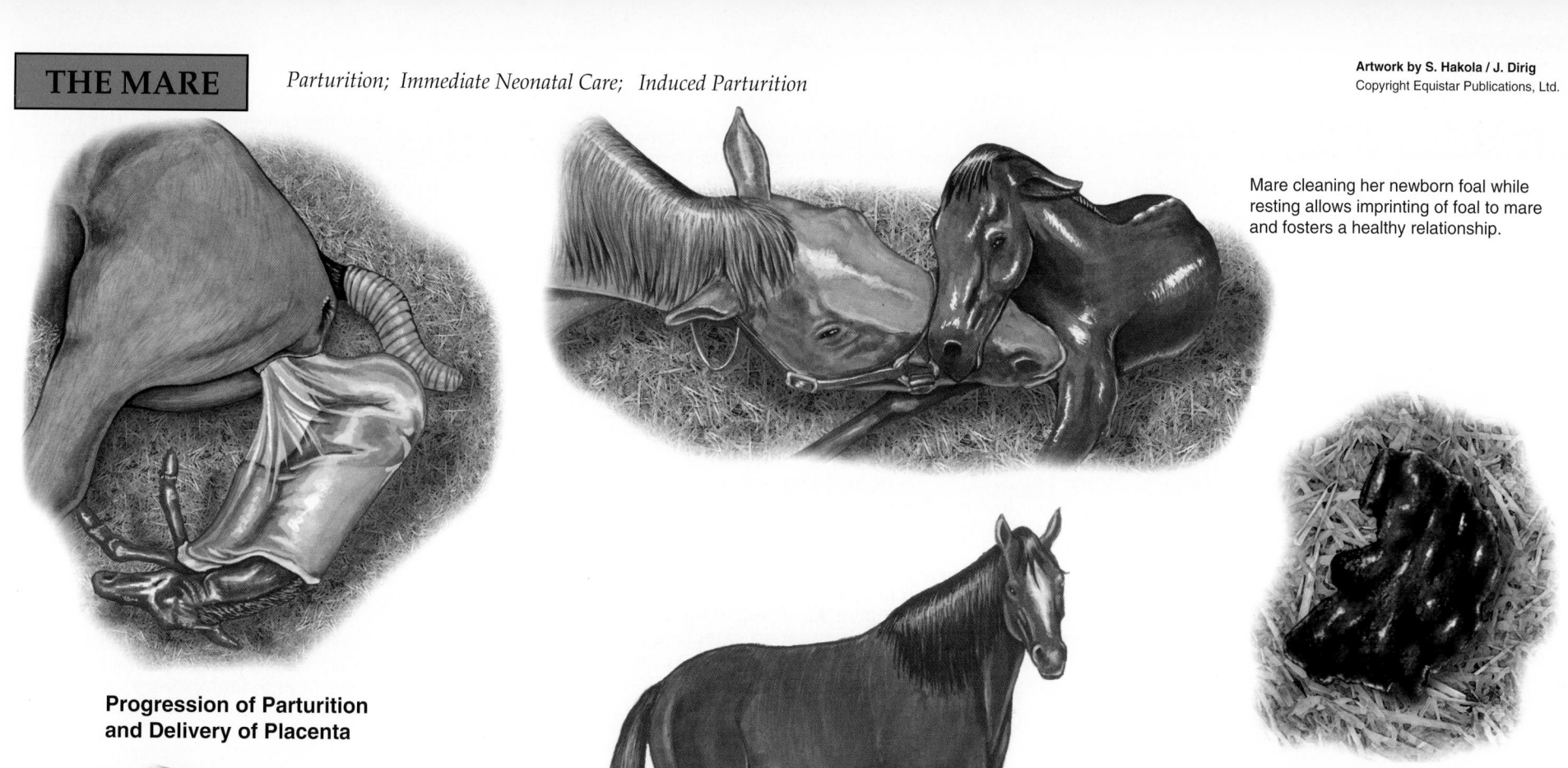

Mare cleaning her newborn foal while resting allows imprinting of foal to mare and fosters a healthy relationship.

Progression of Parturition and Delivery of Placenta

Foal's first meconium

Induction of Parturition Using IV of Oxytocin.

Ingestion of colostrum is essential to the newborn foal.

Third Stage of Parturition

The third stage of parturition encompasses the expulsion of the placental membranes and uterine involution. Once the mare stands, the placenta will be protruding through the vulva. A knot should be placed in the membrane so that it extends no lower than the level of the hocks. This keeps the mare from stepping on the placenta and possibly prematurely tearing it into pieces. The uterus will continue to contract and the placenta will separate from the uterus. It is usually passed within thirty minutes to three hours after foaling. If it has not passed within that three hour period, treatment may be necessary to hasten its expulsion to avoid uterine trauma and possible infection.

While the placental membranes are being expelled, the foaling attendant can quietly check the mare's and foal's vital signs, provide fresh water and fresh hay in the stall, dry off the foal, and disinfect the navel. An enema can be administered with care being taken to be as gentle to the foal as possible.

Immediate Neonatal Care

There are several important observations that should be made in the next 1 - 2 hours after the birth has occurred. The foal should be observed to see that it is normal and not shivering as if cold. Shivering is a natural process for the foal in that it helps establish good circulation. However, there is a limit to the shivering. Common sense will dictate when it becomes excessive, and managerial procedures should come to its aid. Some foals will stand within 20 - 30 minutes after birth, whereas others may take up to 2 hours. Proper footing is essential. In some cases, assistance may be needed to get the foal on his feet. Within the first half hour a suck reflex should be noted with the foal.

Trying to assist a foal to nurse is sometimes the most frustrating event of the whole process. It is frustrating for the mare, the foal, and the attendant. The mare usually has a swollen udder which is very tender. The foal has to gain enough coordination with his nursing reflex and his legs in order to find the nipple and suck. The attendant realizes that without the transfer of colostrum from

the mare to the foal, the essential antibodies that it needs will not be transferred.

A foal cannot survive without the ingestion of colostrum. Antibodies in the colostrum are essential for the foal to fight off bacteria and viruses which cause infection. Most large breeding farms will have a bank of frozen colostrum available so that a mixture from several mares can be administered to the foal usually within an hour of birth. If no such bank exists, it is essential that within two hours of birth, the foal ingest colostrum. It is preferable to have the foaling attendant milk the mare and administer the colostrum orally than have the foal not nurse at all. This managerial step is especially useful when dealing with weaker foals. A normal foal will nurse every 20 - 40 minutes. It is not unusual for the foal to lie down and sleep immediately after nursing.

The last observation that the foaling attendant should make is the passing of the foal's meconium. This is the foal's almost black first manure. If at any time the foal exhibits physical signs that it is struggling to have a bowel movement (i.e.: straining, lying down, and getting up repeatedly), an enema should be administered.

The first twenty-four hours of life are critical. It is essential that both the mare and the foal be observed every 15 - 20 minutes. The foal should be nursing, urinating, and passing fecal material on a regular basis within 12 hours of life. The mare should be eating, drinking, and showing good maternal instincts during this time period. Again, observation does not translate to disturbing the mare and foal. Care should be take to observe their privacy throughout this time period.

INDUCED PARTURITION

Often a mare's owner or client will place pressure on their veterinarian to induce parturition to a mare that is overdue for foaling. The more overdue the mare becomes, the greater the anxiety and the pressure upon the veterinarian. Induction of parturition in the mare can be performed successfully through the use of oxytocin and prostaglandins. Mares should be selected very carefully for this procedure. Above all else, one must insure that the fetus has reached maturity. Communication with the mare's owner is of utmost importance while contemplating this procedure.

Mares that have a history of difficult births, uterine atony, premature placental separation, or any other physical process that may prevent a normal foaling should be considered for induced parturition. Gestation should be at least 335 - 340 days in length, and there should be some relaxation of the pelvic ligament and cervix. Hopefully, there is udder development and a good supply of colostrum apparent within the teats.

Oxytocin is the most frequently used drug for the induction of parturition in the mare. There are various techniques regarding its administration which are all acceptable in accomplishing the end result of the delivery of a foal. It is preferable to mimic the natural birthing process by the administration of oxytocin in low doses given intravenously over a long period of time. A solution can be run intravenously with a dosage rate of 2.5 to 5 IU dripping to the mare continuously. After the first twenty minutes, this dose should be increased or the drip rate increased by 2.5 IU every 20 minutes until the second stage of labor begins. Sometimes it is difficult to calculate how much oxytocin is actually being administered via intravenous methods; however, it should never be greater than 1 - 2 IU of oxytocin per minute.

Artwork by S. Hakola / J. Dirig
Copyright Equistar Publications, Ltd.

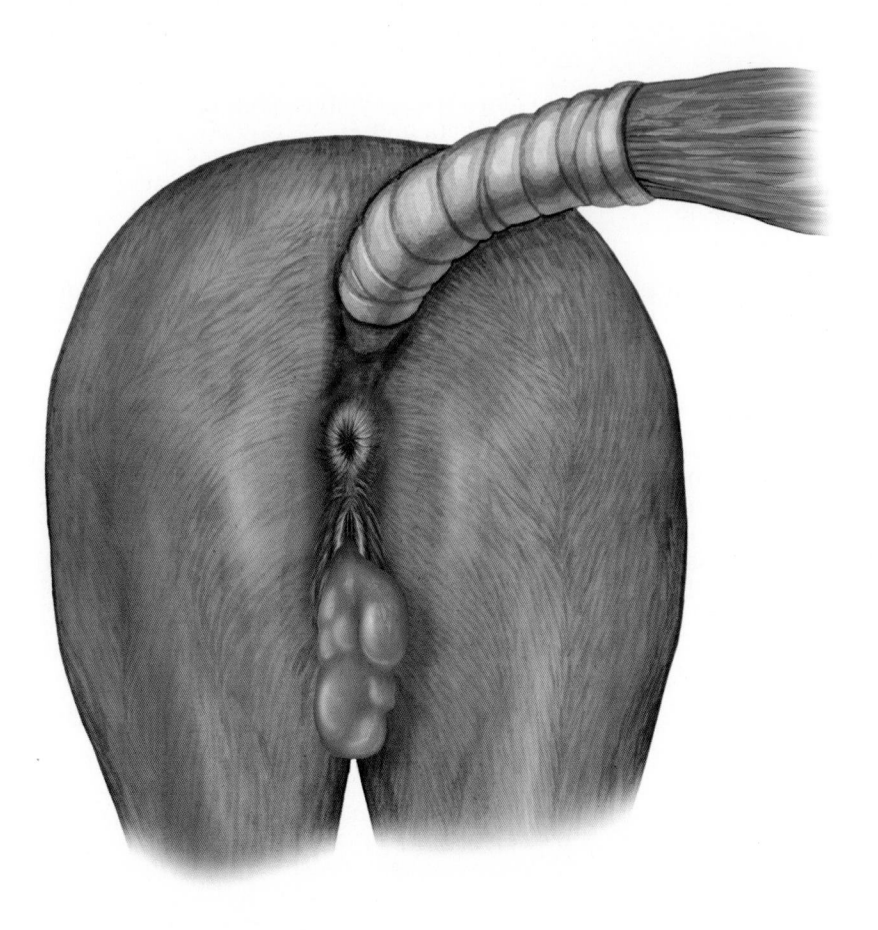

Premature Placental Detachment

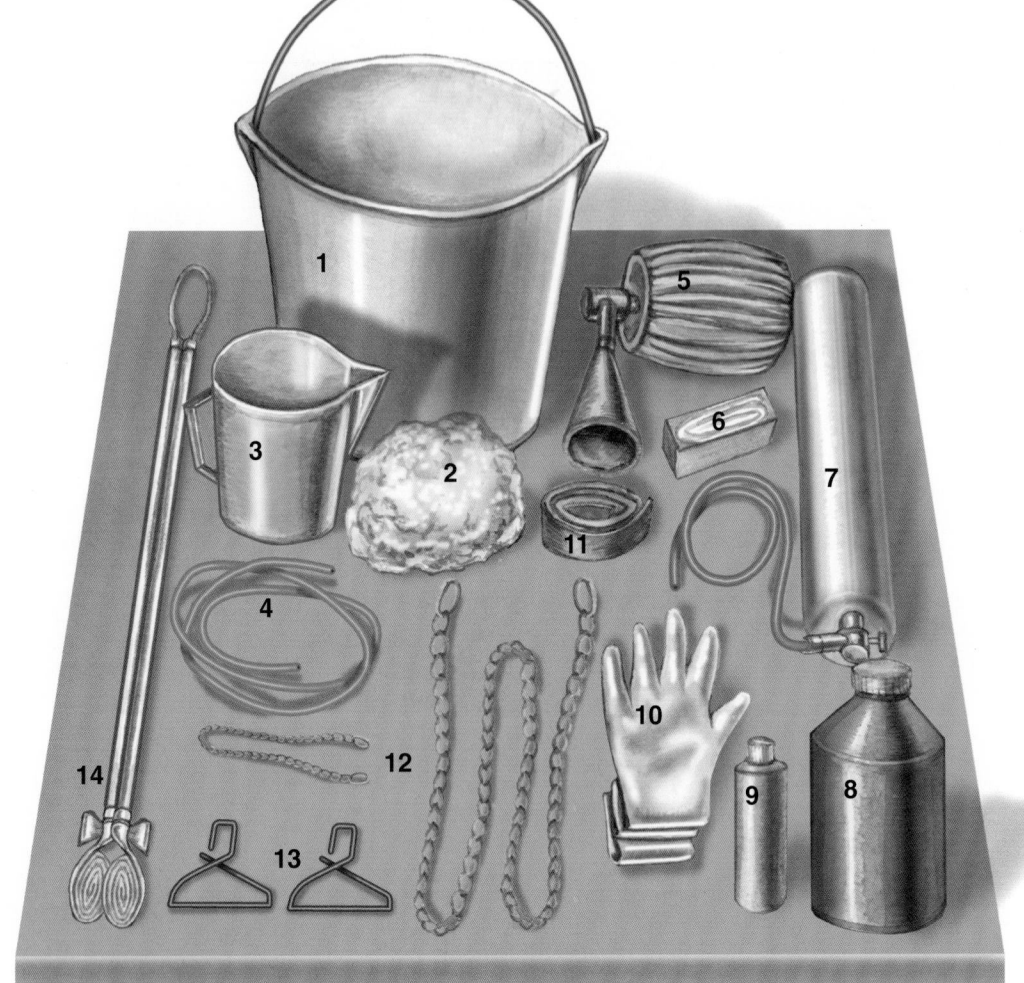

1 - Stainless steel bucket
2 - Cotton
3 - Enema bucket
4 - Enema tubing
5 - Ambu bag

6 - Nasal O$_2$ canula
7 - Oxygen tank
8 - Gallon of lubrication
9 - Disinfectant soap
10 -Exam gloves and sleeves

11 - Obstetrical straps
12 - Obstetrical chains
13 - Handles for chains
14 - Fetotome with coiled wire

Obstetrical Supplies Necessary for Potential Delivery Problems

During the administration of oxytocin, it is not unusual for the mares to become restless and exhibit colic-type symptoms. They will sweat and struggle with all the physical signs of labor occurring very rapidly. If strong abdominal contractions persist for over twenty minutes and there are no visible signs of the chorioallantoic membrane, a vaginal examination should be performed to determine the progress of delivery. The majority of mares will foal within 60 minutes after the initiation of oxytocin administration.

Prostaglandins have also been utilized to induce parturition in the mare. It is important to have a mature fetus before the administration of this medication. The difference with this medication is the variability of the interval for the induction of parturition. The administration of Fluprostenol at 250 mg I.M. will result in the induction of labor 1 to 6 hours after the administration. Numerous complications such as cervical rupture and poor viability of the foal can result utilizing this method.

Before induction is considered, all possible risks should be weighed. All precautions should be made to deal with the possibility of any complication that could arise during the induction process.

PROBLEMS INVOLVING DELIVERY

Delivery problems in the mare consist of premature placental detachment, dystocia, uterine torsion, uterine prolapse, internal hemorrhage, and uterine rupture. Early detection of a delivery problem by the foaling manager is essential to the treatment of any problem. It is usually a very stressful and frightening experience. Any indication that a problem may be present should prompt a call to one's attending veterinarian. It is important to remember that any problem during delivery not only threatens the life of the foal but also that of the mare.

PREMATURE PLACENTAL DETACHMENT

Placental detachment from the uterus before or during the delivery of the foal is commonly referred to as a "red bag" delivery. The side of the placenta that is toward the foal is smooth, shiny, and somewhat greenish-blue or pink in color. The maternal side is blood-red and appears velvety. With a premature placental detachment, the water does not break and a very red sac starts to appear through the vulva. This indicates the placenta has partially or completely detached from the uterus and is moving with the foal rather than remaining attached to the uterus and supplying the foal with oxygen. Therefore, this is an extreme emergency in that the foal no longer receives oxygen from its mother. If the foal is not delivered quickly, the foal will suffocate.

It is important not to panic when this problem is identified. A calm cool head will usually equate into the delivery of a live foal. When the red bag appears in the vulva, the placenta must be opened and the front feet identified. In most cases the placenta can be torn with one's fingers. This opening will release a gush of fluid. The foal's front feet will appear. If they do not, one must reach in through the opening, find the feet, and guide them to the outside. Gentle traction which coincides with the mare's contractions will aid in the delivery of the foal. It is important to make sure that the foal's nose appears shortly after the feet are identified. If the feet are not present, then the foal must be repositioned. The foal has to be delivered as quickly as possible; however, this does not mean that the foal should be traumatically removed from the mare with sheer brute force. As soon as the foal's nose appears, care must be taken to remove the amniotic membrane from the nostrils to allow the foal to breath air as soon as respiration begins.

It is not uncommon with a premature placental detachment that the foal will appear slightly sluggish and have difficulty breathing after the delivery. The nostrils should be cleared of fluid.

The foal may be laid on its side with its hind quarters lifted and the chest off the ground. Then let the head hang down to allow the fluid it has inhaled to clear from the lungs and respiratory passages. After this is done, the foal should be positioned on its sternum, rubbed down briskly with a towel, and covered with a blanket to keep it warm.

DYSTOCIA

The second stage of labor in the mare usually lasts 20 - 30 minutes. If either this or the first stage of parturition is prolonged or nonprogressive, a condition known as dystocia is possible. Literally translated, dystocia means "difficult birth." It can be caused by a large foal (such as in the draft breeds) or more often by an abnormal presentation, position, or posture with the long fetal extremities. Prompt examination and treatment is the only way to save both the life of the fetus and the mare and to prevent injury to the mare's reproductive tract.

Obstetrical instruments and lubricant should be readily available and sterile so that assistance can be offered to the mare and foal. Minimally, this obstetrical equipment should include obstetric chains or straps, handles, a stainless steel bucket, towels, a disinfectant soap, and a gallon of lubricating solution. A preferred lubricating solution consists of polyethylene polymer powder which adheres to the mucosal membranes of the mare's reproductive tract to provide excellent short term lubrication. A carboxy-methylcellulose solution can provide a liquid lubricant that can be pumped into the uterine lumen and around the fetus utilizing a sterile stomach tube. Liquid lubrication can also become a disinfectant through the addition of one tablespoon of chlorhexidine solution to each gallon of lubricating liquid.

Ideally the mare should be standing for an initial examination in order to determine if there is any fetal displacement causing the dystocia. The tail should be wrapped and the perineal area thoroughly scrubbed with an antiseptic soap and rinsed. In most cases, the mare will be laying on her side and an examination must be made in this

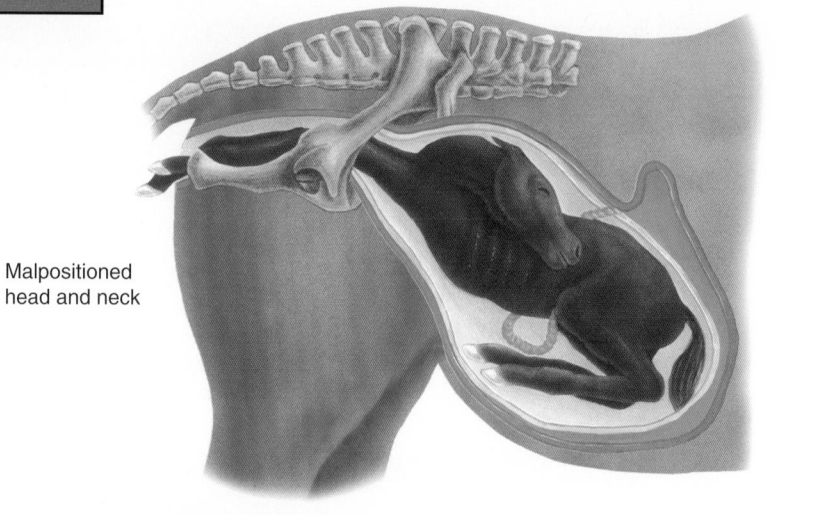

Malpositioned
head and neck

Foreleg reflected down
position frequently
results in fracture

Dystocias

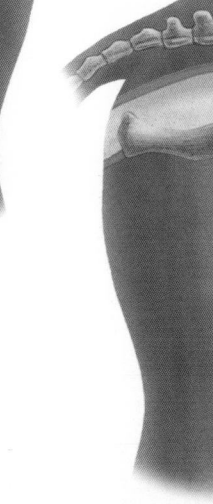

Upside down presentation

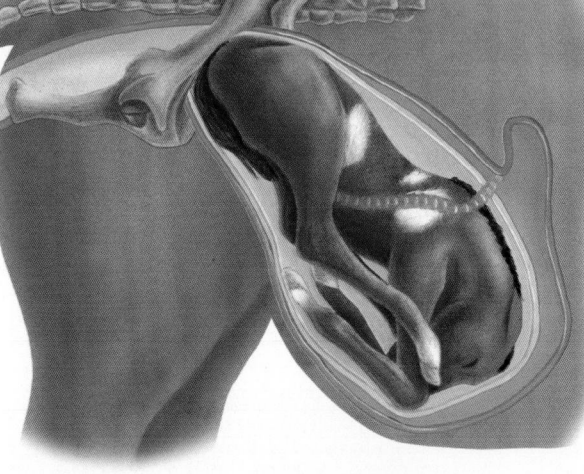

Breech presentation

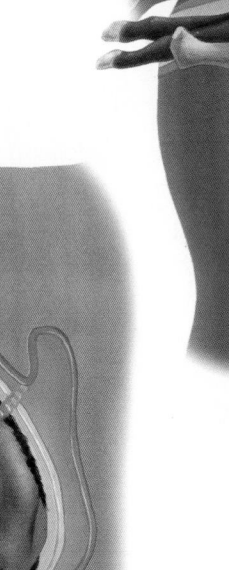

Posterior presentation

position. Care must always be taken to provide a clean environment and as clean an examination as possible. If the mare is straining extremely hard, it may be necessary to administer 1 - 2 cc of a 2% lidocaine solution in the caudal epidural space. A diluted solution of xylazine can also be administered in the caudal epidural space to control straining yet prevent the instability associated with epidural administration of lidocaine.

A scrubbed hand, preferably covered with a sterile plastic sleeve, should be used to gain entry into the birth canal to examine and assess the position of the fetus. Assessment should be made as to the presentation, the position, the size, and the posture of the fetus so that a plan can be formulated for delivery. It is also important at this time to make an attempt to determine if the fetus is still alive by either stimulating a reflex movement or detection of a heartbeat. In some instances, fetal abnormalities, or even trauma to the birth canal or the mare's reproductive tract which predisposes the dystocia, may be discovered at this time.

In most cases, the most common cause of dystocia in the mare is a postural abnormality in the presentation. Any manipulation of the fetus to return it to a normal position of presentation and posture is termed mutation. In many cases, it is necessary to push the fetus from the maternal pelvis back into the abdominal cavity to allow space for repositioning and correction of the fetal malposture. After this repositioning, traction is usually applied and a normal delivery can be accomplished.

A large portion of dystocias with the fetus in an anterior position, occur with the head and neck of the fetus reflected to one side. Usually both feet are noted within the maternal pelvis without the presence of the foal's nose.

Treatment of this problem may be as easy as getting the mare up and walking her for a few minutes or repelling the foal back into the abdominal cavity and repositioning the foal's nose into the correct presentation. If repositioning is unsuccessful and the foal is alive, then a cesarean section should be considered. If the fetus is dead, a partial fetotomy, amputating the head of the fetus, will allow removal of the foal.

If only one front leg and the foal's nose or only the foal's nose appears, then it is likely that one or both of the front legs are reflected down. During the uterine contractions, it is possible that one or both of the forelimbs have hit the rim of the mare's pelvis. The forelimbs are then deflected downward instead of into a normal presentation over the floor of the pelvis and straight ahead. In these cases, the more the mare pushes, the more the foal is jammed into the pelvis with the forelimbs in the down position. At this time, it is necessary to administer an epidural anesthetic before correction and repositioning of the foal occurs. In most cases, one can follow the limb down, grasp it behind the knee, and bring the forelimb up to a normal presentation while being careful to cup one's hand over the hoof to prevent trauma to the mare's reproductive tract. By repelling the head back into the abdominal cavity, this limb can then be extended forward and into the correct presentation. This process is then repeated for the other limb if it is also in a down position. The foal is then delivered through careful traction in a normal manner.

One of the most challenging repositioning tasks is a foal that is presented in an upside down position. Upon examination, both front feet appear upside down in the vulva. It is necessary to confirm on examination that these are in fact the front feet. This presentation predisposes the mare to a rectovaginal laceration. If possible, the mare should be in a standing position to facilitate the foal's rotation back into a proper position. This is sometimes difficult to do but should be accomplished whenever possible. It takes a great deal of strength and perfect timing between contractions to reposition a foal in this upside down presentation. Once the foal is repositioned, careful traction should allow a normal delivery.

There are numerous times when the delivery appears normal with both front feet and the foal's nose appearing through the vulva. However, when a shoulder becomes locked in the pelvis, which happens with a large foal, progress in the birth canal is stopped. In this case a large amount of lubrication should be administered within the birth canal. Traction should be applied first to one leg and then the other. The foal is then worked out through the birth canal small amounts at a time.

Delivery of the foal in a normal presentation can also be impeded when the foal's hips become locked in the pelvis. In this case, a large amount of lubrication should be applied throughout the birth canal. The foal's body should be positioned by pulling downward at a 45 degree angle to facilitate delivery.

Examination of a foal that seems to be in normal presentation but not making any progress through the birth canal may reveal that both hind feet are also in the birth canal approximately at the level of the shoulders. Delivery seems to be proceeding normally, but then the progress suddenly stops when this malposition occurs. In most cases, repelling the foal back into the abdomen will allow repositioning of the feet, and traction can be applied to the forelimbs for a normal delivery.

The first indication that there is posterior presentation of the foal is that the foal's feet are upside down. Examination will then reveal that the foal's hocks are in the birth canal. There are several dangers with this presentation. The first is that the umbilical cord will be pinched off by the pelvis during delivery and the foal will suffocate. Secondly, with the pelvis being the first portion of the foal to be delivered, care must be taken not to traumatize the mare's reproductive tract. Although panic is never the solution, the foal must be delivered rapidly, and the foal's nostrils must be cleared and proper respiration initiated. There is no repositioning needed in this case unless it is an extremely small foal and can be completely turned around. The foal is usually delivered in the posterior presentation by applying traction which coincides with the mare's uterine contractions to facilitate delivery.

Artwork by S. Hakola / J. Dirig
Copyright Equistar Publications, Ltd.

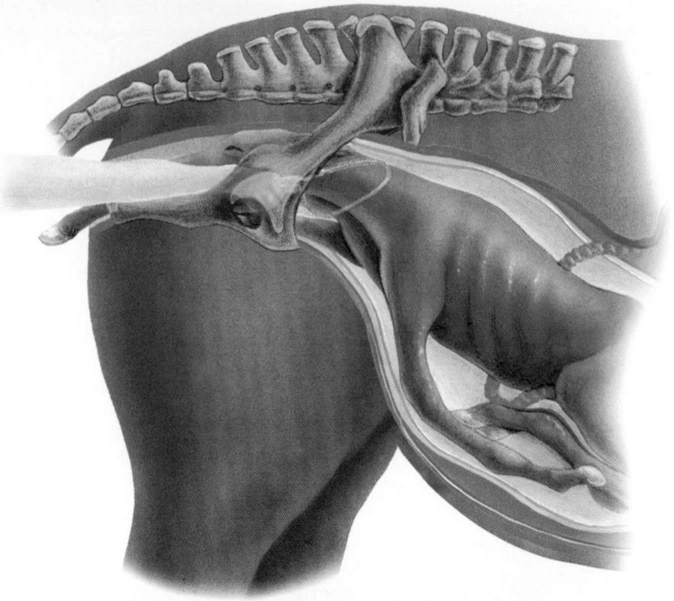

Dystocia Necessitating Fetotomy

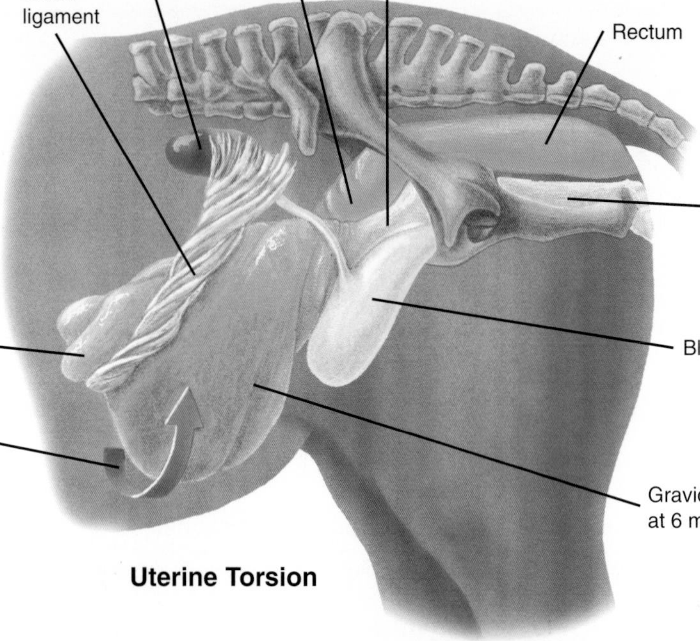

Uterine Torsion

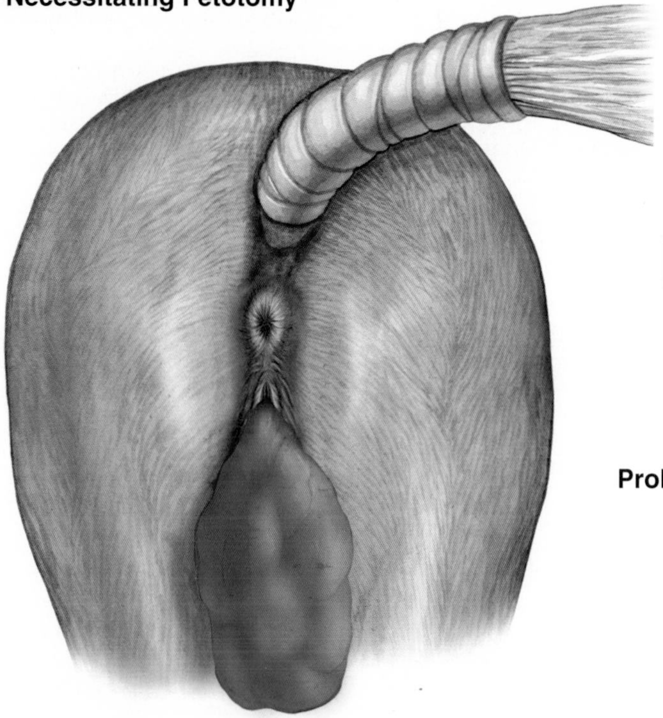

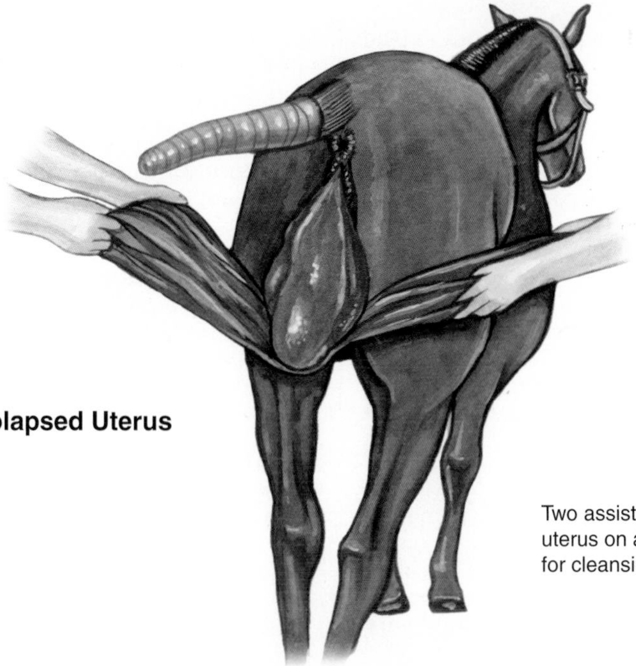

Broad ligament

Kidney

Colon

Cervix

Rectum

Vagina

Bladder

Non-gravid horn of uterus

Direction of torsion

Gravid horn of torsed uterus at 6 months gestation

Prolapsed Uterus

Two assistants holding prolapsed uterus on a garbage bag in preparation for cleansing and reinsertion into mare.

One of the most frightening vaginal examinations during delivery is finding only the foal's tail in the birth canal. This indicates a breech presentation with the hind limbs tucked underneath it and the pelvis of the foal pushing against the mare's pelvis. This is one of the more serious presentations. The foal should be repelled or pushed back down into the mare's abdomen with one hand. The other hand follows the limb down, flexes it, and allows its presentation into the birth canal. Care must always be taken not to allow the foal's limbs to traumatize the mare's reproductive tract. This is often accomplished by cupping one's hand over the foal's hoof to prevent any kind of trauma. This process is then repeated for the other limb. A posterior presentation delivery is then accomplished using normal traction. In print, this procedure sounds extremely simple. In reality, this procedure makes the person delivering the foal wonder how soon one can reach retirement.

Care and patience must always be exercised in all cases of repositioning and application of traction to facilitate delivery. The mare's reproductive tract must always be well lubricated. If straining is a problem, the reproductive tract should be relaxed with an epidural anesthetic. Extreme brute force should never be utilized in the delivery of a foal. In all cases, traction should be synchronized with the mare's abdominal and uterine contractions.

FETOTOMY

If an exam reveals that it is impossible to reposition the foal into a presentation that will allow delivery and the foal is deceased, a fetotomy should be considered. The object of this procedure is to save the mare's life and her subsequent fertility. Special instrumentation and veterinarian assistance is needed to perform this procedure. In special extenuating circumstances, it may be necessary to sacrifice a living fetus through the use of a fetotomy when a cesarean section is not feasible. Special instrumentation such as a fetotome, a wire saw, handles, obstetrical snares, chains, and hooks are needed in order to perform a fetotomy. In all cases, an epidural anesthetic should be given along with large amounts of lubricant.

This procedure involves the separation of the head or specific limbs, through the use of a wire saw, to facilitate more room to allow delivery. A portion of the foal is separated and then removed to allow this delivery. In certain instances, the entire fetus has to be removed piece by piece until the delivery is complete. This procedure is utilized when there is some sort of fetal malformation such as hydrocephalus.

After the procedure is completed, it is normally advantageous to administer systemic antibiotics and oxytocin to allow uterine involution and the passage of the placenta. Antibiotic infusion of the uterus for several days in addition to systemic treatment of the mare is generally indicated after a fetotomy.

UTERINE TORSION

Uterine torsion is an uncommon condition in the mare. It occurs more commonly between months 5 to 8 of gestation than it does in term mares.

Clinically, the mare will appear to be colicky. The symptoms of colic will be unresponsive to medication and rectal palpation will reveal the proper diagnosis. Palpation of the ovaries will reveal the displacement of the ligaments and the direction in which the uterus has twisted.

It is sometimes possible to correct this condition by anesthetizing the mare and placing her in a lateral recumbency on the side of the direction of the torsion. Therefore, a mare with a clockwise or a right directional torsion when viewed from the rear is put in a right lateral recumbency. An assistant then places a 2x12x12 board across the abdomen to hold the uterus in place. The mare is gently rolled onto her other side. A rectal examination will reveal if the torsion has been corrected. Each roll will only reduce the torsion by 180 degrees; therefore, it has to be repeated for any torsion that is 360 degrees or greater.

If the uterine torsion occurs when the mare is term and the cervix dilated, the mare is kept standing and an epidural anesthetic is administered. The

fetus is then grasped ventrally and laterally and then rocked until enough momentum is gained until it can be lifted upward and rotated in the opposite direction of the uterine twist. If the cervix is not dilated and there is a term pregnancy, a cesarean section should be considered.

UTERINE PROLAPSE

Prolapse of the uterus in the mare usually occurs immediately after parturition. There are times when this condition occurs 2 - 3 days after delivery. Usually only one uterine horn prolapses. Prolapse of the equine uterus is an emergency situation and may be complicated by internal hemorrhage, shock, and other difficulties that will endanger the mare's life.

The first step of treatment for a prolapsed uterus is to sedate the mare and then use a caudal epidural anesthetic in order to control the straining. Ideally, the mare should be kept in a standing position. The tail is wrapped and the uterus is gently cleansed with repeated applications of a disinfectant soap. Any tears within the uterine tissue should be sutured, and any hemorrhage should be stopped. If the urinary bladder is distended, it may be necessary to catheterize the bladder and remove the urine before the uterus can be replaced.

After the uterus has been cleansed, it should be lifted to the pelvic level to restore circulation and facilitate replacement. If two assistants are available, it is easy to place the uterus on a plastic trash bag and have an assistant on each side elevate the uterus to the level of the pelvis. This can even be done while the cleansing procedures are being accomplished to help restore circulation. With slow massaging motions, the uterus is replaced through the vagina and back into the body cavity. Care must be taken to completely replace both uterine horns. Once the uterus is replaced, a warm saline solution containing a broad spectrum antibiotic should be infused into the uterus to facilitate complete horn replacement. Excess fluid can then be siphoned out using a sterile stomach tube.

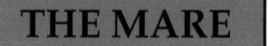
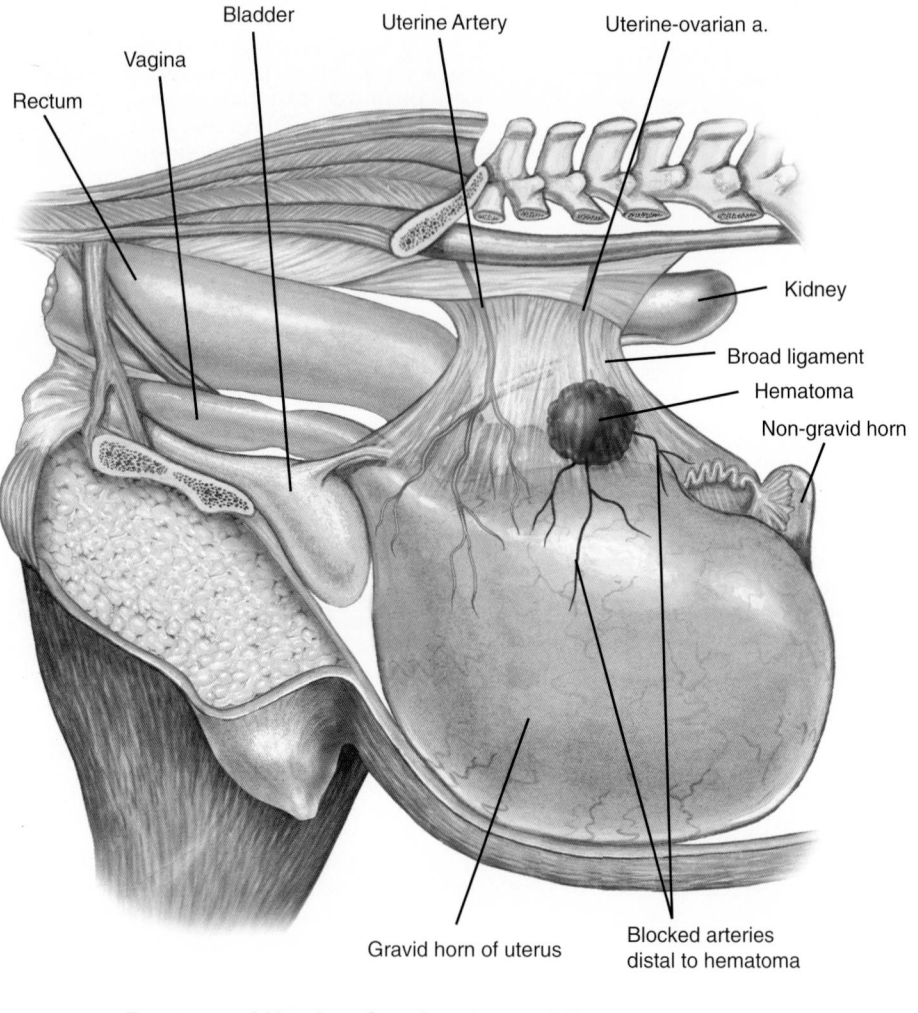

Rectum

Vagina

Bladder

Uterine Artery

Uterine-ovarian a.

Kidney

Broad ligament

Hematoma

Non-gravid horn

Gravid horn of uterus

Blocked arteries
distal to hematoma

**Rupture of Uterine-Ovarian Artery With Loss
of Vascular Flow Distal to Hemorrhage**

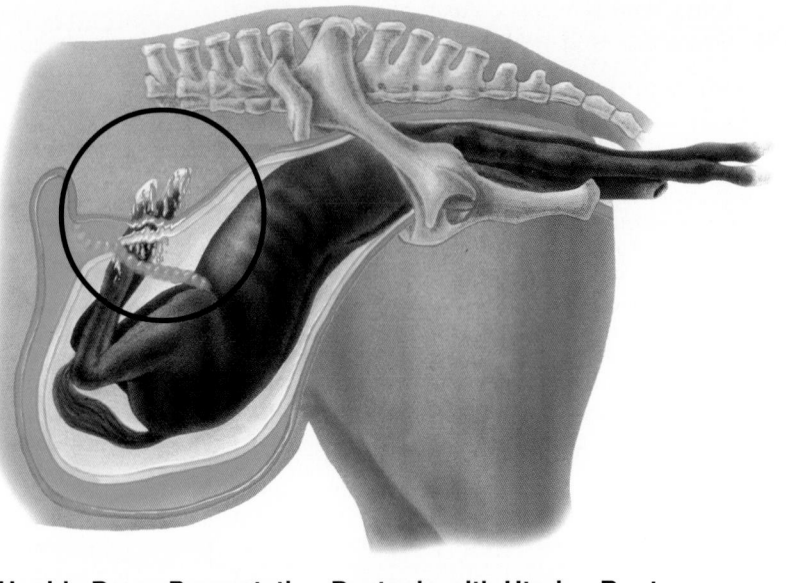

Upside Down Presentation Dystocia with Uterine Rupture

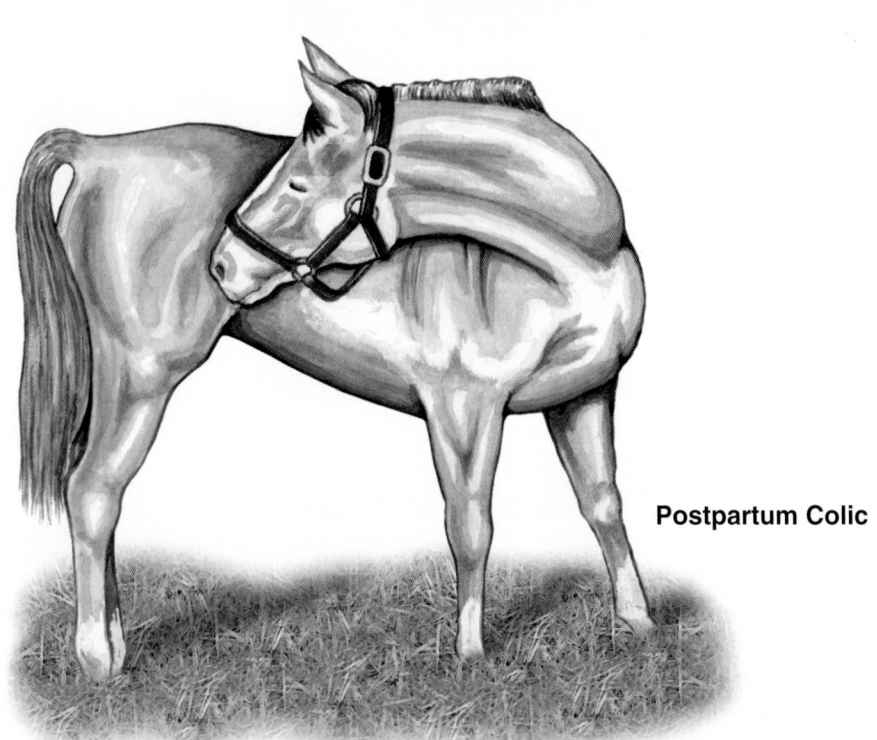

Postpartum Colic

After the uterus has been replaced, 10 - 20 IU of oxytocin should be administered to stimulate uterine contraction and involution. The mare should be placed on a systemic regime of broad spectrum antibiotics for at least 5 - 10 days. In addition, intrauterine infusions are administered with frequency. The type utilized is specific to each case situation. It is also important to provide tetanus prophylaxis to the mare.

Broad sutures placed across the vulva may prevent pneumovagina. Care must be taken in the placement of these sutures in that irritation from them may cause the mare further straining.

INTERNAL HEMORRHAGE

Rupture of the utero-ovarian artery within the broad ligament sometimes occurs during parturition. Other causes of internal hemorrhage may be the result of vascular rupture that occurs concurrently with a uterine prolapse or torsion.

Clinical signs include a nonresponsive colic, an increased pulse and respiratory rate, sweating, and eventually shock. It is quite possible that the mare just appears depressed and may not show any sign of pain. However, when her gums are checked, she will exhibit pale mucous membranes with a very slow capillary refill time.

Unfortunately, treatment of the postparturient mare with internal hemorrhage is limited to analgesic and sedative agents. All efforts should be made to keep the mare quiet and minimize stress. It is possible to confirm the diagnosis of intra-abdominal hemorrhage by an abdominocentesis. If the blood pressure falls and the hemorrhage is stopped, a large hematoma may be detected in the broad ligament of the uterus. If the hemorrhage does not stop on its own, unfortunately, death will result.

If a uterine or broad ligament hematoma is detected during palpation, an ultrasonic exam will determine the extent of its involvement. Careful consideration must be given in the rebreeding of

these mares. They are predisposed to recurrence, and it may even be difficult for them to carry a pregnancy to term.

UTERINE RUPTURE

Rupture of the uterus can occur during a uterine torsion, during manipulation to correct a malposition, during the second stage of labor, and even during vigorous postparturient treatment.

The most obvious clinical sign of a uterine rupture is a hemorrhagic discharge from the vagina. The mare may exhibit signs of colic and usually becomes rapidly depressed or shows signs of shock. Upon a vaginal exam, it is even possible to find a portion of the bowel that has herniated through the uterus and found its way into the vagina or vulvar opening. An abdominocentesis will reveal serosanguineous hemorrhagic fluid.

If the mare has a term pregnancy, immediate treatment with fluid therapy for shock should be initiated. Even though the mare is a poor anesthetic risk, the only chance for her survival consists of the surgical repair of the uterine rupture. A ventral midline incision is utilized with the mare under general anesthetic. The foal is removed from the abdomen and the uterine rupture repaired. The abdominal cavity is then lavaged to remove any source of contamination. Aggressive fluid therapy, systemic antibiotic administration in addition to antiinflammatories, and tetanus prophylaxis should be utilized to facilitate her recovery. In all cases, the prognosis is always very guarded.

COMMON COMPLICATIONS IN THE MARE FOLLOWING BIRTH

Several complications can arise in the postpartum mare. These include simple cramping and colic symptoms, retained placental membranes, uterine infections, and lacerations of the perineal and rectovaginal areas. Very few post-foaling complications occur, but it is necessary to know how to deal with them when they do.

CRAMPING AND GASTRO-INTESTINAL COLIC

It is normal for the mare to have contractions of her uterine tissue after the foal is born. The sole purpose of these contractions is to expel the placental membranes and facilitate an involution of the uterus. This process can occur for 3 - 12 hours following delivery.

The clinical signs of cramping are the same as those as if the mare had a mild case of colic. She will paw the ground and may get up and lay down repeatedly. She may bite at her sides, kick at her belly, or swish her tail. One must always consider that she is in a true gastrointestinal colic if she continues to show signs of abdominal pain 12 hours after she has passed her placental tissues.

Treatment should be as conservative as possible since any medication that is administered to the mare at this time will ultimately end up in the mare's milk and be ingested by the foal. The mare may be continually observed in the hope that she will work through her problem. If the mare is sweating, if respiration and heart rates are increased, and if she is endangering or not letting the foal nurse, then the systemic administration of analgesic agents should be considered. A small amount of flunixin meglumine is administered IV. This is usually enough to provide comfort for the mare and resolve the cramping or mild colic. If the mare is not responsive to this treatment, an accurate diagnosis should be sought.

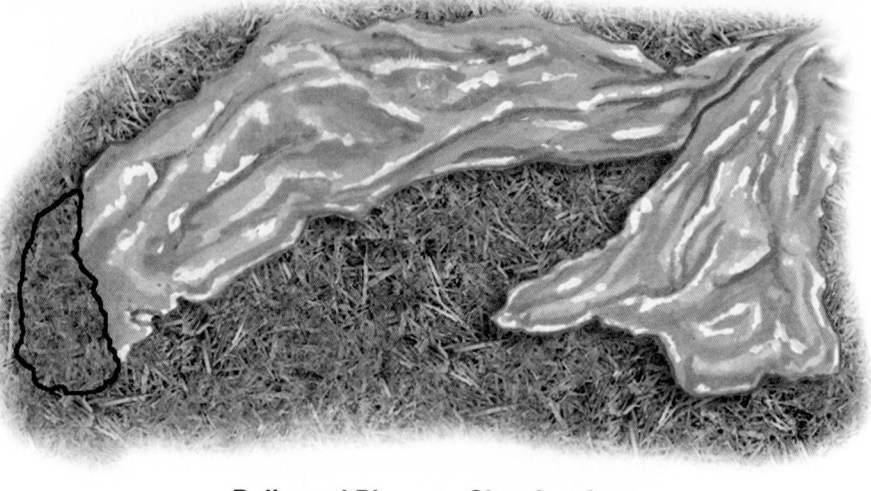

**Delivered Placenta Showing Area
of Torn Placenta Retained in Mare.**

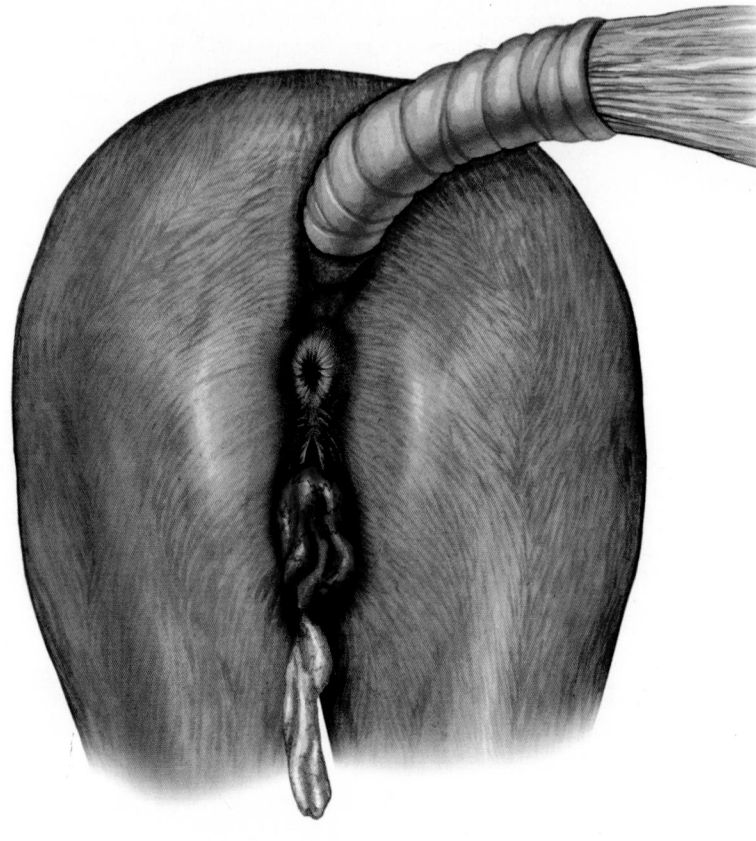

Retained Placenta

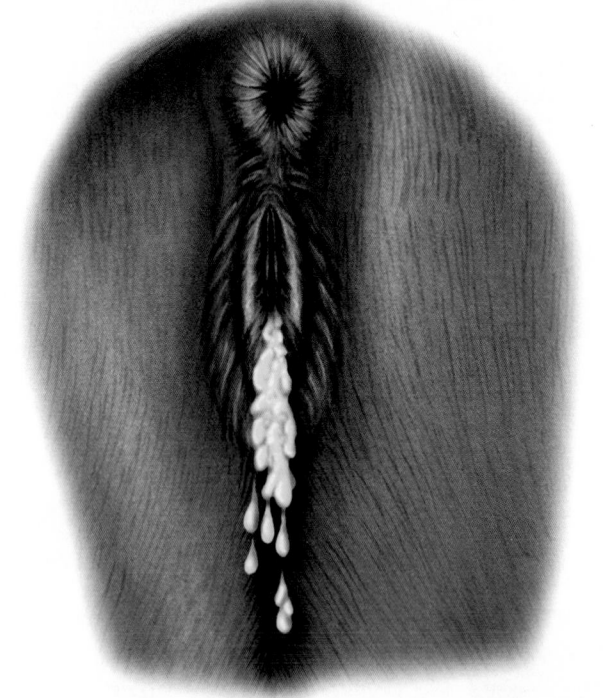

**Bacterial Infection Indicated by
Purulent Vulvar Discharge.**

RETAINED PLACENTAL MEMBRANES

The fetal membranes or placenta ideally should be expelled from the mare within 30 minutes of delivery. These placental membranes are considered retained if they are not expelled within 2 - 3 hours after birth. This retention of the fetal membranes constitutes an emergency situation. The mare can develop a toxic metritis or toxemia and ultimately, laminitis from this condition. Fortunately, only about 5% of the postparturient mares retain their fetal membranes. Etiology of this condition is usually associated with a dystocia, a placentitis, or any disturbance that would occur which inhibits uterine contractions. This inhibition of uterine contractions can occur from an inadequate amount of oxytocin or an inadequate response of the musculature of the uterus to oxytocin.

After the fetal membranes have been expelled, it is important to remove them from the stall in an intact state so that they can be examined throughout their entirety for any missing portions. Any portion of the placenta can break off and remain inside the mare while the remaining membranes are expelled. Most oftentimes, this is a portion of the tip of the placenta contained within the nonpregnant horn of the uterus.

It is very obvious if the entire placenta is retained since part of it will usually be hanging down behind the mare. If a portion or piece of the placenta has been retained, an aseptic intrauterine examination should be conducted.

The entire perineal area should be washed with an antiseptic soap, and a sterile sleeved hand is be introduced into the vagina to determine how tightly the membranes are still attached to the uterus. Traction should never be applied to the retained fetal membranes since this predisposes the tearing off of a piece to be left within the uterus.

If the fetal membranes are not merely knotted at the level of the cervix but are still tightly attached to the uterus, oxytocin therapy should be initiated.

It is advantageous to start an intravenous drip of oxytocin to the mare instead of a large dose administered rapidly. This will stimulate and sustain normal uterine contractions for the passage of the placental membranes. In conjunction with the oxytocin therapy, systemic antibiotics should be started. Uterine lavage would be prudent at this time to help separate the retained membranes and aid in the removal of debris and bacteria from the uterus. Any administration of intrauterine antimicrobial therapy should be coupled with systemic administration of compatible antimicrobials.

If the mare appears toxic from the retention of fetal membranes, immediate treatment should be focused to prevent or correct this toxemia. Fluid therapy should be initiated intravenously. In addition, it is advantageous to administer flunixin meglumine at a level of .025 mg/kg IV every eight hours.

Usually within one hour after initiation of oxytocin therapy, the placental membranes will be passed. The lavage techniques will also aid to separate and facilitate the membrane passage. Intrauterine infusions of antibiotic solutions should also be carried out for several days on any mare that has retained her fetal membranes. Mares that have a history of retaining their fetal membranes should have a dose of oxytocin administered intramuscularly as a preventative measure immediately after foaling.

It is important to treat these mares with retained fetal membranes with great care and patience. However, rigorous overzealous treatment may lead to a tear in the fetal membranes and a possible nidus of infection left within the uterine horn. Overzealous intrauterine lavage may allow for an increased absorption of toxic material, therefore predisposing the mare to toxemia and subsequent laminitis. Conservative treatment and follow-up care over several days is the key to success with the management of retained fetal membranes.

BACTERIAL INFECTIONS

Bacterial infections of the uterus unfortunately are a common complication in the postpartum mare. Etiology behind these infections could be from foaling on sawdust, trauma to the uterine tissue during delivery, a dystocia that was managed with an unsanitary technique, or retained fetal membranes.

The vaginal discharge from mares should be monitored several days postpartum. It is not unusual for the mare to pass a brownish bloody-looking fluid that within a few days would turn clear and be thin in consistency. If this fluid changes color to a yellow or cloudy white thick mucus-like fluid, the mare should be examined for a possible postpartum uterine infection.

If a uterine infection is suspected, a culture should be taken immediately to obtain an accurate diagnosis and guide a proper treatment regime. While the culture results are pending, the mare should be started on systemic broad spectrum antibiotics as well as intrauterine infusions of an appropriate antimicrobial solution. This regime should be maintained for at least 3 - 5 days. After this period of time, the mare should continue to be examined. Subsequent cultures should be done until the mare is given a clean bill of health.

Artwork by S. Hakola / J. Dirig
Copyright Equistar Publications, Ltd.

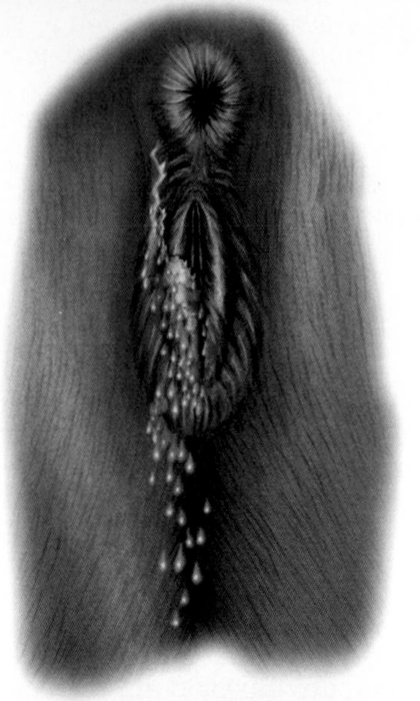

**Perineal Laceration
of Vulvar Lips**

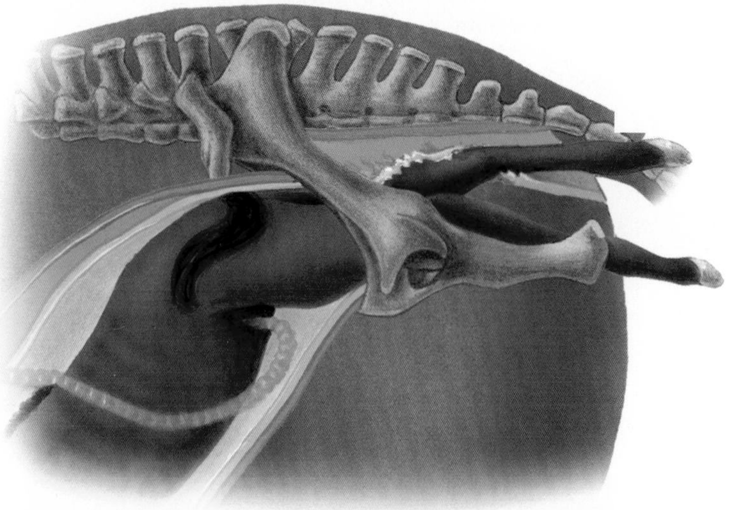

Surgical Repair of Rectovaginal Laceration Performed in Two Stages

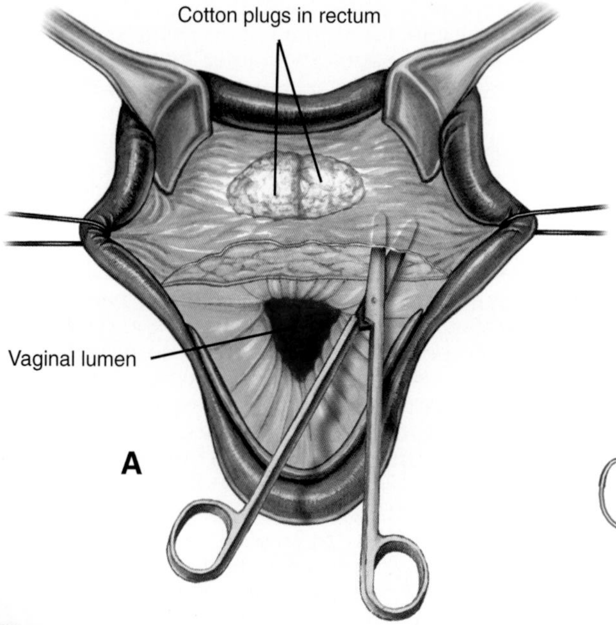

Cotton plugs in rectum

Vaginal lumen

A

Dissection of epithelial scar tissue in a horizontal plane.

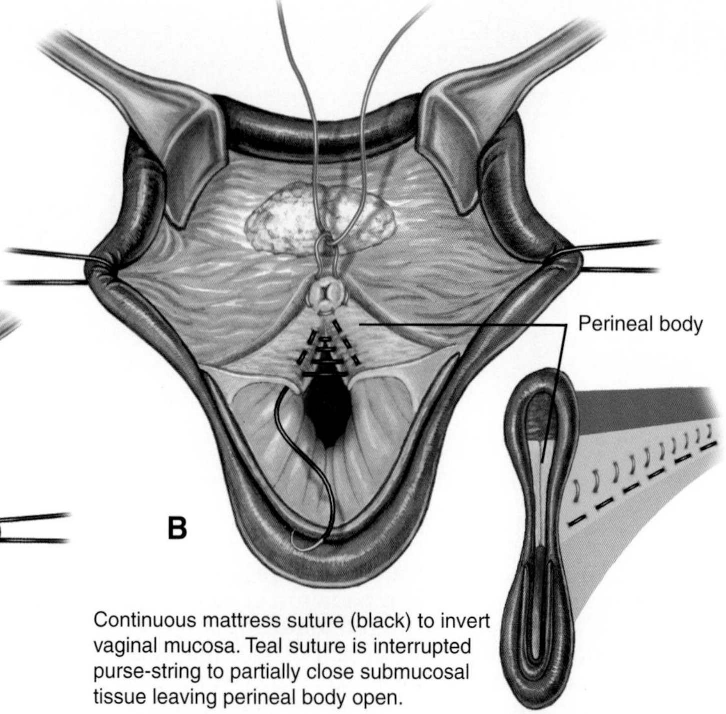

Perineal body

B

Continuous mattress suture (black) to invert vaginal mucosa. Teal suture is interrupted purse-string to partially close submucosal tissue leaving perineal body open.

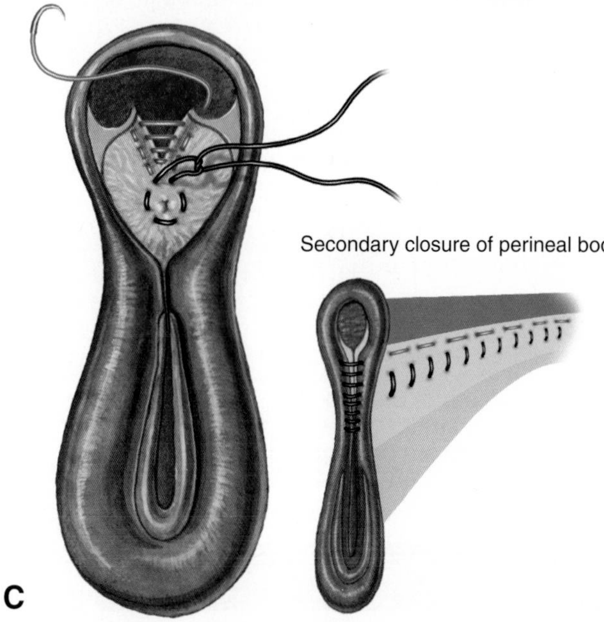

Secondary closure of perineal body.

C

Rectovaginal Laceration

PERINEAL AND RECTO-VAGINAL LACERATIONS

Perineal lacerations occur during delivery. They are usually created from the foal's front feet causing damage or an overstretching of the vulva when the foal's shoulders or pelvis is delivered. These lacerations only involve the mucosal layer and skin of the vulva. They can easily be repaired with a few stitches with subsequent physical therapy techniques to help reduce the swelling.

Rectovaginal lacerations occur when the foal's foot is pushed through the roof of the vagina and inserted completely into the rectum. With the mares next contraction, the foal's leg will tear through the vagina and the rectum simultaneously until it exits out through the anus and perineum. Although serious, this condition is usually not life threatening but needs to be repaired through several steps.

Immediate repair of rectovaginal lacerations is rarely indicated. Because of the traumatic nature of the injury, all swelling and necrotic tissue should be removed before the repair is initiated. It is not unusual for debridement and systemic antibacterial therapy to be done for five days before surgical repair is started. Tetanus prophylaxsis should always be current.

The goal of repair of a rectovaginal laceration should be to reestablish the shelf between the rectum and the vestibule of the vagina and the restoration of a functional perineal body. The surgical procedure is accomplished with the mare in standing position utilizing an epidural anesthetic. The tail should be wrapped and tied out of the way and the entire perineal area prepped for surgery. Cotton should be placed in the rectum to prevent contamination of the surgical site during the procedure. Surgical repair is usually done in two stages. The first step is to reconstruct the rectovestibular shelf without closure of the perineal body. Three to four weeks later, the second step is accomplished which involves the closure of the remainder of the perineal body.

Debridement of all necrotic tissue should be accomplished before actual closure begins. The section of the tissues that are to be closed are dissected free so that they can be apposed with minimal tension to them. The vestibule is closed on the midline using a continuous suture pattern with absorbable material. It is advisable that this pattern invert the vestibular mucosa into the vestibule. Submucosal tissue layers are also closed to eliminate dead space. As the suturing progresses, sutures can be placed in a purse string fashion so that they can later be closed to eliminate dead space in the newly created rectovestibular shelf. Sutures are then placed in a sagitally oriented manner within the boundaries of the purse string sutures to appose the rectal and vestibular submucosal tissues. This manner of closure with the remainder of the submucosal tissues occurs caudally to the level of the cutaneous perineum.

In approximately 3 - 4 weeks, the epithelium is removed from the surface of the remaining perineal body, and the submucosal tissues are then apposed on the midline. An absorbable suture material is used within the rectum as the epithelial tissues are apposed in a continuous fashion. It is advantageous at this time also to perform a Caslick vulvoplasty.

It is possible to get these mares in foal after this traumatic injury. Cultures and treatments should be done in a timely manner until a clean culture has resulted. Artificial insemination techniques should be utilized when breeding these mares since natural service is not recommended for at least 90 days after this surgical repair is completed. Common sense dictates that a decision should be made in the rebreeding of these mares since they are going to require close management upon their next delivery.

Gravid horn

Incision line in
uterine horn

Peritoneal
cavity

A

**Elevation of Gravid Uterine
Horn Containing Extremities**

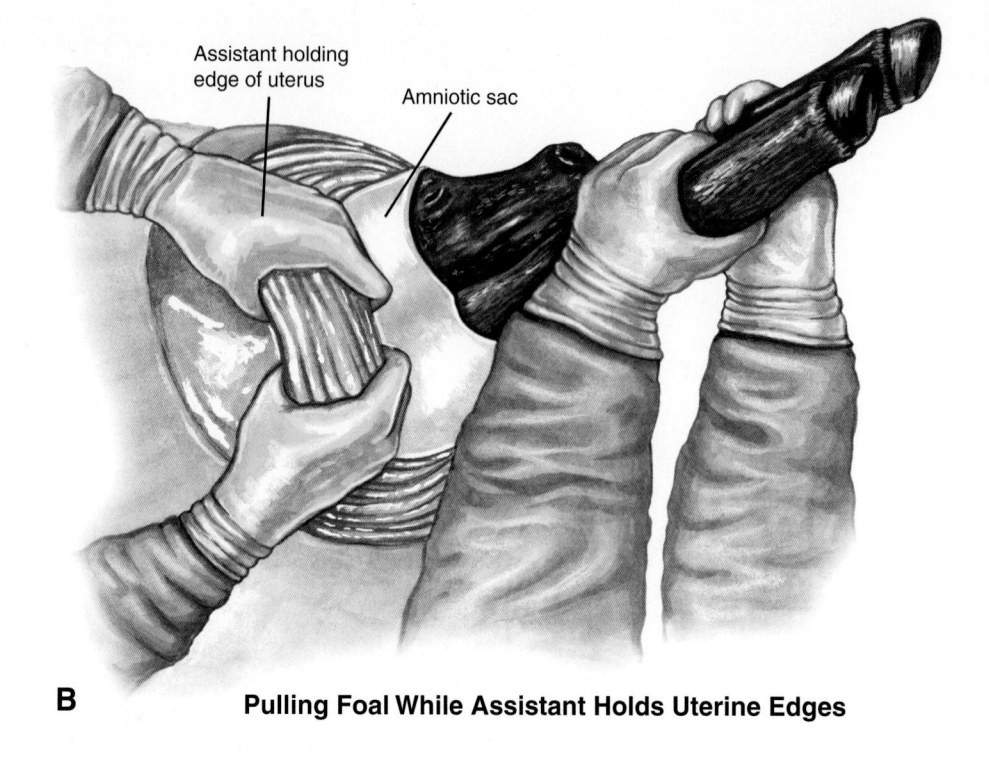

Assistant holding
edge of uterus

Amniotic sac

B   **Pulling Foal While Assistant Holds Uterine Edges**

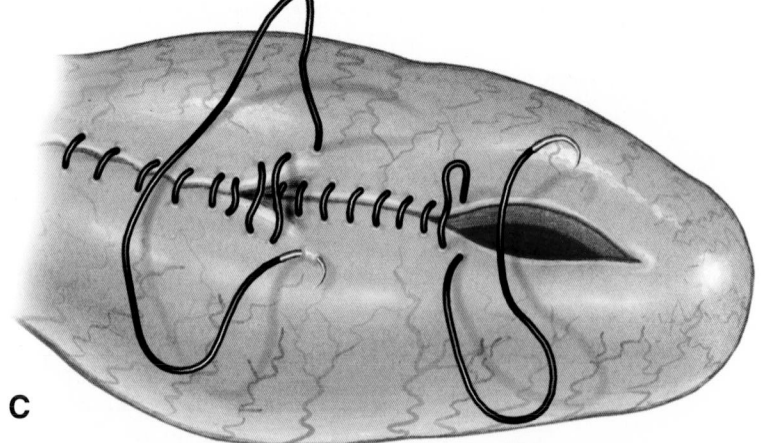

C

**Double Closure of Uterus:
Initial Continuous Suture Line
is Oversewn with a Cushing's
Suture Pattern**

CESAREAN SECTION

A cesarean section is the surgical delivery of a foal that is undertaken if a vaginal delivery is not possible. There are numerous reasons for consideration of a cesarean section. It may be required during a dystocia that cannot be repositioned, in certain cases of uterine rupture, and when there is a uterine torsion that cannot be corrected by either rolling the mare under anesthesia or a detorsion of the uterus through a flank laparotomy.

Once the decision is made to perform a cesarean section, all efforts to enhance the mare as a favorable surgical candidate should be undertaken. The mare should be immediately started on intravenous fluids and systemic antibiotics. The anesthetic that is used will be determined by the viability of the foal. If the foal is dead, one does not have to consider the pharmacological effects of the anesthetics on the foal. If the foal is alive, gas anesthesia using methoxyflurane or isoflurane are preferable since they are short acting and do not enhance uterine bleeding.

There are two approaches that are used for cesarean delivery. One approach is a low oblique flank incision and the other involves a ventral midline approach. In the low oblique flank approach, it is preferable to use the left flank to avoid the cecum which is present in the right flank region. The incision begins just caudal to the midcostal region and extends caudoventrally to just below the fold of the flank. The incision is extended through all the numerous muscle layers and fat until the peritoneum is reached and incised. The incision line is then retracted to allow exposure of the gravid horn of the uterus. The only problem with this approach is the closure of the numerous muscle layers which predisposes dehiscence of the incisions.

It is preferable to approach the cesarean section through a midline incision. In utilizing this approach, there are no muscle bellies encountered which keeps hemorrhage to a minimum. This incision should be begun just cranial to the

mammary glands and extend cranially for approximately 35 centimeters along the ventral midline. A midline approach allows good exposure to the uterine horn as well as easy entry into the abdominal cavity for manipulation of the uterus if needed.

Once the gravid uterine horn is isolated, it is important to prevent the uterine fluid from within it to contaminate the abdominal cavity. Proper draping and pads should be employed to prevent this occurrence. An incision is then made through the uterine tissue over the greater curvature of the gravid horn. The placenta and amnion are then incised with a scalpel or scissors, taking care to avoid any large vessels. After the uterus is opened, the fetus is extracted usually with the aid of an assistant.

It is important to allow the foal time to begin respiration before the umbilical artery is cut. This will usually take place within five minutes after withdrawal from the uterus. Once breathing is established, the umbilical cord may be broken a few centimeters from the navel. It is helpful to apply a hemostat and possibly a ligature before the artery is severed.

The fluid that remains in the uterus should be suctioned off to reduce the chances of abdominal cavity contamination. Any portion of the placenta that remains attached should be carefully removed. The cavity of the uterus itself can be lavaged with a physiological saline solution containing a dilute antiseptic such as a povidone-iodine solution. Hemostasis should be established throughout the procedure. Each vessel should be ligated individually so as to control as much hemorrhage as possible during the procedure.

The first layer of closure is a simple continuous pattern using a very strong absorbable suture material. This suture line should be very tight since this will also help control hemorrhage. The uterus is then closed using a two layer inverting pattern such as a continuous Cushing or a continuous Lembert suture pattern, again using a heavy absorbable material. It is preferable after the first layer of closure to cleanse the incision line with an antimicrobial solution of choice or a

physiological saline solution containing a dilute antiseptic. It is also necessary to check the entire uterus for any tears which should be repaired before the uterus is replaced within the abdomen.

The completely sutured uterus should be replaced within the abdominal cavity. At this point, oxytocin should be added to the intravenous fluids to encourage involution of the uterus. Each layer of the skin incision is then closed in the normal manner ensuring that all layers are properly apposed.

Postoperative care of the cesarean section patient should be aggressive in nature. Fluid therapy should be maintained until the patient is stable. Systemic antibiotics should be administered for at least 5 - 10 days along with a nonsteroidal anti-inflammatory such as flunixin meglumine. It is also important to make sure that the tetanus prophylaxis is current. Subsequent intrauterine infusions and cultures should be undertaken until all evidence of a bacterial metritis is eliminated.

Most mares, with proper surgical procedure, will survive a cesarean section. Due to the stress in the administration of anesthetics, foal survival rates from a cesarean section range from about 10 - 30%. If the cesarean section was an elective instead of an emergency situation, over half of the mares will again conceive and become pregnant. If a vaginal delivery is going to be very traumatic to the mare, do not delay in the decision to consider a cesarean section. Even though this seems to be a harsh step, the survivability of the mare through this procedure may depend on the prompt decision and action by the staff at the breeding farm.

Artwork by S. Hakola / J. Dirig
Copyright Equistar Publications, Ltd.

Initial Neonatal Examination

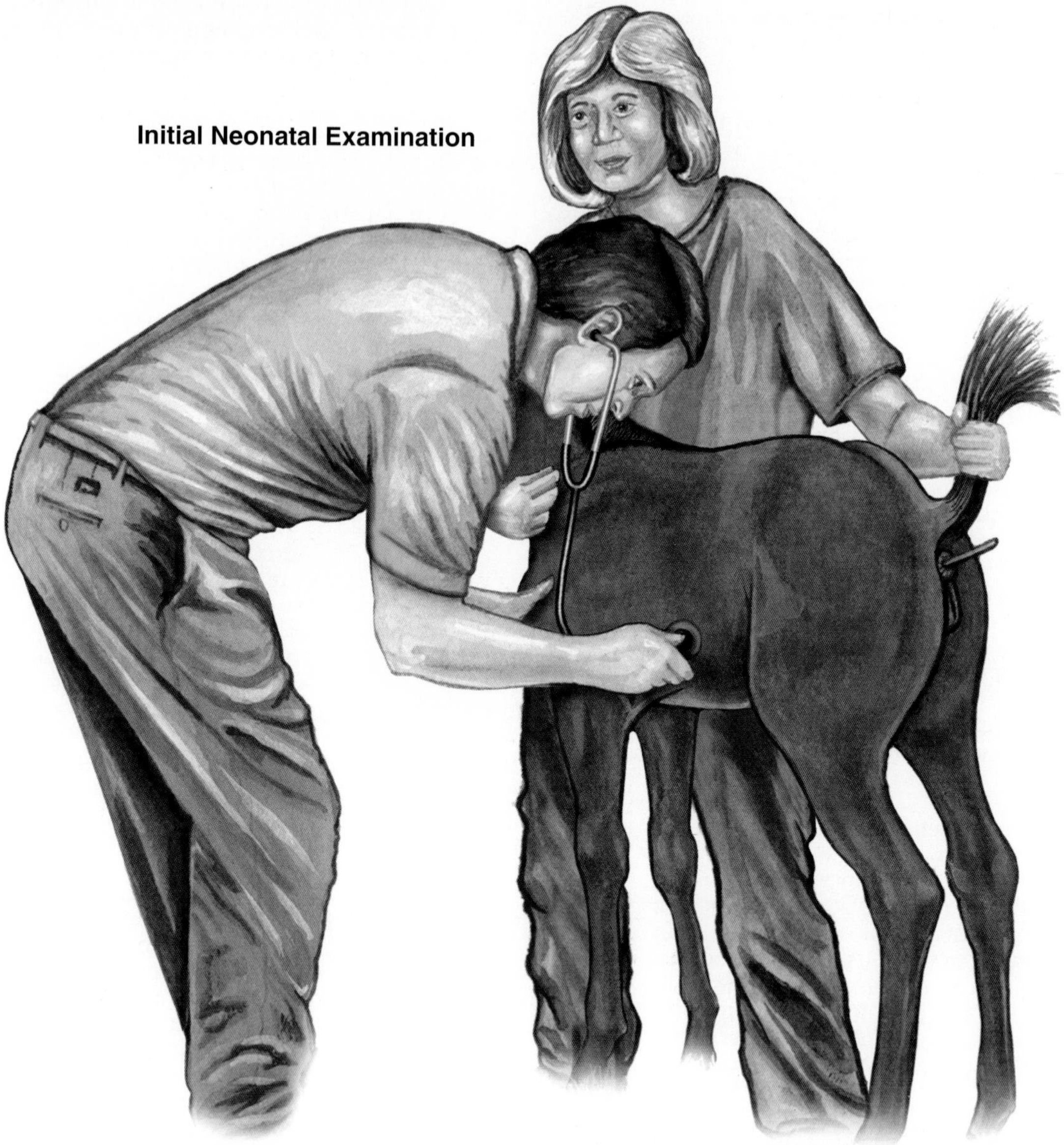

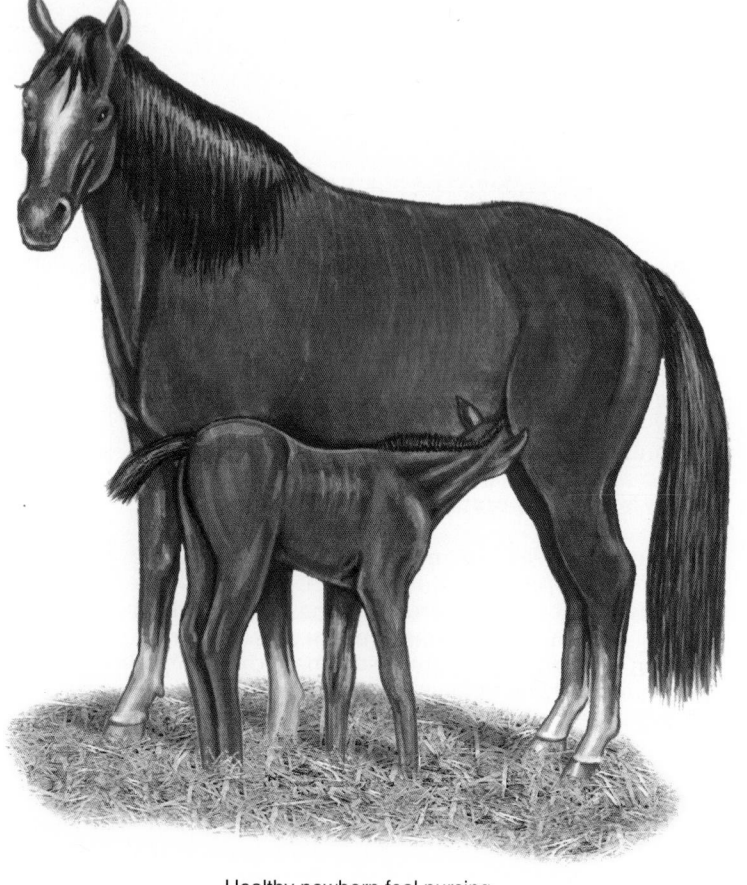

Healthy newborn foal nursing

Initial neonatal examination with assistant properly restraining newborn foal.
Veterinarian is auscultating the bowel soundswhile a rectal temperare is being taken.

3

Foal Disorders

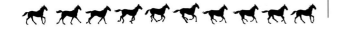

INITIAL NEONATAL EXAM

During parturition, the neonatal foal emerges from a protected intrauterine fluid environment to an external gaseous environment. This change of environment challenges the foal's ability to survive. Numerous common disorders in the foal are made evident during this neonatal pediatric period. These disorders can involve the immune system, the gastrointestinal system, and the musculoskeletal system. The foal will be challenged by numerous viruses and bacteria. Neurological problems may become evident during this initial time frame of life. Urinary tract disorders and respiratory disorders will also be manifested. Congenital malformation or deformities of the limbs may be obvious. Early recognition of these different disorders and their proper diagnosis will be vital to proper management of these problems.

It is important to evaluate the foal immediately after birth with a thorough physical exam. Proper restraint of the foal is done by placing one arm around the chest and simultaneously pulling the tail up over the back. With a minimal disturbance, this will allow sufficient restraint to perform a thorough physical examination.

Both eyes should be checked for any evidence of any congenital ocular problems. Entropion, or turning in of the lids, will sometimes be noted. This is a common finding when the foal is slightly dehydrated. Congenital cataracts are probably the most common problems noted within the eye of a newborn foal. These may be caused from trauma, infection, nutritional, or even hereditary causes.

The mucous membranes within the oral cavity should be checked and capillary refill time should be normal (within one or two seconds.) The oral cavity should also be inspected for any malocclusions or evidence of a cleft palate.

The heart should be auscultated. Normal heart rate should range from 60 - 110 beats per minute, but this level could be elevated due to the stress of restraining the foal. It is not uncommon to auscultate a systolic heart murmur even up to two months after birth. This is considered to be a normal finding.

Auscultation of the lungs is very difficult because there may be some fluid retained within the pulmonary cavity immediately following birth. During the first hour after birth, it is typical for the respiratory rate of the foal to reach 70 breaths per minute. Usually an hour after parturition, this rate has fallen to 25 or 30 breaths per minute in the unstressed foal.

The abdomen should be palpated and auscultated to determine normal gastrointestinal movement. Discovery of a tender abdomen may be the first sign of a gastrointestinal impaction or a urinary tract problem.

Normal rectal temperature for the foal is 100 - 102.5 degrees Fahrenheit. This range is normal from birth to 4 - 5 days of age. Any rectal temperature reading above this should be investigated further as to its cause. Subnormal temperatures below 99.5 degrees are definitely cause for concern.

It is normal for a foal to not pass urine up to six hours after birth. Frequent urination and dilute urine is also normal in a newborn foal. An observation should be made to ensure that there is no communication between the urinary bladder and the umbilicus.

The entire musculoskeletal system should be examined. Any evidence of congenital disorders should be diagnosed and treated accordingly.

DISORDERS OF THE IMMUNE SYSTEM

When the foal enters the world, his immune system is totally naive and vulnerable to all of the pathogens within its environment. Mother nature has provided a way of temporarily protecting the newborn foal against those pathogens by providing him with passive immunity from the mare's colostral immunoglobulins. This temporary

Failure of Passive Transfer of Immunoglobulins; Neonatal Isoerythrolysis

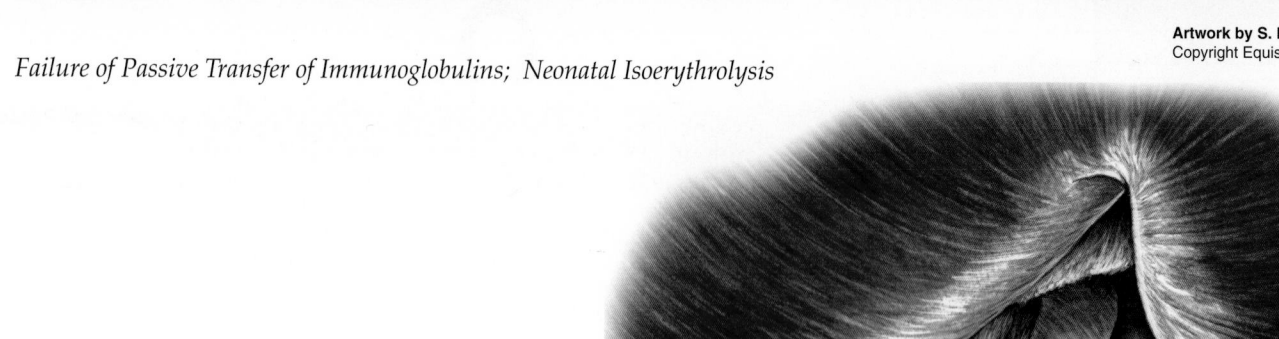

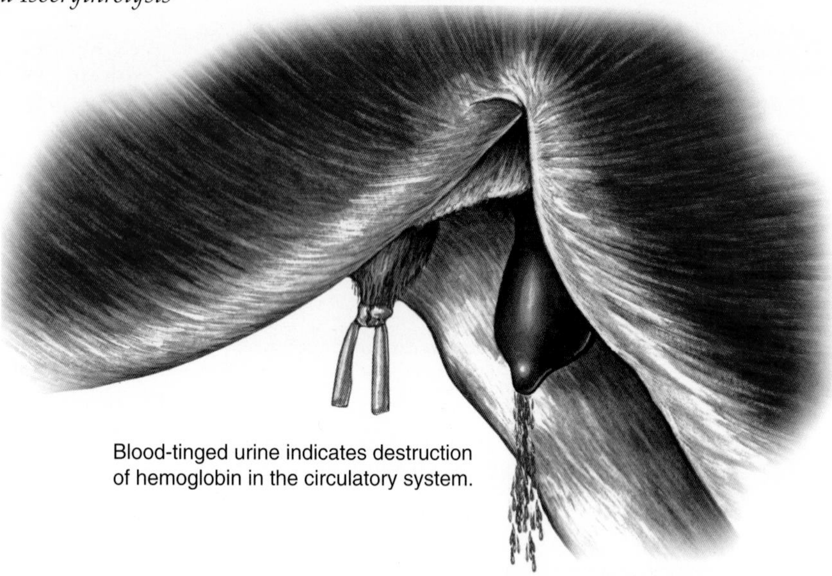

Blood-tinged urine indicates destruction of hemoglobin in the circulatory system.

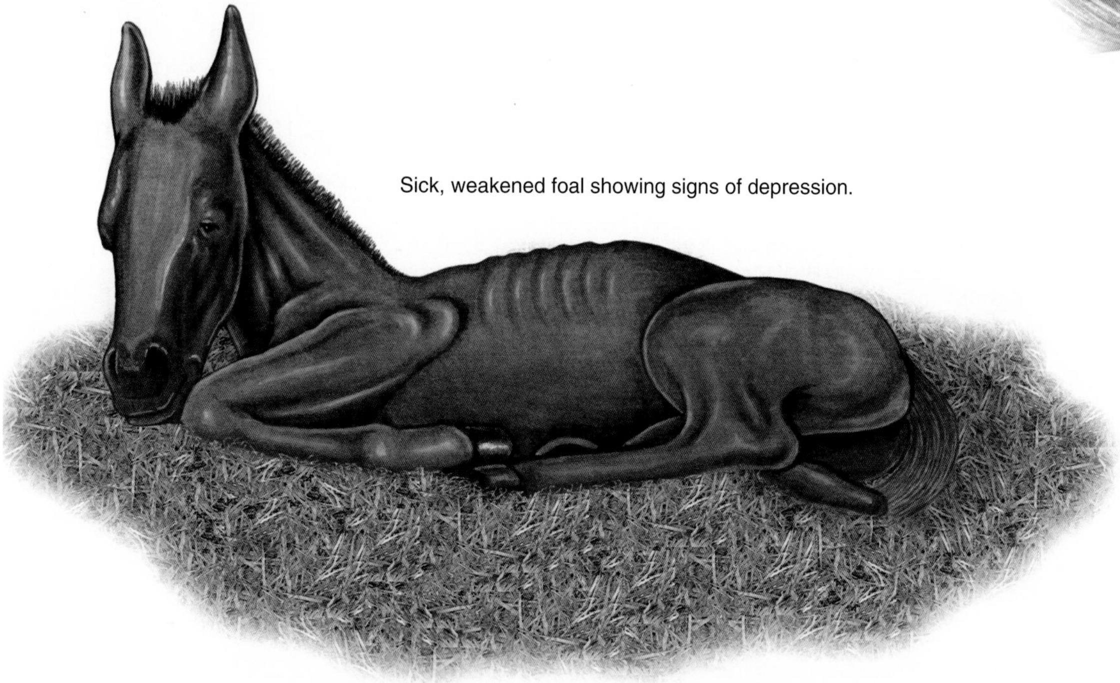

Sick, weakened foal showing signs of depression.

Neonatal Isoerythrolysis

Failure of Passive Transfer of Immunoglobulins

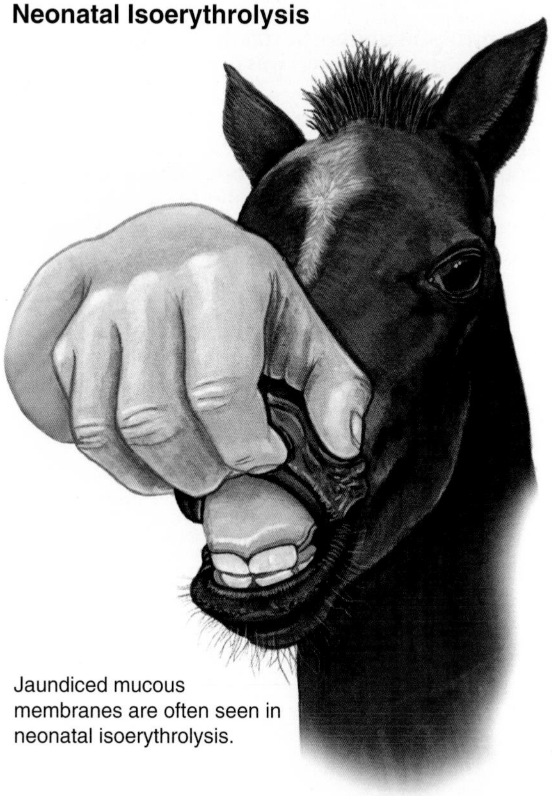

Jaundiced mucous membranes are often seen in neonatal isoerythrolysis.

immunity will protect the foal until its own immune system can mature sufficiently to meet the environmental challenges. Any deficiencies in the colostral antibodies or failure of this passive transfer of immunoglobulins exposes the foal to the pathogens within its environment.

In addition to providing the foal with passive transfer of immunity, the colostrum from the mare may contain antibodies to the foal's red blood cells. This disorder is termed neonatal isoerythrolysis.

Combined immunodeficiency is a hereditary disorder that occurs primarily within the Arabian breeds. The incidence of this immunodeficiency is low because it is an autosomal recessive trait. Both parents have to be carriers for the manifestation of this disorder to be present. Approximately 25% of the Arabian horses in this country may be carriers. This condition results from the failure of production of both T and B lymphocytes.

FAILURE OF PASSIVE TRANSFER OF IMMUNOGLOBULINS

During the first 6 - 12 hours after birth, the foal receives his immunity from the colostral immunoglobulins. It has been estimated that between 8 - 12 hours after birth the foal will consume 1 - 2 liters of colostrum. On most large farms, it is advantageous to maintain a colostrum bank where colostrum collected from numerous mares is dated and frozen to be used when needed. Colostrum from several different mares can be combined and administered orally to the foal approximately 6 hours after birth. This provides a smorgasbord of immunity from several different mares.

Clinical Signs

Clinical signs that the foal has had a failure of passive transfer includethe following: foals with slightly elevated temperatures, foals that are weak, and foals that are presenting signs of early

septicemia. The mare's udder should be examined and a determination should be made whether the foal has suckled in a timely fashion or not.

Diagnosis

Diagnosis can be made through the use of a blood test to detect a failure of passive transfer. A blood sample should be obtained from the foal between 18 - 24 hours after birth. This test will determine the level of immunoglobulin G (IgG) within the foal's plasma. Any blood sample that has less than 800 mg/dL indicates failure of passive transfer. Values that are less than 400 mg/dL reflect an almost total failure of passive transfer, whereas those levels between 400 - 800 mg/dL are considered suboptimal predisposing the foal to an infection from a variety of bacteria.

Treatment

Treatment of passive transfer failure involves providing this foal with immunoglobulins. Colostrum can be administered orally or via a nasogastric tube if the foal is resistant. Commercially available lyophilized equine IgG can also be administered orally. If the foal is more than 12 hours old, oral supplementation of colostrum or serum will usually be ineffective because the gastrointestinal tract has closed itself off to immunoglobulin transfer.

When a failure of passive transfer has been detected on a foal older than 12 hours, serum transfusion of immunoglobulins may be indicated. Commercially available products of normal equine plasma can be administered very slowly intravenously. A sufficient volume of this plasma should be given to achieve the desired concentration of immunoglobulins in the foal. Constant testing should be undertaken to determine the level of IgG within the foal's circulatory system to ensure adequate concentrations of IgG.

When failure of passive transfer of immunoglobulins has been diagnosed, the foal should be immediately started on systemic antibiotic therapy. Care should be taken to not be

too overzealous in this endeavor since constant antimicrobial use will lead to development of resistant strains of bacteria or cause other gastrointestinal problems.

NEONATAL ISOERYTHROLYSIS

Etiology

This condition results in the destruction of the foal's own red blood cells by colostral maternal antibodies. After these antibodies are absorbed, they attack and destroy the foal's red blood cells. This condition occurs more commonly in mares that have had numerous foals.

Clinical Signs

The onset of clinical signs are variable depending on the amount of antibody that is ingested and absorbed from the mare. The foal will usually start to appear listless and have a decreased appetite. Respiratory and heart rates will be elevated, but the rectal temperature of the foal will remain normal. There may be a change in color in the foal's urine because the hemoglobin from the destroyed red blood cells is being passed through the urinary system. As the condition progresses, the mucous membranes will appear jaundiced. A blood sample from the foal will reveal a packed cell volume of less than 22%, and the plasma will appear icteric.

Diagnosis

Diagnostic tests for neonatal isoerythrolysis must demonstrate the presence of maternal anti-red blood cell antibody. This anti-red blood cell antibody can be detected in the mare's plasma, serum, or colostrum. A direct Coomb's antiglobulin test can be performed on the foal's blood to detect the presence of antibody on the foal's red blood cells.

Neonatal Isoerythrolysis

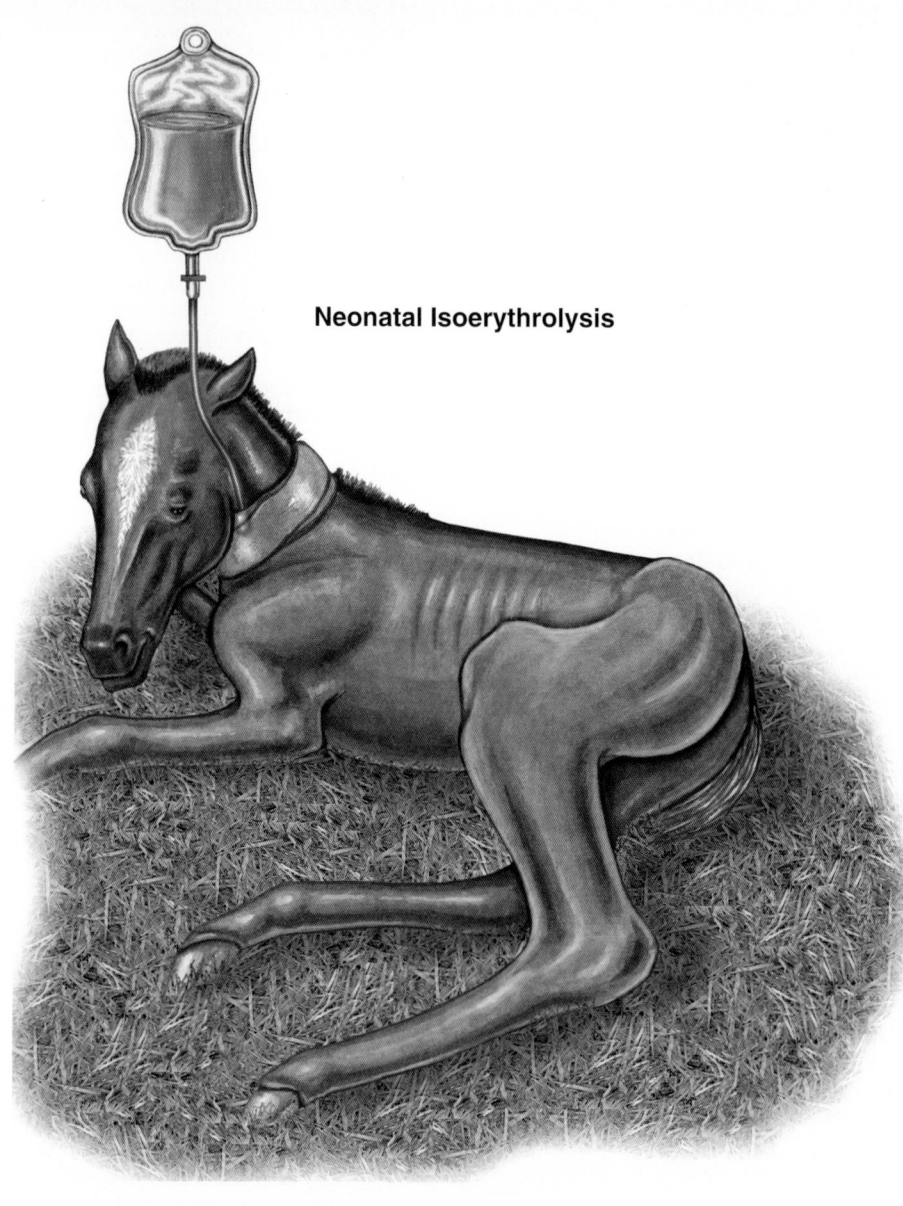

Treatment of neonatal isoerythrolysis with blood transfusions.

Meconium Retention

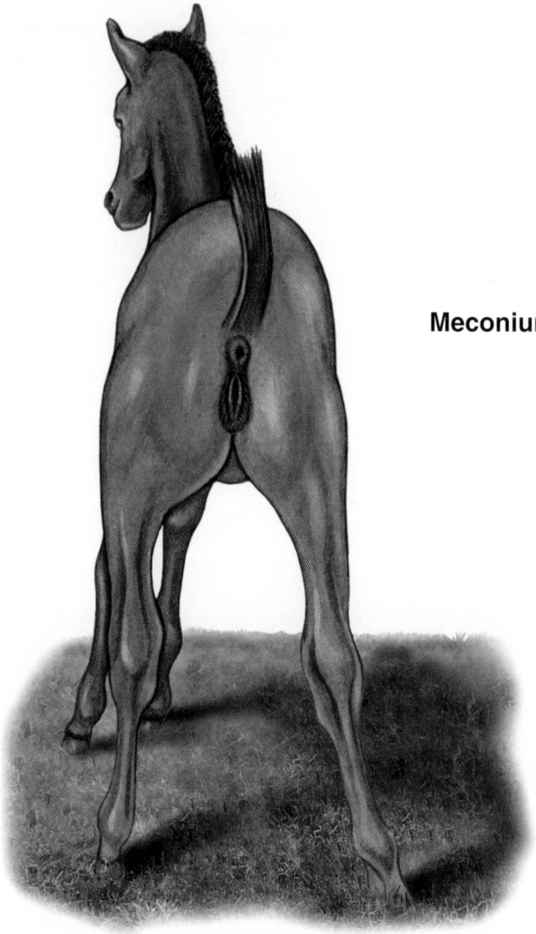

Foal straining to pass meconium.

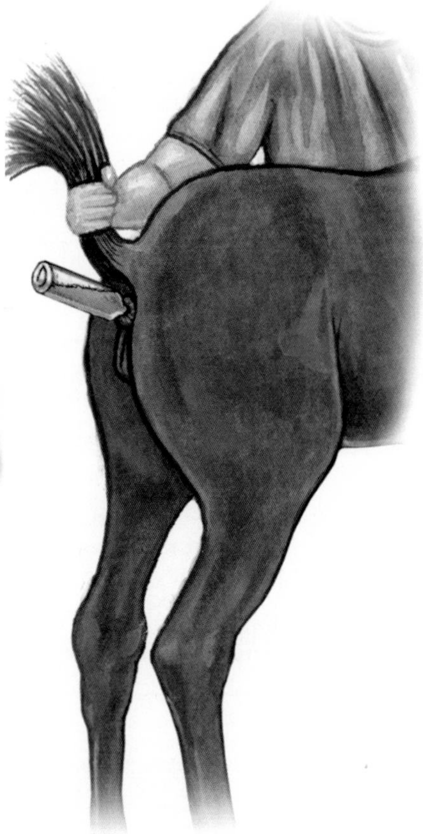

Enema administration in lower meconium retained cases.

Treatment

Treatment of affected foals involves the provision of intensive supportive care and a transfusion of red blood cells from an appropriate donor. Intravenous fluid therapy should be initiated with a combination of balanced electrolytes and glucose. Systemic antimicrobial therapy as well as nursing care to the foal should also be initiated.

Cross matching with a donor mare should be undertaken to provide an appropriate source of blood for the foal. An appropriate donor mare should be identified, and 4 - 8 liters of blood should be collected from her. The donor's red blood cells can then be washed using a 3.8% sodium citrate or acid citrate dextrose solution using one part solution to each nine parts of blood. This procedure is accomplished through the use of a centrifuge. The red blood cells and plasma are separated and the RBCs are harvested. The red blood cells are then washed and administered intravenously to the foal through the use of an administration set with a filter. It is important to perform an IgG test to determine if there is also a concurrent failure of passive transfer in these foals.

COMBINED IMMUNODEFICIENCY

Combined immunodeficiency is a lethal hereditary disorder that primarily occurs within the Arabian or part Arabian breeds. This is actually a failure of the immune system. It is an inherited condition where both the sire and the dam of an infected foal are carriers of this genetic trait. Unfortunately, there are no available tests to identify this genetic trait until a specific mating produces an afflicted foal.

These foals appear normal at birth. They have a passive immunity transfer from the colostrum and the IgG levels do not decline until the foal is about 2 - 3 months of age. This condition results in the failure of the foal to produce T and B lymphocytes which provide him with immunity.

The foal that suffers with combined immunodeficiency will usually present at 2 - 3 months of age with a nonresponsive respiratory condition that just does not seem to improve. Unfortunately, other than a bone marrow transplant, there is no treatment for this disorder. Early diagnosis can save expense to the owner. Proper histopathologic examinations of the thymus, lymph nodes, and spleen will identify this foal as suffering from combined immunodeficiency. Subsequent matings between this particular mare and stallion can then be avoided.

DISORDERS OF THE GASTROINTESTINAL SYSTEM

The three most common disorders occurring within the gastrointestinal system of the foal are retention of the meconium, diarrhea, and gastroduodenal ulcers. If the foal exhibits any symptoms of abdominal pain, it is important to obtain an accurate diagnosis and proceed with the correct treatment of the problem. With any disturbance of the gastrointestinal tract in the foal, it is always important to assess the hydration level of the foal immediately and administer appropriate fluid therapy to correct any deficiencies.

MECONIUM RETENTION

The meconium is the light brown to greenish - black contents within the bowel of the newborn. While the foal is suspended within the fluid environment of the mare, it ingests amniotic fluid, glandular secretions, and mucus. Under normal conditions, the newborn foal will pass this substance from the bowel usually within 2 - 3 hours after birth.

Clinical Signs

Initially the foal will appear restless. Observation will reveal a straining to defecate in which the foal will arch his back and walk around the stall with its tail elevated. Both the heart and respiratory rates will be increased. Auscultation of the abdomen will reveal a lack of intestinal sounds in some areas and hyperperistalsis in other areas. As the condition worsens, the foal will exhibit abdominal pain much as an adult horse would with colic. The foal will repeatedly lie down and get up or may even roll and place itself in an upside down position.

Diagnosis

Diagnosis is based on a digital rectal exam, reflux through the nasogastric tube, abdominocentesis, and possibly an ultrasonographic examination of the foal's abdomen. A differential diagnosis should be made between a simple meconium retention, a colon torsion, an intussusception, a ruptured urinary bladder, or a diaphragmatic hernia.

Treatment

If the meconium retention occurs within the lower portion of the bowel, treatment usually consists of 1 - 2 pints of an enema-type solution administered rectally. A soft flexible tube should be gently inserted into the rectum as far as possible and the enema administered through gravity flow. Another technique involves the use of a foley catheter. A size thirty French foley catheter is inserted into the rectum approximately 2 inches and the 30 cc balloon is then inflated. Approximately 8 - 12 ounces of an enema-type solution is administered and allowed to remain in the bowel for approximately 20 - 30 minutes. The balloon is then deflated and the catheter removed to allow the foal to defecate. Unless the foal is uncontrollable, it is inadvisable to use any type of sedation during this procedure since sedation will also have a depressive effect on the musculature of the bowel.

If meconium retention has occurred in the upper part of the bowel, it is necessary to pass a nasogastric tube to the stomach of the foal. A solution of mineral oil and electrolytes (approximately 8 - 12 ounces) should then be administered via the nasogastric tube. Systemic intravenous fluid therapy should also be utilized in a high meconium retention case. One to two liters

Diarrhea

Artwork by S. Hakola / J. Dirig
Copyright Equistar Publications, Ltd.

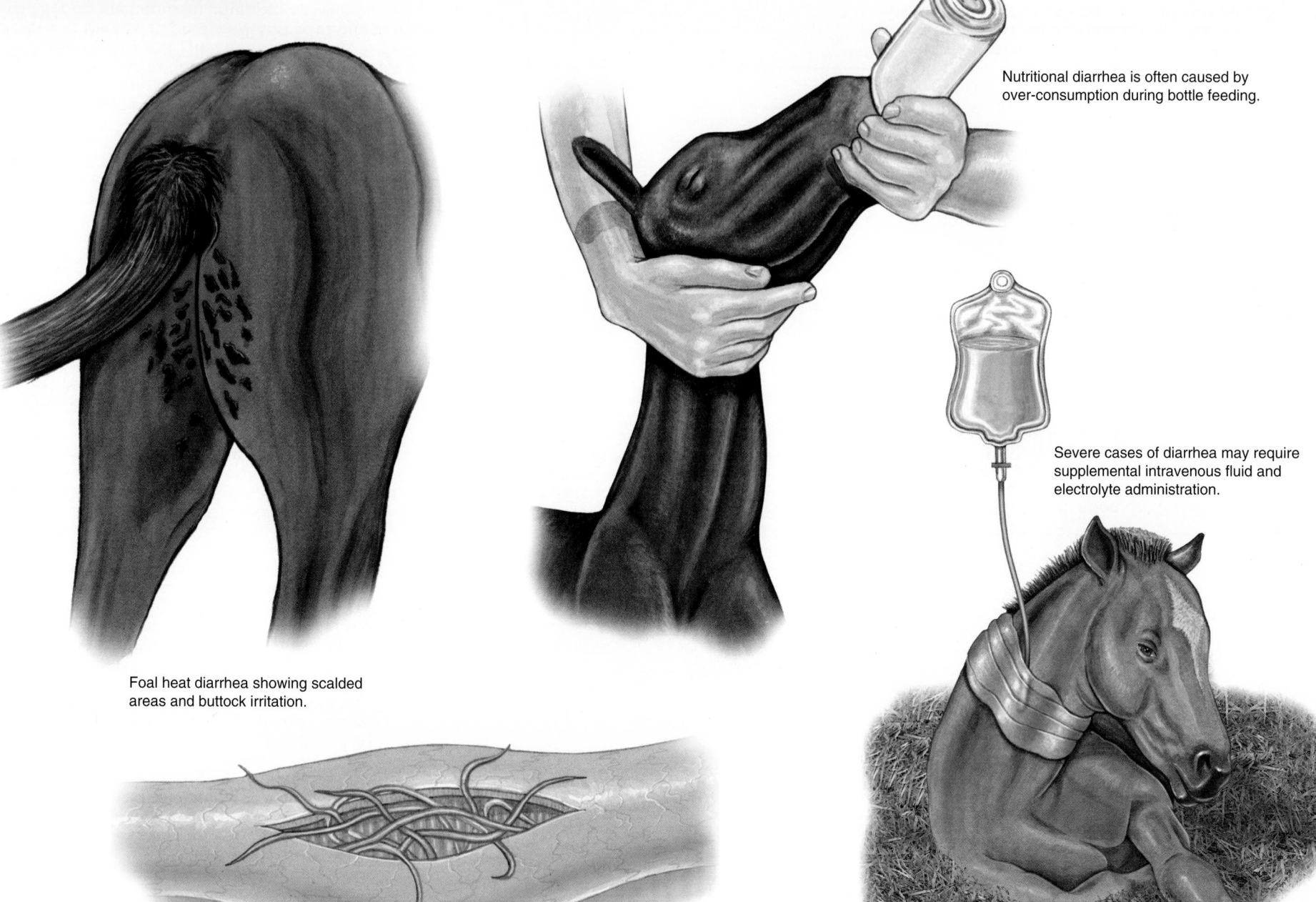

Nutritional diarrhea is often caused by over-consumption during bottle feeding.

Severe cases of diarrhea may require supplemental intravenous fluid and electrolyte administration.

Foal heat diarrhea showing scalded areas and buttock irritation.

Parascaris infestation of the small intestine.

of a warm lactated Ringers solution should be administered slowly intravenously.

Most meconium retentions can be prevented through the administration of a small enema shortly after birth. This will soften the initial stool and prevent many of the lower retained meconiums. In all cases, hydration of the foal should be monitored closely. Any imbalances should be corrected through appropriate fluid therapy.

DIARRHEA

Etiology

Diarrhea in the foal can be caused by nutritional factors, parasites, bacteria, viruses, and "foal heat". In all cases of diarrhea in the foal, it is necessary to assess the hydration state of the foal and provide appropriate fluid therapy when needed. A thorough physical examination is important when dealing with diarrhea in the foal to determine whether it is a systemic septicemia, a nutritional problem, or parasitic in nature. This examination should include blood work, blood cultures, and fecal examinations.

Foal Heat Diarrhea

Foal heat diarrhea occurs most frequently between 5 - 10 days of age and usually corresponds to the mare's first postpartum estrus. Clinically, the foal is bright and alert and shows no sign of any discomfort. The rectal temperature of the foal is normal as is any blood work that is taken on the foal. This diarrhea usually lasts 2 - 5 days then disappears. The only treatment that is required is to cleanse the perineum of the foal and apply a soothing ointment to these tissues.

Nutritional Diarrhea

A nutritional cause of diarrhea in the foal most commonly occurs when the foal has consumed an excessive amount of milk. This occurs when the foal has been separated from the mare for a period of time, an overfeeding, or when a change in milk replacer in ill or orphaned foals has taken place. A nutritional diarrhea may also occur in the foal when there is a major change in the diet of the mare (such as a change of the type of pasture used or an abrupt change in grain.) Foreign material such as sand or dirt can be ingested by the foal and may cause a transient diarrhea to occur. This can be easily determined by a fecal exam for grit or sand. In almost all cases of these nutritional diarrheas, maintenance of the foal's hydration, possible oral administration of electrolytes, and something to coat the bowel may be all that is needed to treat these cases. Kaolin and pectin can be administered at a dose rate of 4 ounces / 45 kilograms orally every 2 - 3 hours and usually is sufficient to provide a protective bowel coating.

Parasitic Diarrhea

Three parasites can be responsible for causing diarrhea in the foal. They are *Strongyloides westeri, Parascaris equorum,* and *Cryptosporidium spp.* In the case of *Strongyloides westeri,* diarrhea in the foal occurs at 1 - 4 weeks of age. Transmission consists of larvae being passed in the mare's milk at approximately four days postpartum with a peak at 10 - 12 days. A diagnosis is obtained by flotation of a fresh fecal sample obtained from the foal at approximately 24 - 30 days of age. Treatment consists of worming the foal with an appropriate commercially available wormer. It has been documented that the administration of an Ivermectin wormer to the mare on the day of parturition usually prevents transmission of this parasite to the foal. Infestations of *Parascaris equorum* occurs when the foal is just a few weeks of age. Heaviest infestations of this parasite occurs when the foal is about to be weaned. In some cases of heavy infestation, diarrhea from this parasite is possible. When a foal has a failure of passive transfer of immunoglobulins or suffers from an immunodeficiency, *Cryptosporidium spp.* can manifest itself as a diarrhea in the foal. Diagnosis is made through a fecal float with a sugar solution searching for the *Cryptosporidium spp.* oocysts. Supportive treatment is the only treatment available with the *Cryptosporidium spp.* parasite.

Bacterial Diarrhea

E. coli, Salmonella spp., Clostridium perfringens (type C), Clostridium difficile, and *Rhodococcus equi* bacteria are common causes of foal diarrhea. In almost all cases of bacterial diarrhea in the foal, a septicemia and/or endotoxemia occurs. In each case, a diagnosis can be made through the use of a fecal culture which will also determine which antibiotic is necessary to stop the infection. These foals will appear severely depressed, anorexic, and septicemic. Aggressive fluid therapy combined with oral and systemically administered antibiotics are necessary to successfully treat these foals. Intensive aggressive treatment and nursing care around the clock are necessary to provide supportive care to these foals.

Viral Diarrhea

The most common viral cause of diarrhea in foals is that caused by rotovirus. This virus can effect a foal that is only 1 - 2 days old and typically occurs when the foal is less than 2 months of age. It is usually seen in numerous foals within the same barn. Treatment of a viral induced diarrhea is no different than that caused from other etiologies. Rehydration should be accomplished using both oral and intravenous administration routes along with any supportive care that is needed. Antibiotics should be used judiciously to protect against a secondary bacterial infection. The bowel can be coated to help protect it through the use of kaolin, pectin, bismuth subsalicylate, and even the administration of activated charcoal.

Gastroduodenal Ulcers; Fetal Circulation

Artwork by S. Hakola / J. Dirig
Copyright Equistar Publications, Ltd.

Gastroduodenal Ulcers

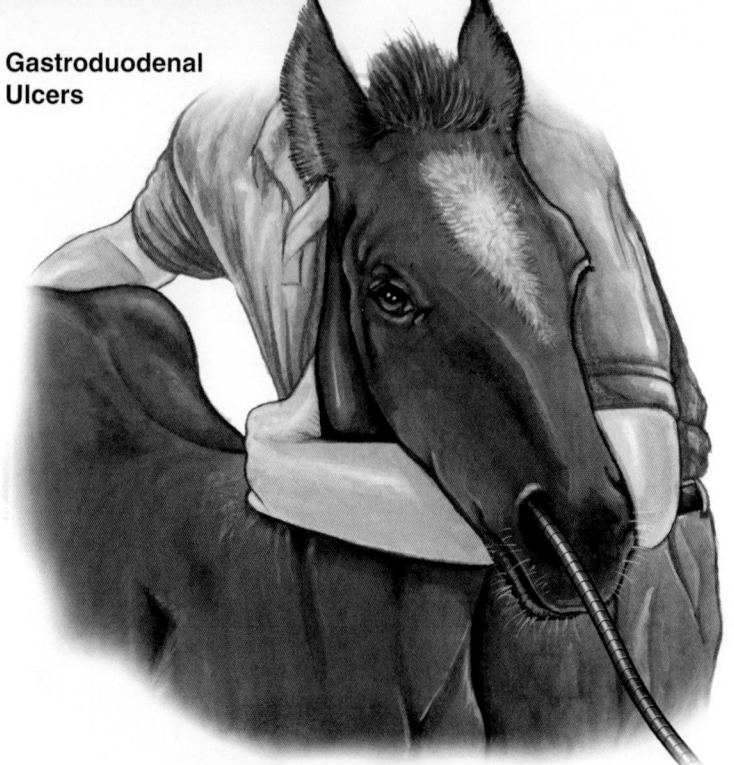

Foal undergoing gastric endoscopic examination while being properly restrained.

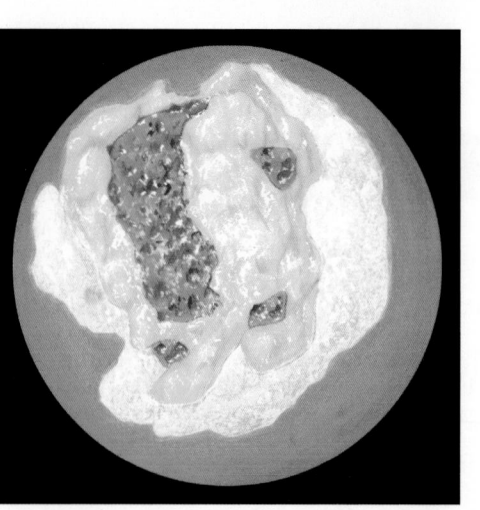

Gastroduodenal ulcer in a 7 day old foal as seen through the visual field of the scope.

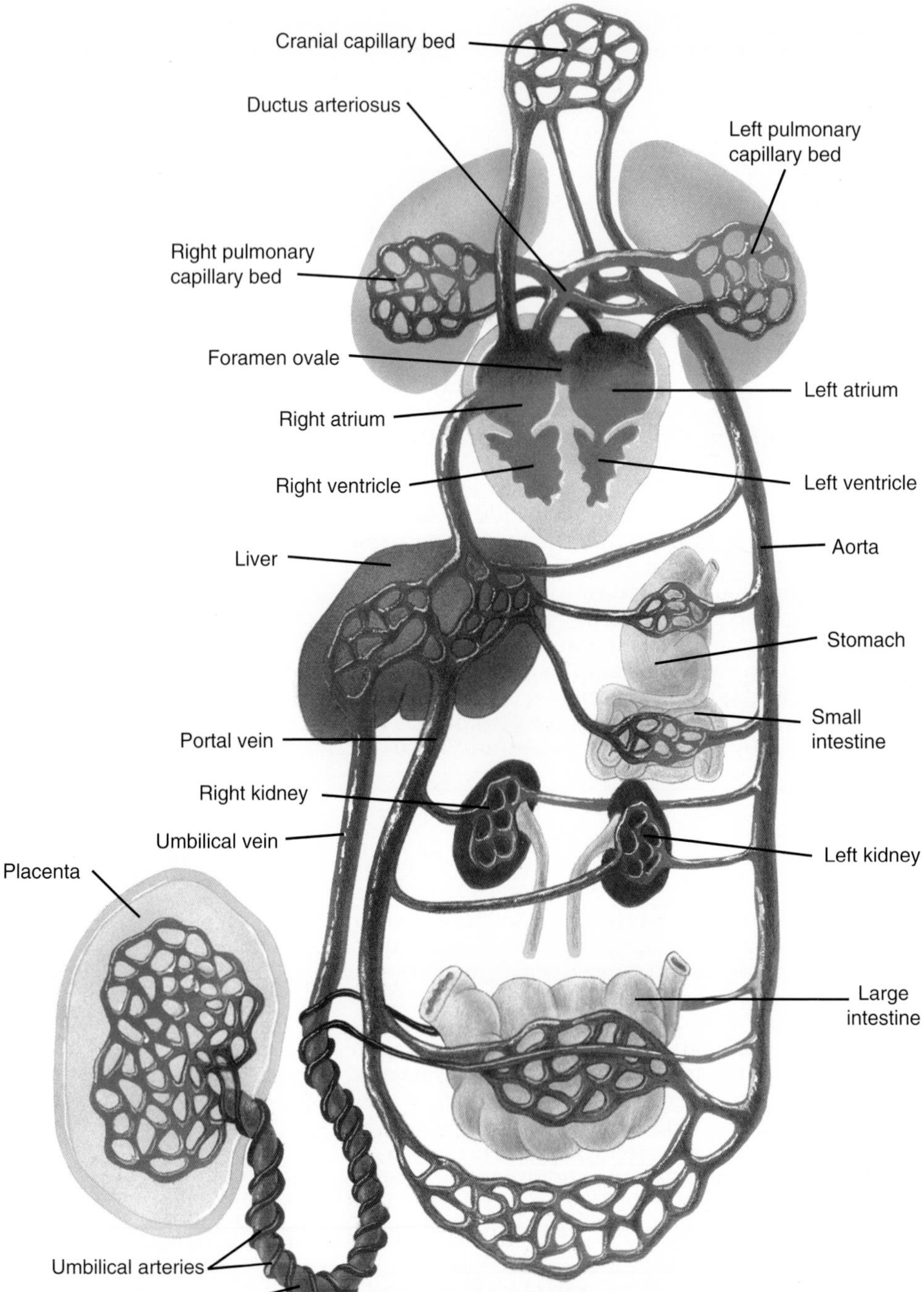

Cranial capillary bed

Ductus arteriosus

Left pulmonary capillary bed

Right pulmonary capillary bed

Foramen ovale

Left atrium

Right atrium

Right ventricle

Left ventricle

Liver

Aorta

Stomach

Portal vein

Small intestine

Right kidney

Umbilical vein

Left kidney

Placenta

Large intestine

Umbilical arteries

Umbilical cord

Schematic Rendering of Fetal Circulation

GASTRODUODENAL ULCERS

Etiology

The exact cause is unknown, but gastroduodenal ulcers may occur as sequelae to various bacterial infections or viruses. It is possible that these ulcers are simply due to a stress such as transporting or surgery. A history of nonsteroidal anti-inflammatory drug administration is commonly found in foals with gastroduodenal ulcers.

Clinical Signs

Clinically, diarrhea is the most common sign. The foal may excessively salivate and grind its teeth. There may be a slightly elevated temperature and a decrease in appetite. The foal may also appear to be in pain although it is not necessarily a colic-type pain that is manifested.

Diagnosis

The diagnosis is based on clinical signs, gastric reflux, gastroendoscopy, and sometimes contrast radiography. When a nasogastric tube is passed to the foal, a foul smelling hemorrhagic fluid may be refluxed out through the tube. Gastroendoscopy will provide a way of directly visualizing the ulcers. Radiographic findings may include delayed gastric emptying and a large gastric silhouette on the film.

Treatment

The goal of treatment of these ulcers is to decrease the gastric acid secretion, provide an antacid for the gastrointestinal environment, and protect the mucosa. Pharmaceuticals such as Cimetidine and Ranitidine can be utilized to decrease the gastric acids. Mylanta II and Maalox can be used to provide an antacid for the stomach environment and Carafate can be administered 2 - 4 times a day orally to help protect the mucosa. Hydration should be assessed on a regular basis and any deficiencies should be corrected through the use of intravenous fluid therapy.

FETAL VERSUS NEONATAL CIRCULATION

The fetus lives in the aqueous environment of the uterus. Upon delivery, this neonate takes its first few breaths which results in a transformation from an aqueous environment to that which is gaseous. The neonate must now adapt a circulatory system to transport oxygen and nutrients from its gaseous environment to all the structures within the body.

Fetal Circulation

The circulatory system within the fetus is characterized by multiple adaptations which minimize the blood flow through the nonfunctional vascular beds. In the fetus, the functions of the neonatal lung tissues and the liver are accomplished by the placenta. Therefore, these two organ systems in particular are relatively nonfunctional in the uterus and require minimal circulation.

The terms vein and artery with reference to fetal circulation need clarification. Arteries usually carry oxygen-enriched blood while veins carry oxygen-depleted blood. Therefore, arteries carry blood from the heart while veins carry blood to the heart. In the fetal tissue structures, the lungs are nonfunctional. Gas transport is carried out within the placental tissues. Oxygenated fetal blood is carried by veins to the heart, whereas deoxygenated blood is transported via the umbilical arteries to the placenta.

One of the first structures that can be noted utilizing ultrasonography is the beating fetal heart. The heart originates from the fusing of two tubes within the embryo's chest. Eventually this muscular structure is partitioned into four chambers: the right and left atria and the right and left ventricles. The umbilical vein transports oxygenated blood from the placenta into the right atrium. It is here that the foramen ovale allows approximately 2/3 of the blood to pass out of the right atrium into the left atrium. This allows delivery to the heart, the head, and the upper torso of the fetus. The remaining 1/3 of the blood passes

through the right ventricle and is shunted across the ductus arteriosus which feeds into the descending aorta to profuse the abdominal viscera and lower extremities. These two shunts allow blood to be diverted away from the nonfunctional pulmonary circulation into systems requiring circulation within the fetus.

Neonatal Circulation

Immediately after parturition, the foal gasps and respiration within its gaseous environment begins. The foal now has to adapt to a gaseous exchange across the lung tissue instead of through the placental membranes. There is a dramatic increase in pulmonary blood flow that coincides with a decrease in pulmonary vascular resistance. Circulation throughout the placenta is eliminated, and the vascular resistance increases throughout the systemic neonatal circulation. The blood that is returning to the right atrium now flows through pulmonary circulation rather than across the ductus arteriosus. The foramen ovale closes when the left atrial pressure exceeds the pressure within the right atrium. Some blood leaving the left ventricle will still encounter a patent ductus arteriosus. The ductus arteriosus will usually close by day four or five of age.

Immediately following birth, the newborn's heart rate will range 40 - 80 beats per minute. Within the first few hours of birth, that heart rate will increase to 120 - 150 beats per minute. During the first week of life, the heart rate will then plateau to approximately 80 - 100 beats per minute. It is not unusual to detect the presence of a sinus arrhythmia immediately following birth. This should disappear within the first 24 hours. As the ductus arteriosus closes, a systolic murmur that may range in intensity from a grade one to a grade four may be detected during the first week of life. If a cardial murmur persists after one week of age, one should suspect a congenital cardiac defect.

Artwork By S. Hakola / J. Dirig
Copyright Equistar Publications, Ltd.

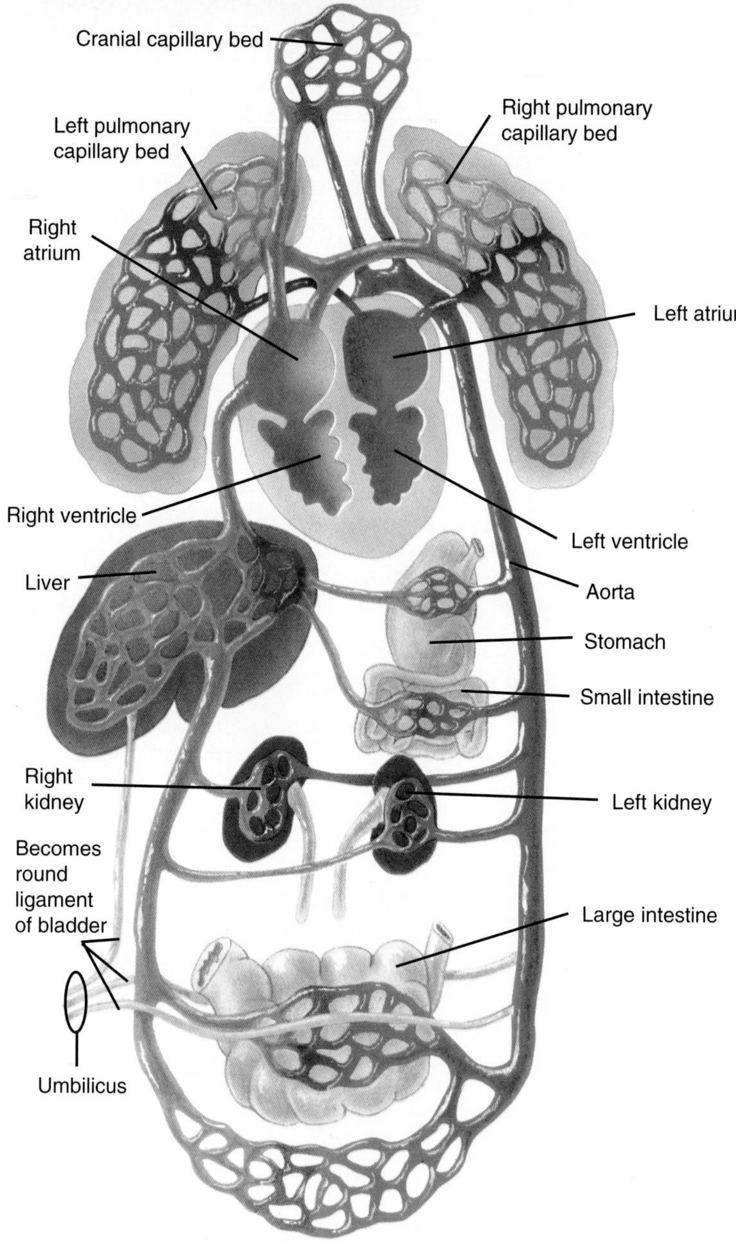

Cranial capillary bed

Left pulmonary capillary bed

Right pulmonary capillary bed

Right atrium

Left atrium

Right ventricle

Left ventricle

Aorta

Liver

Stomach

Small intestine

Right kidney

Left kidney

Becomes round ligament of bladder

Large intestine

Umbilicus

Schematic Rendering of Neonatal Circulation

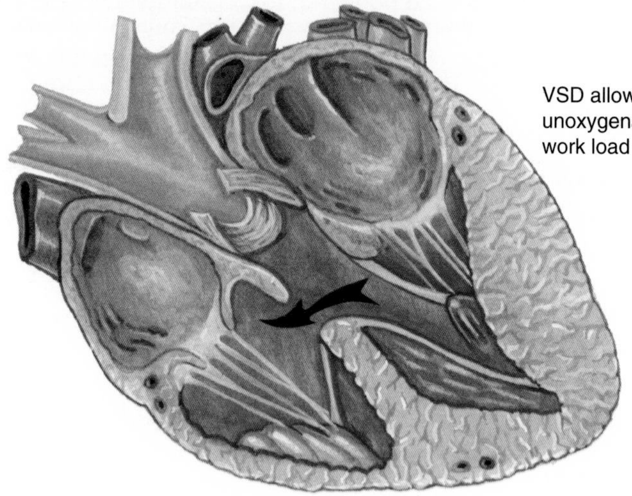

VSD allows oxygenated blood to mix with unoxygenated blood and increases the work load on the right side of the heart.

Ventricular Septal Defect

ASD allows mixture of unoxygenated blood with oxygenated blood in the left atrium.

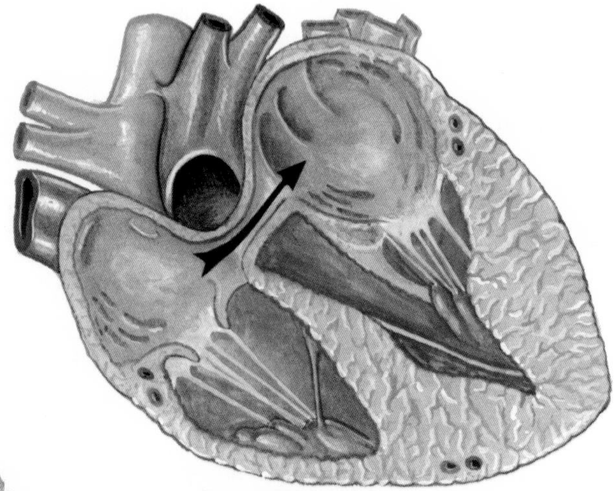

Atrial Septal Defect

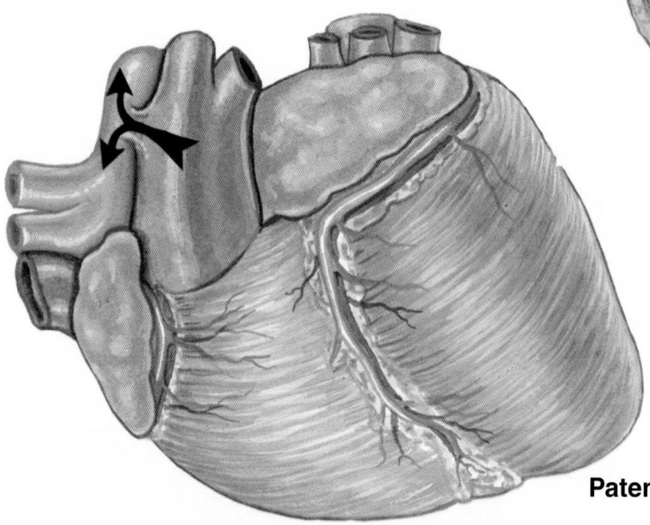

PDA allows unoxygenated blood supposedly going to the lungs to mix with oxygenated blood being transported throughout the rest of the body.

Patent Ductus Arteriosus

CONGENITAL CARDIAC ABNORMALITIES

Congenital cardiac deformities can be simple and include a ventricular septal defect, a patent ductus arteriosus, a patent foramen ovale, or an atrial septal defect. Complex defects such as tetralogy of Fallot and tricuspid atresia can also be noted. Vascular anomalies which include a persistent right aortic arch and anomalous coronary arteries can also be diagnosed. An accurate diagnosis usually requires a combination of a thorough physical exam of the cardiovascular system and diagnostic aids such as electrocardiograms, thoracic radiographs, echocardiography, and cardiac catheterization or angiography.

Ventricular Septal Defect

This congenital cardiac disorder can occur by itself or in conjunction with other defects such as tetralogy of Fallot. Upon physical exam, a loud holosystolic murmur is usually detected over the left heart base. The electrocardiogram is often normal or only contains small defects. The echocardiogram may also be normal or have only small defects within it. Larger septal defects produce an increased diastolic dimension or volume of the left atrium and both left and right ventricles. Cardiac catheterization can confirm the diagnosis of ventricular septal defect in that the oxygen saturation in the pulmonary artery and right ventricle is greater than that in the right atrium or great veins. Foals that have a 5 - 6 mm ventricular septal defect usually carry a good prognosis for a normal life. Any foals that have a larger defect have a poor prognosis for survival and are always predisposed to left heart failure.

Patent Ductus Arteriosus

The ductus arteriosus shunts blood from the pulmonary artery to the aorta. Therefore, a continuous murmur can be localized over the left heart base between the third and fourth intercostal spaces. A right heart catheterization will reveal an increased pressure within the right ventricle. An injection of radiopaque contrast medium at the aortic root will result in opacification of the aorta and pulmonary artery. This can be detected utilizing radiography. The degree of shunting within the ductus arteriosus dictates the prognosis of these foals.

Tetralogy of Fallot

There are four defects of the heart that exist concurrently which comprise the tetrology of Fallot: a ventricular septal defect, a repositioning of the aorta to override the ventricular septal defect, a hypoplastic pulmonary artery, and secondary right ventricular hypertrophy. Auscultation of the heart will reveal a systolic ejection murmur along the left heart base. A simple physical exam will reveal a slight jugular venous pulse. Radiographs will depict a mild to moderate enlargement of the heart and decreased pulmonary vascularity. The electrocardiogram will reveal a right ventricular hypertrophy which is indicated by negative QRS complexes on leads I,II, and VF. Echocardiography will reveal a right ventricular dilation, a ventricular septal defect, and an overriding aorta. Survival for foals with tetrology of Fallot is very difficult. If an accurate diagnosis is obtained, euthanasia is usually the most rational recommendation.

Tricuspid Atresia

A symmetrical cyanosis is noted upon physical exam either at rest or following a very mild exertion. Those foals are dyspniec and have a weak pulse. There is a holosystolic murmur along the left heart base. An electrocardiogram usually results in an increased p-wave amplitude and increased QRS amplitudes due to left ventricular enlargement. Radiographs are typically normal. Echocardiography will usually reveal an enlarged left ventricle, a very small right ventricle, and a ventricular septal defect. In all cases, if the diagnosis is accurate, euthanasia is recommended.

Atrial Septal Defect

Foals that suffer from atrial septal defect usually exhibit no outward clinical signs. This defect is caused by a failure of the closure of the foramen ovale. Anatomically, the foramen ovale closes within 15 days to nine weeks after birth. The lack of closure produces the atrial septal defect and permits blood to shunt left to right in the area of the foramen ovale. This defect overloads the pulmonary valve and in extreme cases, may produce a holosystolic murmur. Echocardiography can distinguish the presence of an atrial septal defect. There is a bright echo perpendicular to the site of discontinuity of the atrial septum. Angiography will reveal an opacification of the right atrium following venous administration of radiopaque contrast material.

Atrial septal defects along with other cardiac defects carry a hereditary nature with their occurrence. Even though these animals may survive to adulthood, breeding affected animals should be avoided. There is no successful surgical correction of this defect. Foals that are afflicted must be monitored closely and recommendations should be made according to all of the clinical signs.

Respiratory Distress Syndrome; Bacterial Pneumonia

Increased breathing effort is seen in the flared nostrils and use of neck and abdominal musculature during inspiration.

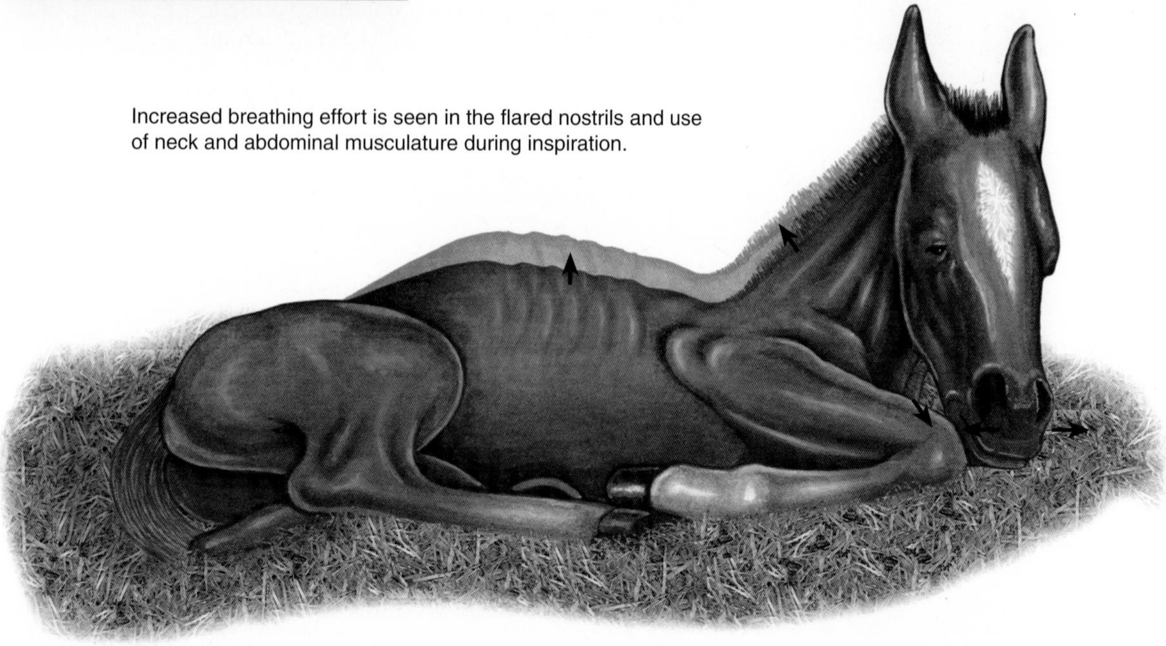

Oxygen administration using a small bucket around the foal's rostrum secured with a towel to keep a seal. IV fluids with antimicrobials may be administered.

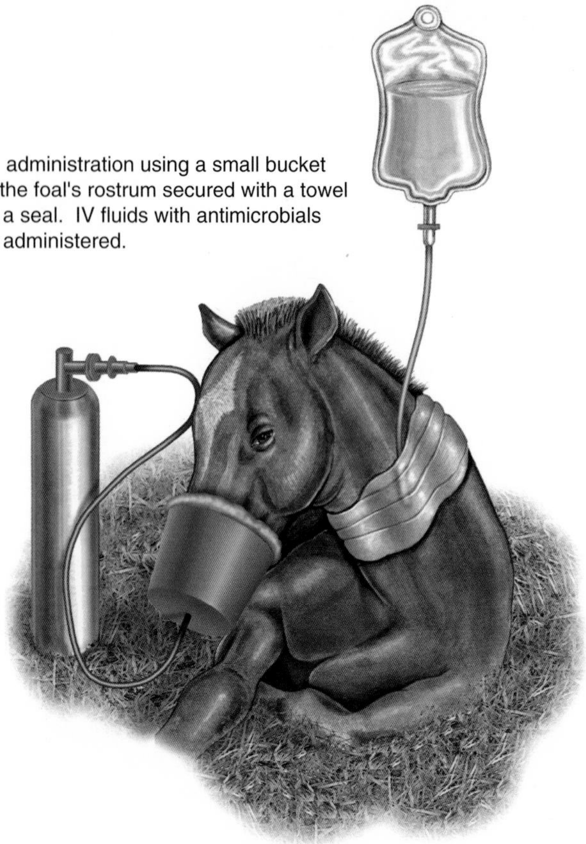

**Respiratory Distress Syndrome
Bacterial Pneumonia**

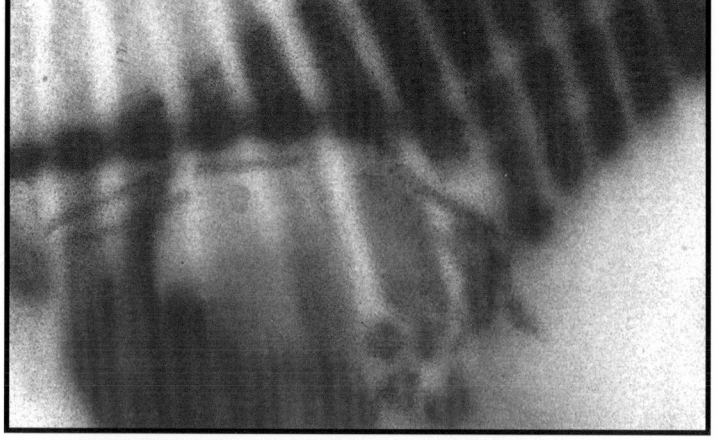

Thoracic radiograph reveals consolidation of ventral lung tissue with alveolar infiltration as seen in bronchopneumonia.

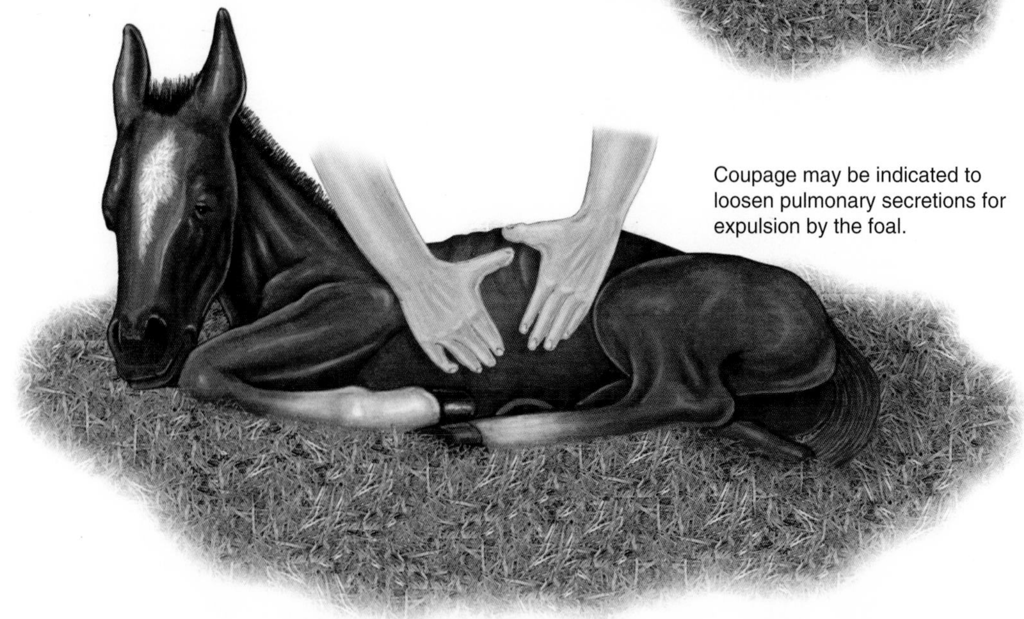

Coupage may be indicated to loosen pulmonary secretions for expulsion by the foal.

RESPIRATORY DISTRESS SYNDROME

Etiology

There are a number of factors that can predispose the foal to the condition known as respiratory distress syndrome. This syndrome features the impairment of the lung's ability to adequately exchange gases at the alveolar level. This produces hypoxemia and carbon dioxide retention. This is commonly found in premature foals. Other causes of respiratory distress syndrome include a bacterial or viral pneumonia, a premature placental separation, a dystocia condition, or any long term condition of infection.

Clinical Signs

Clinically, these foals exhibit similar symptoms as those seen with pneumonia. The foal will be making a concerted effort to breathe. The nostrils will be flared and breathing will be rapid. Auscultation will reveal a poor entry of air into the lungs. The foal may exhibit grunting sounds while breathing. In severe cases, cyanosis may be present on the mucous membranes.

Treatment

Treatment of respiratory distress syndrome focuses on supporting the respiratory system and possibly correcting a predisposing factor such as an infection. The foal should be maintained in a sternal recumbent position if possible. This improves the oxygenating efficiency of the lung tissue. Warm humidified oxygen can be provided as ventilation therapy. In extreme cases, it may be necessary to monitor blood gases and correct any acidotic condition with appropriate fluid therapy.

BACTERIAL PNEUMONIA

Etiology

Bacteria are a common cause of respiratory disease. These bacteria gain entry into the foal's system while the foal is still enclosed in an infected placenta, during parturition, through the umbilicus, or through inhalation of potential pathogens. Remember that the foal is born with an immature immune system. If there are any inadequacies with the protection provided by the mare's colostral immunoglobulins, then the foal is predisposed to bacterial pneumonia. The most common bacteria that cause foal pneumonia are *E. coli, Klebsiella spp., Salmonella spp., Actinobacillus spp., Pasteurella spp.,* and *Streptococcal spp.* All of these organisms can infect the foal during the birthing process and immediately postpartum. *Rhodococcus equi* is a bacteria that usually infects foals that are older than 2 - 3 weeks of age.

Clinical Signs and Diagnosis

Usually the first clinical sign that these foals are in a condition of respiratory distress is depression within the foal. This is usually coupled with a decreased appetite. The mare will often have a distended udder which indicates that the foal is not nursing as regularly as before. The foal may have a fever, and the respiration rate may be rapid. In many cases, the foal will have a productive cough which could supply a sputum specimen.

Auscultation of the lung will reveal fluid sounds and "crackles". If possible, thoracic radiographs should be taken to reveal the extent of the problem and provide baseline data for future evaluation.

Treatment

The first step of treatment of a foal with bacterial pneumonia should be an evaluation of the foal's immune system. Foals that have a serum IgG concentration below 800 mg/dL should be treated intravenously with hyperimmune plasma at a rate of 20 - 50 ml/kg. The foal should be immediately started on broad spectrum antimicrobial therapy.

Usually a combination of drugs is utilized to achieve maximum antibiotic therapy. When possible, a culture should be obtained via a trachial wash to determine specific antibiotic treatment. Antimicrobial therapy should be continued for at least 2 - 3 weeks to ensure that the infection is eliminated.

Treatment of *Rhodococcus equi* should be handled differently than other bacterial pneumonias. When untreated, this bacteria forms abscesses within the pulmonary tissue. Therefore, the foal should be treated a minimum of 8 - 12 weeks with appropriate antibiotic therapy. The most commonly used antibiotic treatment of *Rhodococcus equi* is Erythromycin estolate at 20 - 30 mg/kg orally every 6 hours coupled with Rifampin at 5 - 10 mg/kg orally every 12 hours.

Physical therapy should not be overlooked as a complimentary treatment of any foal suffering from bacterial pneumonia. The foal should be kept in sternal recumbency. This will minimize pressure on the down lung and allow better oxygenation efficiency for the pulmonary tissues. Coupage can be performed on the chest with a cupped hand positioned over the intercostal spaces. Massage of the musculoskeletal system and stretching will promote more circulation to the muscle tissues in a foal that is severely depressed and sick. Nebulization with warm moist air containing bronchodilators as well as antibiotics may help alleviate some of the pulmonary distress.

VIRAL PNEUMONIA

Etiology

The most common viral pathogens that cause pneumonia in foals include the Influenza virus, the Adenovirus, Equine Herpes virus type I, and Equine Arteritis virus.

Equine herpes virus can attack the foal while it is still within the maternal tissues. The foal may be born live and appear healthy. However, the foal will develop signs of respiratory distress within a few hours of birth. Equine herpes virus may also

FOAL DISORDERS

Bacterial and Viral Pneumonia; Ruptured Bladder

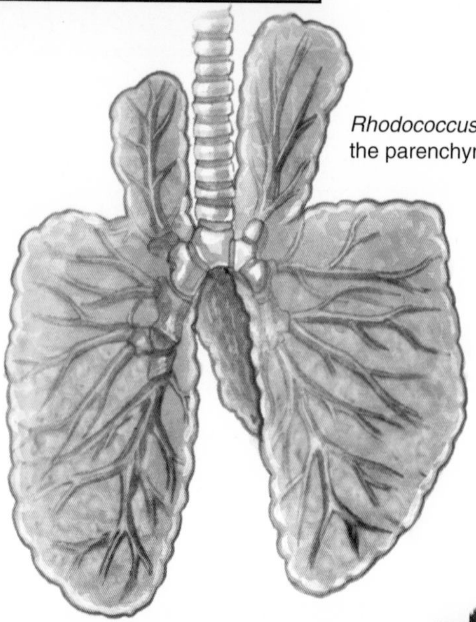

Rhodococcus equi abscesses in the parenchymal lung tissue.

Pneumonia

Sternal recumbent position with nebulization using warm moist air containing bronchodilators.

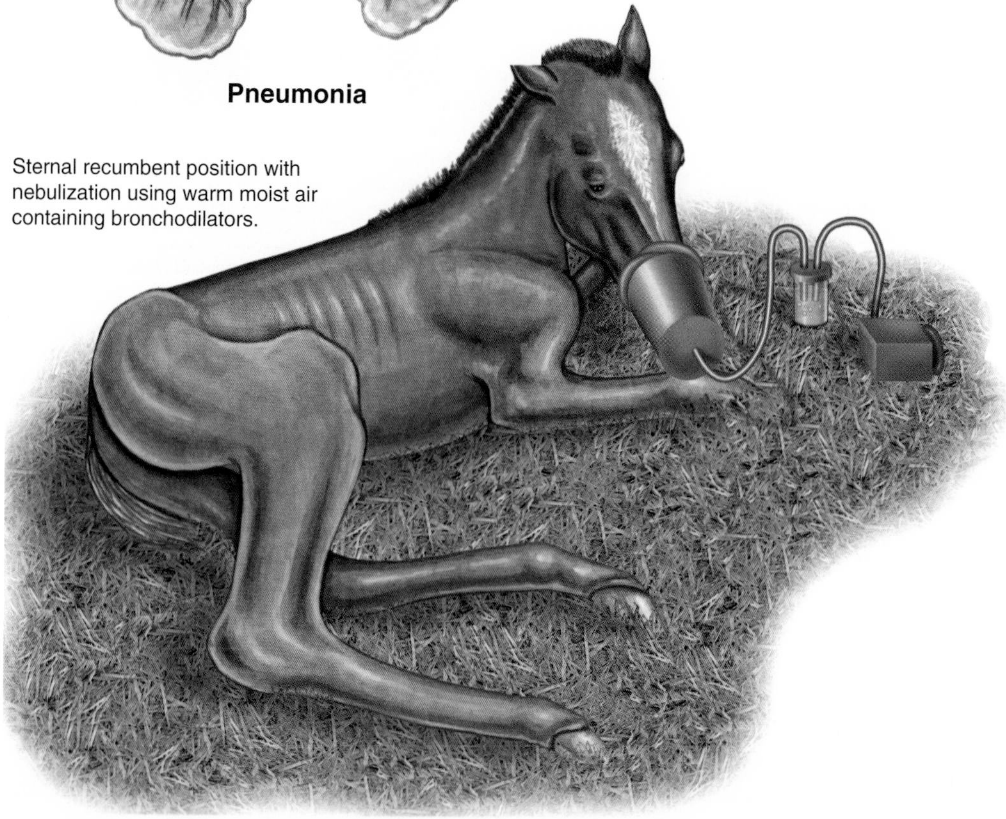

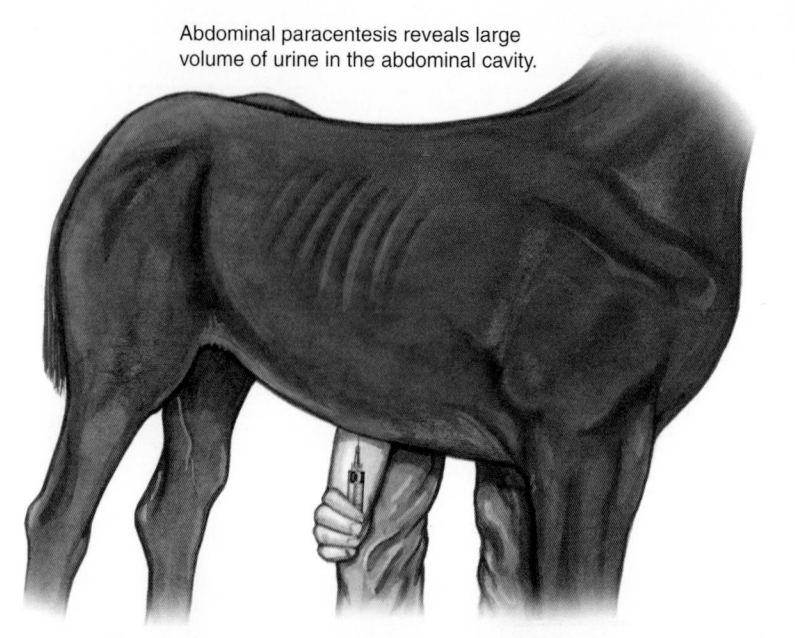

Abdominal paracentesis reveals large volume of urine in the abdominal cavity.

Ruptured Bladder

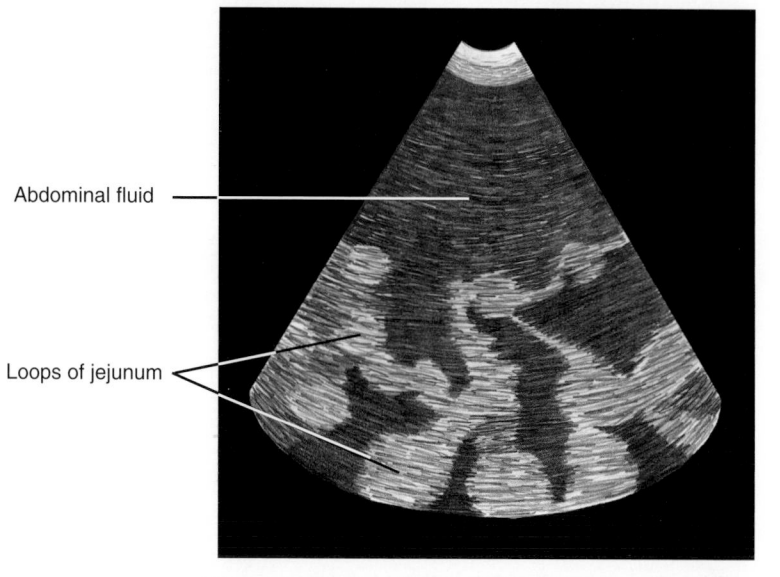

Abdominal fluid
Loops of jejunum

Ultrasound showing abdominal fluid with no intact bladder seen.

be one of the first viral pathogens to attack any foal that is immunodeficient. This usually occurs within the first 24 - 48 hours after birth.

Another cause of interstitial type pneumonia in neonatal foals is the influenza virus. It is less common than the herpes virus type I. Foals usually develop symptoms to this within the first 48 hours of life.

Combined immunodeficiency that is observed in Arabian foals usually has the sequela of adenovirus pneumonia. This condition produces an anorexia, a polypnea, and usually both nasal and ocular discharge. Most foals will recover from this if they are not severely immunodepressed.

Another cause of interstitial pneumonia in the foal is Equine arteritis virus. These foals can be born either weak or healthy and usually develop signs within the first 48 hours of life.

Diagnosis

Diagnosis of a viral pneumonia in foals can be confirmed with virus isolation techniques. Unfortunately, it is very difficult to obtain a specimen and transport it to the laboratory to confirm the virus.

Treatment

Treatment of a viral pneumonia involves aggressive supportive care to the foal and broad spectrum antimicrobial administration to prevent secondary bacterial infections. In severely infected cases, fluid therapy is essential for any degree of success. Antimicrobial therapy should always be continued in these cases for 2 - 3 weeks to ensure an adequate duration of therapy to prevent bacterial recurrence. Sternal recumbency, nebulization, and physical therapy techniques should also be utilized in the treatment of these viral pneumonia foals.

Etiology

Urinary disorders within the equine neonate effect the kidney tissue and the bladder. The most common disorder that effects the kidney tissue is a lack of an adequate amount of blood flowing through the functional kidneys due to dehydration. This dehydration may be caused from a number of factors such as diarrhea or infection. Disorders of the neonatal kidney also occur from a secondary colonization of bacteria that which happens in a generalized septicemia. Neonatal isoerythrolysis can produce a hemoglobin nephrosis within the neonatal kidney tissue. Even the overzealous administration of Tetracycline, utilized in the treatment of contracted tendons, can cause damage to the functional neonatal kidneys.

Clinical Signs and Diagnosis

The decreased production of urine, termed oliguria, is uncommon with acute renal failure in neonatal foals. Normally, foals will produce 6 ml/ kg of urine per hour. Specific signs of a urinary disorder within the foal may not be present; however, a generalized septicemia or dehydration within the foal should prompt consideration of the renal tissues when determining treatment. It is important to remember that any BUN levels taken from the foal on the first 1 - 2 days of life will usually reflect those BUN levels of the mare.

Specific urinalysis levels within the foal are quite different from those found in adult urine. For example, normal foal urine contains protein for the first 36 hours of life. The urine should carry a pH of 6 - 7 and specific gravity of 1.001 to 1.012.

Treatment

Treatment of any renal problem in the foal is usually accomplished through appropriate fluid therapy via an oral or intravenous route. Periodic blood samples should be taken to constantly assess the hydration levels within these patients.

Potassium should be avoided since the foal has a limited ability to excrete that ion. Carefully monitored use of aminoglycoside antibiotics is indicated as they can cause urinary damage in the neonate.

Clinical Signs

This is a disorder that usually occurs in male foals less than seven days of age that appear normal at birth. Clinically, the foal will start to exhibit signs after day two of age. The foal will appear depressed and will exhibit mild abdominal pain. The abdominal cavity may appear distended due to the build up of urine within it.

Diagnosis

Diagnosis is made through the use of an abdominal paracentesis and abdominal ultrasonography. Fluid gathered on the abdominocentesis will be large in volume and may carry an ammonia-type smell. Abdominal ultrasonography will reveal fluid within the abdomen and there will be an inability to visualize an intact bladder.

Treatment

Ideal treatment involves immediate surgical correction of the bladder rupture. An incision is made 2 - 3 centimeters paramedian to the prepuce or along the midline allowing reflection of the preputial tissues. The bladder is located and the tears are repaired surgically. It is advantageous to place a urinary catheter within the bladder. It can be left in the foal 2 - 3 days following the surgery. The urine is drained out of the abdominal cavity and closure is accomplished through normal suturing procedures.

Systemic antibiotics and fluid therapy is begun immediately. These foals require intensive nursing care and careful monitoring of their hydration levels and blood electrolyte values.

Artwork By S. Hakola / J. Dirig
Copyright Equistar Publications, Ltd.

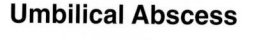

Umbilical Abscess

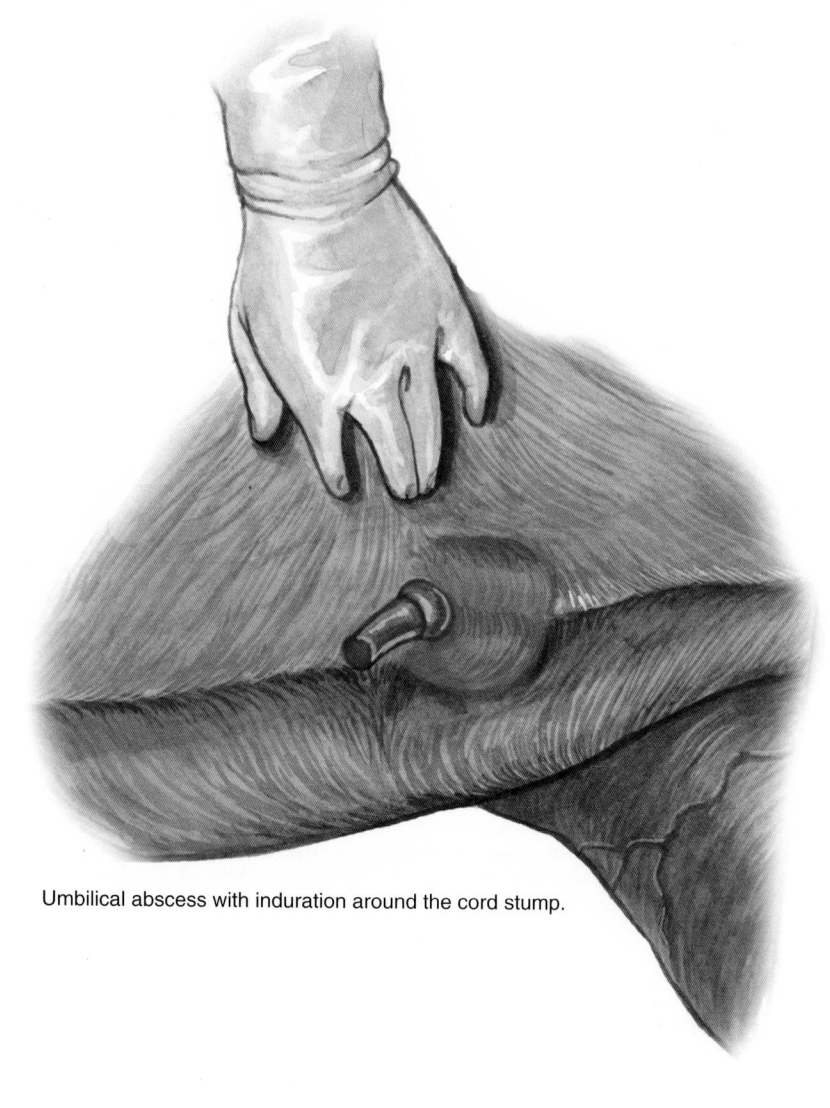

Umbilical abscess with induration around the cord stump.

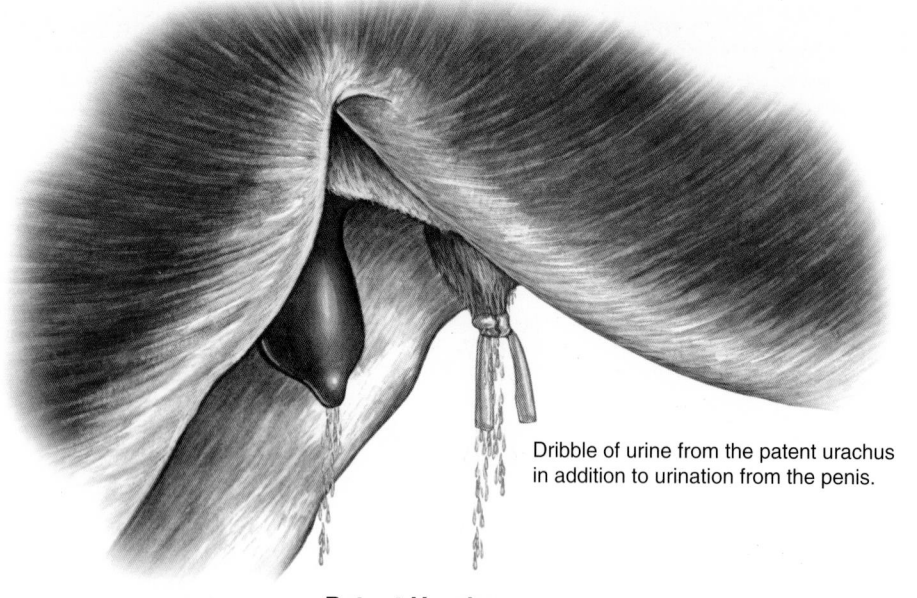

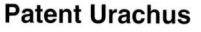

Dribble of urine from the patent urachus in addition to urination from the penis.

Patent Urachus

Umbilical Hernia

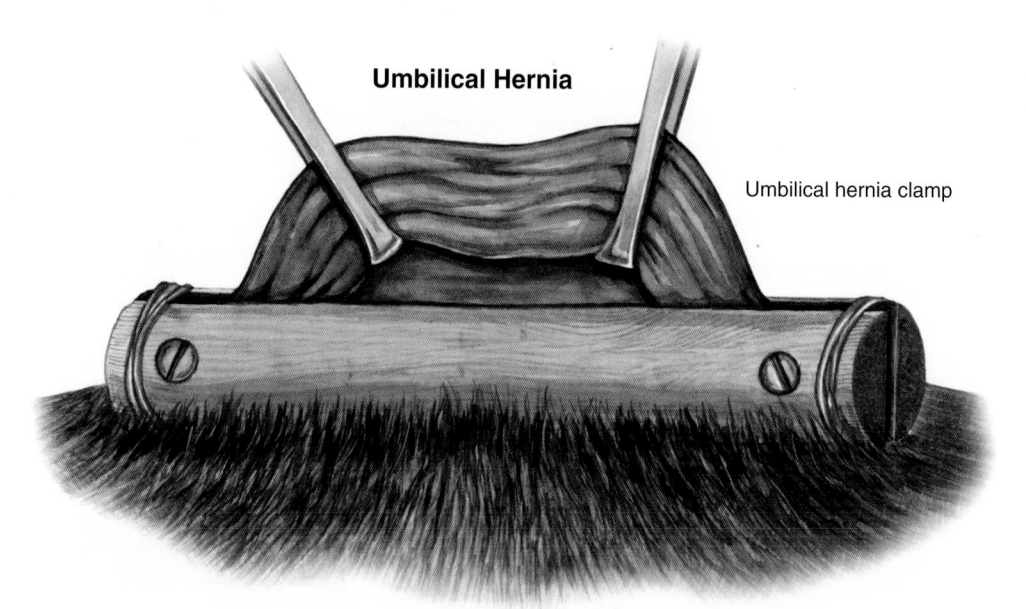

Umbilical hernia clamp

UMBILICAL DISORDERS

Umbilical problems in the foal can consist of an abscess, a swollen umbilicus, a patent urachus, and umbilical hernias. The umbilicus of a neonatal foal consists of two umbilical arteries, an umbilical vein, and the urachus. These structures change from their function while the foal was in utero to that in the neonate. The umbilical arteries, before parturition, connected the internal iliac arteries. After birth, the umbilical arteries regress to become the round ligaments of the bladder in the foal. The umbilical vein which connected the placenta to the liver and portal cava before birth becomes the round ligament of the bladder after birth. The urachus connected the fetal bladder to the allantoic cavity before the foal was born.

There are several methods available to diagnose umbilical disorders within the foal. The easiest method relies on digital palpation of the umbilical area; hernias are readily diagnosed using this technique. Ultrasonography may be utilized for the diagnosis of any abscesses or fluid enlargements within the umbilicus.

UMBILICAL ABSCESSES

These abscesses usually occur outside the abdominal cavity in the foal. Clinically, an enlarged naval is visualized which is swollen and painful upon palpation. This usually occurs in foals that are older than one week of age. Diagnosis is based on a digital palpation and/or an ultrasound exam of that anatomical area.

Both medical and surgical methods can be utilized in the treatment of an umbilical abscess. Applications of hot packs to the area and establishment of drainage may be the appropriate treatment of choice. If there is any suspicion of a systemic infection, administration of systemic antibiotics should be considered. If the foal is nonresponsive to the topical medical treatment, it may be necessary to anesthetize the foal and perform surgery to establish proper drainage.

PATENT URACHUS

This disorder is manifested by a dribble of urine from the umbilicus during urination. This leakage of urine may be very subtle and may appear as only a small amount of moisture around the umbilicus. Foals usually appear absolutely normal except for this unusual urination.

The cause of this is merely a lack of closure between the bladder and the umbilicus. These tissues may have closed and then reopened due to a trauma to that area. This can occur during aggressive handling of the foal or even from a very aggressive mare that paws at the foal.

Treatment of a patent urachus is focused on the closure of these tissues and prevention of a systemic infection. A caustic solution of iodine can be applied repeatedly to the umbilicus. Chemical cautery can be accomplished through the use of silver nitrate sticks that are inserted into the first 1 to 2 centimeters of the urachus. Surgery should be performed to close the tissues between the bladder and the urachus in those cases where cautery does not gain a response.

UMBILICAL HERNIAS

Although some umbilical hernias are evident immediately at birth, most umbilical hernias are noticed several weeks after foaling. Digital palpation will reveal the size of the opening. The decision whether to surgically repair these hernias rests on this determination. If the opening is very small and allows only the passage of two fingers, repair can be accomplished when the foal is older. If the hernia is large enough to allow a small portion of the bowel or omentum to pass through it, then a repair with either the application of hernia clamps or surgery should be considered very soon. In the rare case of a strangulated hernia in the foal, surgical repair should be done immediately.

NEUROLOGICAL DISORDERS

Most neurological disorders of the foal first illicit themselves as a depression, a decreased suckling activity, an independence or lack of affinity for the mare, and an increased amount of time that is spent lying around the stall. One should avoid the general term of a "dummy foal". A neurological examination should be done on the foal and an actual diagnosis determined.

Within twenty minutes of birth, most foals will exhibit a suckle reflex. The foal should stand and nurse within the first hour or two following birth. Even though the first movements are awkward, the foal should make an attempt to follow the mare very closely. The foal should be alert and respond to any stimulus in its environment. Any deviation from these normal behaviors signal the need for a complete physical examination to determine if there are any problems present.

A neurological examination of the foal should begin with the head and involve all the reflexes and range of motion in the limbs. The eyes should be examined for any abnormality and the presence of the foal's head should be normal. Foals will usually carry their head in a fixed position and have very abrupt movements in response to the stimulation from their environment. Restraint attempts on the foal should illicit either a flight response from the foal or cause it to relax and collapse slowly in one's arms. The stimulation of any nerves should elicit a response in them. The patellar reflex can be obtained. Typically, it is almost to the point of being hyperexaggerated. All limbs should have normal to wide range of motion. It is not unusual for a foal to exhibit a pacing gate rather than a trot.

FOAL DISORDERS

Neonatal Maladjustment Syndrome; Seizures; White Muscle Disease

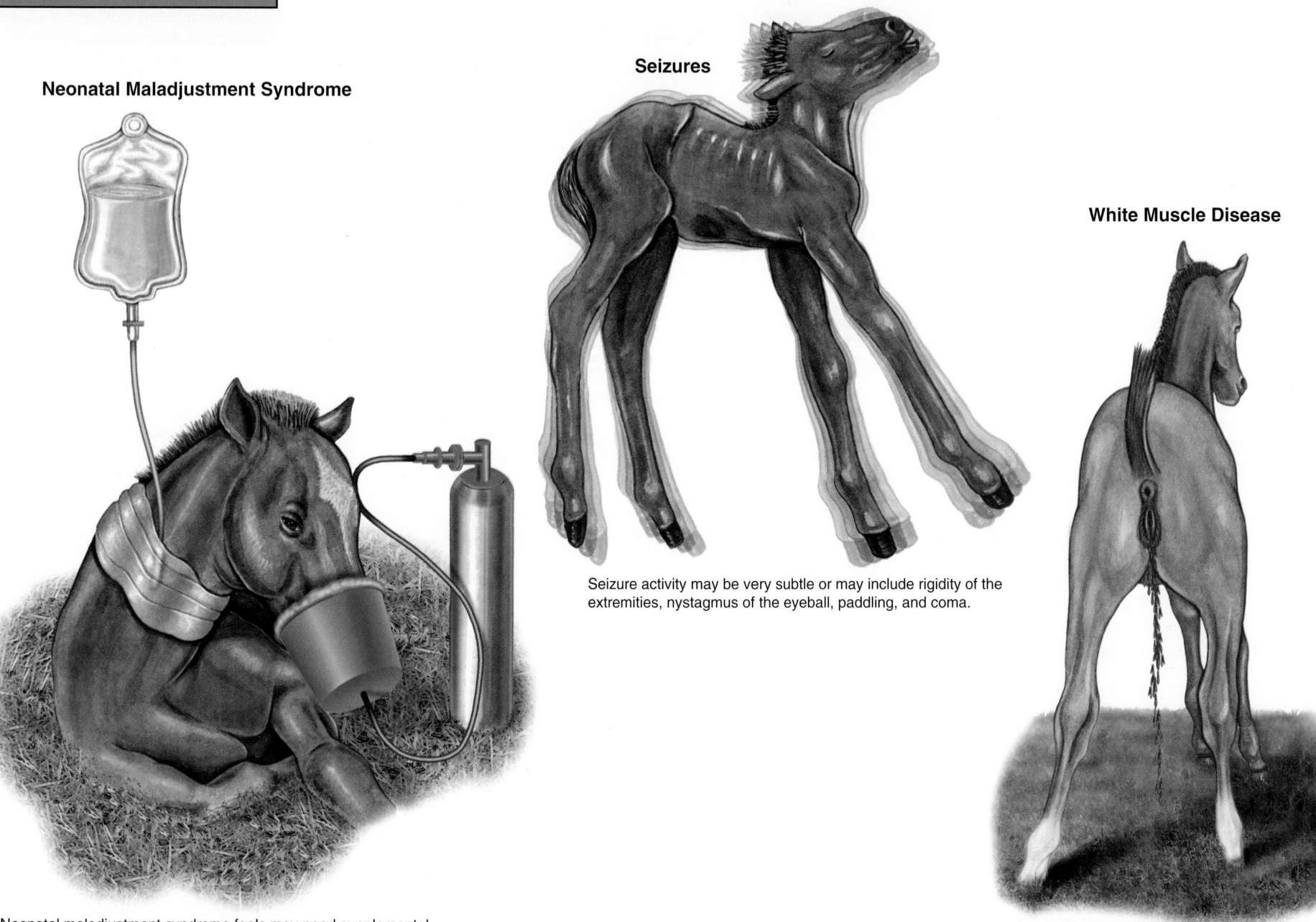

Neonatal Maladjustment Syndrome

Seizures

White Muscle Disease

Seizure activity may be very subtle or may include rigidity of the extremities, nystagmus of the eyeball, paddling, and coma.

Neonatal maladjustment syndrome foals may need supplemental oxygen support. IV fluids with medications for reducing cerebral edema, antiinflammatories, and/or antibiotics may be indicated.

White muscle disease must be considered when myoglobulinuria is seen in the foal.

NEONATAL MALADJUSTMENT SYNDROME

Etiology and Clinical Signs

This is a noninfectious neurological disorder of newborn foals and is characterized by gross disturbances within the foal's normal behavior. This disorder usually occurs within 24 hours after birth. Most affected foals are full term and usually have had some degree of dystocia during parturition. The foal is typically of normal weight and size. These foals stop suckling and become increasingly depressed. The foal will gradually lose recognition of the mare and begin a wandering type behavior. The foal may "bark" which is really an abnormal grunting respiratory sound. Most foals will exhibit a degree of dypsnea and in some cases, appear to be blind.

Diagnosis

It is important to eliminate a septicemia as a possible differential diagnosis immediately upon recognition of these clinical signs. This can best be done through a monitoring of rectal temperature and blood work. Other important etiologies to eliminate would include a central nervous system hemorrhage or edema, a metabolic problem, or hypoxia at birth.

Treatment

Paramount to treatment of these foals is the provision of adequate nursing care and constant monitoring of the hydration status. Foals that suffer from hypoxia can be provided with intranasal oxygen administration. Nutritional support is essential if the foal has ceased all suckling response. When cerebral edema is suspected, administer an IV solution of DMSO at a dose rate of .5 gm/kg in a 20% solution. (A 50 kg foal will require the addition of 45 ml of 90% DMSO solution into 500 ml of 5% dexstrose.) Mannitol solutions can be administered at .25 gm/kg IV every 6 - 8 hours for the first 24 - 48 hours. Flunixin meglumine at 1 mg/kg every 12

hours for 24 - 48 hours will be of antiinflammatory benefit. Antimicrobial pharmaceuticals should be administered to prevent a possible septicemic condition or a secondary bacterial infection.

Only 50% of foals survive this disorder. When compounding factors are present in these cases, the survival rate falls even below this number. The prognosis of these foals is extremely poor if there is no response from the foal after 36 - 48 hours.

SEIZURES

Etiology

The most common cause of seizures in the foal is some degree of metabolic abnormality. This could be as simple as a hypoglycemia or it may be more involved, such as a complication from a septicemia or meningitis. In the Arabian breeds, epilepsy should also be considered.

Clinical Signs

Seizures in the foal can be very subtle illiciting only abnormal jaw movement or salivation. More severe seizures may be manifested by muscle twitching. Generalized severe seizures are unmistakable with rigid extension within the comas, nystagmus, and paddling.

Treatment

Diazepam is a safe drug that should be immediately used to control the seizures. Up to 5 - 10 mg /45 kg should be administered intravenously in a slow drip. Care must be taken to not administer diazepam too rapidly which could result in respiratory or cardiac arrest. Other medications such as phenobarbital or phenytoin can be utilized when satisfactory results from diazepam are not achieved.

WHITE MUSCLE DISEASE

Selenium deficiencies occur along the east and west coasts in addition to most of the midwestern states. This creates a degeneration within the muscle tissues and is termed white muscle disease.

Clinical Signs and Diagnosis

Initially these foals appear weak and are reluctant to rise. They seem to be in a generalized state of pain and are reluctant to walk or nurse. Care must be taken not to evaluate these foals as a colic or seizure case when they make repeated attempts to get up.

Those familiar with this condition will usually make a diagnosis based on clinical signs. Blood work will reveal an elevation in the serum creatine kinase and astartate aminotransfer levels. There is usually a myoglobulinuria present at some stage of this disorder.

Treatment

A commercially available vitamin E and selenium preparation should be administered at a dose rate of 1 mg / 45kg of body weight. This dosage should be repeated in 3 days and again at approximately 2 weeks. Proper nursing care and good utilization of physical therapy techniques will aid in the recovery of foals suffering from this disorder.

Artwork By S. Hakola / J. Dirig
Copyright Equistar Publications, Ltd.

Botulism

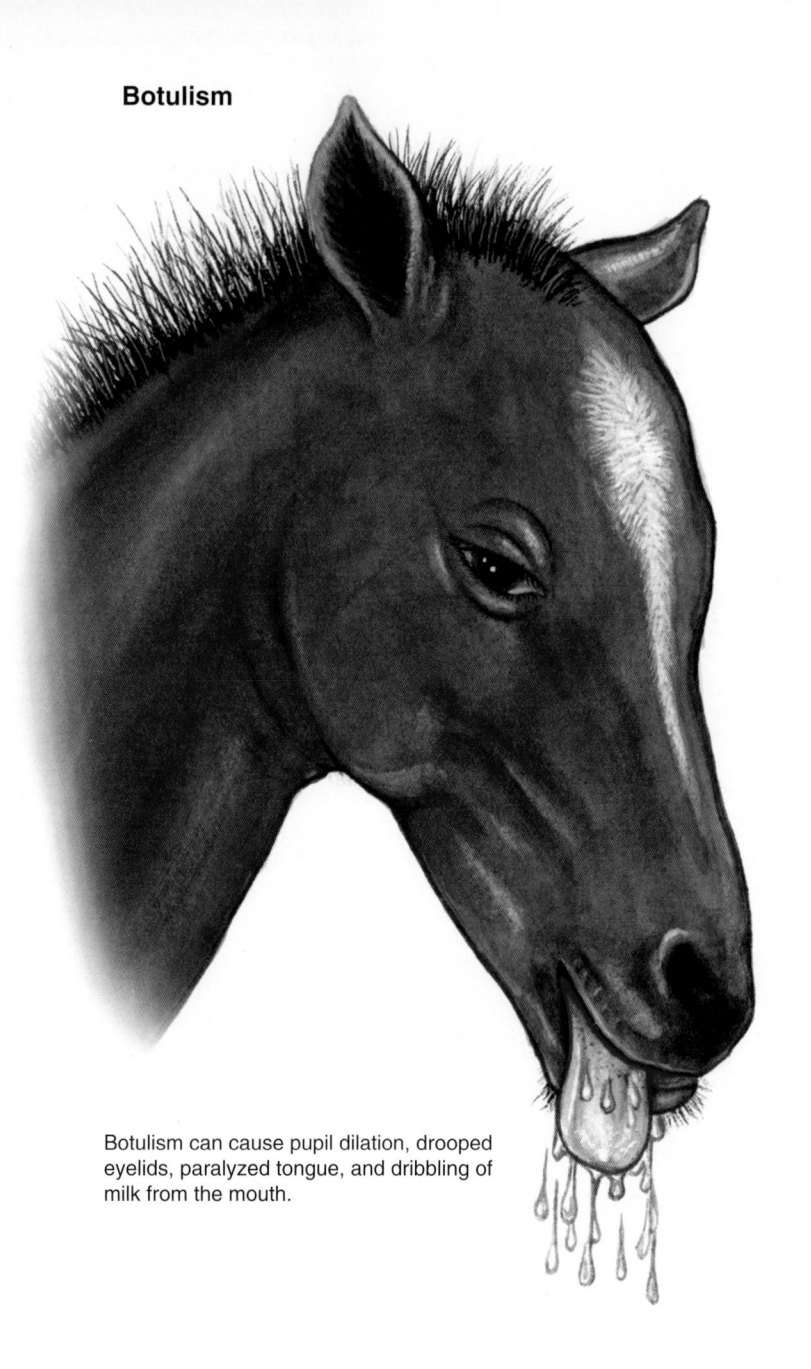

Botulism can cause pupil dilation, drooped eyelids, paralyzed tongue, and dribbling of milk from the mouth.

Tetanus

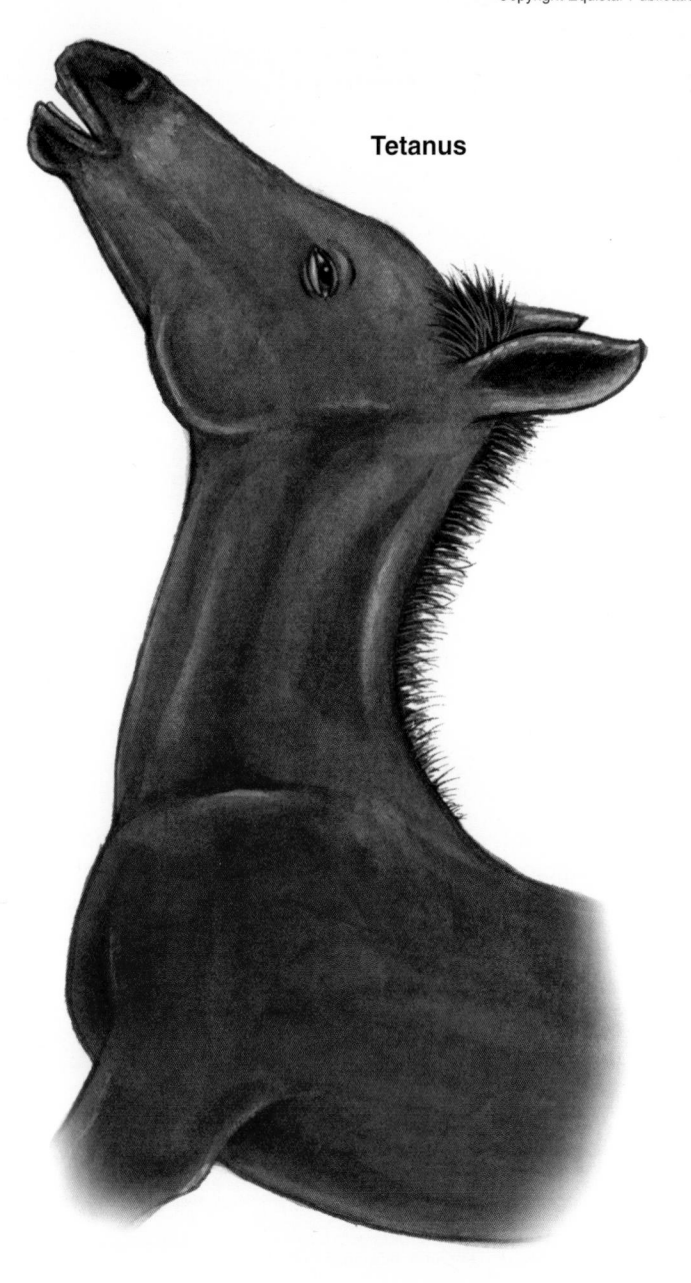

Prolapsed third eyelid, flared nostrils, and rigid arched head and neck as seen in tetanus.

BOTULISM

Etiology

Botulism in the foal is a neurological syndrome caused by *Clostridium botulinum* type B. It is commonly referred to as "Shaker Foal Syndrome". The exotoxin from this bacteria causes this disorder usually at 2 - 4 weeks of age. However, it can be manifested even during the first week of life.

Clinical Signs

Clinically, the symptoms of this disorder can have a very slow or gradual onset of 2 - 4 days or can appear to affect the foal within a mere 24 hours. The first sign that is usually noted is a weakness or depression within the foal. The foal's pupils are typically dilated, and it will dribble milk because it is unable to swallow. The eyelids and tail will both lack tone and begin to droop. The muscle will visually fasciculate and the foal will ultimately collapse and be unable to stand.

Diagnosis

An early diagnosis is often critical since treatment needs to be initiated immediately in order to have any degree of success. The toxins can be isolated from the intestinal tract but their isolation takes up valuable time. A diagnosis has to be made through the elimination of the other differentials. Other possible disorders to consider are simple cases of hypoglycemia and hypocalcemia, septicemia, and white muscle disease.

Treatment

Treatment consists of an aggressive administration of potassium penicillin IV along with a polyvalent equine type B antitoxin. Nursing care is essential in the recovery of these foals.

Fortunately this problem can be prevented with the administration of botulism type B toxoid to pregnant mares three times before parturition. The last dose administered to these mares should be 2 - 3 weeks before foaling.

TETANUS

Etiology

The *Clostridium tetani* organism will cause this disorder in neonatal foals. It most commonly occurs when the foal has suffered a failure of passive transfer of immunity from the mare. It is also seen in foals from mares that are not vaccinated for tetanus in the last trimester of their pregnancy. Tetanus is a common secondary occurrence when there is a puncture wound or infection of the umbilical stump.

Clinical Symptoms

One of the first clinical signs that is manifested in the neonatal foal is a prolapse of the third eyelid. These foals are stiff and reluctant to move. Any noise such as clapping of the hands will produce tetanic muscle spasms. The foal's nostrils are usually flared with the head tilted backwards and the tail partially elevated, a position termed "opisthotonos." These foals will also have difficulty in swallowing which is called "dysphasia."

Diagnosis

A differential diagnosis will include hypocalcemia, hypoglycemia, meningitis, white muscle disease, and even strychnine poisoning. Diagnosis should be made upon the vaccination history of the mare and clinical signs.

Treatment

Treatment of these foals is challenging. Potassium penicillin should be administered intravenously at a high dose. Ten thousand IU of tetanus antitoxin should be administered four times a day for several days. Sedation and muscle relaxation administration should be administered if the muscle spasms are severe. Intensive nursing care and nutritional support will have to be provided in almost all cases.

Prevention of this disorder can be accomplished through the vaccination of the mare with tetanus toxoid 3 - 4 weeks prior to foaling. Foals of any unvaccinated mares should receive 1500 IU of tetanus antitoxin at birth. This provides approximately 45 days of protection once administered.

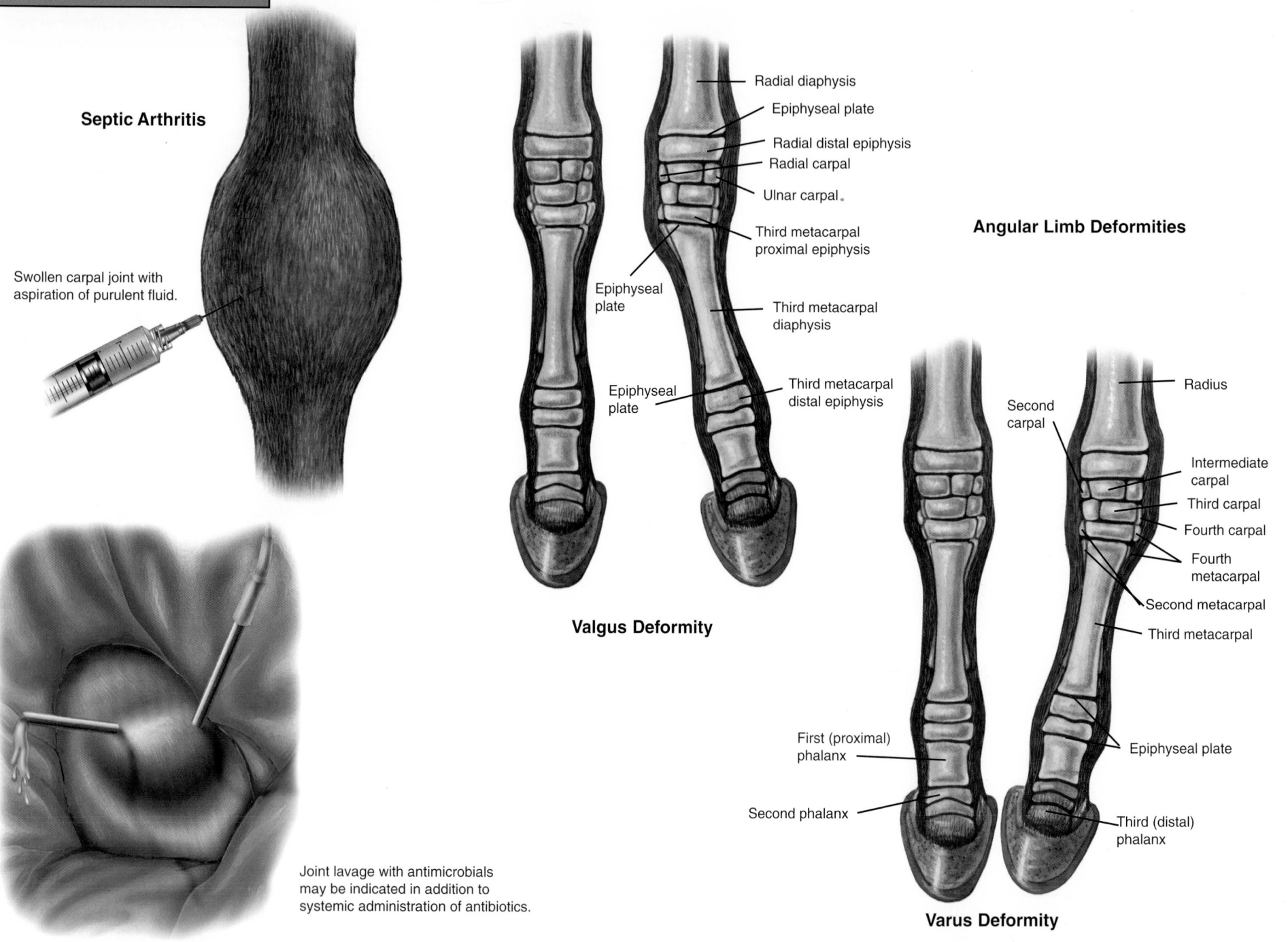

FOAL DISORDERS

Septic Arthritis; Angular Limb Deformities

Septic Arthritis

Swollen carpal joint with aspiration of purulent fluid.

Joint lavage with antimicrobials may be indicated in addition to systemic administration of antibiotics.

Angular Limb Deformities

Radial diaphysis

Epiphyseal plate

Radial distal epiphysis

Radial carpal

Ulnar carpal

Third metacarpal proximal epiphysis

Epiphyseal plate

Third metacarpal diaphysis

Epiphyseal plate

Third metacarpal distal epiphysis

Valgus Deformity

Radius

Second carpal

Intermediate carpal

Third carpal

Fourth carpal

Fourth metacarpal

Second metacarpal

Third metacarpal

Epiphyseal plate

First (proximal) phalanx

Second phalanx

Third (distal) phalanx

Varus Deformity

MUSCULOSKELETAL DISORDERS

The disorders involving the musculoskeletal system in the newborn foal are usually not fatal but they are detrimental to the athletic potential. These disorders include septic arthritis and osteomyelitis, angular limb deformities, and flexor and extensor limb deformities, and clubfeet.

SEPTIC ARTHRITIS AND OSTEOMYELITIS

Etiology

These bone and joint infections are usually a consequence to some type of general septicemia within the foal. They are commonly called joint IU, naval IU, infectious arthritis, and septic polyarthritis. This condition usually occurs in foals that are less than 30 days of age. A rapid diagnosis and aggressive therapy are important in preventing irreversible damage due to this condition.

The four common causes of septic arthritis and osteomyelitis in the foal include the following: 1) a failure of passive transfer that results in a current bacteremia; 2) a respiratory infection caused by bacteria which result in a systemic infection that involves the joints and bone structures; 3) an umbilical infection that has gone systemic and localized itself within the joint and bone structures; and 4) a systemic bacteremia that has resulted from a condition of diarrhea or enteritis within the foal.

Clinical Signs

Clinically, most of these foals will appear ill and show signs of a systemic infection. They will be depressed, have a lack of appetite, and have a fever. These foals will exhibit some sort of lameness with or without a distention of the joint.

Diagnosis

A diagnosis of septic arthritis and osteomyelitis is usually made when presented with the appropriate clinical signs. Confirmation of this disorder with a joint that is not particularly swollen can be made through a synovial fluid exam which will contain a high number of white blood cells, usually greater than 10,000 with 70% of the white blood cells being neutrophils. Normal white blood cell content of synovial fluid is approximately 800 per microliter with only 8% of those being neutrophils. Bacteria may be found in the synovial fluid and are visible under the microscope. There is an increase in protein content in the synovial fluid, and the color of the fluid is usually cloudy or turbid in nature. Cultures can be prepared utilizing both aerobic and anaerobic techniques. A series of radiographs may be necessary to further evaluate the joint.

Treatment

Treatment of septic arthritis and osteomyelitis is an emergency situation. The foal should be immediately placed on systemic broad spectrum bactericidal antimicrobials. A combination of ampicillin and Amikacin sulfate is usually effective on most of these bacteria. One should not wait for culture results to initiate antimicrobial therapy, because bacteria will cause damage within the joints during the time of the pending culture. Intraarticular administration of antibiotics should also be considered and combined with systemic antimicrobial therapy. This administration of intraarticular antibiotics can be combined along with lavage and drainage of the joint. Gentamicin sulfate can be administered at a rate of 15 - 25 mg/day per joint. It is also important to monitor the immunoglobulin level (IgG) within the foal and provide adequate serum levels if needed. In certain instances the joint may have to be immobilized through the use of splints and support wraps. If the foal is in a great deal of pain, it may be advantageous to administer a nonsteroidal antiinflammatory medication such as flunixin meglumine. Care must be taken to prevent any overdose of this drug. If the joint is flushed and lavaged, it may also be advantageous

to administer hyaluronic acid intraarticuarlarly to compliment the procedure which will provide antiinflammatory relief. Since this disorder is usually a sequela to some other septic condition, it is important to also correct that condition.

ANGULAR LIMB DEFORMITIES

Most foals are born with crooked legs. These legs typically correct themselves spontaneously within the first few days after birth. This emphasizes the importance of exercise in the first few postpartum days. Several deformities correct themselves very slowly but are usually corrected within the first thirty days of life. An evaluation should be made in each individual case and treatment should be recommended on conservative levels since many of these disorders may correct themselves spontaneously.

There are two terms which are important in angular limb deformities in the foal: 1) a valgus deformity which is any lateral deviation of the distal portion of the limb, and 2) a varus deformity which is any medial deviation of the distal portion of the limb. Any rotational deformities of the limb usually improve as the chest cavity expands on the foal.

Etiology

The cause of these deformities is not always inherited. The most common cause to an angular limb deformity is an abnormal position in the uterus. There may be a hormonal imbalance in the mare which results in a deformity. Any ingestion of toxins by the mare such as a poisonous plant could result in an angular limb deformity in the foal. There may be an incomplete ossification of the bones within the foal which would result in an angular limb deformity. Nutritional imbalances within the pregnant mare's diet may also result in an angular limb deformity within the foal.

Diagnosis

It is important to radiograph all limbs that are involved with an angular limb deformity. This procedure will identify any musculoskeletal

Treatment of Angular Limb Deformities

Flexor Deformities

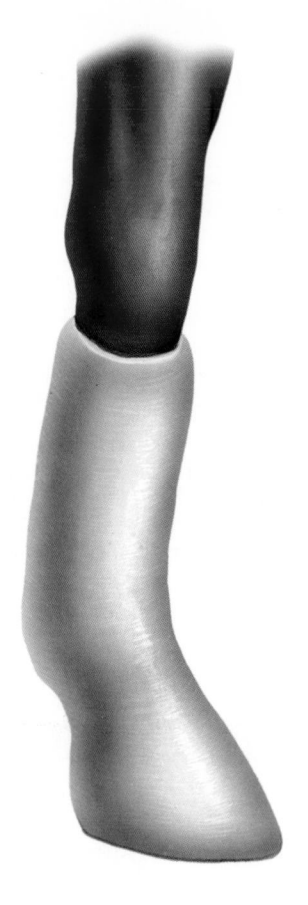

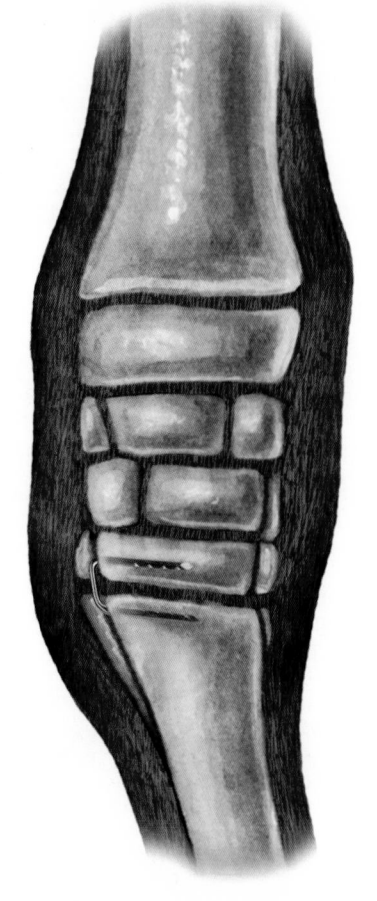

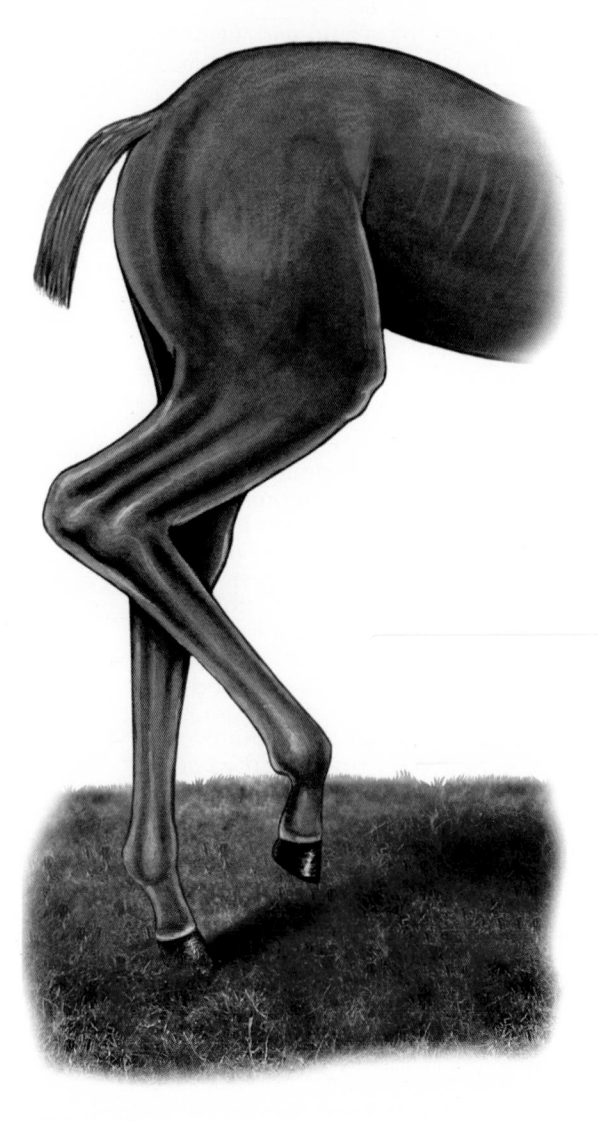

Hoof trimmed with application of fiberglass tube cast.

Transphyseal staple inserted to force contralateral growth of the physis.

Flexor deformity of the hock joint where the foal is unable to extend the hock joint and straighten the hind limb.

abnormalities which may contribute or coexist with an angular limb deformity. These abnormalities include degenerative joint disease, dysplasia of the epiphyseal ossification, acute physical trauma, or overloading of the limb. The density of the bone can be evaluated with radiographic techniques. The severity of the angle can be assessed through these radiographs and progress can be monitored through subsequent radiographic films.

Treatment

Treatment of these angular limb deformities may be as conservative as a stall confinement or as complex as a surgical technique. Any angular limb deformity that is greater than a 15 degree angle should warrant immediate aggressive treatment. When a deviation is between 6 - 15 degrees, conservative treatment can include hoof trimming, exercise, physical therapy, and external supports such as tube casts. Severe cases may involve periosteal stripping or transphyseal bridging. Periosteal stripping was first introduced in the 1980's and is merely a transection of the periosteum at the physis which releases the physis from restrictive forces by the fibroelastic periosteum. This surgery can be repeated if needed. Transphyseal bridging involves the placement of screws, wires, plates, or staples across the physis to retard growth asymmetrically. The success of this surgery depends on the compensatory growth of the contralateral side of the physis. Therefore, this procedure must be performed while the physis still has sufficient growth potential which will allow the limb to then become symmetrical.

FLEXOR / EXTENSOR LIMB DEFORMITIES

Etiology

This deformity disorder of the limb exists in the cranial/caudal plane of the carpus, fetlock, or pastern. It is usually caused genetically or from a malposition of the foal within the uterus. Clinically, it can vary in degree from a slightly raised heel to extreme flexion at the carpus so that the foal cannot rise.

Treatment

Mild cases will respond to exercise, proper nutrition, and physical therapy. Severe cases will require exercise, physical therapy, and shoes with heel extensions. This heel extension on the shoes will reposition the weight bearing surface on the ground and change the entire angle of the fetlock. Older foals should have their heels trimmed to restore the weight bearing surface to the flat surface of the hoof. In these older foals, shoes can actually be applied to their feet to correct this problem. Tape is used in younger foals to avoid nailing.

CONTRACTED FLEXOR DEFORMITIES

These flexor contraction deformities can include deformities of the carpus, tarsus, fetlock, and pastern. This deformity is characterized by a flexed position and the inability of the foal to straighten the involved joint. These deformities can vary in severity from mild where the joints just begin to knuckle, to moderate where the foal knuckles over when standing, to severe where the foal cannot stand at all.

Etiology

These flexor contraction deformities usually result from soft tissue structure abnormalities. If the contracture is not corrected, damage to the bony structures will result because of the imbalance on the weight bearing limb. These flexor contraction deformities can also be acquired when the foal is in the recumbent position for a long period of time due to an illness.

Treatment

Treatment of mild flexor deformities usually involves physical therapy techniques coupled with bandages or splints. These foals are typically recumbent. They have straight fetlocks and pasterns and the distal joints will just begin to knuckle. Massage and manipulation of the limbs through normal range of motion is excellent therapy for these recumbent foals. If the foal is able to stand, bandages or splints can be applied to provide relaxation to the tendons.

If the foal knuckles over when standing, this is a moderate flexor contraction deformity. In these cases a splint, cast, or orthopedic brace must apply counter tension to the contraction. It is advantageous to be able to remove the splints or the braces periodically to allow physical therapy techniques to speed the healing. If a cast is used, care must be taken to prevent any pressure sores or any complications involved with casting.

A severe flexor contraction deformity occurs when the foal cannot stand unassisted. In these cases surgery must be performed to transect the soft tissue structures until a normal posture can be obtained. A thorough evaluation of these patients must occur and a humane consideration of the patient should be considered before surgery is undertaken.

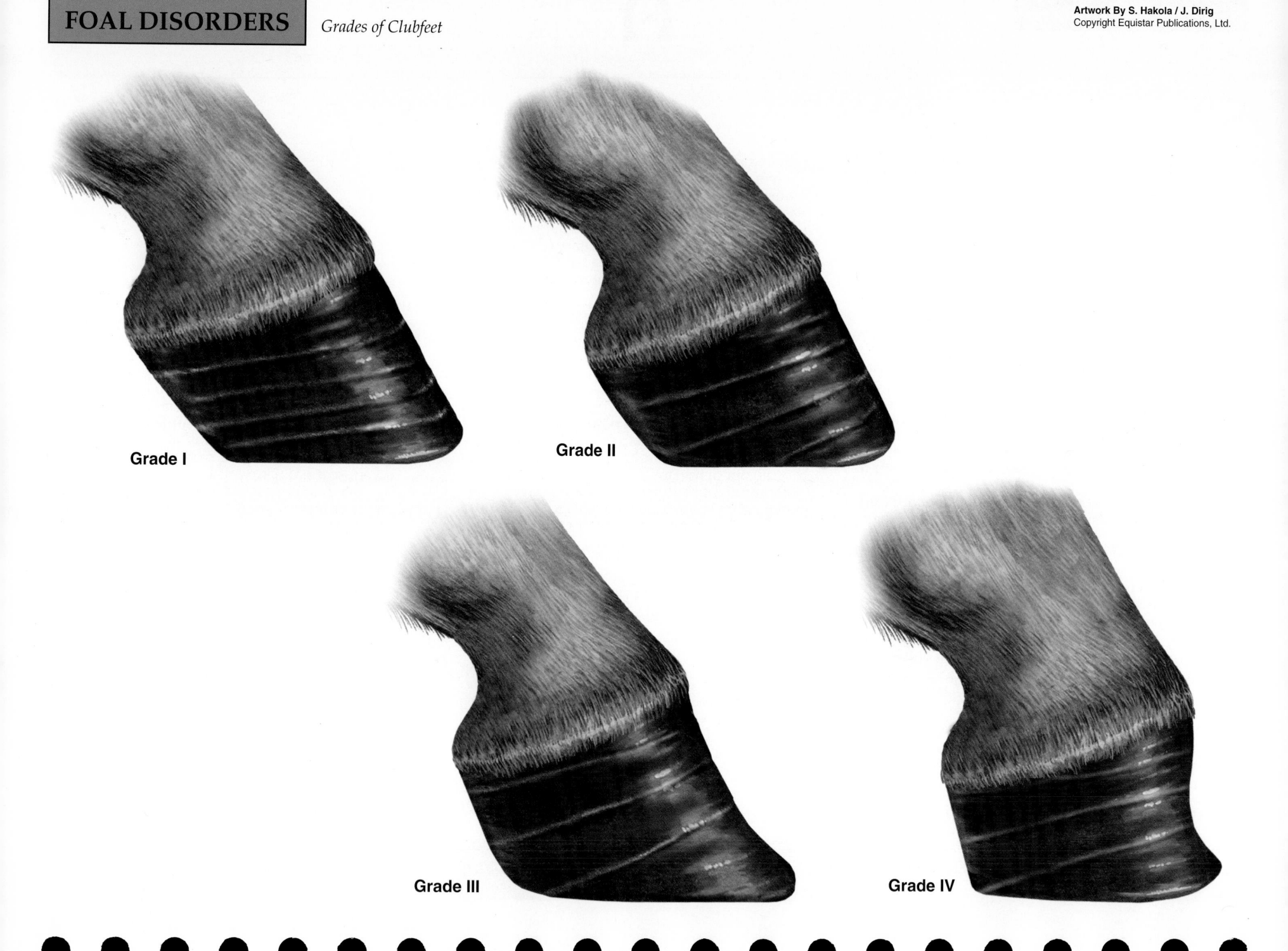

Grade I

Grade II

Grade III

Grade IV

CLUBFEET (CORONOPEDAL DEFORMITY)

When the equine hoof has an angle of 60 degrees or more, it is described as a clubfoot. Terms such as contracted foot or flexural deformity are also used synonymously with the clubfoot syndrome. This condition is usually confined to the forefeet and it may effect either or both feet. In severe cases, there is a marked "dish" shape to the dorsal hoof wall.

Etiology

Contracted feet or clubfeet can either be a congenital or an acquired condition. Other factors that can contribute to this clubfoot syndrome include nutritional considerations, heredity, and any lameness condition that results in pain such as osteochondrosis. When the pathogenesis for clubfeet is congenital, it is often bilateral. This may arise from a uterine malposition, an injury immediately following birth, or as a result of a genetic defect. In most cases the cause is unknown, but it usually involves a flexor deformity of the superficial and deep digital flexor tendons and the suspensory ligaments.

Acquired clubfeet or acquired flexural deformity can occur in sucklings and weanlings at 8 - 12 months of age. The pathogenesis of the acquired clubfoot syndrome may be nutritional, but is most commonly the result of some extended period of lameness. Bearing of weight by the foot is the stimulus for hoof expansion. Acquired clubfeet syndrome is the result of a reduction of weight on the weight-bearing surface of the foot which leads to the horn conforming to a smaller diameter.

Clinical Signs

In all cases, the affected foot or feet are smaller in diameter and have a hoof axis of 60 degrees or greater. The animal will often walk on its toe. This will predispose it to an excessive amount of weight within the toe which results in abscesses and additional pain. One foot is usually worse than the other. As the condition progresses, this small hoof will have an elongated heel and a dished dorsal hoof wall.

Grades of Clubfeet

Clubfeet can be categorized into four different grades. They are as follows:

Grade One: merely a mismatching of the feet with the hoof angle of the clubfoot being 5 degrees greater than its opposite.

Grade Two: this hoof is characterized by not only being 5 - 8 degrees higher than the opposite foot, but also has growth rings which are wider at the heel than at the toe. If the foot is trimmed to its normal length, the heel will not touch the ground.

Grade Three: the dorsal hoof wall of this foot will have the characteristic dished appearance. There is usually sole bruising due to the sole having a weight bearing property. Radiographically, there will be lipping along the coffin bone.

Grade Four: the hoof wall of this foot will be greater than 80 degrees. The sole will be a weight bearing structure, and the dorsal hoof wall will have a heavy dished appearance. Radiographics of the distal phalanx will show several degrees of rotation and will be demineralized.

Diagnosis

When establishing a diagnosis of clubfeet, it is important to also consider the possibility of contracted heels and some degree of laminitis. The etiology of the problem should be discerned so that the proper treatment can be initiated. A radiographic study should be performed to determine the involvement of the pedal bone and also whether there is a physitis, an osteochondrosis, or a degenerative joint disease problem. The position of the pedal bone should be established radiographically relative to the dorsal aspect of the hoof wall. Often the pedal bone will appear misshapened and new periostal bone formation will occur at the tip of the bone on a lateral radiograph.

Treatment

If a newborn foal can walk without knuckling forward, the congenital clubfoot syndrome will usually spontaneously correct itself within 2 - 3 days after birth. If this upright conformation condition persists in the foal, it has proven to be therapeutic to administer intravenous oxytetracycline to facilitate relaxation of the tendons. This administration of oxytetracycline may be contraindicated if it causes diarrhea. Corrective trimming of a very young foal will also help alleviate this condition. The heels should be lowered and frog pressure should be established.

If the clubfeet or flexural deformity is the result of a nutritional problem, then the diet should be assessed with deficiencies and imbalances immediately corrected. In most cases, the nutritional cause for this is overfeeding and imbalances in the mineral content of the diet due to excessive supplementation.

Although the cause is usually unknown, a ruptured common digital extensor tendon will cause the foal to knuckle over at the fetlock and appear over at the knee. A temporary splint is usually applied to these animals to prevent knuckling over which allows a more even weight-bearing surface to the foot.

When there is a congenital flexural deformity of the deep digital flexor tendon, the foal will usually stand on his toe and knuckle forward at the level of the fetlock. In some cases, the superficial flexor tendon is also involved. Conservative treatment for these animals involves splinting the legs back into a normal position.

If conservative treatment by splinting of the limbs is non-rewarding after 30 days, an inferior check ligament desmotomy should be considered. This involves cutting of the check ligament just below the knee. By transecting the check ligament, the tendon is released and allowed to lengthen. Before this procedure is accomplished, the owner should be forwarned of the potential for a blemish at the surgical sight where the desmotomy is performed.

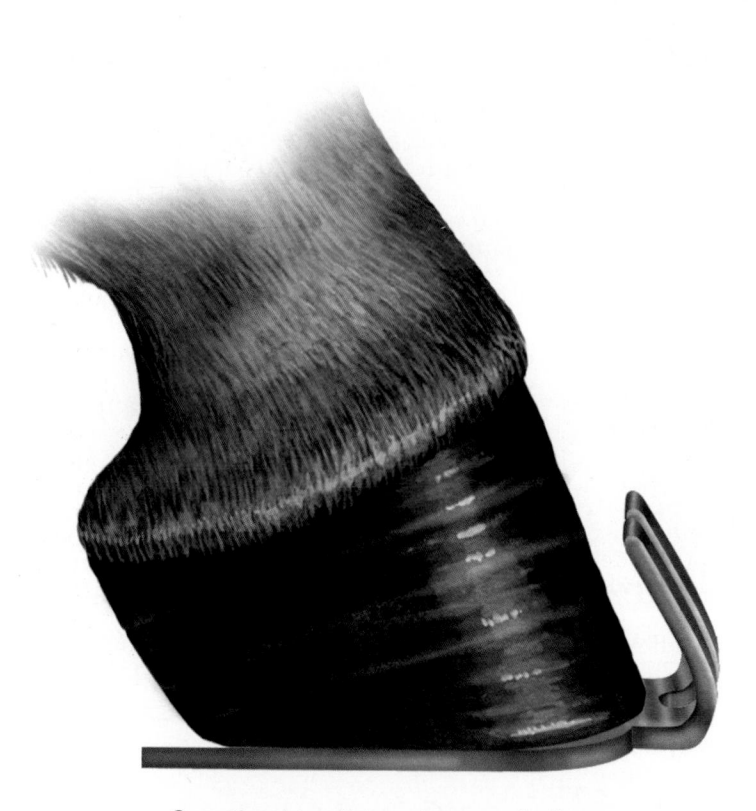

Corrective shoe with toe extension redistributes weight so that sole abscesses and bruises can be eliminated or prevented.

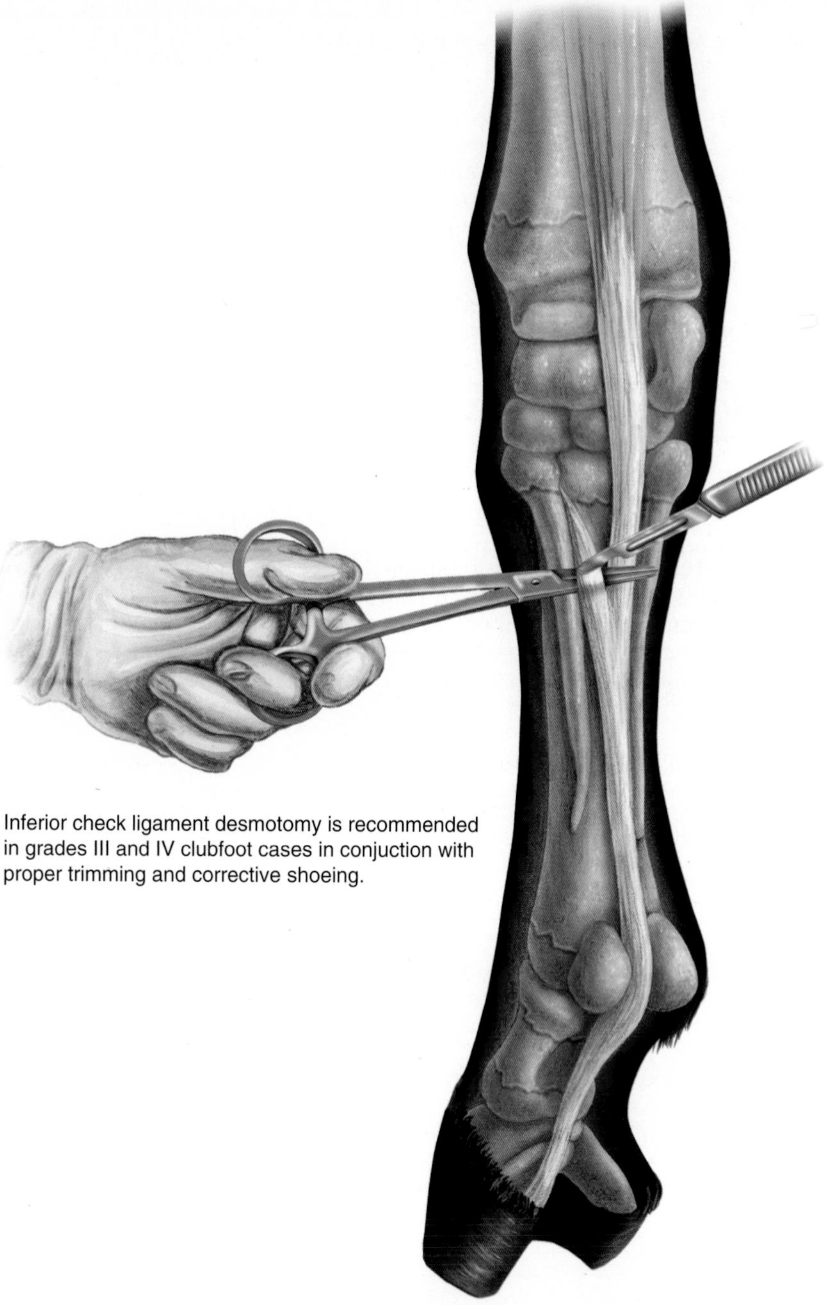

Inferior check ligament desmotomy is recommended in grades III and IV clubfoot cases in conjuction with proper trimming and corrective shoeing.

Treatment of acquired flexural deformity involves the alleviation of pain, an examination of the nutritional plane involved with this animal, surgery, and corrective shoeing. If the cause of contraction of the deep digital flexor tendon is the result of the lameness problem, then that lameness problem should be alleviated. This might involve the treatment of OCD lesions, a joint infection, or any other acute trauma to the tissues. If the flexural deformity is the result of a high plane of nutrition, this must be evaluated and corrected.

A corrective shoe with an extended toe should be applied in an attempt to realign a normal hoof-pastern axis. The heels should be lowered in conjunction with this corrective shoeing. The theory behind the shoe is to prevent excessive wear to the toe and to mechanically stretch the deep digital flexor tendon. These shoes are successful in treating grade one cases. When the treatment involves corrective shoeing of clubfeet, it is important to examine and trim the feet every 2 - 3 weeks.

Grade two cases are less likely to respond merely to corrective shoeing and often require splinting and surgery. Grade three clubfeet should initially be trimmed and shod using a toe extension shoe. The inferior check ligament should be surgically severed after the shoe has been applied and in place for at least a week to ten days. Grade four clubfeet require aggressive treatment to achieve any degree of success. A toe extension shoe is applied. The deep digital flexor tendon is surgically severed around the middle range of the cannon bone. In these severe cases the inferior check ligament desmotomy does not allow for enough laxity in a deep digital flexor tendon to provide results. Usually this aggressive procedure is a salvage operation involving long months of stall rest, hand walking, and a fairly sound horse.

Artwork By S. Hakola / J. Dirig
Copyright Equistar Publications, Ltd.

Sagittal Section Through the Head

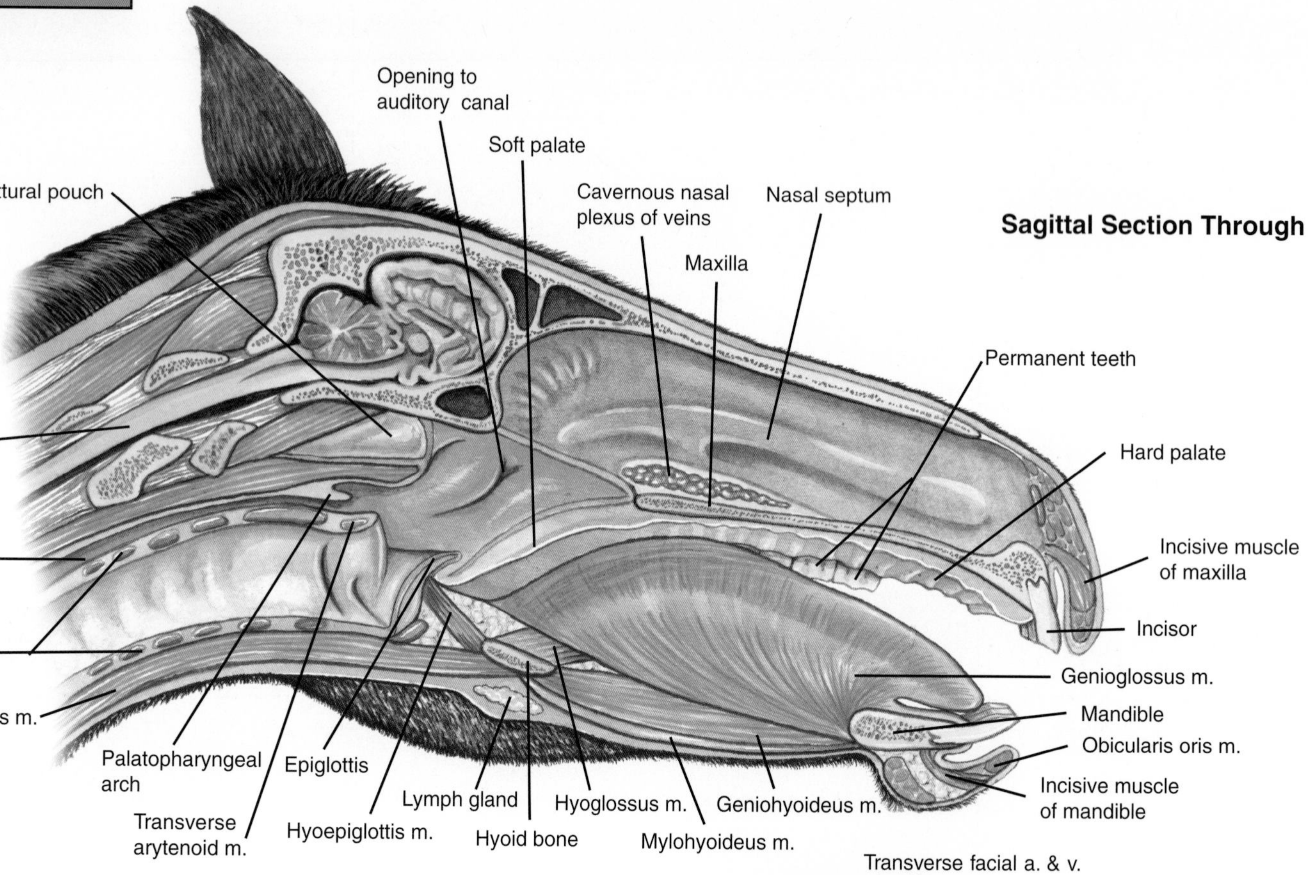

Opening to auditory canal

Soft palate

Septum over guttural pouch

Cavernous nasal plexus of veins

Nasal septum

Maxilla

Permanent teeth

Hard palate

Spinal cord

Incisive muscle of maxilla

Esophagus

Incisor

Tracheal rings

Genioglossus m.

Sternohyoideus m.

Mandible

Obicularis oris m.

Incisive muscle of mandible

Palatopharyngeal arch

Epiglottis

Lymph gland

Hyoglossus m.

Geniohyoideus m.

Transverse arytenoid m.

Hyoepiglottis m.

Hyoid bone

Mylohyoideus m.

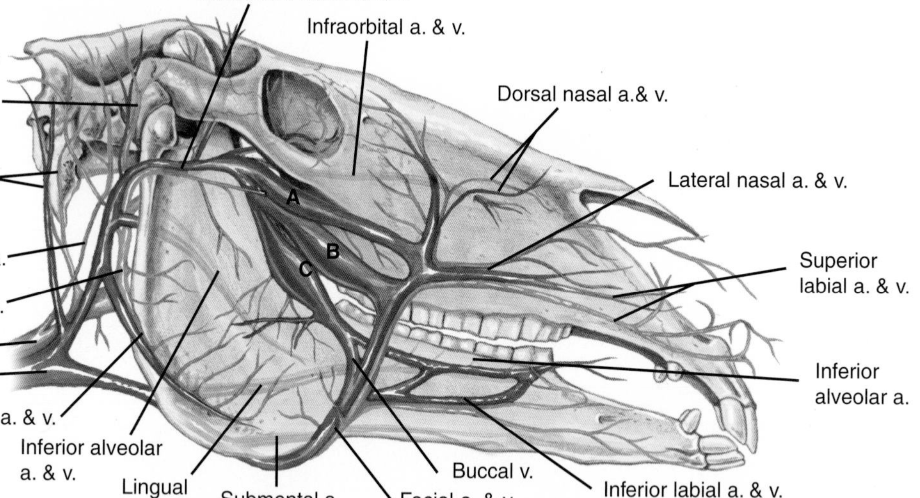

A = Dilation of transverse facial v.
B = Dilation of deep facial v.
C = Dilation of buccal v.

Transverse facial a. & v.

Infraorbital a. & v.

Rostral auricular a.& v.

Dorsal nasal a.& v.

Occipital a. & v.

Lateral nasal a. & v.

Internal carotid a.

External carotid a.

Superior labial a. & v.

Common carotid a.

External jugular v.

Inferior alveolar a.

Masseteric a. & v.

Inferior alveolar a. & v.

Lingual a. & v.

Submental a. & sublingual v.

Buccal v.

Facial a. & v.

Inferior labial a. & v.

Vascular Anatomy of the Skull

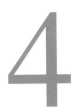

The Oral Cavity

ANATOMY OF THE ORAL CAVITY

The oral cavity or mouth of the horse is the first portion of the alimentary canal. This cavity is often one of the most neglected areas concerning the health of the horse, yet it is one of the easiest areas to examine. Common problems such as head shaking, biting, loss of appetite, excessive salivation, poor body condition, and riding difficulties can all be traced to problems within the oral cavity.

Anatomically, the oral cavity of the horse is bounded laterally by the cheek, dorsally by the palate, ventrally by the mandible, and caudally by the soft palate. Examination of this area can include direct observation, palpation, radiography, and endoscopy. It is often necessary to use an oral speculum to allow visual observation of the oral cavity. Coupled with tranquilization, this instrumentation will allow a thorough visual and physical examination of the oral cavity without endangering either the patient or the examiner.

Continuous at the margin of the lips with the common integument are the mucous membranes. These membranes should be pink in color, although in certain areas, the membrane color is difficult to determine due to pigmentation. When digital pressure is applied to these membranes, the pink color should disappear and reappear in a matter of seconds which indicates capillary refill time.

The opening of the horse's mouth is surrounded by two musculomembranous folds which are called lips. Externally these lips are covered by skin which contain long tactile hairs in addition to normal fine hairs. Internally these lip structures are covered with mucous membranes which may or may not be pigmented. Between this external skin layer and the internal mucous membrane layer are muscle tissues, glands, blood vessels, and nerves. The labial glands are more numerous on the upper lip than the lower lip. The superior and inferior palatolabial arteries provide arterial blood to the lip structures. Venous drainage is provided through the external maxillary vein. Sensory nerves originate from the trigeminal nerve, and motor nerve supply arises from the facial nerve.

Forming the sides of the mouth are the cheeks. These structures are comprised of a skin layer, which is thin and pliable, a muscular/glandular layer, and an inner mucous membrane. The buccinator muscle is the primary muscle tissue composing the muscle layer; however, there are several other small muscles also contained within this anatomical area. The superior and inferior buccal glands comprise the glandular layer. The mucous membranes that line the cheek are usually pink in color and commonly depict pigmented areas. The mucous membrane is continuous above and below with the gums and intersects with the mucous membrane of the soft palate. Opening opposite the third upper cheek tooth is the parotid duct. Vascular supply to the cheek arises from the facial and buccinator arteries, and drainage is supplied by veins of the same name. Sensory innervation arises from the trigeminal nerve and the motor nerves arise from the facial nerve.

The gum tissue of the oral cavity is comprised of dense fibrous tissue that is continuous with the periosteum of the alveolar processes. The gums are devoid of all glandular tissue and characteristically have a low degree of innervation and sensation. The gum tissue is covered by a smooth mucous membrane.

Bounded in the front and laterally by the teeth and the alveolar processes is the hard palate. At approximately the level opposite the second to last cheek tooth, the hard palate continues as the soft palate. The base of the hard palate is formed by the premaxilla, maxilla, and palatine bones. The hard palate is covered by a smooth mucous membrane and is attached to these bones by a submucosa which is very vascular in its anterior portion. The surface of the hard palate is divided into two equal portions by a central ridge or raphe. Each portion contains eighteen transverse curved ridges. The palatine arteries and veins supply the blood to the hard palate and form a generous venous plexus, particularly in the rostral portion. The trigeminal nerve provides the innervation.

THE ORAL CAVITY

Anatomy of the Oral Cavity

Artwork By S. Hakola / J. Dirig

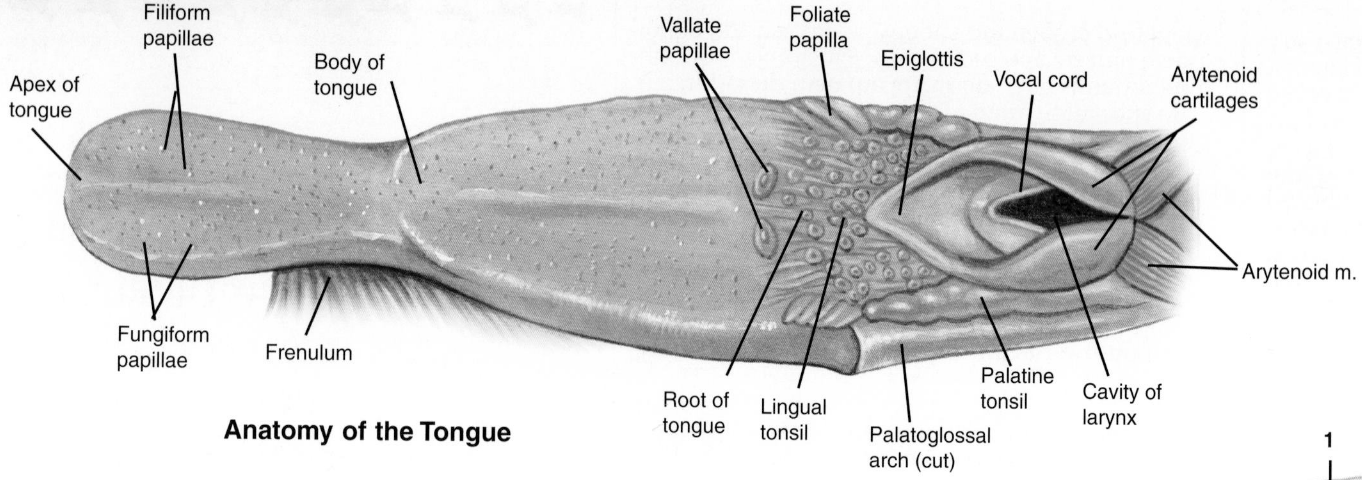
Apex of tongue
Filiform papillae
Body of tongue
Vallate papillae
Foliate papilla
Epiglottis
Vocal cord
Arytenoid cartilages
Arytenoid m.
Fungiform papillae
Frenulum
Root of tongue
Lingual tonsil
Palatoglossal arch (cut)
Palatine tonsil
Cavity of larynx

Anatomy of the Tongue

1- Peripheral cement
2- Peripheral enamel
3- Central cement
4- Central enamel
5- Infundibulum (cup)
6- Dentin
7- Dental star (secondary dentin deposited into pulp cavity)
8- Remains of Infundibulum (mark)
9- Pulp cavity containing blood vessels and nerves
10- Bone

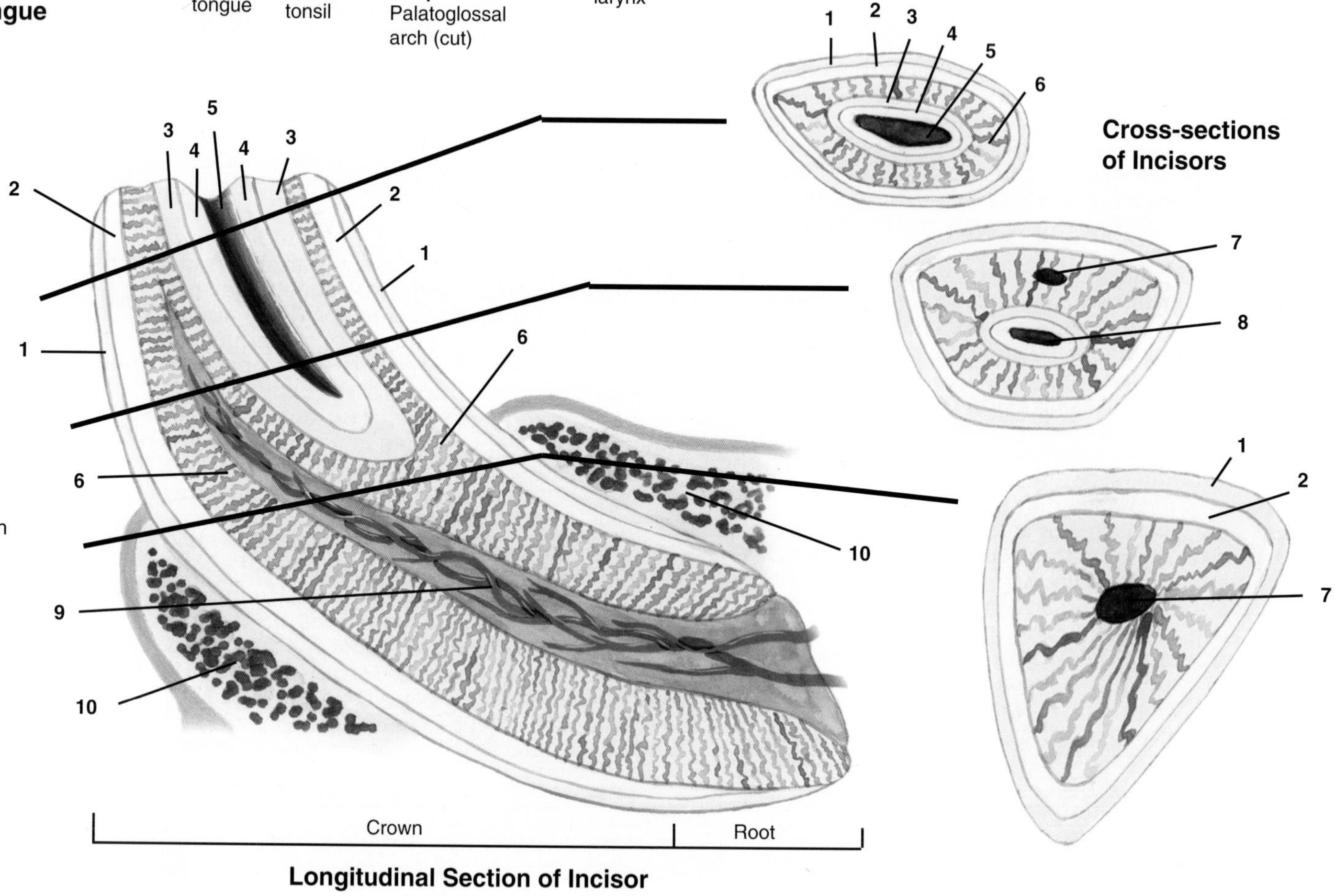
1
2
3
4
5
6
7
8
9
10
Crown
Root

Cross-sections of Incisors

Longitudinal Section of Incisor

The soft palate, which is continuous with the hard palate, is comprised of muscular membranous tissue that separates the cavity of the mouth from that of the pharynx except during swallowing. It is remarkably elongated and hangs down with a free margin in front of the epiglottis. This anatomical relationship between the soft palate and the epiglottis explains the inability of the horse to resort to oral breathing during respiratory distress. Also, on the rare occasion when a horse vomits, the ingesta is denied access to the mouth by the soft palate, and therefore has to pass into the nasopharynx and outward through the nasal cavity.

There are actually four layers of the soft palate. Superficially, the mucous membrane covers the soft palate and is continuous with the mucous membranes of the hard palate. Deeper there is a glandular layer approximately 1/2 inch in thickness which contains the palatine glands. This is followed by a muscular layer. Lastly, the pharyngeal mucous membrane layer is continuous with the mucous membranes of the nasal cavity. The blood supply of the soft palate arises from the internal and external maxillary arteries and venous drainage is provided by the corresponding veins. Innervation arises from the trigeminal, vagus, and glossopharyngeal nerves.

The floor of the oral cavity anteriorly is formed by the body of the mandible simply covered by mucous membranes. The remaining floor is occupied by the tongue, which if manually displaced to one side, the caruncula sublingualis can be visualized as a papilla opposite the canine tooth. It is through this structure that the duct of the mandibular gland empties into the oral cavity. The ventral surface of the tongue contains a medium fold mucous membrane termed the frenulum linguae. Laterally, the sublingual fold extends from the frenulum to the level of the fourth cheek tooth and contains numerous small papillae.

The tongue can be anatomically described in three areas: the root, the body, and the apex. The root is the most posterior portion and is attached to the hyoid bone, the soft palate, and the pharynx. The body has three free surfaces with only the ventral portion attached to muscular tissues. A free

spatula-shaped anterior portion is termed the apex. It has free upper and lower surfaces and a rounded border.

There are four layers throughout the entire anatomical structure of the tongue. The mucous membranes vary in thickness and cover all of the structure except the ventral surface of the tip and the lower portions of the lateral surfaces of the body. Four types of papillae cover the mucous membranes. The filiform papillae are located on the dorsal surface and the tip but are absent on the root. Fungiform papillae are large and can be seen with the naked eye over the free end and the lateral sides. The vallate papillae are 1/4th inch in diameter and are located on the posterior part of the median plane, one on each side, and about one inch apart. The foliate papillae are found in front of the anterior pillars of the soft palate. Taste buds are located throughout the fungiform, vallate, and foliate papillae.

The lingual follicles and glands are contained within the numerous folds and elevations along the root of the tongue. These follicles are basically lymphoid tissue which are inside crypts and collectively are called the lingual tonsil. Lingual and mucous glands are located along the sides and dorsal surfaces of the tongue. The muscle layer of the tongue consists of the styloglossus, the hyoglossus, and the genioglossus muscles. These are integrated systems of muscular fibers that allow retraction, depression, and protrusion of the tongue. Arterial supply to the tongue is provided by the lingual and sublingual branches of the external maxillary artery. Venous drainage is provided by the internal and external maxillary veins. Sensory innervation arises from the lingual and glossopharyngeal nerves with the muscles being innervated by the hypoglossal nerve.

THE ANATOMY OF THE TOOTH

Changes in the anatomical composition of the occlusal surface of the tooth provides an aid in the determination of the horse's age. These changes occur because of the abrasiveness of the fodder on the occlusal surface of these teeth. Each permanent

incisor is 5 - 7 cm in length and has a single root. The occlusal surface is a transverse oval that is encased by a hard enamel ring. There is an inner enfolding enamel ring that is partially filled with cement. The small cavity remaining on the occlusal surface is referred to as the cup. The cementum and dentin are worn away faster than the enamel during mastication.

The inner enamel ring which forms the infundibulum is partially filled with cement. This cup readily fills with deposits of food and turns black. As the horse ages, the wear on the occlusal surface causes the cup to disappear and all that remains is a dental spot in the center of the tooth. As the incisor continues to wear away, one would think that eventually the actual pulp of the tooth would be exposed. However, the formation of darker secondary dentin (known as the dental star) occurs.

There are six incisors in the mandible and maxillary arches. From an anterior to posterior view they are referred to as the central, intermediate, and corner incisors. When in contact with the labial surface, these arches are convex. As they grow out to compensate for wear, the arches become flattened and are almost straight when the animal reaches 20 yearsof age. Geometrically, when the animal is 8 years old, the angle between the upper and lower incisors is approximately 180 degrees. As the horse ages, the lower arch begins to straighten. The upper arch straightens at a slower rate resulting in an angle of approximately 135 degrees. When the animal reaches 25 years old, this angle decreases to almost 90 degrees.

The canine teeth form in both sexes, although they are rarely seen in mares due to rudimentary development and failure to erupt. They occur in the area known as the diastema in a closer proximity to the corner incisor than to the first premolars. They are conical in shape with the roots being much larger than the exposed crowns. The canine teeth can erupt as early as 3 1/2 years of age but generally erupt around 4 years. Some canine teeth erupt as late as 5 years of age.

The first premolar is referred to as the "wolf tooth". This tooth is usually vestigial and occurs just

THE ORAL CAVITY

Anatomy of the Oral Cavity, The Dental Examination

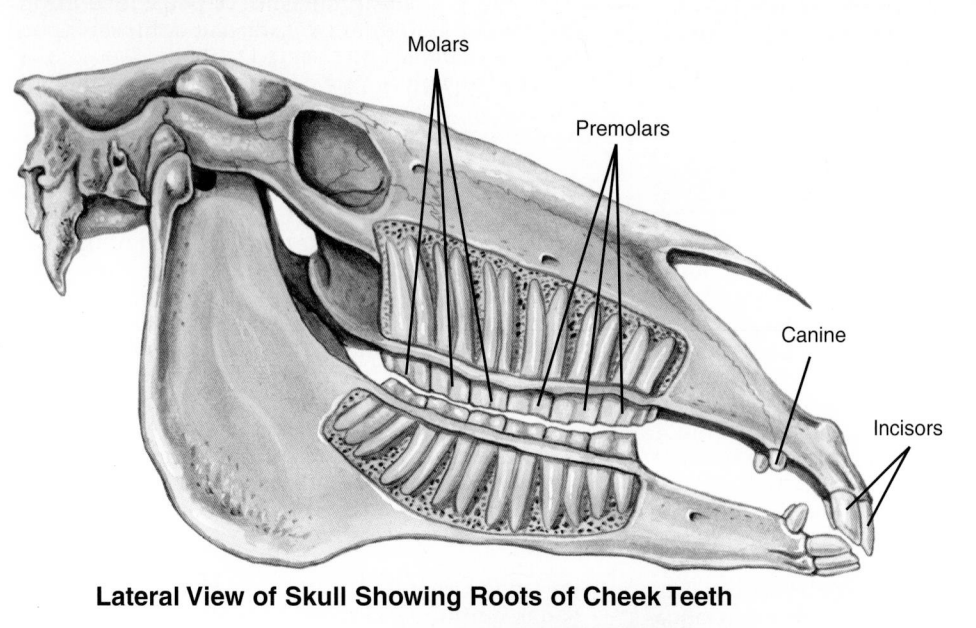

Molars
Premolars
Canine
Incisors

Lateral View of Skull Showing Roots of Cheek Teeth

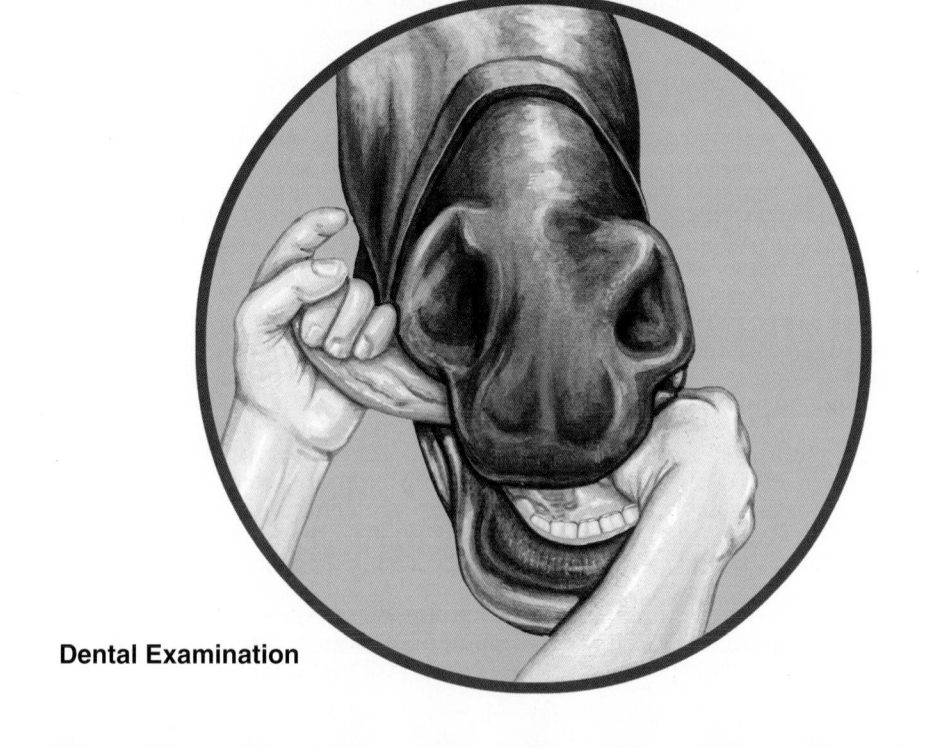

Dental Examination

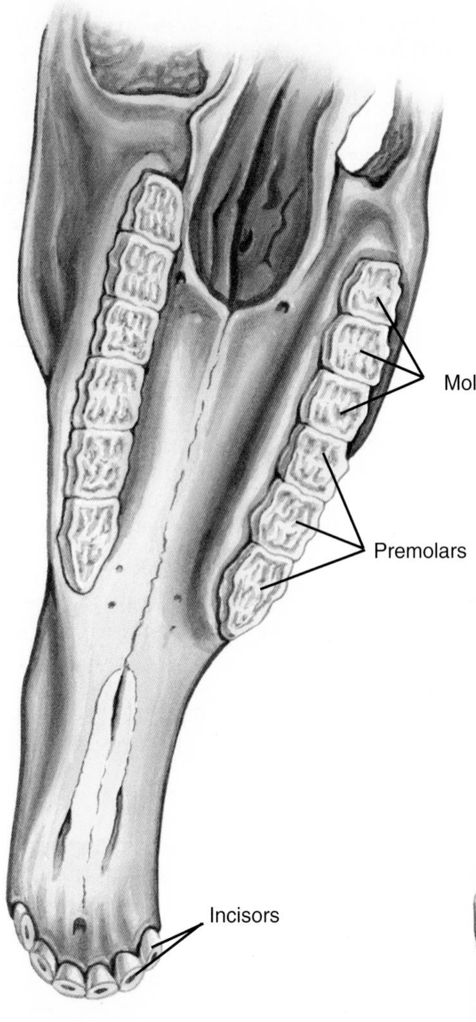

Molars
Premolars
Incisors

Ventral View of Maxillary Arch

Mandibular Arch

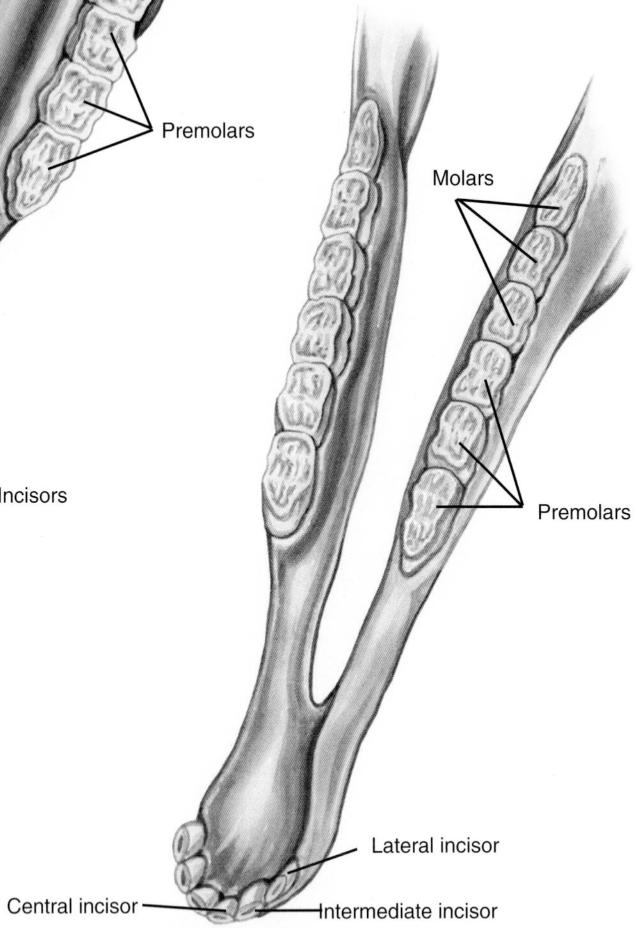

Molars
Premolars
Lateral incisor
Central incisor
Intermediate incisor

medial to the second premolar on the upper jaw. The wolf tooth is routinely extracted.

There are three more premolars that occur in a row that is continuous with the three molars. There are several major differences anatomically between the upper and lower sets. The upper premolars and molars have three and four roots, whereas the lower premolars and molars only have two roots each. The upper cheek teeth are wider and consist of a more convoluted enamel folding which forms two separate infundibulae that fill with cement before eruption. There are no infundibulae with the enamel folds of the lower cheek teeth. On the upper cheek teeth, the area outside the infundibulum fills with dentin out to the enamel casing. The dentin and cement wear faster than the enamel, and the occlusal surfaces develop a rasp-like quality to aid in mastication.

THE DENTAL EXAMINATION

Through evolution, the equid has become a flight creature. One cannot properly examine the oral cavity of the horse without first gaining the confidence of the horse or applying sufficient restraint techniques. A thorough history should be taken to discover the type of diet the animal partakes, any problems the horse exhibits, and any objectionable oral habits it may have. One can often reach a differential diagnostic list from these three facts and focus the dental examination in this direction. The fecal material should be examined to determine if the food particles are over one quarter to three eighths of an inch in length. If this is the case, the animal is having occlusal problems within the molars.

The patient should be relaxed and calm. The use of a mild injectionable tranquilizer such as Detomidine hydrochloride or xylazine may be necessary to gain this state so that a methodical exam technique can be followed. An external exam of the general conformation of the entire head should be done initially, because any abnormalities that appear externally could have an internal origin. The position of the jaws should be noted as

well as any swelling or abnormal lumps of either the maxilla or mandible. The lips should be retracted to examine the incisors. It should be noted if the incisors are deciduous or permanent, whether there is a normal number, the current placement and direction of the incisors, and whether they correspond with one another reciprocally. Most genetic abnormalities such as "parrot mouth" can be easily detected.

After this initial visual examination is finished, a more thorough exam of the buccal cavity must be completed both visually and manually. Either the right or left hand should be inserted through the interdental space on one side of the mouth. The tongue should be grasped firmly and brought laterally to a position on that side. The other hand is then free to examine the teeth and the dental arcades on the opposite side from which the tongue is being held. Care should be taken so as not to traumatize the frenulum on the ventral surface of the tongue which would also cause the animal to resist the examination. The goal of this technique is to hold the tongue between the teeth to prevent the examiner's hand from being bitten.

The incisors should be examined to determine their eruption time, their occlussal surfaces for wear, and their shape and length. The canine teeth should be observed for wear, their eruption time, and their length. The molars and premolars should be examined on both sides. First, the examination of one side occurs. Then the grasp of the tongue is transferred to the opposite side to facilitate a manual examination of that side. The cheek teeth should reveal their state of dentition, the structure of their occlusal surfaces, the length and direction of each tooth, and the health status of the buccal mucosal membranes and gingiva.

There are times when a mouth gag or a full mouth speculum is helpful. A simple mouth wedge can be inserted and attached to the halter. A flashlight or other light source is also a great aid in the visualization of all the surfaces that require examination. Radiographs form an important diagnostic aid in the dental examination. Oblique views are especially desirable in assessing the roots and the paranasal sinuses. In most cases, some degree of anesthesia is indicated to obtain good diagnostic films.

The frequency of routine dental examinations is determined by a number of factors. The primary factors are the breed, the age of the animal, the general conformation of the head, and the occlusion of the teeth within the mouth. Performance demands, type of feedstuffs fed, and housing (stabled versus pasture care) also determine the amount of wear upon the teeth and the need for dental care.

Artwork By S. Hakola
Copyright Equistar Publications, Ltd.

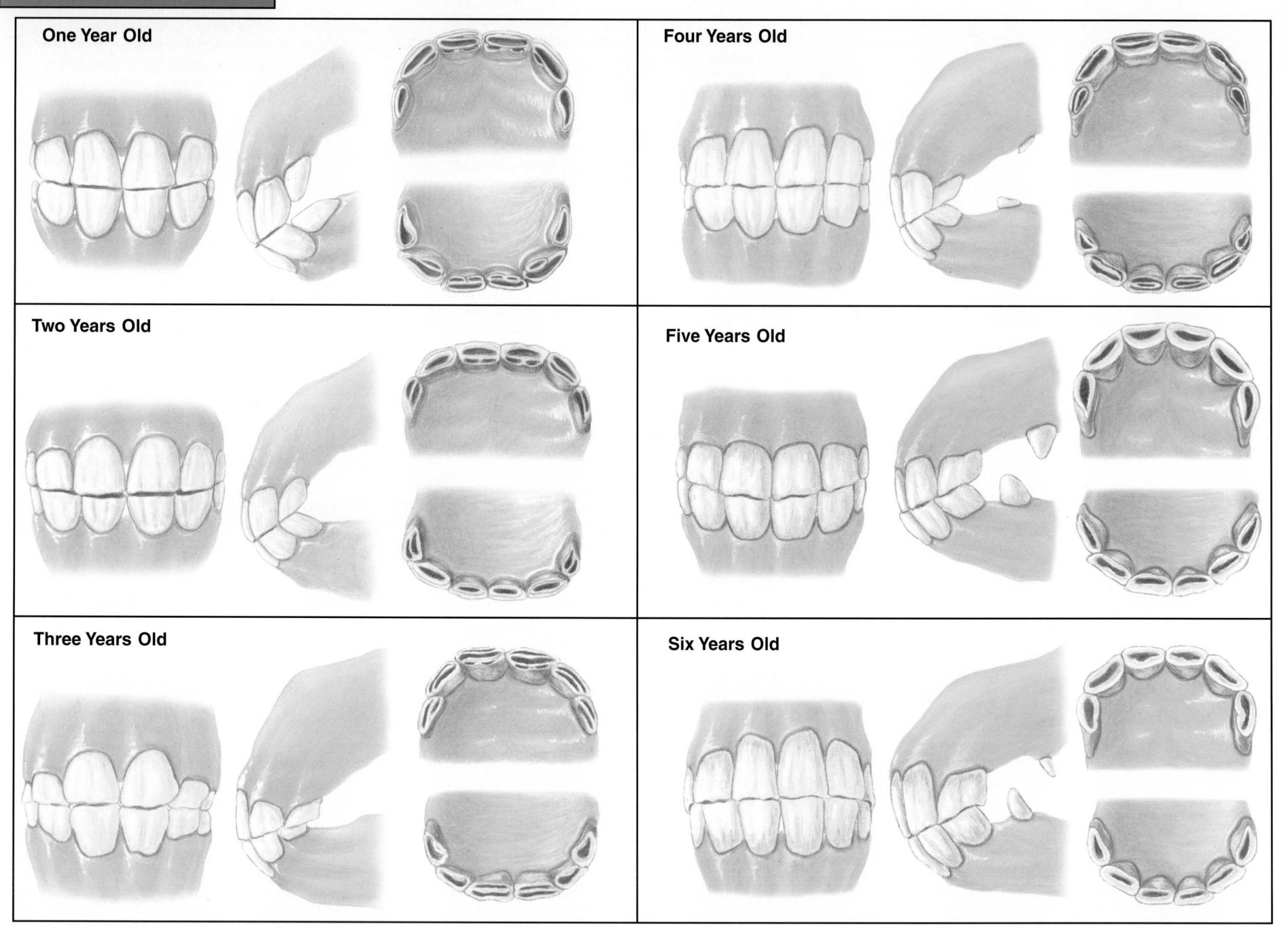

One Year Old

Two Years Old

Three Years Old

Four Years Old

Five Years Old

Six Years Old

THE DETERMINATION OF THE HORSE'S AGE

The determination of the age of the horse can be fairly accurate when certain characteristics are examined. The following nine characteristics give an accurate depiction of age up to 10 years:

1) The eruption of the deciduous teeth: the central at 6 days, the intermediate at 6 weeks, and the corner at 6 months.

2) The eruption of the permanent incisors: the central through corner erupt at 2.5, 3.5, and 4.5 years.

3) The infundibulum cup disappears with wear. The deciduous cup disappears at ages 1, 1.5, and 2. The permanent cup disappears at 6, 7, and 8 years of age.

4) The occlusal surfaces change shape.

5) The arch formed by the incisors changes angle.

6) The wear on the entire tooth. This is subjective, but the teeth are in full wear 6 months posteruption.

7) The angular profile of the incisors when viewed laterally.

8) The seven year hook on the corner incisor.

9) Galvayne's groove on the corner incisor appears at the gum line at 10 years, proceeds distally until 20 years of age, and then recedes until the horse is 30 years old.

One Year Old

When viewed from the front, the true yearling at 12 months old will have all of the deciduous teeth erupted and in wear. Laterally, the corner incisors from the upper and lower arcade will not be in contact. The central and intermediate incisors will have a longitudinal dental star, whereas the corner incisor will not. The first permanent molars may start to appear at this time.

Two Year Old

When the animal reaches two years of age, the central incisor is removed from the gum in preparation for the eruption of the central permanent incisor. The occlusal surfaces of the central and intermediate incisors are level, smooth, and show considerable wear. The corner incisor is in wear and depicts a dental star. The second permanent molar erupts, and care should be taken to see that the deciduous caps are removed from them.

Three Year Old

The three year old shows all four central incisors completely erupted and in wear. Each one of these central incisors will have a deep cup since the infundibulum has just started to wear. The intermediate incisor and corner incisor will have a long neck and appear ready to be replaced by the permanent incisors. The "wolf teeth" should be easily visible. The second and third premolars erupt and the deciduous caps are shed.

Four Year Old

The central and intermediate permanent incisors are in firm contact and wear in the four year old horse. The remaining deciduous corner incisors appear smaller in comparison. The canines may erupt at 3 1/2 years of age but are more likely to erupt at age four. The dental cup is still deep on the central incisor, whereas the intermediate incisor has a sharp surface. The fourth permanent premolar and molar should erupt at this time.

Five Year Old

All of the permanent dentition is complete in the five year old and all of the teeth are in wear. The jaws are convex when viewed anterior to posterior. The canine teeth should have erupted completely. All of the incisors should have a dental cup, but the central incisors will show considerable wear.

Six Year Old

In the sixth year, the cup will be gone on the central incisor. The intermediate incisor will show distinct cups and the corner incisor will be completely in wear. Viewed anterior to posterior, the mouth will appear as it did as a 5 year old. The canine teeth are usually at full length.

Artwork By S. Hakola
Copyright Equistar Publications, Ltd.

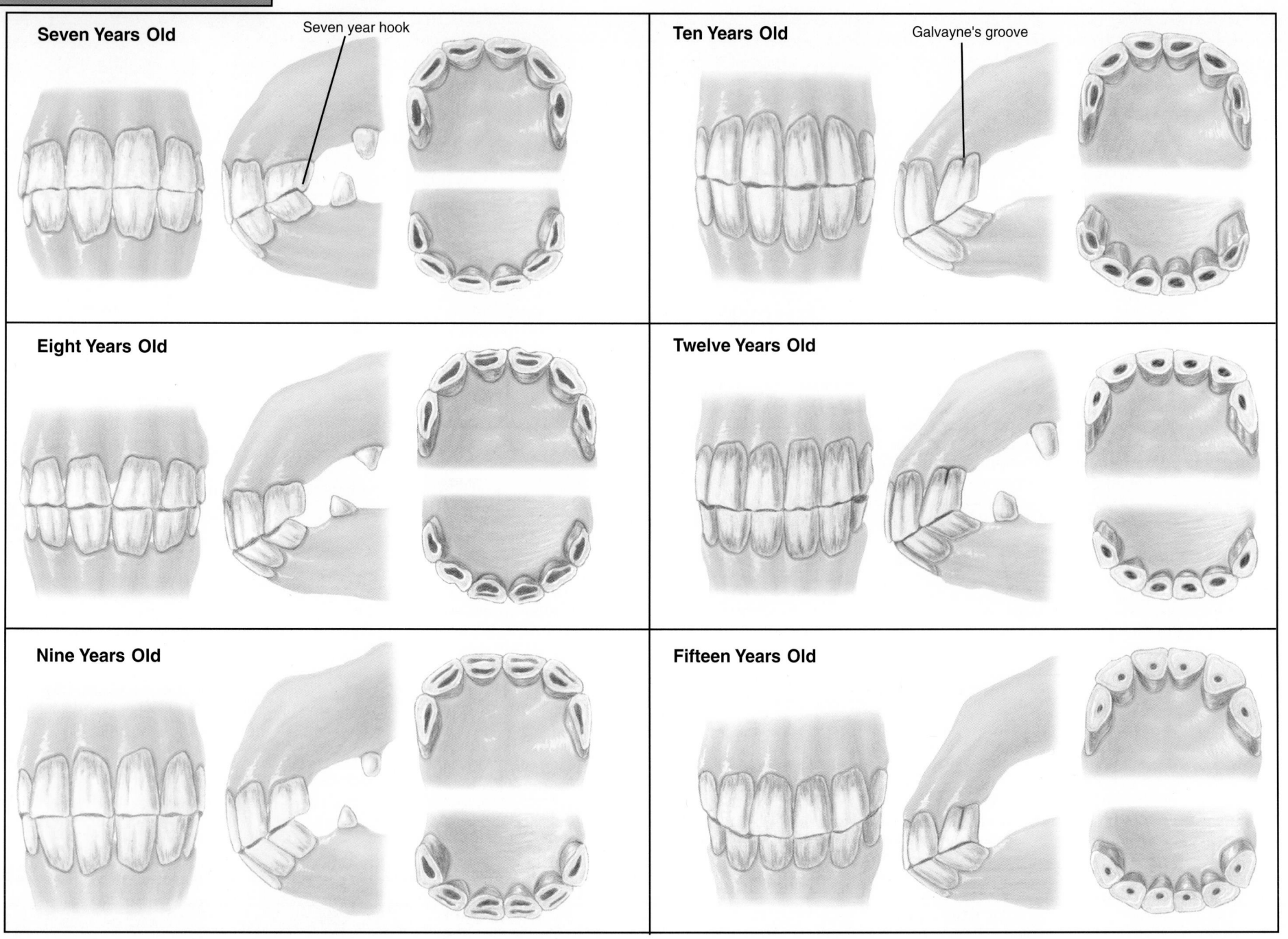

Seven Years Old — Seven year hook

Ten Years Old — Galvayne's groove

Eight Years Old

Twelve Years Old

Nine Years Old

Fifteen Years Old

Seven Year Old

A seven year hook is present on the caudal occlusal surface of the corner incisor at seven years of age. The occlusal surface of the central incisor is level. On the intermediate incisor, the cup is gone. The dental cup is still present on the corner incisors only.

Eight Year Old

The first dental star appears on the central incisor when the horse is 8 years old. In some instances, the first stages of a dental star (a dark yellow or brownish-yellow line) appears on the occlusal surface of the intermediate incisor. When viewed laterally, the upper and lower incisors are at a more oblique angle than before.

Nine Year Old

The shape of the incisors and the occlusal surfaces distinguish the nine year old. The central incisors are round, and they have a distinct dental star in the center. The intermediate incisors are becoming round and the corners are oval. The seven year hook has usually disappeared from the upper corner incisors by the ninth year.

Ten Year Old

The ten year old horse has the distinction of Galvayne's groove starting to show on the labial surface of the upper corner incisor. The distal end of this groove should just protrude through the gum line at this age. The central and intermediate incisors are round and the dental stars on the occlusal surfaces should be in the center of the teeth.

Twelve Year Old

At 12 years of age, the angle of occlusion of the incisor arch becomes prominently oblique. All of the occlusal surfaces of the incisors are round. The dental stars are merely small yellow dots near the center of each tooth. Galvayne's groove is progressing posteriorly approximately 1/4 of the way down the labial surface of the corner incisor.

Fifteen Year Old

Galvayne's groove should extend approximately halfway down the labial surface of the corner incisor on the 15 year old horse. The central incisor should be triangular in shape, with the intermediates round to triangular. The dental star in the center should be almost round in shape on all of the incisor occlusal surfaces.

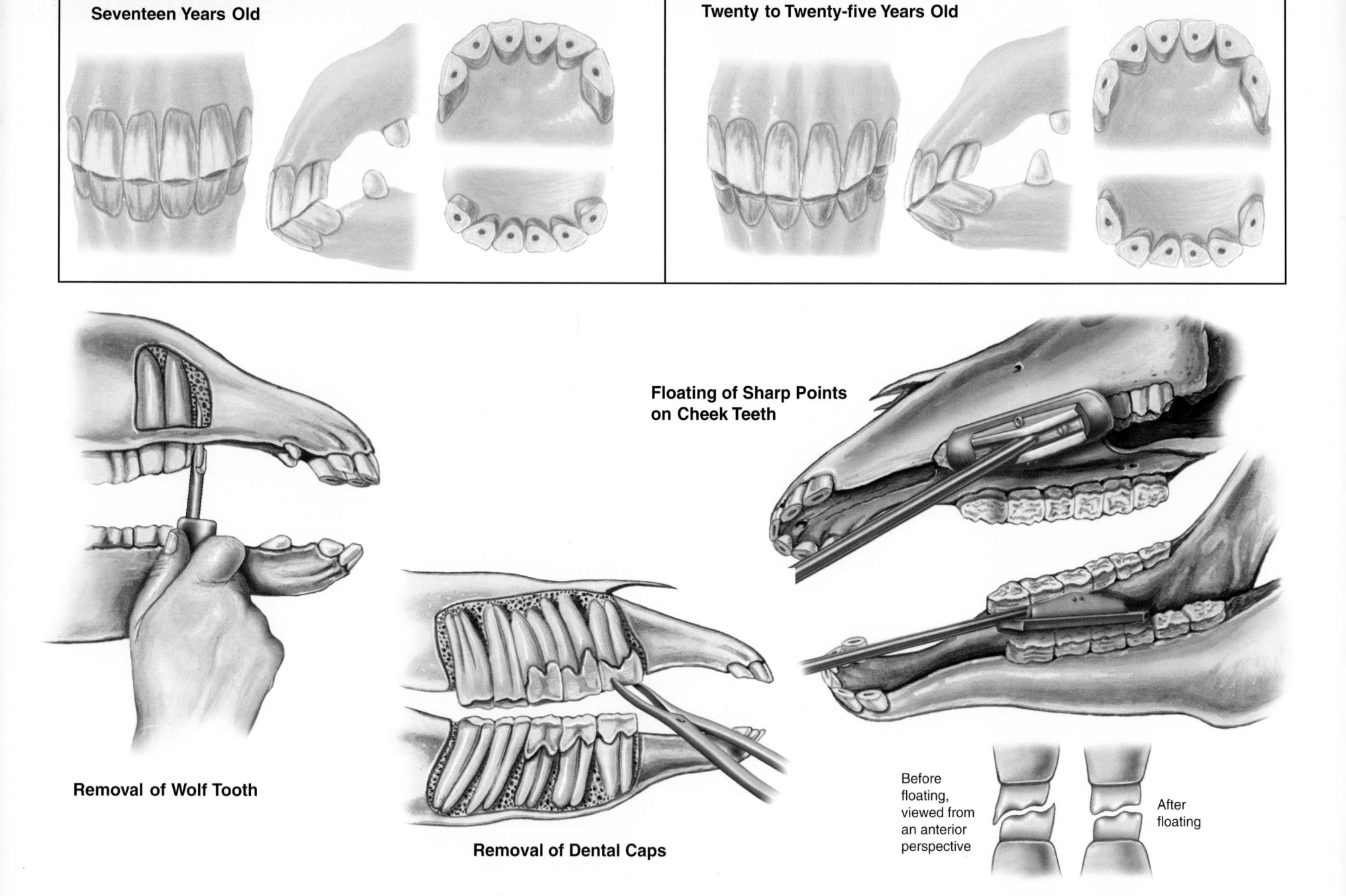

Seventeen Years Old

Twenty to Twenty-five Years Old

Floating of Sharp Points on Cheek Teeth

Removal of Wolf Tooth

Removal of Dental Caps

Before floating, viewed from an anterior perspective

After floating

Seventeen Year Old

At 17 years of age, all of the incisors should be triangular in shape and all of the dental stars round. Galvayne's groove should extend distally 3/4 of the way down the corner incisor.

Twenty Year Old

Galvayne's groove extends the entire labial surface length of the upper corner incisor of the 20 year old horse. The occlusal surfaces of the lower arches should all be worn and compressed. The upper and lower incisors will meet in a very oblique arch.

DENTAL ERUPTION TABLE

Deciduous Teeth

Central incisors	Present birth to one week
Intermediate incisors	4 1/2 to 6 weeks
Corner incisors	6 to 9 months
Premolars	Present at birth to first 2 weeks

Permanent Teeth

Central incisor	2 1/2 years
Intermediate incisor	3 1/2 years
Corner incisor	4 1/2 years
Canine	3 1/2 to 5 years
1st Premolar (wolf tooth)	6 months to 3 years
2nd Premolar (cheek)	2 to 3 years
3rd Premolar	3 years
4th Premolar	4 years
1st Molar	9 to 12 months
2nd Molar	2 years
3rd Molar	3 to 4 years

WOLF TOOTH EXTRACTION

There are many ways to extract the first premolar or wolf tooth. Often, these teeth are large and lay in direct contact with the second premolar. These are the most difficult to extract because it is important to remove all of the accompanying root as well as the erupted crown. The key to extraction of the wolf teeth lies in the use of the dental elevator to loosen the tooth from surrounding gum tissue and maxilla. The teeth are then easily removed with forceps.

REMOVAL OF THE DENTAL CAPS

Removal of the dental caps, or deciduous teeth of the premolars, is sometimes indicated when these caps are impeding the eruption of the underlying permanent tooth. Usually when this condition arises, there is a swelling over the maxillary sinus due to the impacted permanent tooth.

Removal of the caps is facilitated by the use of a simple mouth wedge or speculum. This allows easy palpation of the teeth and a visualization of the dental arcade. A simple heavy-duty pair of forceps merely clasps the cap and frees it from the underlying tissues. There have been times in practice where a bone elevator, a long shafted screwdriver, and even a small pair of hoof testers have been utilized to remove dental caps.

"FLOATING THE TEETH"

Where did the term "floating" have its origin? Dental prophylaxis to the horse is anything but "drifting through the air like a feather on a light summer breeze." Rasping or filing of a horse's teeth is known as floating. The object of this routine biannual procedure is to maintain normal dental occlusion and prevent gingivitis or buccal mucosal irritation.

Horses in their typical grazing environment, continuously feeding and browsing, wear down their teeth normally. Stabled horses eat only a small part of the day and their feedstuffs of processed grains are softer than the normal grass. This type of husbandry allows the teeth to become excessively long and to wear unevenly.

Sharp edges are found on the buccal borders of the upper arcade and on the lingual borders of the lower arcade of all the cheek teeth. The routine removal of these edges can be accomplished without any anesthesia or the use of a mouth wedge or gag. The halter is usually loosened so as not to restrict the movement of the float between the teeth and the buccal membranes.

The dental float is inserted over the sharp edges of the upper arcade at approximately a 60 degree angle. The lingual sharp edges are removed in the same fashion. Long smooth strokes with an angled float insure fast removal of the points and a minimum amount of trauma to the mucosal membranes.

In finishing the procedure, the sharp edges that occur on the rostral edges of the second premolar should be removed by a small file or float. This float should have a 45 degree angle to the head and be positioned in a way that is close to the animal's head. When numerous sharp edges occur over the cheek teeth, the animal usually shows reluctance to respond to the bit and the horse allows food to fall from its mouth while feeding. This spillage is referred to as "quidding."

The goal for the entire dental procedure is to gain a balance to the animal's teeth and have 70% or more occlusion of the premolars and molars during the mastication cycle. The wolf teeth should be removed along with any caps. Tartar should be removed, especially around the canine teeth. The gums, palates, and cheeks are inspected for any injury or trauma. Proper dental prophylaxis will free the animal from any existing or potential pain which will allow the animal to achieve maximum performance and condition.

THE ORAL CAVITY

Cheek Teeth Extraction; Dental Disorders and Malocclusions

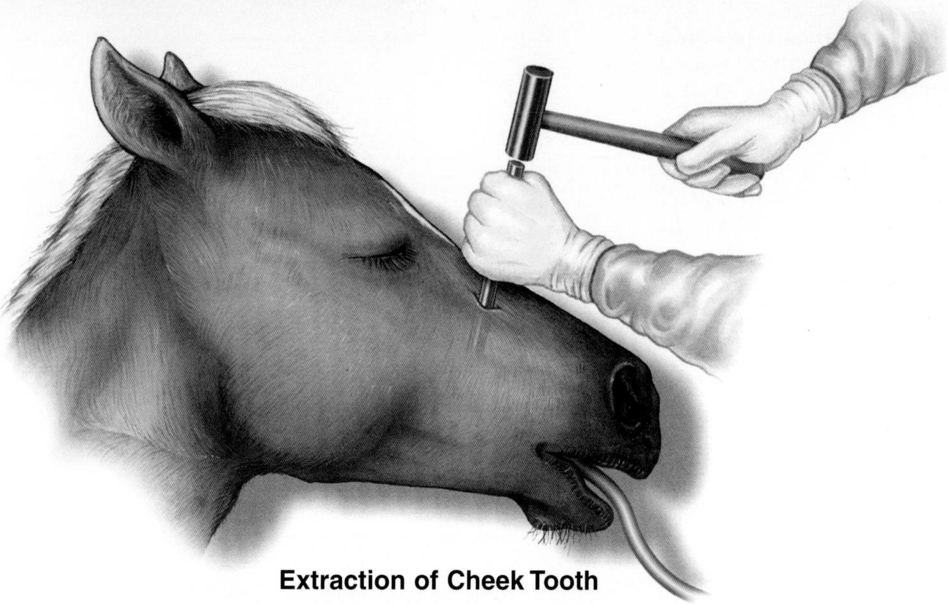

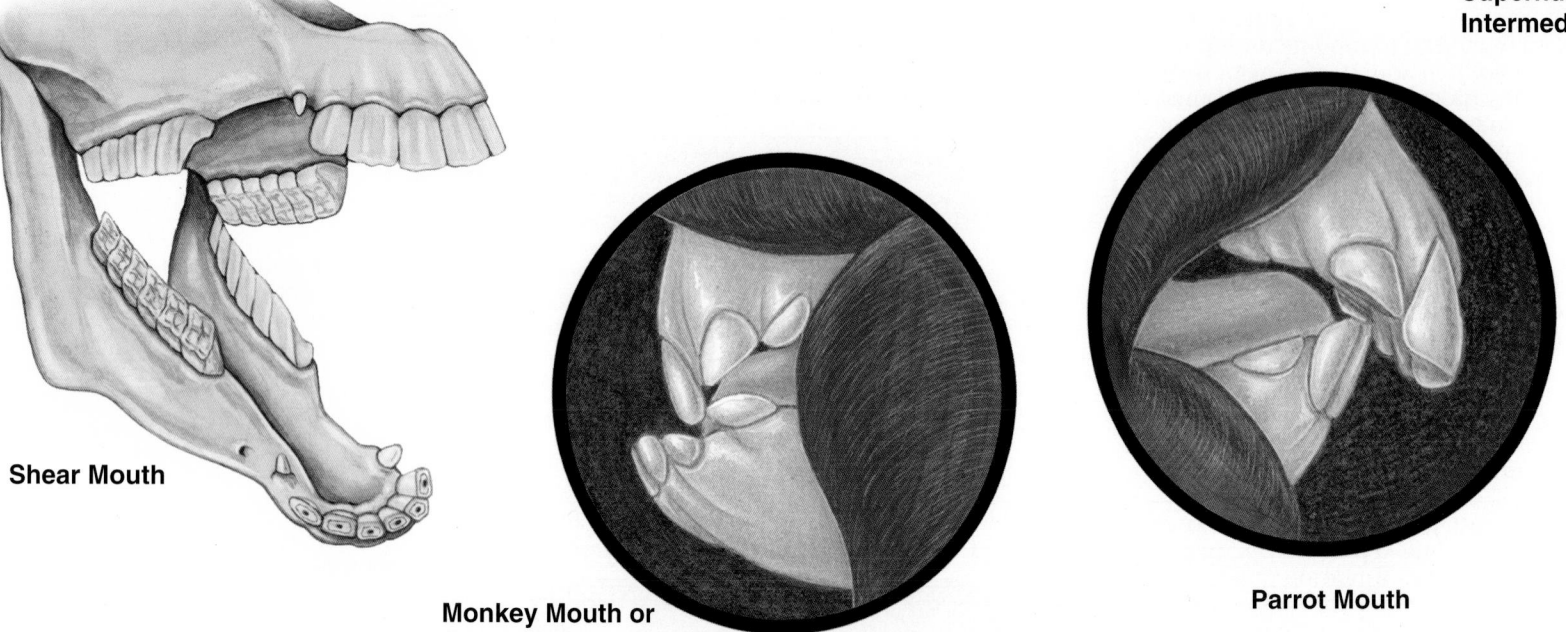

Extraction of Cheek Tooth

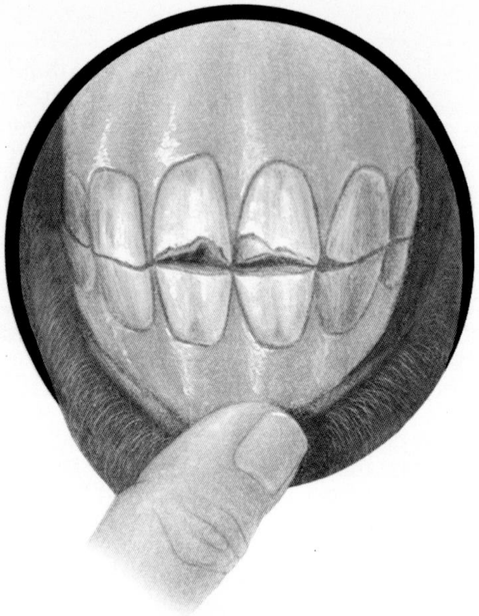

Cribbing

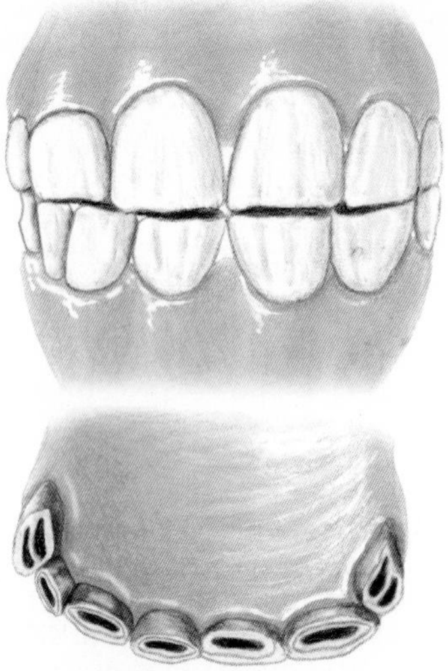

Supernumerary Intermediate Incisor

Shear Mouth

Monkey Mouth or Sow Mouth

Parrot Mouth

EXTRACTION OF THE CHEEK TEETH

Extraction of the cheek teeth is indicated in cases of severe periodontal disease with abscesses within the roots. The patient should be placed under general anesthesia and intubated. Radiographs should be taken to visualize the involvement of the roots and the surrounding tissues. If the tooth is loose enough from the surrounding gums and boney structures, one can merely grasp it with a forceps to remove it. Use of another float instrument on the occlussal surface of the next rostral tooth as a fulcrum will facilitate the extraction.

When extraction is unsuccessful, repulsion of the tooth is the alternate approach. Simply stated, repulsion is the removal of the cheek tooth by gaining access to the roots. By using a punch and mallet, the tooth is driven from the socket without fracturing the jaw. Each tooth has its own root. An incision is made through the skin over the corresponding area which is identified by radiographs. A trephine opening is made to expose the roots so that a punch and mallet can be used. The tooth is loosened with an elevator before being driven out with the punch.

After the tooth is removed and the socket is cleaned, the skin should be approximated and sutured back in place. The socket should be disinfected daily and the animal started on systemic antibiotics. Postoperative care should be that for any surgical procedure. An alternative to this is to not suture the skin, insert a drain, and allow for healing by second intention.

COMMON DISORDERS AND MALOCCLUSIONS

Cribbing

If excessive wear is noted on the incisors, it may not be due to foraging on abrasive surfaces but due to a behavioral neurosis known as cribbing or crib-biting. There is a characteristic pattern of wear on the rostral margin of the upper central incisors. This pattern is determined by the age of the horse (such as foals with deciduous teeth learning the behavior from the dam) and the duration of the behaviorial pattern.

Supernumerary Teeth

When the dental bud is split during development, the uncommon genetic abnormality of supernumerary teeth develops. This is usually seen within the incisors and results in a dental crowding of these teeth. Gaps can occur between the teeth with resultant gingivitis, periodonitis, osteitis, and/or malocclusion This malocclusion then results in possible ulceration of the corresponding hard palate or the tongue. The treatment for this is removal of these teeth and frequent floating to correct the malocclusion.

Parrot Mouth (Overbite)and Monkey Mouth (Underbite)

The most common inherited disorder involves the maxilla and/or the mandible and is referred to as "parrot mouth." In this case, the upper jaw is longer than the lower jaw (maxillary brachygnathia.) Conversely, mandibular brachygnathia refers to the lower jaw being longer than the upper. This is commonly called "monkey mouth" or "sow mouth." Both conditions result in abnormal wear to the incisors. Affected horses are generally considered unsound. The only treatment available is a regular program of rasping the incisors to prevent incisor overgrowth.

Overjet and Underjet

These are terms that are used to describe the partial displacement of the incisor teeth front-to-back. This partial overlay of the incisor teeth results in a malocclusion of the incisors.

Shear Mouth

"Shear mouth" is a condition that exists when the maxilla is wider than the mandible. Even if this is slight, the resultant change to the occlusal surfaces is drastic. The sharp edges of the buccal surfaces of the upper arch and the lingual surfaces of the lower arch are greatly exaggerated. Consequently, the movement within the temporomandibular joint is affected. This results in a degenerative joint disease leading to osteoarthritis. Treatment of this condition involves rasping the sharp edges off or actually cutting them so as to realign the occlussal surfaces. In a mild case this has some merit, but a severe case is nonrewarding.

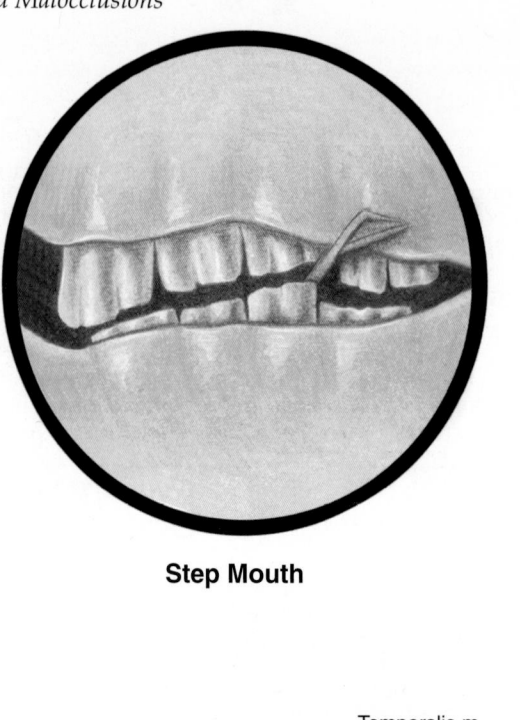

Step Mouth

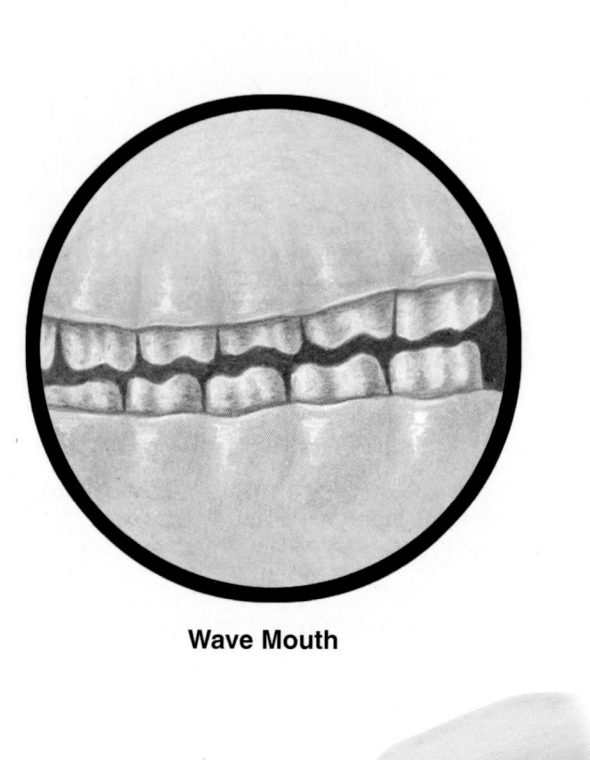

Wave Mouth

Smooth Mouth

Temporalis m.

TMJ Articular disc

Deep muscles of mastication are exposed after removal of mandible ramus to show anatomy medial to the mandible.

Lateral pterygoid m.

Medial pterygoid m.

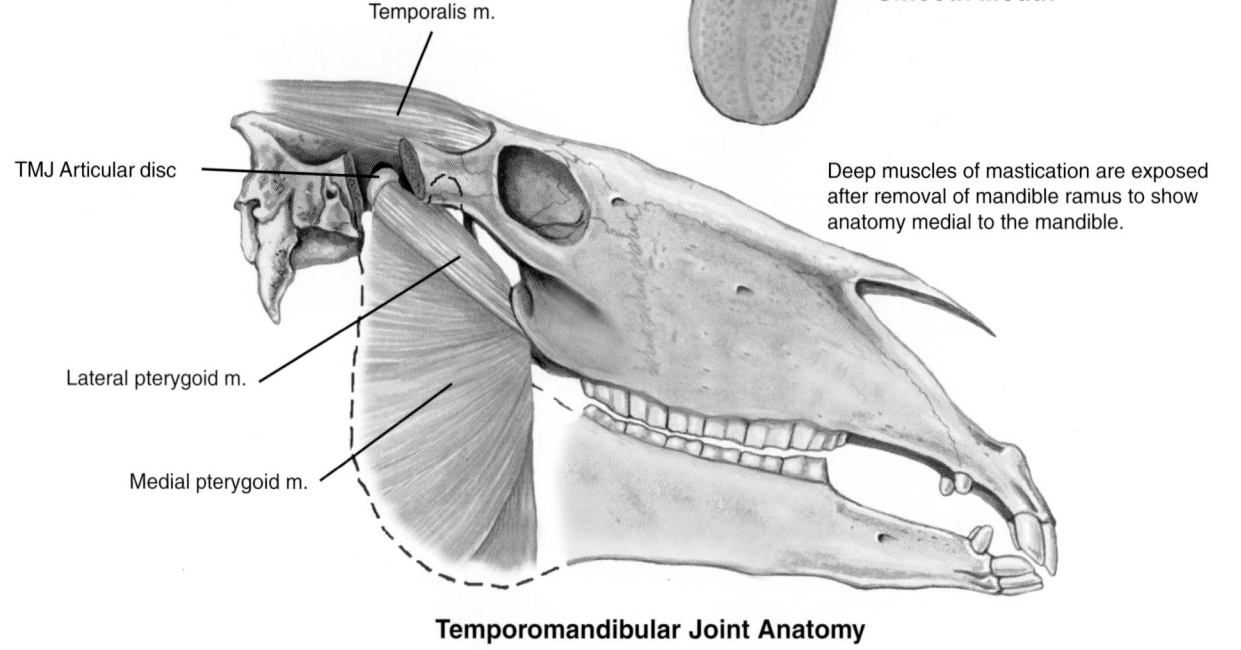

Tartar and Gingivitis

Temporomandibular Joint Anatomy

Wave Mouth and Step Mouth

When a series of waves develops on the occlusal surface of the cheek teeth, the horse is said to possess a "wave mouth." This is believed to be caused by a stereotypical chewing behavior. The entire arch is involved with a matching wave on the opposing occlusal surfaces. "Step mouth" occurs when only one tooth is involved with excessive wear or when a tooth is missing. Routine floating may help both the step mouth and wave mouth conditions. The step mouth condition is much harder on the animal and requires constant vigilance and appropriate care.

Smooth Mouth

When one performs dental exams on extremely old horses, one will note that most of the horses will have a characteristic "smooth mouth." There is excessive wear to all the premolars and molars sometimes down to the gingiva. This results in pain, incomplete mastication and digestion, and resultant weight loss. Treatment other than feeding mashes and soft pellets is unfortunately useless.

Lampas, Tartar, and Gingivitis

Lampas is any edema or congestion within the lining of the roof of the horse's mouth. The most common occurrence anatomically is just behind the incisors. This condition occurs when there is an injury to the tongue which results in an irritation of the lining of the mouth from the unmasticated feedstuffs that is not reaching the molars. Tartar is formed from calcium phosphate, mucus, and saliva and deposited on the teeth. Routine prophylaxis should include the removal of this substance. Gingivitis is caused from a number of factors that result in the inflammation of the gums. Whatever cause is precipitating this inflammation should be rectified.

The Temporomandibular Joint and Corresponding Muscle Mass

Palpation of the temporomandibular joint (TMJ) will reveal the placement of this joint. Proper placement of the TMJ will indicate the placement of the mandible. If there is a displacement to one side, this indicates the presence of a dental problem or an injury to the area. Whenever there is a displacement within the temporomandibular joint, there will be a variation within the temporal and masseter muscles. These muscles will be overdeveloped on the side where most of the mastication is taking place and atrophied on the side of little use.

ROUTINE DENTAL CARE

Yearlings

Time and patience are of utmost importance since during this formative time, the animal should be initiated into routine dental prophylaxis. Premolars should be floated and proper occlusion attained. Wolf teeth should be removed when appropiate.

Two Year Old

The premolars and permanent molars should be floated to obtain ideal occlusion. The eruption of the first permanent molars should be visualized. Extraction should be performed on any wolf teeth present.

Two and One - Half Year Olds

The premolars and permanent molars should be floated to gain occlusion. Any retained premolar or incisor caps should be removed. The eruption of any permanent molars or incisors should be checked visually and any wolf teeth should be removed.

Three Year Old

Both the premolars and permanent molars should be floated to occlusion. The third premolar cap should be checked for retention and removed if necessary. Eruptions of the incisors and second permanent molar should be checked.

Three and One - Half Year Old

Occlusion should be gained through floating of the premolars and permanent molars. Eruptions of the permanent molars and incisors should be checked. Removal of any retained second incisor caps or number four premolar caps should be done at this time.

Four Year Old

All retained molar caps should be removed with any retained cap slivers or splinters. The molars should be floated to gain optimal occlusion. The eruption of the third permanent molar should be visualized. The incisors should be inspected for any deciduous incisor root fragments which might remain.

Four and One - Half Year Old

All of the molars should be floated and any retained caps should be removed. The eruption of the third permanent molars should be checked in addition to the canine eruption in the male horses. The third incisor should be checked for the presence of a retained cap.

Five Year Old and Older

Routine dental floating should be done twice a year to maintain a balanced mouth and good occlusion.

Artwork by S. Hakola / J. Dirig
Copyright Equistar Publications, Ltd.

Lateral View of Esophagus

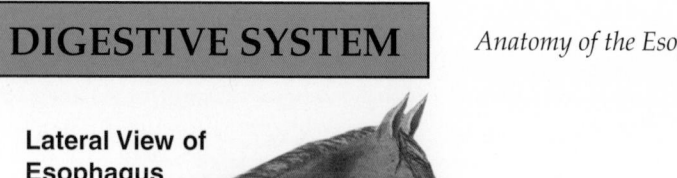

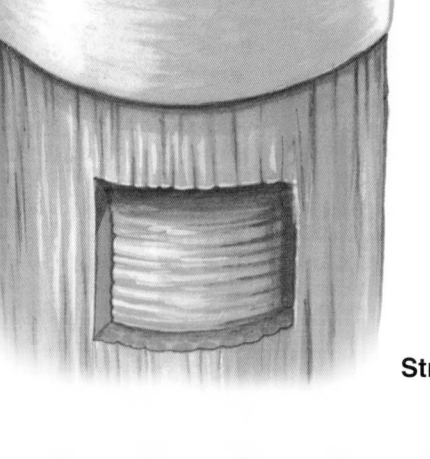

Longitudinal muscle layer

Circular muscle layer

Submucosa

Mucosal layer

Exterior Wall

Structure of the Esophageal Wall

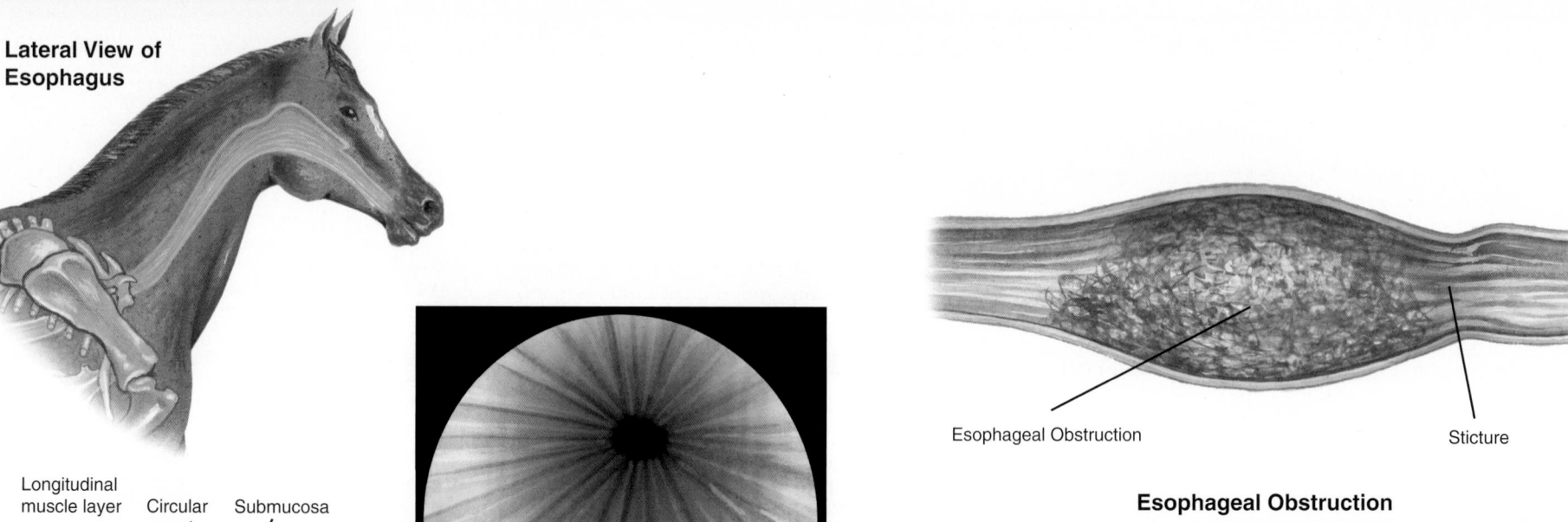

Endoscopic View of the Normal Esophagus

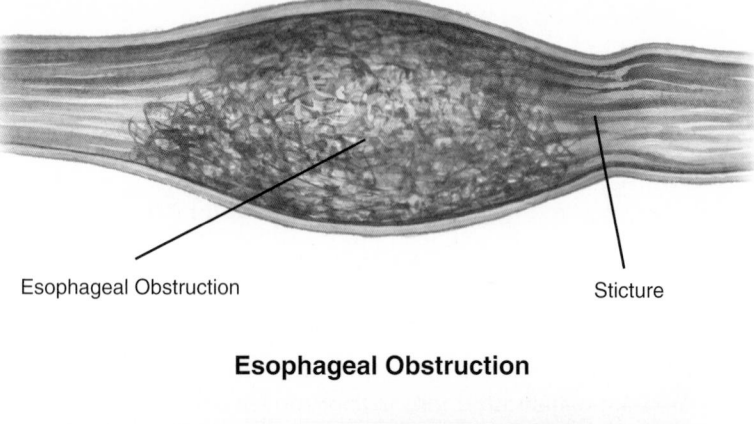

Esophageal Obstruction

Sticture

Esophageal Obstruction

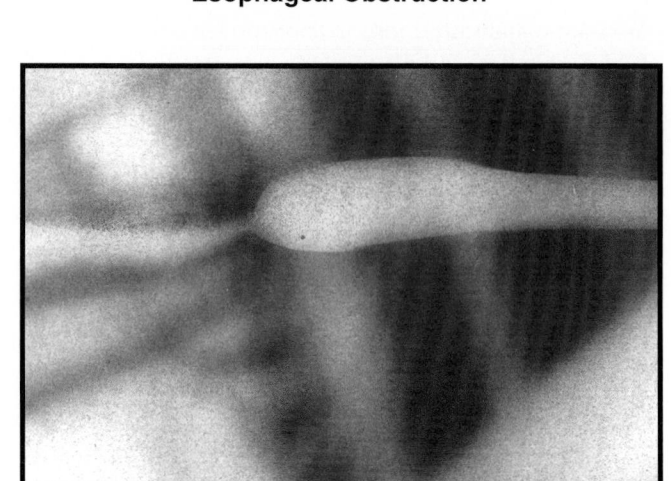

Contrast radiograph of esophageal stricture

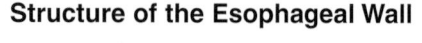

5

The Digestive System

THE ESOPHAGUS

Extending from the pharynx to the stomach is a musculomembranous tube, about 125 - 150 cm in length which is termed the esophagus. Passing on the left side of the trachea, the esophagus extends from the fourth cervical vertebra to the area of the third thoracic vertebra. It is oriented ventrally to the trachea at the posterior end of the sixth cervical vertebra where it then passes dorsally and caudally through the thoracic inlet along the mediastinum until it reaches the diaphragm. After it passes through the diaphragm, the esophagus terminates into the cardiac orifice of the stomach at approximately 10 - 12 cm ventral to the vertebral end of the fourteenth rib.

The musculomembranous wall of the esophagus consists of four layers. There is a fibrous sheath termed the tunica adventitia covering the outer most surface. A muscular layer consists of both striped and unstriped muscles.   The striped version extends from the pharynx to the base of the heart where the musculature changes to the unstriped type which continues on to the stomach. This muscular layer is thick and firm and consists of two layers of fibers arranged spirally or elliptically that intercross both dorsally and ventrally. The submucous layer serves as an attachment for the mucous membrane lining that surrounds the lumen.

Blood supply to the esophagus is supplied from branches of the carotid, the bronchoesophageal, and the gastric arteries. Nerve supply is supplied to the structure via the vagus, the glosso-pharyngeal, and the sympathetic nerves.

CHOKE
(ESOPHAGEAL OBSTRUCTION)

Etiology

The most common cause of esophageal obstruction is the ingestion of food of an abnormal consistency or from a foreign body. Personal experience has shown that the majority of the choke cases have been caused by the ingestion of entire ears of corn or corn cobs.

Clinical Signs

The animal will be in pain and make repeated attempts to swallow. There will be neck extension accompanied by an arching of the neck and squealing. The animal will exhibit profuse salivation and may even appear to have a nasal discharge that consists of saliva mixed with food particles. The esophagus may be visibly distended, or the distention can be easily recognized with digital palpation. In cases that are not acute, the horse may exhibit halitosis. It is always an amazement to note how well these horses tolerate this condition. In most cases the horse continues to eat which compounds the problem by filling the entire esophageal lumen with ingesta.

Diagnosis

A case of esophageal obstruction can be diagnosed from the clinical signs. A nasogastric tube is passed where it will meet with resistance at the site of obstruction. If a foreign body is suspected, it is possible to take plain radiographs of the throat and cervical region to help identify the problem. Esophagoscopy using an endoscope can provide visualization of the obstruction and possibly the complications involved.

Differential Diagnosis

1.) Stomatitis
2.) Gastroduodenal Ulcerations
3.) Dental Problems

Treatment

The first step in resolving a case of choke is to sedate the animal and provide relief from pain. This can be done with the administration of sedatives, muscle relaxants, and nonsteroidal anti-inflammatories. A nasogastric tube is then passed to the point of obstruction and a lavage technique is initiated with warm water mixed with a light grade of mineral oil. While the lavage process is

DIGESTIVE SYSTEM

Anatomy of the Digestive System; Stomach Anatomy

Artwork by S. Hakola / J. Dirig
Copyright Equistar Publications, Ltd.

Right Lateral View

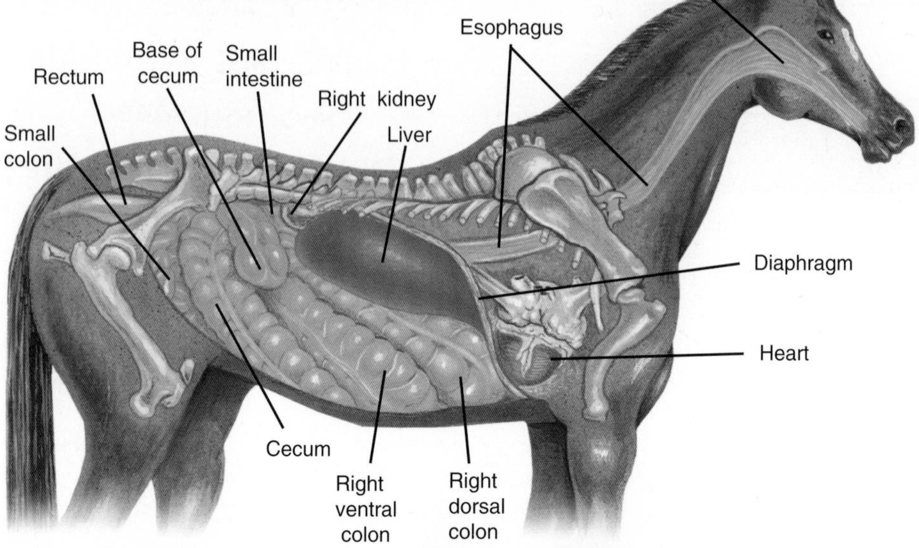

Pharynx

Esophagus

Rectum

Base of cecum

Small intestine

Right kidney

Liver

Small colon

Diaphragm

Heart

Cecum

Right ventral colon

Right dorsal colon

Left Lateral View

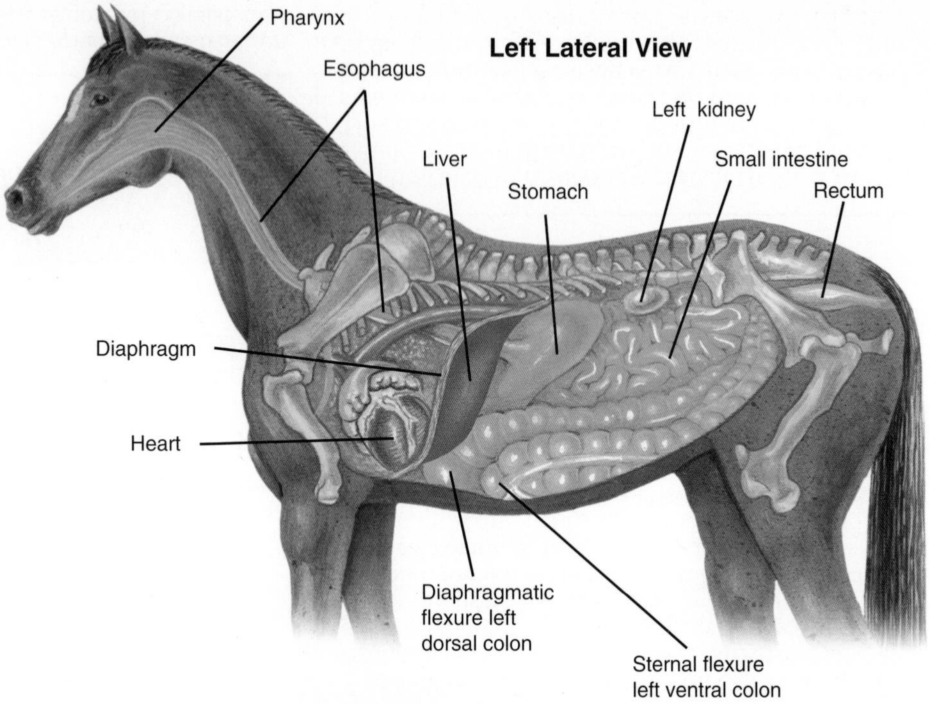

Pharynx

Esophagus

Liver

Left kidney

Small intestine

Rectum

Stomach

Diaphragm

Heart

Diaphragmatic flexure left dorsal colon

Sternal flexure left ventral colon

Ventral View

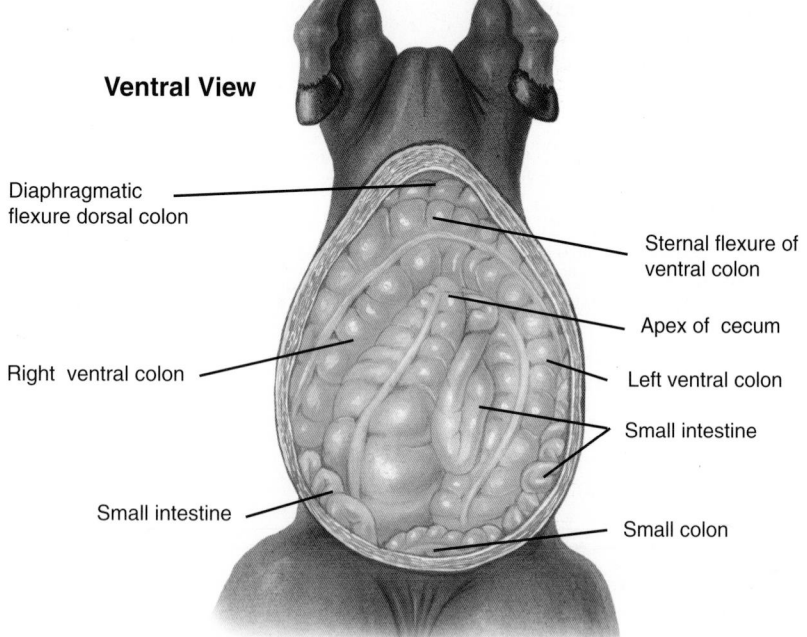

Diaphragmatic flexure dorsal colon

Sternal flexure of ventral colon

Apex of cecum

Left ventral colon

Right ventral colon

Small intestine

Small intestine

Small colon

Median Section of the Stomach

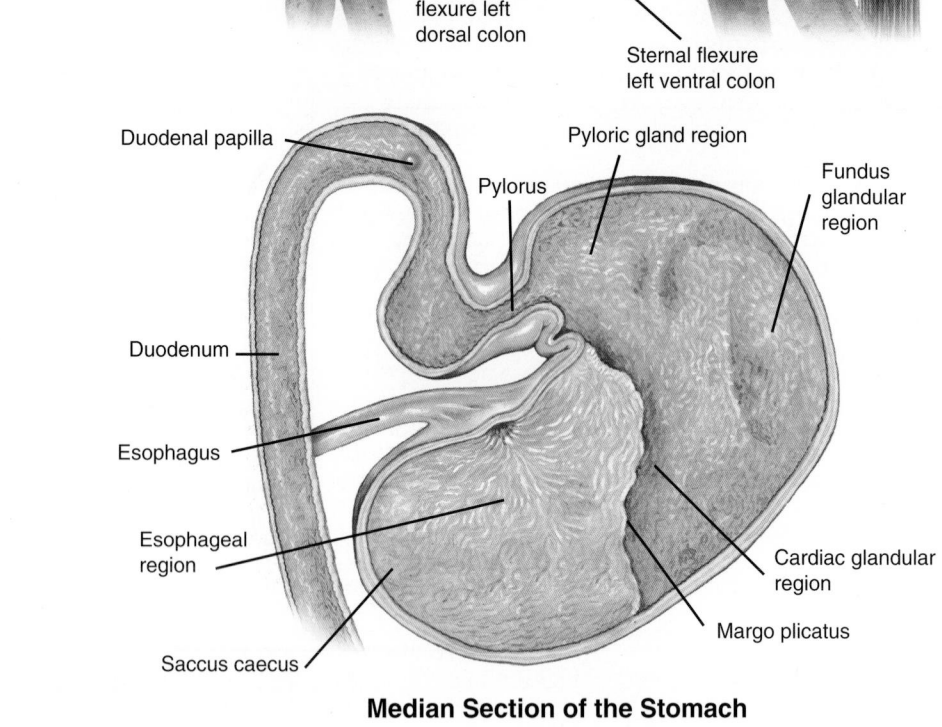

Duodenal papilla

Pylorus

Pyloric gland region

Fundus glandular region

Duodenum

Esophagus

Esophageal region

Cardiac glandular region

Margo plicatus

Saccus caecus

undertaken, digital massage of the esophageal mass may have some merit in alleviating the obstruction.

In instances where conservative lavage therapy is unsuccessful, the horse should be placed under general anesthesia to allow further muscle relaxation and possible resolution of the obstruction. If this is still unsuccessful, an esophagostomy should be considered, but only as a last resort.

After the relief of a mild obstruction, feed should be withheld for approximately 12 - 24 hours to allow the mucosal lining to heal. Alfalfa and bran mashes are then slowly introduced to avoid the obstruction from recurring. The horse should be placed on antibiotics and treated with nonsteroidal antiinflammatory medications such as phenylbutazone or flunixin meglumine. If an esophagostomy was performed, the wound is allowed to heal by second intention. Initially, fluid and nutritional support may have to be provided through the use of a nasogastric tube. Supportive therapy such as systemic administration of IV fluid therapy and broad spectrum antibiotics are indicated.

There are several complications that can occur with choke. An obstruction can produce mucosal ulceration, fibrous strictures, and esophageal dilations. Each one of these complications should be diagnosed and treated accordingly.

THE STOMACH

The equine stomach is the large dilation of the alimentary canal that occurs between the esophagus and the small intestine. It is remarkably small in size relative to the size of the animal with a capacity of 5 - 15 liters. It is sharply curved almost configuring to the letter "J" with the right part being shorter than the left. The left portion is larger and comprises the fundus, whereas the right portion of the stomach is termed the pyloric portion. It occurs within the left half of the abdomen and remains within the protection of the rib cage. Ordinary techniques of clinical

examination per rectum do not allow examination of the stomach. When the stomach is moderately distended after a meal, the fundus extends under the upper part of the fifteenth rib, and the pyloric portion reaches the ventral areas of the ninth and tenth rib. Therefore, any enlargement of the stomach after feeding distends the stomach mainly downward and forward.

Anatomically, the stomach contains two surfaces, two curvatures, and two extremities. The convex surface, which is termed the parietal surface, is directed forward, upward, and to the left. This surface usually directly opposes the diaphragm and liver. The other convex surface faces in the opposite direction and is termed the visceral surface. It comes in contact with the large colon, the pancreas, the small colon, the small intestine, and the greater omentum. These surfaces exhibit borders which are termed curvatures. The short, or lesser, curvature extends from the termination of the esophagus to the junction of the small intestine. The greater curvature of the stomach is much larger. It extends from its most cranial portion dorsally and curves over the left extremity where it descends, passes to the right, crosses the median plane, and curves upward to end at the pylorus. Along the left portion of this curvature, there is opposition to the spleen, whereas the ventral portion is opposed to portions of the great colon. The left extremity of the stomach is termed the saccus caecus, lies ventral to the left crus of the diaphragm, and is beneath the dorsal portion of the sixteenth and seventeenth ribs. It is opposed to the pancreas and in contact with the great colon behind the base of the spleen. The right extremity is smaller and is continuous with the diaphragm. It occurs just right of the median plane and is opposed to the visceral surface of the liver.

Internally, the stomach consists of a large nonglandular region which occupies the fundus and part of the body, and a glandular region which occupies the lumen within the rest of this structure. The nonglandular region occurs just within the cardiac sphincter at the entrance from the esophagus. This portion of the stomach has almost the same mucosal lining as that of the esophagus. The glandular portion of the stomach consists of the cardiac fundus and pyloric glandular zones.

These zones are ill-defined with the fundic glandular zone being somewhat darker and redder than the reddish-colored cardiac and pyloric zones.

The cardiac sphincter which governs the entrance of the esophagus is well developed. This is the structure that is responsible for the horse's reputed inability to vomit. The pyloric sphincter is the orifice that exits the stomach and enters the duodenum.

The stomach receives its arterial blood supply from all the branches of the celiac artery. The gastric veins drain the blood from the stomach into the portal vein. Nerve supply to the stomach is derived from the vagus and sympathetic nerves.

THE INTESTINAL TRACT

The intestinal structures occupy most of the abdominal cavity. The small intestine connects the stomach with the large intestine. It averages approximately 70 feet in length and has a capacity of approximately 40 - 50 liters. The large intestine extends from the ileum of the small intestine to the anus. It is approximately 25 feet in length and is divided into the cecum, great colon, small colon, and rectum. The large intestine is the reservoir for the microbial fermentation of the ingesta.

THE SMALL INTESTINE

The small intestine is divided into the duodenum, the jejunum, and the ileum. The duodenum is a relatively short structure that is only 3 or 4 feet in length. It is shaped somewhat like a horseshoe with the convex surface being directed toward the right. It directly opposes the middle and right lobes of the liver as it ascends dorsally. The second portion is opposed to part of the colon, the right lobe of the liver, and the right kidney. The last portion passes from right to left behind the attachment at the base of the cecum. About 5 or 6 inches from the pylorus is a pouch termed the diverticulum duodeni. It is here that the pancreatic and hepatic ducts open.

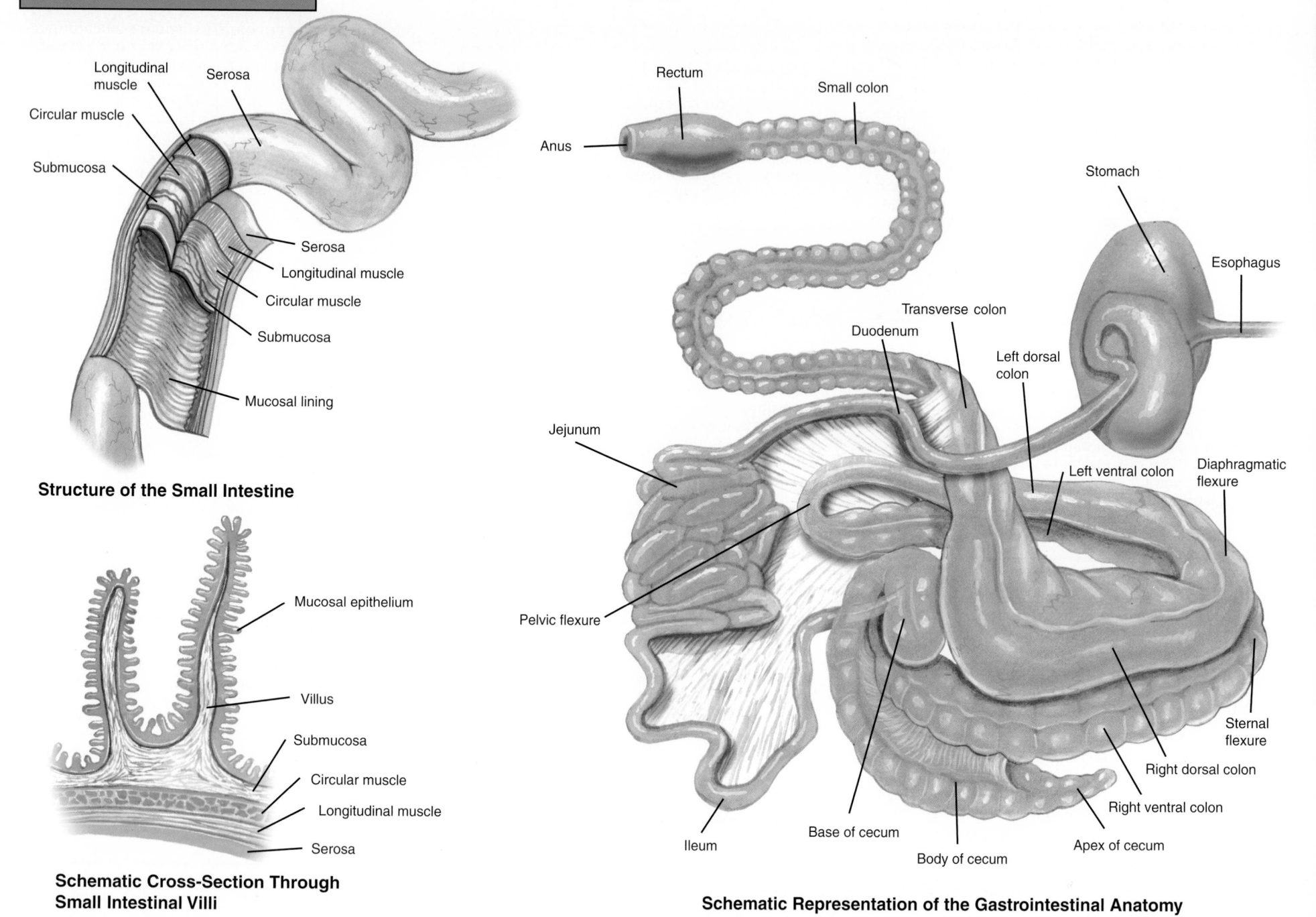

Longitudinal muscle
Serosa
Circular muscle
Submucosa
Serosa
Longitudinal muscle
Circular muscle
Submucosa
Mucosal lining

Structure of the Small Intestine

Mucosal epithelium
Villus
Submucosa
Circular muscle
Longitudinal muscle
Serosa

**Schematic Cross-Section Through
Small Intestinal Villi**

Rectum
Small colon
Anus
Stomach
Esophagus
Transverse colon
Duodenum
Left dorsal colon
Jejunum
Left ventral colon
Diaphragmatic flexure
Pelvic flexure
Sternal flexure
Right dorsal colon
Ileum
Base of cecum
Body of cecum
Apex of cecum
Right ventral colon

Schematic Representation of the Gastrointestinal Anatomy

The remainder of the small intestine consists of the jejunum and ileum. There is no distinct point where the jejunum divides into the ileum. The long coils of this structure are usually located in the left dorsal portion of the abdomen where they mingle with those coils of the descending colon. The average diameter of the jejunum and ileum is approximately 6 - 7 cm. The last meter of this structure is slightly thicker in structure, and this characteristic defines it as the ileum. The last portion of the small intestine projects slightly into the cavity of the cecum and is bounded by the ileocecal valve.

The structure of the small intestine consists of four layers: the serous, the muscular, the submucosal, and the mucosal layers. The serous coat surrounds the bowel exteriorly except at the mesenteric edge where the blood vessels and nerves reach the bowel. The muscular coat consists of two layers. There is an external longitudinal and an internal circular layer of muscles. Along the last few feet of the small intestine, this muscular layer thickens which allows this portion to be demarcated as the ileum. The submucosal layer consists of areolar tissue into which the blood vessels and nerves ramify. This layer also contains duodenal glands and lymph nodes. The mucous membrane lines the lumen of the small intestine and is soft and velvety in appearance. This area is very vascular and thick with villi which are small projections of the mucous membrane into the lumen. Each villus is relatively short and thick and contains a central lymph vessel surrounded by capillaries, lymphoid tissue, and unstriped muscle fibers. These villi structurally increase the surface area of the lumen which allows absorption of nutrients from the contents within the intestine.

There are two kinds of glands within the small intestine: the intestinal, and the duodenal glands. The intestinal glands are present throughout the small intestine and are simple tubular glands which open between the villi. The duodenal glands are present within the first 20 feet of the bowel and are branched in structure. These glands are situated within the submucosa so that their ducts perforate both the muscle layer and the mucous membrane.

Arterial blood supply arises from the celiac and anterior mesenteric arteries. Venous drainage is deposited within the portal vein. Nerve supply to the small intestine arises from the vagus and the sympathetic nerves.

THE LARGE INTESTINE

The large intestine has an enormous capacity. It has a sacculated appearance which occurs from the shortening of muscle bands consisting of external longitudinal muscles and elastic fibers at certain positions on the circumference of the bowel. It is divided up into the cecum, the great colon, the small colon, and the rectum.

THE ANATOMY OF THE CECUM

The cecum consists of an expanded dorsal base, a curved tapering body, and a blind ventral apex. It is a cul-de-sac between the small intestine and colon. It has a capacity of approximately 25 - 30 liters of fluid. The cecum is curved in structure somewhat like the comma punctuation mark.

The base of the cecum lies on the right dorsal portion of the abdomen partially against the flank and partially under cover of the ribs. It extends from the abdominal roof and sublumbar areas of the fifteenth rib to the coxae tuber. Dorsally, it opposes the region of the pancreas and right kidney. The body of the cecum extends downward and forward from the base and is opposed to the ventral wall of the abdomen. The apex lies on the abdominal floor just right of the median plane and usually about a hand's length behind the xiphoid cartilage.

The cecal base attaches dorsally to connective tissue and the peritoneum. It opposes the ventral surface of the pancreas and the right kidney. Medially, the base attaches to the terminal portion of the great colon and ventrally to the origin of the great colon. The apex of the cecum is free which allows it to vary in position within the abdomen.

The cecum contains four longitudinal bands which results in four rows of sacculations. These bands are situated on the dorsal, ventral, right, and left surfaces.

The ileocecal orifice occurs on the lesser curvature of the base, within the cecum, approximately 5 - 7 1/2 cm to the right of the median plane. The cecocolic orifice is small in relation to the size of the cecum and colon. It is lateral to the ileocecal orifice with only 5 cm between them. It is, however, separated by a large fold of tissue which projects into the anterior portion of the cecum.

ANATOMY OF THE GREAT COLON

The great colon is approximately 10 - 12 feet long with an average diameter of 8 - 10 inches. It has the capacity of approximately 50 - 60 liters of ingesta. It begins at the cecocolic orifice and terminates in the small colon behind the saccus cecus of the stomach.

The great colon consists of four parts. The right ventral colon begins at the base of the cecum and forms an initial curve which is directed upward and backward. This portion of the great colon is in direct opposition to the upper part of the right flank. When it reaches the xiphoid cartilage, it bends sharply to the left and backward forming the sternal flexure. The second portion of great colon is termed the left ventral colon. It passes backward on the abdominal floor to the left of the right ventral colon and cecum. When this portion reaches the pelvic inlet, it bends sharply dorsally and forward forming the pelvic flexure. The third portion of the great colon is the left dorsal colon which passes forward dorsally. This is lateral to the left ventral portion and upon reaching the diaphragm, turns to the right and backward forming the diaphragmatic flexure. The fourth portion of the great colon is the right dorsal colon. It travels backward dorsally until it reaches the medial surface at the base of the cecum. It then turns to the left and dorsally to pass behind the left sac of the stomach where it decreases in size and

Artwork by S. Hakola / J. Dirig
Copyright Equistar Publications, Ltd.

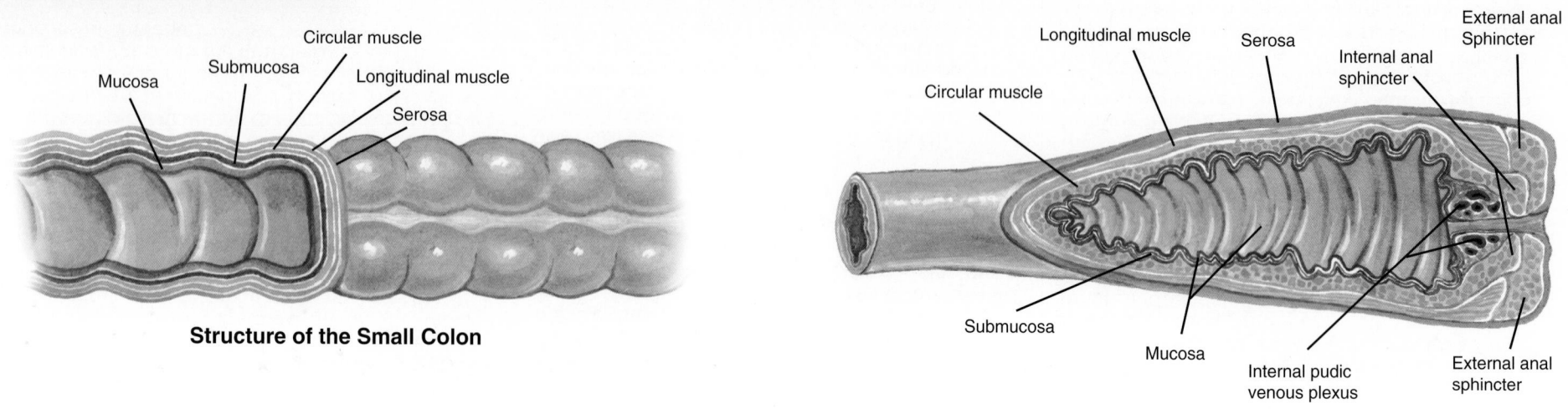

Mucosa

Submucosa

Circular muscle

Longitudinal muscle

Serosa

Structure of the Small Colon

Circular muscle

Longitudinal muscle

Serosa

Internal anal sphincter

External anal Sphincter

Submucosa

Mucosa

Internal pudic venous plexus

External anal sphincter

The Rectum and Anus Viewed in a Sagittal Section

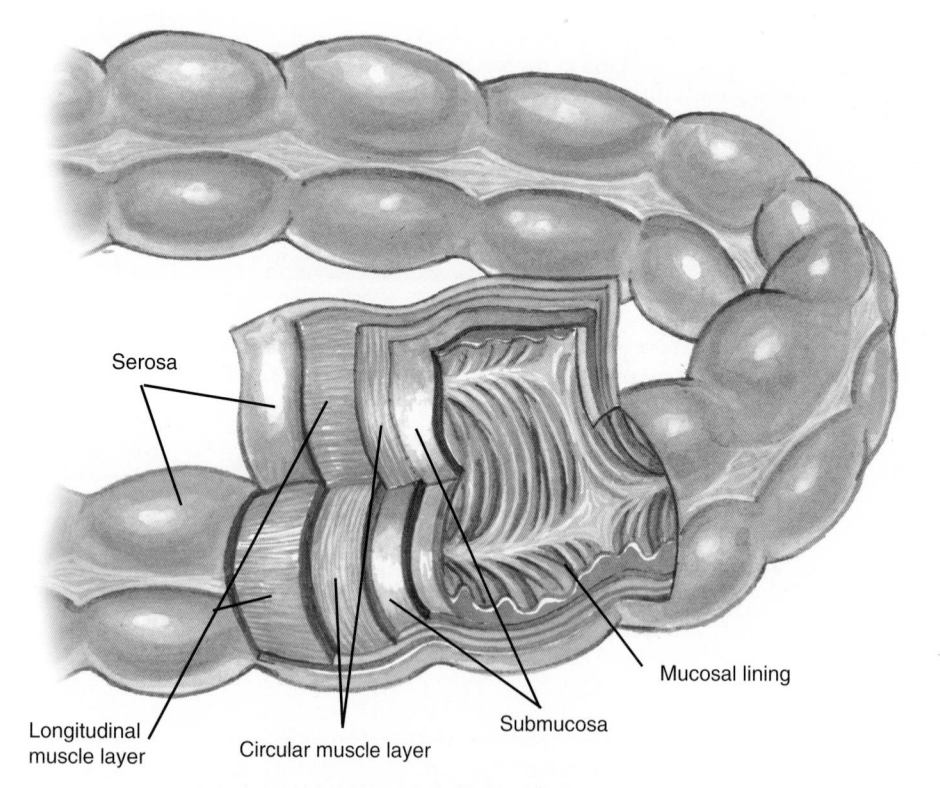

Serosa

Mucosal lining

Submucosa

Longitudinal muscle layer

Circular muscle layer

The Large Intestinal Wall and Lumenal Surface

joins the small colon below the left kidney.

The relationships of the location of the great colon within the abdominal cavity are very complex. The ventral portions of the great colon have extensive contact with the abdominal wall ventrally and laterally. On the right side of the horse, the great colon is usually not in contact with the flank because of the cecum. On the left side of the horse, it lies against the ventral portion of the flank. Dorsally, the great colon comes in contact with the stomach, duodenum, liver, pancreas, small colon, small intestine, aorta, posterior vena cava, and portal vein. The pelvic flexure is variable in its position but is usually directed against the posterior portion of the right flank or lies in the right inguinal region.

Portions of the great colon are distinguishable by palpable bands that vary in number on the different anatomical areas on the large colon. The ventral portions of the large colon have four palpable bands of tissue. The pelvic flexure has a band that occurs on its lesser curvature. The left dorsal colon has at first only one band which is a continuation of the proceeding one. Further forward along the left dorsal colon, two other bands appear and the three are continued onto the right dorsal portion. The ventral portions of the great colon have alternate constrictions and sacculations.

ANATOMY OF THE SMALL COLON

The small colon can be divided up into a transverse portion and a descending portion. It begins at the termination of the great colon behind the saccus caecus of the stomach, travels ventral to the left kidney, and terminates into the rectum at the pelvic inlet. It is approximately 10 - 12 feet long and varies in diameter from 7 1/2 - 10 cm.

The transverse portion is short and passes from right to left in front of the root of the mesentery. Characteristically, it carries two bands of tissue and terminates into the smaller diameter descending

colon. The descending portion is narrower than the transverse portion and occurs mainly within the dorsocaudal and left portion of the abdomen. It is usually located within the pelvic region and characteristically has two prominent bands of tissue. Rectal palpation will usually reveal dry fecal balls within this structure.

ANATOMY OF THE RECTUM

The rectum begins around the pelvic inlet and terminates in the anus. It is usually about one foot in length and may approach the rectum directly or occur at a slightly oblique angle. The first portion of the rectum usually lies along the left wall of the pelvic cavity and is related to coils of the small colon, the pelvic flexure of the great colon, and ventrally to the bladder or uterus.

INTERNAL ANATOMY OF THE LARGE INTESTINE

The large intestine is comprised of four layers. The serous layer covers different portions of the large intestine in various degrees. It does not cover the large intestine where the opposed surfaces of the cecum and colon lie between the layers of cecocolic fold and the mesocolon. It is also incomplete in the anatomical areas where there is parietal attachment of the cecum and colon and where the retroperitoneal part of the rectum is located. The muscular layer contains both longitudinal and circular fibers. Even though these longitudinal and circular fibers exist, the bands within the cecum and ventral portions of the great colon consist largely of elastic tissue. The dorsal portions of the colon contain a large portion of muscular tissue, whereas those of the small colon vary in the muscular content within this layer. The submucosal layer is prevalent throughout the large intestine, but is well defined in the wall of the rectum. This anatomical characteristic allows the mucous membrane to be loosely attached to the muscular layer, thereby forming folds when the bowel is empty. The mucous membrane of the

intestine contains no villi or duodenal glands but does contain large semilunar folds that correspond to the external constrictions of this structure. There are large and numerous intestinal glands throughout the large intestine. Within this mucous membrane layer, aggregated lymphatic tissues exist at the apex of the cecum, in the pelvic flexure, and throughout the left dorsal part of the colon.

Arterial blood supply arises from both the anterior and posterior mesenteric arteries and internal pudic artery. Venous drainage is accomplished through the portal and internal pudic veins. Innervation is derived from the mesenteric and pelvic plexus of the sympathetic nervous system.

THE ANUS

The anus is the terminal structure of the digestive system. It is located externally just beneath the root of the tail where it forms a projection with a central depression. Externally it is covered by a thin hairless integument that contains numerous sebaceous and sweat glands. A mucous membrane that is glandless and covered by thick squamous stratified epithelial tissue lines the lumen of the anal canal. Contraction at the end of defecation within this structure is made possibly through the use of two sphincter muscles: the sphincter ani internus and the sphincter ani externus. The retractor ani muscle is located between the rectum and the sacrosciatic ligament. This ligament helps control the prolapsing of the tissues within the anus as the animal undergoes defecation. The blood supply to the anus arises from the internal pudic arteries with venous drainage to the internal pudic vein. Innervation to this anatomical area arises from the pudic nerve.

Artwork by S. Hakola / J. Dirig
Copyright Equistar Publications, Ltd.

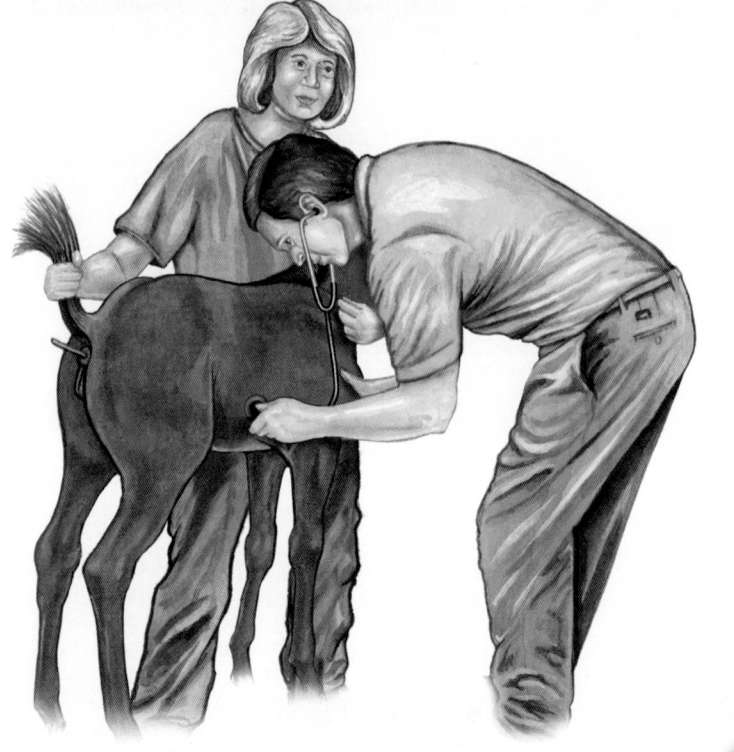

Auscultation of the Bowel in the Neonatal Foal

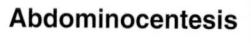

Abdominocentesis

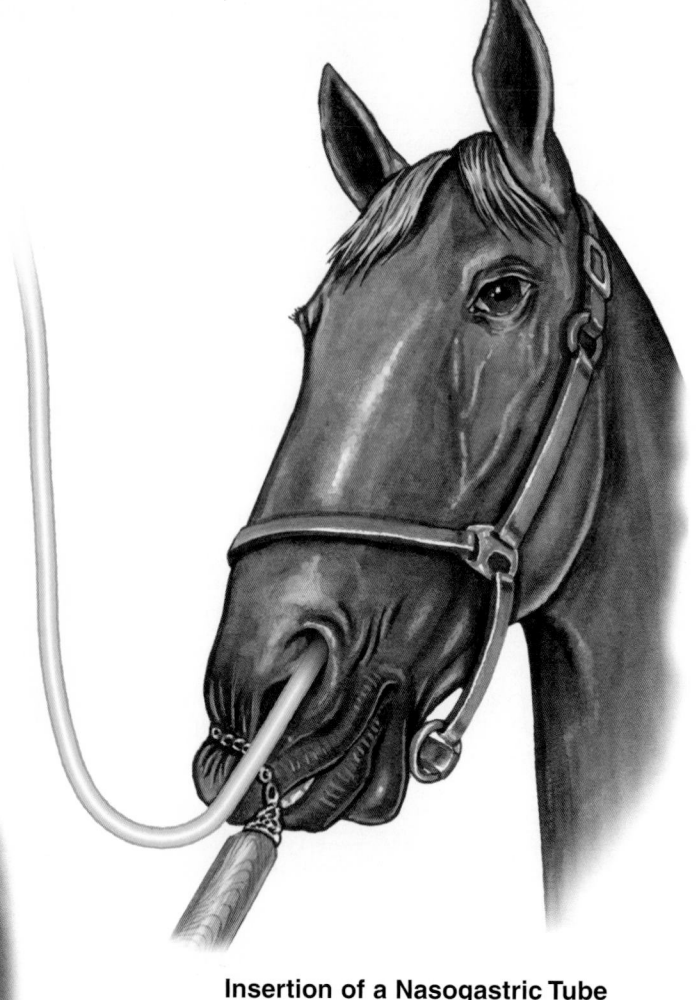

Insertion of a Nasogastric Tube

EXAMINATION OF THE DIGESTIVE TRACT

Whenever there is an animal that has a suspected gastrointestinal tract disorder, a comprehensive careful examination of the digestive tract is essential. This examination should include a patient history, a physical exam, auscultation, nasogastric intubation, a rectal exam, abdominocentesis, ultrasonography, and blood work.

The patient history should include general historical data, recent events, and questions that will reveal the current state of a possible disorder. General patient history should include a numeration of the current feed stuffs, the daily routine of the horse, the use of the horse, the environment, and current parasite control. Current data should include questions that pin point the last time the horse was fed, the current consumption of both feed and water, any change in feed, water, housing, and bedding, and any recent administration of a deworming compound. The pregnancy status of the animal should be noted in addition to any current treatment regimes that are being administered. Numerous questions should be asked to evaluate any historical data that directly relates to a gastrointestinal disorder: When was the last defecation from the horse? Does the horse salivate excessively when eating? Is there any evidence of acute weight loss? Is there any evidence of any abdominal pain or change in degree of pain that the animal is experiencing? Does the animal paw, roll, or kick at its abdomen, stare at its flank, or simply stay recumbent? Does walking help alleviate the animal's distress? Has there been any previous episode of the disorder or recent surgery involving the digestive tract?

A thorough physical exam should be conducted which involves an evaluation of all physical parameters and end with nasogastric intubation. The pulse rate and quality, rectal temperature, respiration rate and effort should be the first signs evaluated in compiling base line data. The animal's attitude should be noted for signs of depression, hyperexcitability, and alertness. Any physical sign of pain and its severity should be evaluated. Determine if the pain is continuous or intermittent in duration. Mucous membranes should be observed for color and capillary refill time. All of this data should be gathered so a decision can be made regarding the next step to be undertaken in the evaluation of the digestive system.

Nasogastric Intubation

Passive passage of a nasogastric tube is a vital part in the evaluation of the digestive system. The tube will readily identify a possible obstruction, will provide decompression of the proximal gastrointestinal tract, and will allow for the administrations of fluids and medications. The tube is introduced via the ventral nasal meatus, into the pharynx and the esophagus. Patience is essential for proper placement of the tube. Expertise should be gained in this procedure to allow quick placement with minimal distress.

There are several techniques involved that insure the proper placement of the nasogastric tube. When the nasogastric tube is in the esophagus, it is both visible and palpable on the left side of the neck. The exception to this is when the esophagus is located on the right side of the trachea. As the tube is advanced, there is slight resistance to its passage. Blowing into the end of the tube meets with a slight resistance within the esophagus or gurgling within the stomach and a reflux of stomach gases. Within the trachea, there is no resistance to passage or blowing into the end of the tube. The animal will sometimes cough and synchronized breaths can be detected.

Auscultation of the Abdomen

Auscultation of the abdomen is then performed. This procedure should take at least five minutes. A stethoscope should be applied to at least 4 sites throughout the upper and lower paralumbar regions. Normal characteristic sounds such as rumbling, bubbling, and splashing should be heard on either side of the abdomen along the ventral surface. Sounds of gas intermixing with fluid should arise mostly from the large colon and cecum. The small intestine can have normal motility with no sound at all being referred to the external abdominal wall.

Along the right paralumbar fossa, ileocecal sounds can be heard. These sounds are hard to describe, but should be higher pitched and sound like water rushing down a drain pipe. When the horse has not recently eaten, these sounds should occur at least one to three times per minute. Low pitched fluid sounds, which are referred to as borborygmi, often occur on the lower part of the abdomen. In general, mixing sounds should occur 2 - 4 times per minute and progressive sounds, meaning ingesta moving in an orderly fashion towards the rectum, should be heard once every 2 - 4 minutes. These progressive sounds are usually differentiated from mixing sounds by their cyclic pattern and longer duration.

Many pharmaceutical products cause the bowel sounds to be reduced or even cease after the drug is administered. The administration of atropine, xylazine, butorphanol, and detomidine all reduce bowel sounds for about sixty minutes. Care must be taken when administering these drugs since some of them, atropine in particular, can result in a long term ileus, which will result in bowel stasis and distention of the abdomen.

Whenever there is a moderate to severe case of abdominal pain, most progressive sounds within the bowel are reduced. In cases of severe abdominal pain, most sounds from the abdomen will be absent. If the horse is walked, bowel fluid and gas will be mixed. Upon auscultation, bubbling and pinging sounds will be heard. These should not be misinterpreted as progressive movements within the bowel. Increased sounds can also be heard, which are referred to as spasms. These may be due to a parasite irritation, an area of severely compromised bowel, or numerous contractions against an impaction. Sand can be heard during large colon movement through auscultation on the ventral abdomen. Sounds that resemble sand pouring on itself in a sand pile with a hissing or high frequency grinding sound can be heard when sand is present in large quantities.

DIGESTIVE SYSTEM

Examination of the Digestive System by Rectal Palpation

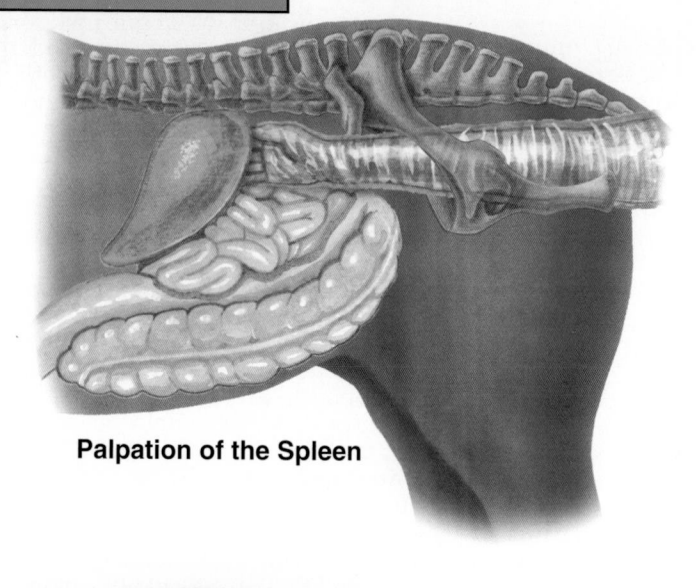

Palpation of the Spleen

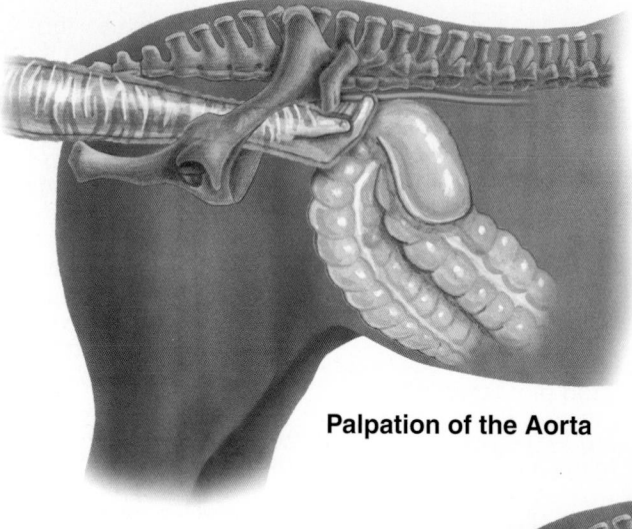

Palpation of the Aorta

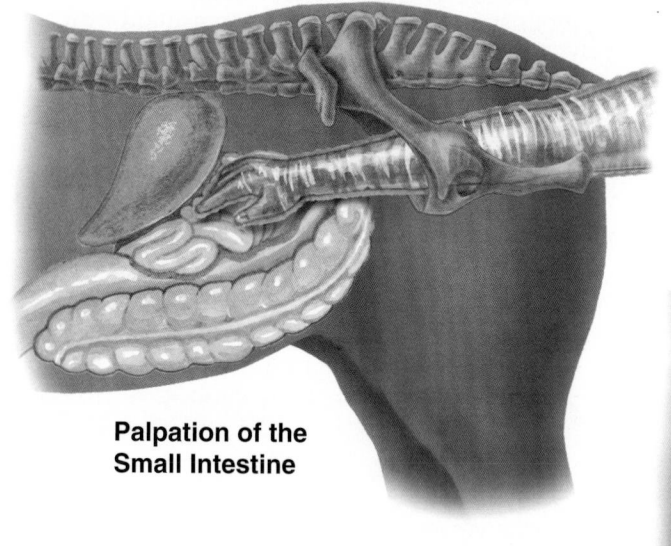

Palpation of the Small Intestine

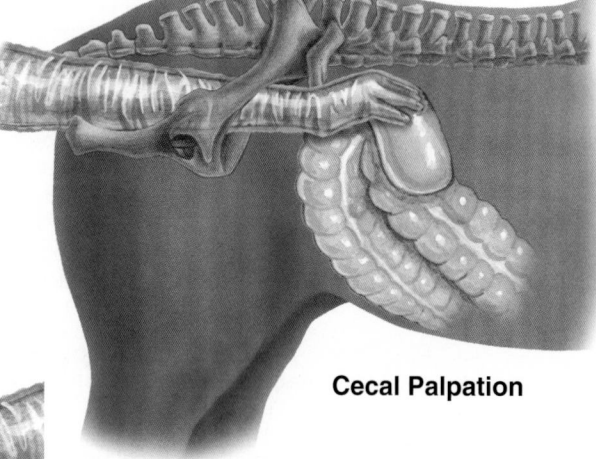

Cecal Palpation

Palpation of the Pelvic Flexure

Rectal Examination

A rectal examination should be performed whenever a suspected gastrointestinal tract disorder exists. One can sometimes diagnose from rectal palpation and possibly provide early determination regarding the need for surgery. The animal should be carefully restrained, and care taken to minimize the risk to both the horse and the examiner. A twitch should be applied and chemical sedation or hobbles may be needed to allow a complete and systematic rectal examination.

A rectal sleeve is put on along with copious lubrication such as methyl cellulose or KY jelly. If the animal is straining excessively, 60 milliters of lidocaine can be administered into the rectum to help control the straining. Slow entry is gained to the rectum until the entire arm is advanced to its full length. Keeping one's arm still within the rectum should allow relaxation within these structures. It is not unusual for relaxation to occur after 30 - 45 seconds.

A sequential thorough examination should be undertaken so that no areas or lesions are missed. The abdomen should be divided into quadrants with the left dorsal quadrant being identified by the presence of the spleen and left kidney. From this point, the examiner's arm is moved to the right and extended forward to the midline until the mesenteric stalk is identified. The base of the cecum may be identified through the presence of the cecocolic artery. Dorsal to the base of the cecum is the attachment of the duodenum. The cecum itself can be palpated in the right dorsal quadrant. The ventral and median bands should be identified. These should not be tight or stretched. The cecum can then be followed forward on the ventral midline of the floor of the abdomen. The palpator's hand is then moved ventrally and caudally to the pelvic brim. The large colon, filled with soft ingesta, can usually be identified in the left ventral quadrant on the midline just below the pelvic brim. The small colon should be filled with fecal balls and can be found in several positions around the abdomen with the most common location being within the left ventral quadrant.

The following structures should be evaluated with their unique characteristics during the course of the rectal examination:

Feces: The consistency of the stool should be examined in addition to the content. Any evidence of blood, mucus, or sand should be noted.

Inguinal rings: These are usually located approximately 10 cm lateral to the midline on the pelvic brim. These should be checked for the presence of any loops of bowel entrapped within them.

Spleen: This structure should be near the level of the last rib and on the left side of the abdomen next to the abdominal wall.

Small intestine: This structure is usually very difficult to palpate or examine. If distended loops of bowel are found in the central portion of the abdomen, this could indicate an intussusception of the small intestine or other possible disorders.

Small colon: This structure should have formed fecal balls within its lumen. Abnormalities within the small colon would indicate the presence of an impaction or gas distention.

Pelvic flexure: This flexure should be palpable within the caudal ventral portion of the abdomen near the midline. This is one of the most common sites of impaction. In most cases, firm masses can easily be identified within the pelvic flexure.

Large colon: Any gaseous distention within this structure will result in taut bands of tissue and may indicate the presence of a large colon torsion or malposition.

Right dorsal colon: This structure is usually difficult to palpate but may be distended due to gas or fluid. One of the most common causes of this distention is the presence of an enterolith within the lumen of the small colon.

Cecum (ventral band): This structure descends dorsally and ventrally on a right to left diagonal path within the abdomen. The base and body of the cecum are easily palpated when it is distended

with gas or ingesta. When the cecum becomes impacted, digital palpation will usually reveal a very firm doughy mass.

Abdominocentesis

An evaluation of the abdominal fluid can provide clarification as to the type of disorder and the severity of that disorder within the abdomen. This technique is performed utilizing an 18 gauge 1 1/2 inch needle placed through a surgically prepped site on the ventral midline of the abdomen. After placement of the needle, abdominal fluid should be collected into one tube containing EDTA or another anticoagulant and a sterile tube that can be submitted for bacteriological growth and examination. This abdominal fluid should be examined for the presence of red blood cells, other nucleated cells, and total protein content.

Special Techniques

Several specialized techniques can be utilized to help diagnose gastrointestinal disorders. Ultrasonography and endoscopy are two of the more common techniques utilized to further evaluate the gastrointestinal tract. Complete blood counts and blood chemistry values are utilized extensively to evaluate the alimentary canal.

Artwork by S. Hakola / J. Dirig
Copyright Equistar Publications, Ltd.

**Typical "Dog-Sit Position"
Seen in Gastric Dilation
and Rupture**

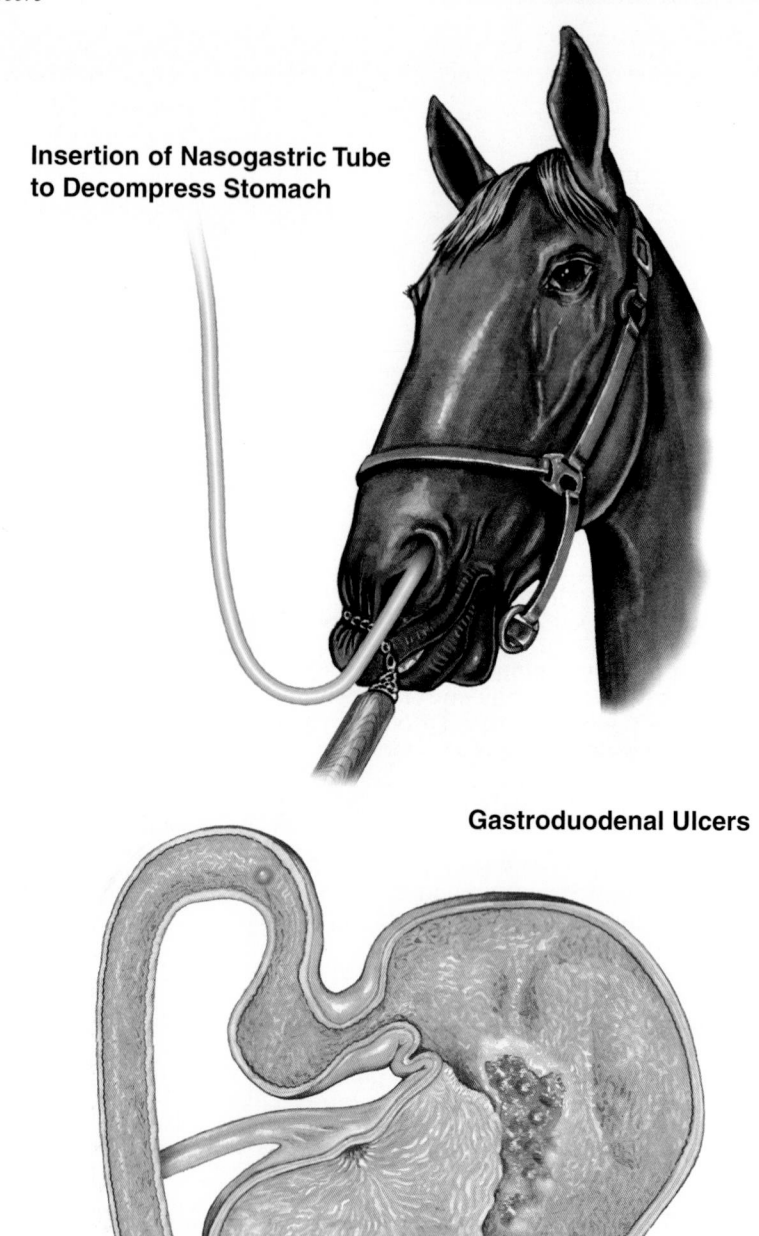

**Insertion of Nasogastric Tube
to Decompress Stomach**

Gastric Dilation and Rupture

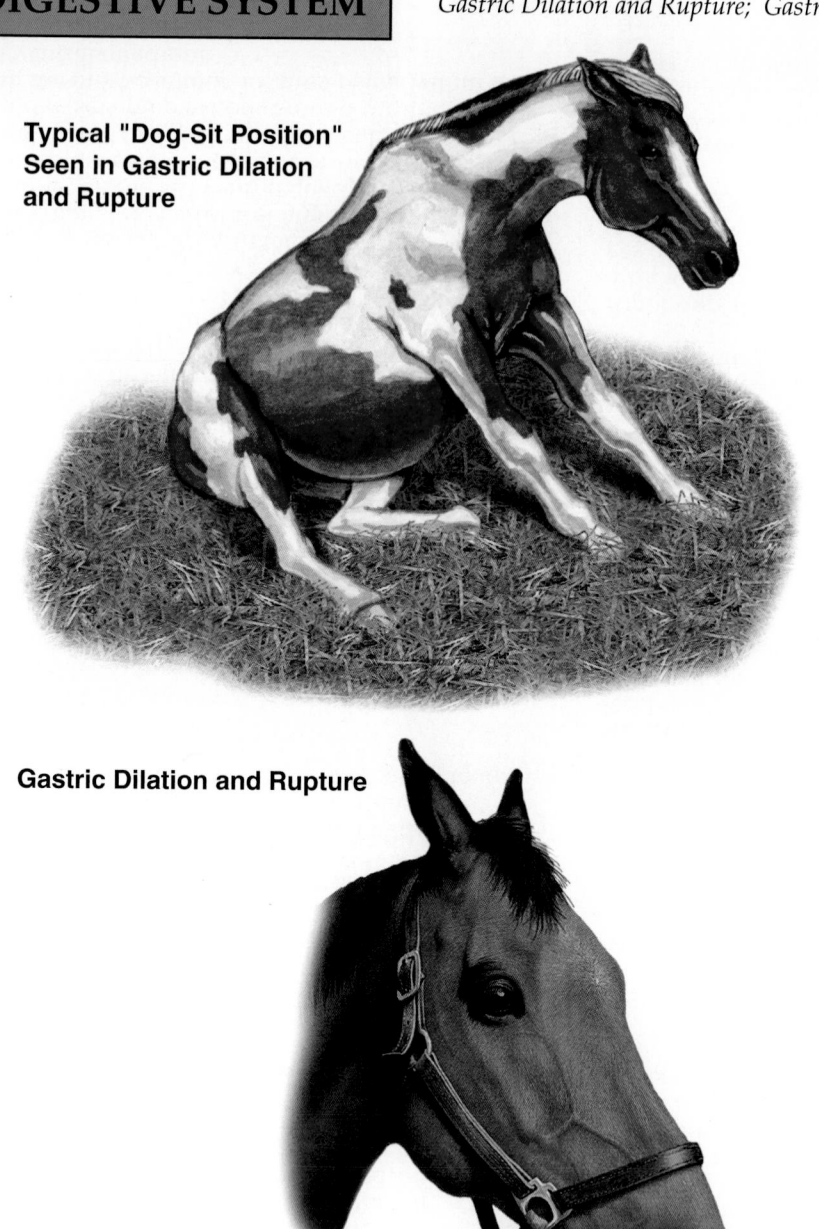

**Gastric Obstruction Resulting
in Saliva and Foodstuffs Around
Nostrils and Oral Cavity**

Gastroduodenal Ulcers

**Large Chronic
Stomach Ulceration**

GASTRIC IMPACTION, DILATATION, AND RUPTURE

Etiology

The consumption of low quality food stuffs by the horse predisposes it to a stomach impaction. This commonly occurs when an animal is first bedded on straw versus its normal bedding of sawdust. Impaction of the stomach can also occur when roughages are poorly masticated when there is poor dentition or another problem within the oral cavity. Dilatation of the stomach occurs as a primary event in which only the stomach is affected or arises as a sequela from an obstruction further down the digestive tract that restricts the flow of gastric contents. Primary gastric dilation occurs from the ingestion of an excessive amount of grain or hay, an excessive and rapid intake of water, or even intake of air in a horse that cribs. Secondary gastric dilation results when there is an obstruction involving the small intestine. Because horses are unable to vomit, the stomach will rupture if the dilation becomes excessive.

Clinical Signs

When a horse suffers from impaction or dilation of the stomach, it may will "dog sit" to decrease the pressure on the stomach. This characteristic posture is an attempt by the horse to relieve the abdominal pain resulting from this disorder. The pain can be very mild to extremely severe. The animal may exhibit increased salivation and may have ingesta present within the nares. If clinical symptoms of retching and vomiting occur, it is usually a sequelae to a terminal event. Vital signs all show an animal in distress in addition to dehydration and possible shock.

Differential Diagnosis

1.) An obstruction of the bowel
2.) An anterior enteritis
3.) Colic as a result of other causes

Treatment

The passage of a nasogastric tube is always indicated. Gastric fluid is siphoned off which reduces the chance of a gastric rupture. A nasogastric tube with numerous holes is preferable since a gastric lavage should be undertaken to remove as much of the grain and ingesta as possible. Lavage coupled with a removal of the gas provides gastric decompression. The inciting cause of the impaction or dilatation should also be corrected. Systemic intravenous fluid therapy is indicated to correct any deficit in the animal's hydration. Analgesics should be administered to help control abdominal pain.

GASTRODUODENAL ULCERATION

A large number of foals, yearlings, and adult horses are affected by gastric ulceration. Ulcers within the duodenum primarily occur within foals and on a rare occasion, the yearling. One seldom finds a duodenal ulcer in the adult horse.

Etiology

Different pathogenic mechanisms result in various anatomical locations of the ulcers. When there is an excessive acidity, the gastric squamous mucosa exhibits a lesion. When there is defective mucosal production, gastric glandular lesions will result. A predisposition to the formation of ulcers occurs whenever there is an incidence of delayed gastric emptying and prolonged gastric contractions.

Excessive acidity can result in a very short period of time. With a diet that contains high levels of concentrates and low levels of roughage intake, acidity quickly becomes excessive. Those horses that are turned out on pasture full time can be examined with an endoscope and typically have no gastric lesions. These animals have a very high intake of roughage and no ingestion of concentrates.

The administration of nonsteroidal anti-inflammatory drugs promotes pathogenic gastric ulceration through the inhibition of local mucoprotective mechanisms. Toxicity levels of these pharmaceuticals also results in colon mucosal lesions.

Clinical Signs

Clinical signs include recurring colic, poor appetite, weight loss, inappetence, and diarrhea. These signs of ulceration can be very benign with the only symptom being that of poor racing or athletic performance. The animal's history should be examined for the administration of nonsteroidal antiinflammatory medications given either recently or periodically over a long period of time.

Diagnosis

Diagnosis of gastric ulceration involves the characteristic clinical signs and endoscopic examination which will determine the location and the severity of the ulcers, and provide enough information to establish a prognosis. Examination of the stool sample for occult blood and the use of contrast radiography are both unreliable diagnostic tools for gastric ulceration.

Treatment

Treatment should be focused on alleviating stress from the animal, reducing or neutralizing acid secretion, and promoting gastric mucosal epithelial healing. Gastric acid secretion can be reduced through the administration of cimetidine or ranitidine. Both of these medications inhibit gastric acid secretions. Treatment of gastric ulceration with antacids will effectively reduce gastric acidity, but will, unfortunately, do it for a very short period of time. These compounds are usually composed of aluminum and/or magnesium suspensions. Unfortunately, they have to be administered approximately every two hours. A sulfated polysaccharide is utilized in the treatment of peptic ulcers in humans. This compound is thought to adhere itself to damaged gastric mucosa and stimulate local blood flow and mucous secretion. This is particularly effective treatment in horses that develop squamous mucosal lesions.

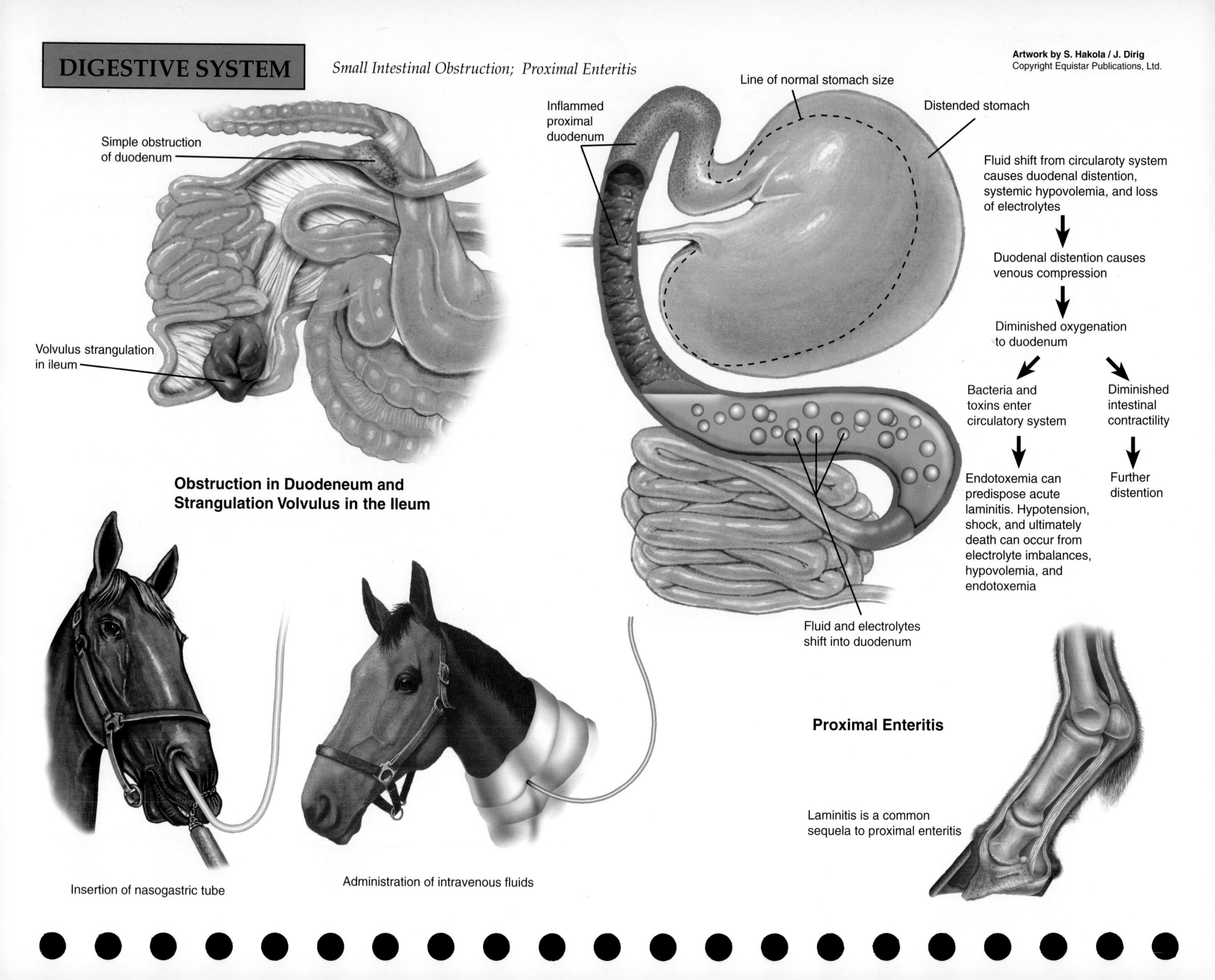

Simple obstruction of duodenum

Volvulus strangulation in ileum

Obstruction in Duodeneum and Strangulation Volvulus in the Ileum

Insertion of nasogastric tube

Administration of intravenous fluids

Inflammed proximal duodenum

Line of normal stomach size

Distended stomach

Fluid shift from circularoty system causes duodenal distention, systemic hypovolemia, and loss of electrolytes

Duodenal distention causes venous compression

Diminished oxygenation to duodenum

Bacteria and toxins enter circulatory system

Diminished intestinal contractility

Endotoxemia can predispose acute laminitis. Hypotension, shock, and ultimately death can occur from electrolyte imbalances, hypovolemia, and endotoxemia

Further distention

Fluid and electrolytes shift into duodenum

Proximal Enteritis

Laminitis is a common sequela to proximal enteritis

Gastrointestinal motility can be increased without the increase of gastric acid output through the administration of bethanecol. Care must be taken, however, to not administer this drug in extremely high doses since one of the side effects is diarrhea.

If medical treatment proves nonrewarding, gastroenterostomy may be required. This decision must be carefully considered, as these horses will still require treatment with acid suppressive and gastrointestinal stimulatory drugs postoperatively.

SMALL INTESTINAL OBSTRUCTION

Obstruction within the small intestinal tract can be characterized as simple or strangulating, and high (proximal), or low (distal). A simple obstruction of the small intestine involves intraluminal blockage without strangulation. When an intestine is twisted on its own axis, strangulation occurs which obstructs the small intestinal tract. An obstruction that occurs in the proximal portion of the small intestine at the level of the duodenum will result in a metabolic alkalosis. An obstruction that occurs more distally in the small intestine usually produces metabolic acidosis. When an obstruction is caused by a strangulation, the blood supply to the area of the bowel is compromised which creates a life threatening emergency.

Etiology

Simple obstructions may be caused from the following disorders:
1.) Intussusception
2.) Foreign bodies
3.) Adhesions from a previous surgical procedure or from peritonitis
4.) Intestinal stricture
5.) Ileal impaction
6.) Non-strangulating infarction from verminous arteritis

Strangulating obstructions result from:
1.) Inguinal hernias
2.) Strangulating umbilical hernias
3.) Mesenteric herniation
4.) Volvulus and herniation through the epiploic foramen.

Clinical Signs

Abdominal pain exhibited by these obstructed animals varies from very mild with resultant depression to that of severe, where the animal is uncontrollable. The horse may exhibit profuse sweating, constant rolling, and pawing in response to the distress. Systemically, there is an increased heart rate, injected or inflamed mucous membranes, and an increase in the packed cell volume and total plasma protein values. Rectal examination will usually reveal multiple distended loops of the small intestine. Fluid is typically recovered after the passage of a nasogastric tube into the stomach. An abdominocentesis will usually reveal an increase in the total nucleated cell count and protein content. If the bowel is strangulated, there will be a serosanguineous appearance to the fluid.

Differential Diagnosis

These clinical signs are exhibited with other abdominal disorders: anterior enteritis, colitis, large bowel obstruction, displacement, peritonitis, and any other cause of colic. These disorders should all be considered when the above listed clinical signs are noted.

Treatment

Mild or simple obstructions may respond to medical treatment which should include pain control through the use of nonsteroidal antiinflammatory drugs, decompression of the stomach through the use of a nasogastric tube, and restoration of fluid balance within the horse. If a foreign body can be palpated, it is of therapeutic benefit to administer laxatives and lubricants as well as electrolyte solutions via the nasogastric tube. Fluid therapy should be administered in large volumes so that the cardiovascular functions are assisted, and there is an increased volume of fluid within the gastrointestinal tract. The administration of laxatives such as mineral oil are contraindicated in any of the strangulating obstructions of the small intestines.

Any simple nonresponding or strangulating obstruction will require surgical intervention. Exploratory surgery should be done as soon as possible to avoid deteriorization of those portions of compromised bowel.

PROXIMAL ENTERITIS

Proximal enteritis is also referred to as duodenitis anterior enteritis, or duodenitis/proxmial jejunitis syndrome. This disorder is characterized by an inflammatory reaction within the small intestine that results in excess fluid and electrolyte secretion by the small intestine which in turn produces large volumes of enterogastric reflux. Proximal enteritis usually occurs in horses that are greater than three years old. Because of the acute abdominal pain that is involved with this syndrome, horses affected by this disorder are usually taken to surgery because they show signs similar to small intestinal obstruction. At surgery, no obstruction is found, but the small intestine is severely inflamed and distended The etiological agent for this disorder has not been identified, although *Salmonella* and *Clostridium* species have been recovered from enterogastric reflux.

Clinical Signs

Proximal enteritis exhibits similar clinical signs to those found in small intestinal obstructions. The animal is usually in a severe amount of pain. When a stomach tube is passed, there is a large volume of fetid nasal gastric reflux which flows from the tube following passage. The severe pain that these animals experience is temporarily relieved following gastric decompression. These horses are often severely depressed, dehydrated, febrile, and an increased heart rate and injected mucous membranes. Neutophilia will be seen on a complete blood count. Rectal examination will reveal small intestinal distention and inflammation. Auscultation of the abdomen will reveal depressed or absent borborygmi.

Differential Diagnosis

Proximal enteritis can be tentatively differentiated from a strangulated obstruction of the small

Impaction Colic of the Large Intestine

Artwork by S. Hakola / J. Dirig
Copyright Equistar Publications, Ltd.

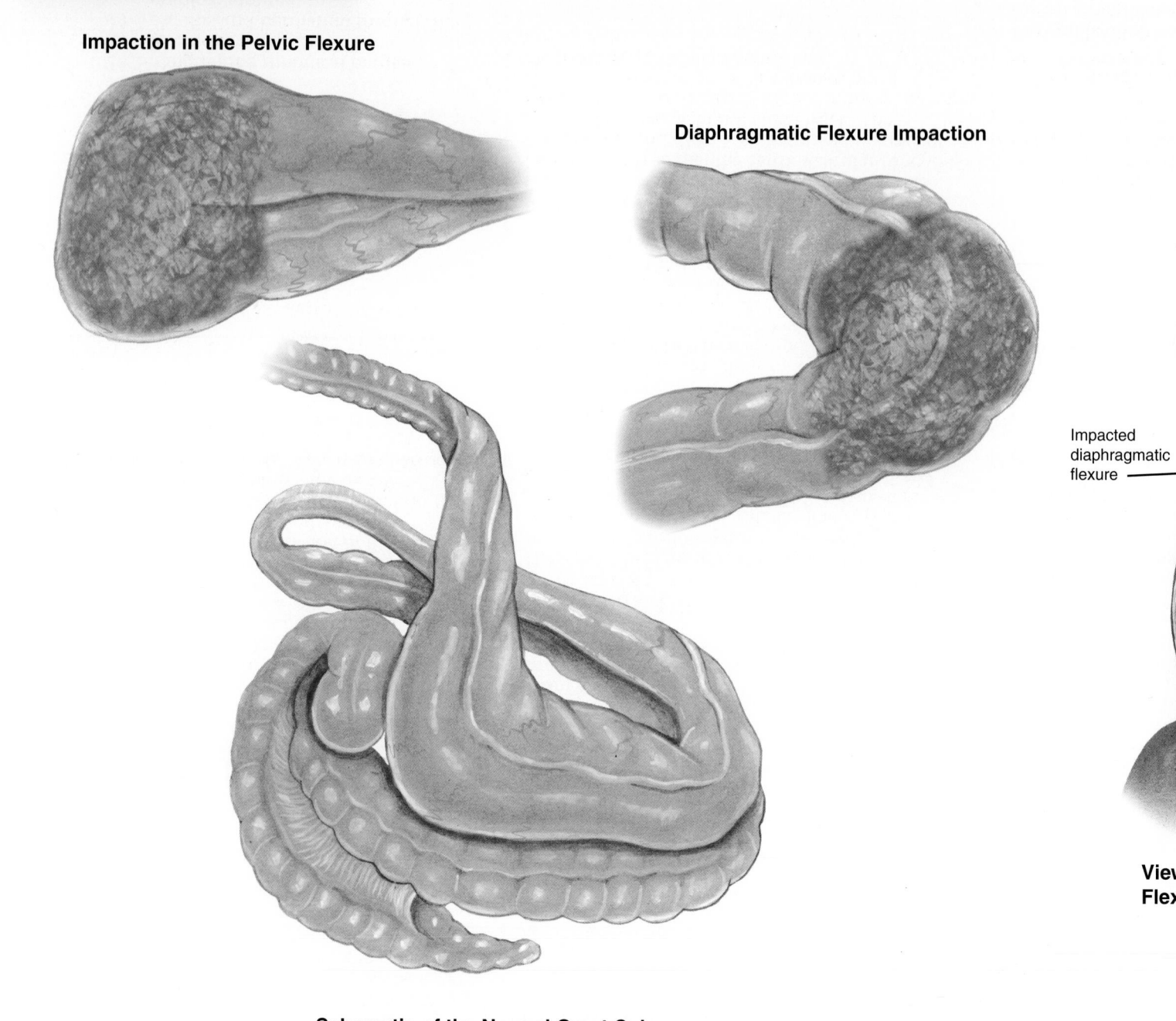

Impaction in the Pelvic Flexure

Diaphragmatic Flexure Impaction

Impacted diaphragmatic flexure

View of Impacted Diaphragmatic Flexure of the Dorsal Colon

Schematic of the Normal Great Colon

intestine from the fact that there is a significant reduction in pain following gastric decompression. Strangulating obstructions are not alleviated after gastric decompression. These animals will still be severely depressed. The most difficult thing to differentiate from proximal enteritis is that of the small intestinal obstruction or strangulation. All causes of abdominal pain should be considered when these clinical signs are presented, including colon colitis, large intestinal obstructions, and peritonitis.

Treatment

Since the causative agents of proximal enteritis are unknown, aggressive supportive therapy is the treatment of choice. This treatment may be required for three to four days or sometimes as long as ten days. The goal of the treatment is to provide gastric decompression, to relieve pain, to prevent gastric rupture, and to allow the small intestine to heal and return to function.

Nasogastric intubation is usually left dwelling or at least repeated every one to two hours. This reduces the risk of gastric rupture and helps control pain. During the initial intubation, it is not unusual to recover six to ten liters of reflux fluid. Continuous intravenous administration of balanced electrolyte solutions are required to maintain renal function, treat hypovolemia, and to restore an electrolyte balance. In the acute stage, it is not unusual to administer over fifty liters of intravenous fluids through both jugular veins. Careful attention should be paid to the levels of potassium, calcium, and magnesium during long term fluid therapy.

Parenteral nutritional support should be administered to these animals since these horses should receive nothing orally until the small intestine has had some chance to repair. These solutions should contain glucose, balanced amino acid solutions, lipid emulsions, trace minerals, and vitamins.

There has been some evidence that the intravenous administration of DMSO in a ten to twenty percent solution will assist in the reduction of the inflammatory process within the bowel. This is administered slowly intravenously and may decrease other complications such as laminitis.

Nonsteroidal antiinflammatory therapeutic agents such as flunixin meglumine are indicated to provide analgesia, to decrease endotoxemia, and as a prophylactic measure for laminitis. Broad spectrum antimicrobial therapy should be administered. Since the *Clostridium* species is a suspected etiological agent, penicillin administered at the rate of 15,000 to 20,000 IU/kg intramuscularly every twelve hours plus an aminoglycoside or third generation cephalosporin therapy should be considered.

Since laminitis is a common sequela to proximal enteritis, preventative foot care is indicated. These animals should be stalled in deep wood shavings or in sand if possible. This will help provide sole and frog support. If this is not possible, sole and frog pressure can be applied by using a role of gauze or gauze sponges that are held in place with elastic bandages.

DISORDERS OF THE LARGE INTESTINES

Disorders of the large intestine produce the most common causes of abdominal pain in the horse. The large intestines are very mobile and, based on volume, constitute the major portion of the gastrointestinal tract of the horse. Any disorder within the large intestine will result in pain, a change in hydration and electrolyte balance within the horse, and cause the accumulation of gases. Disorders of the large intestine can be divided into those that are obstructive and those that are inflammatory in nature.

OBSTRUCTIVE DISORDERS OF THE LARGE INTESTINE

Impaction within the large colon of the horse is the most common form of colonic obstruction and therefore, a frequent cause of colic.

Etiology

The causes for impaction in the colon are numerous, and the actual etiological agent is not always known. The physical obstruction caused by the accumulation of ingesta can be predisposed by a coarse feed, poor dental health, foreign substances within the feed, stress, decreased water intake, and dysfunctional bowel motility. The impaction usually occurs at the two anatomical sites where the bowel narrows. The pelvic flexure and the transverse colon are both sites where the intestine narrows and where motor centers can induce ingesta retention to facilitate further mixing of the food. Those animals that have poor dentition and those that are older and subjected to colder weather with low water intake are usually predisposed to colon impaction.

Clinical Signs

These horses usually exhibit intermittent colic that gradually worsens. Initial signs of colic may be as subtle as the animal turning and staring at the abdomen or simply pawing. There may initially be only mild abdominal pain, but this usually progresses to severe pain over a period of time. The animal's heart rate, mucous membranes, and hydration levels are initially normal. Ausultation of the bowel will usually reveal increased peristaltic movement against an obstruction. Typically, there is a moderate to severe decrease in other gastrointestinal sounds throughout the abdomen. A rectal examination will reveal a firm mass within the pelvic flexure; however, a mass within the transverse colon may go undetected due to the difficulty of its palpation.

Differential Diagnosis

1. Small intestinal obstruction or strangulation
2. Other causes of large colon impaction such as enteroliths or sand
3. Large colon displacement or torsion
4. Colitis
5. Peritonitis

Enteroliths; Sand Impaction

Artwork by S. Hakola / J. Dirig
Copyright Equistar Publications, Ltd.

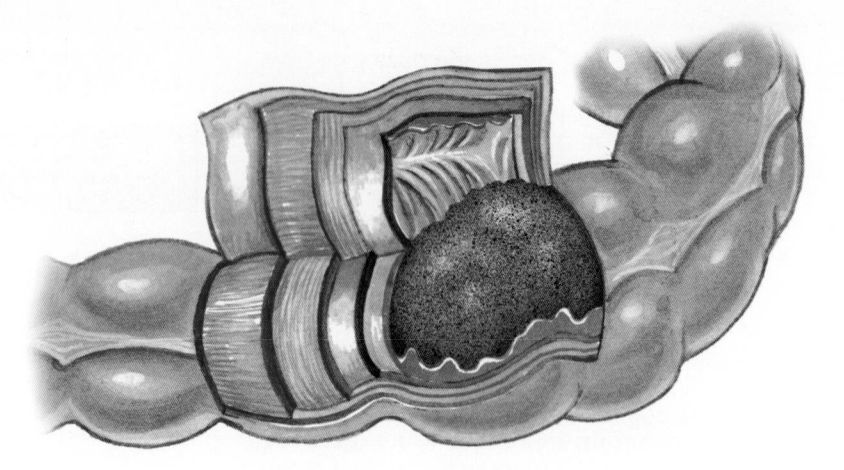

Sand Impaction in the Great Colon

Enteroliths in the Pelvic and Diaphragmatic Flexures

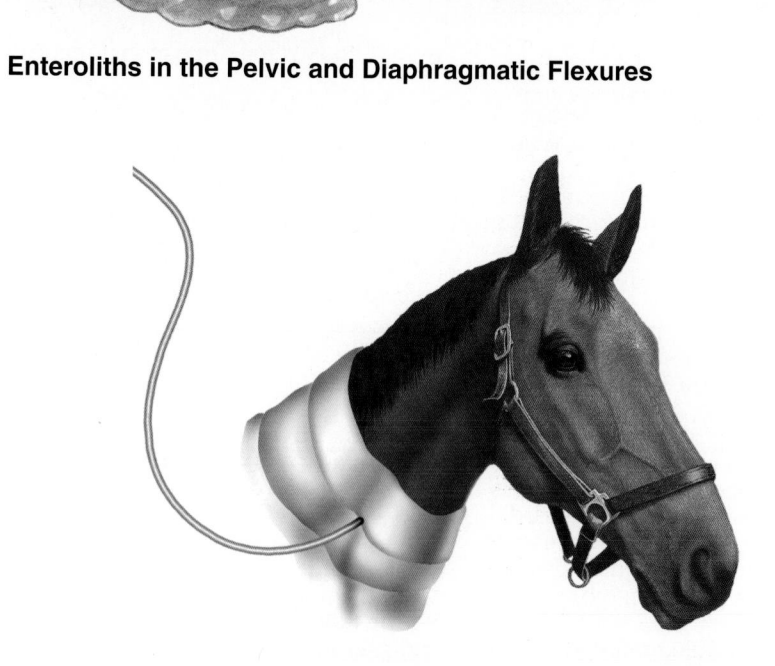

Administration of intravenous fluids

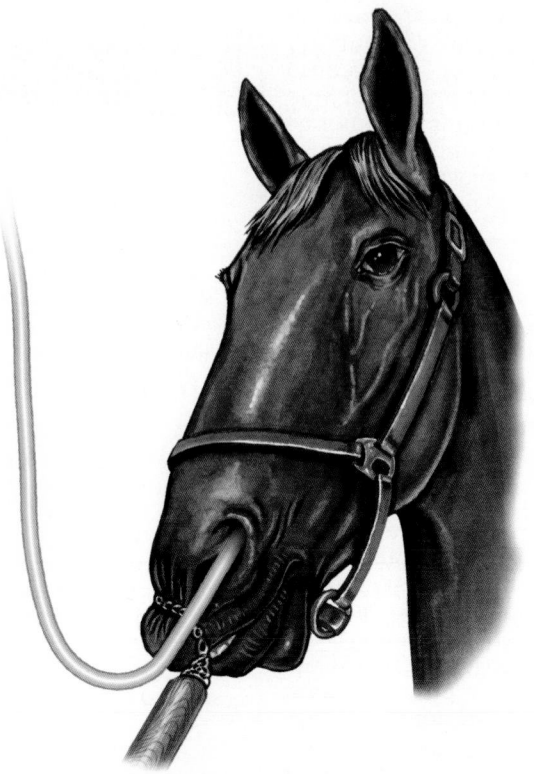

Nasogastric intubation

Treatment

Medical treatment consisting of the administration of oral laxatives and fluids, intravenous fluid therapy, and analgesia will usually correct a simple impaction within the large colon. Low doses of flunixin meglumine can be used to provide pain relief and protect against endotoxemia. Oil mixed with an oral electrolyte solution is administered via a nasogastric tube. Aggressive balanced fluid therapy should be administered intravenously at a rate of approximately fifty liters within a twenty-four hour period. This will aid in softening the mass and maintaining bowel motility. In those animals where medical treatment does not resolve the impaction, surgical intervention is the only choice.

ENTEROLITHS

Etiology

Enteroliths are mineral concretions usually composed of magnesium ammonium phosphate which forms around a nidus within the large intestine. The highest incidences of these mineral concretions is found on the coasts in California and Florida. All breeds are affected by this disorder, but Arabians seem to have the highest incidence. The nidus within the center of the concretion usually includes hair, metal, or another foreign material such as silicon dioxide which is a flint-like stone.

These intestinal calculi can be located in several anatomical areas within the intestinal tract. The large calculi usually occur in the right dorsal colon. The transverse colon and the descending colon are usually the sites for smaller calculi. These small calculi may be single or may be found in groups of just a few calculi to actually hundreds. These multiple small calculi can cause pain without causing an obstruction due to the irritating affects and stretching on the walls of the colon.

Clinical Signs

These animals usually exhibit a progressive anorexia and depression. The amount of pain that is evident can be dependent upon the degree of obstruction and the amount of distention within the bowel. Auscultation of the abdomen will reveal decreased frequency within the progressive motility. When many small calculi are present, a characteristic gravelly sound can be heard in the ventral abdomen. Rectal palpation will reveal a distention within the bowel and on rare occasions, the enterolith itself can be palpated.

Treatment

Most cases will require surgical removal of the enterolith. This is accomplished under general anesthesia. Medical management is similar to that in the treatment of a primary impaction of the large intestine. Analgesia is provided in addition to administration of large volumes of intravenous fluids. Oral laxatives and electrolyte solutions may facilitate the removal of very small calculi.

SAND IMPACTION

Etiology

This disorder is common within horses that live in areas where there is loose sandy soil. This affects horses of all ages, and occurs when the animal is fed off the ground or inadvertently consumes sand due to short or nonexistent grass within the pasture. The pathogenesis is similar to that of an impaction resulting from an accumulation of normal ingesta. Fine sand accumulates in the ventral colon while coarse sand has a predominant accumulation within the dorsal colon.

Clinical Signs

Clinical signs of sand impaction are very similiar to those produced from other large colon impactions. The animal will exhibit intermittent signs of mild to moderate pain. These symptoms usually respond immediately to the administration of analgesic agents. The horsess appear to be in pain, will stand stretched out, or may just lay down for longer periods of time than normal. The pulse rate and hydration is usually normal. Rectal palpation may reveal a sand impaction within the ventral colon but may not detect sand or an impaction at all. Auscultation of the abdomen may reveal the sound of sand, such as sand pouring upon itself. Small amounts of sand may be found in the stool sample.

Differential Diagnosis

1. Small intestinal obstruction and strangulation
2. Other causes of colon impaction such as feed
3. Colitis
4. Peritonitis
5. Large colon displacement or torsion

Treatment

Medical management is centered around providing analgesia, intravenous fluid therapy, and the oral administration of laxatives. Administration of flunixin meglumine should be done to provide analgesia. Intravenous fluid therapy should be administered at the rate of at least 25 - 50 liters of fluid within a 24 hour period of time. The laxative of choice for sand impactions is psyllium hydrophalic mucilloid at a dose of .25 - .5 kg per 500 kg of weight. This psyllium product is mixed with 4 - 8 liters of water and administered through a nasogastric tube. This product can also be mixed with mineral oil and the solution that contains mineral oil, water, and psyllium can be given through the nasogastric tube. Those animals that do not respond to medical treatment will require surgical intervention.

As in all disorders, prevention is the key to the management of horses that are predisposed to sand impactions. Animals should not be fed off the ground. Pasture should be provided that is not overgrazed or short. Dry psyllium can be given periodically at 1 - 2 cups per 500 kg daily for 2 - 3 weeks to provide relief to initial clinical signs. The psyllium can also be fed routinely 1 - 2 cups per 500 kg for a week every 4 - 6 weeks to prevent sand accumulation.

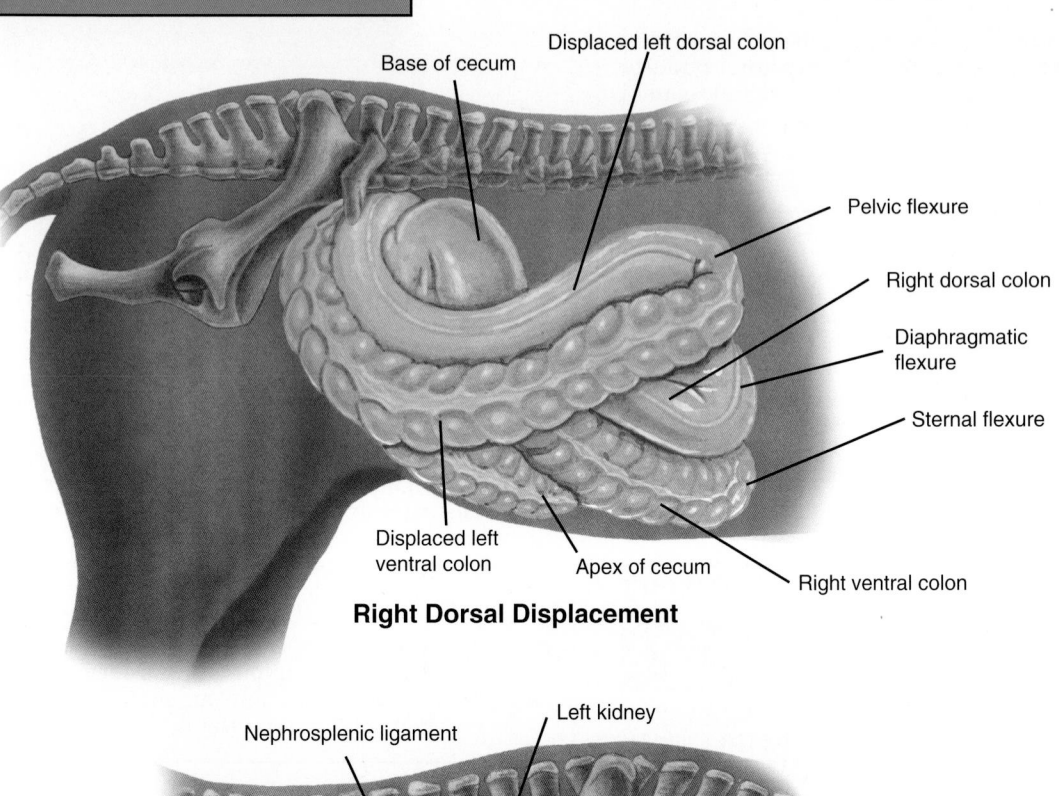

Base of cecum
Displaced left dorsal colon
Pelvic flexure
Right dorsal colon
Diaphragmatic flexure
Sternal flexure
Displaced left ventral colon
Apex of cecum
Right ventral colon

Right Dorsal Displacement

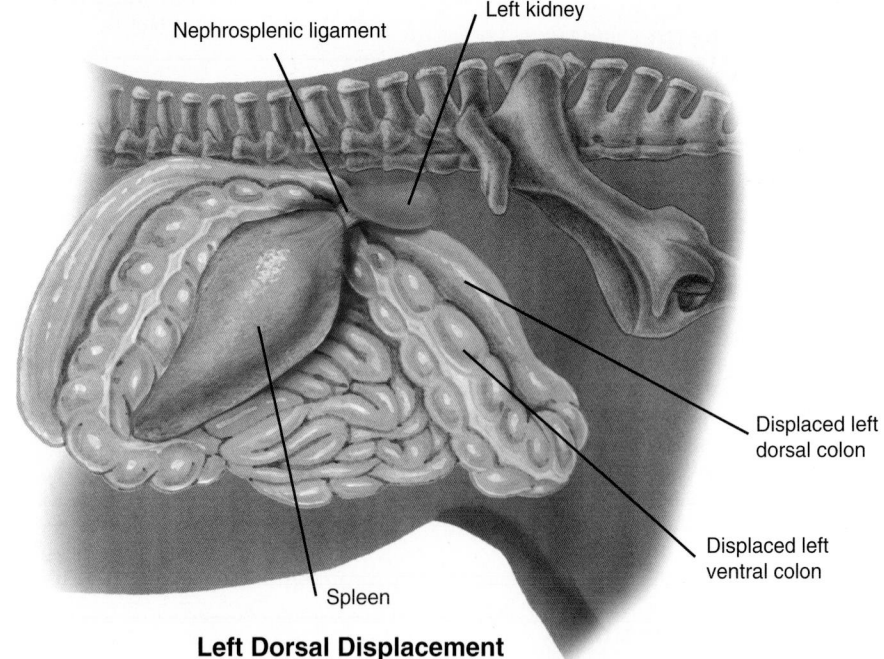

Nephrosplenic ligament
Left kidney
Displaced left dorsal colon
Displaced left ventral colon
Spleen

Left Dorsal Displacement

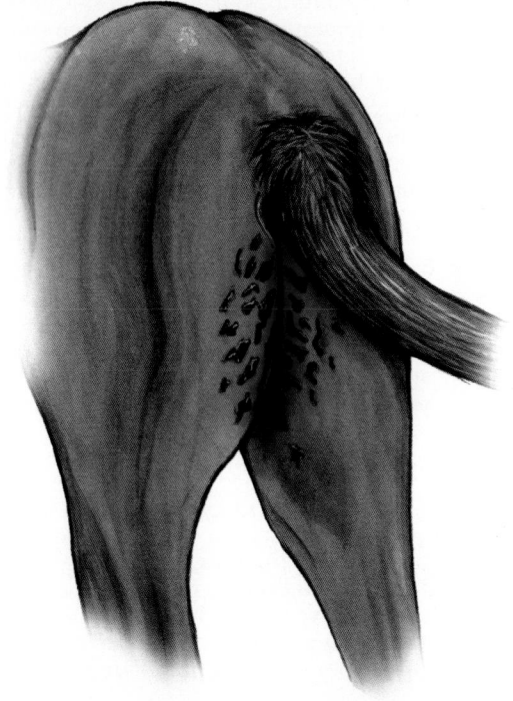

Diarrhea with perineal scalding

Salmonellosis

Salmonella gram stain

RIGHT DORSAL DISPLACEMENT

Etiology

Right dorsal displacement of the colon is a malposition of the left colon to the right of the cecum. Either a hypomotile or hypermotile state produces accumulation of gas, fluid, or ingesta which results in the aberrant movement of the colon within the abdominal cavity. Large breed horses such as Belgians, Percherans, and warmbloods seem to have a higher incidence of this disorder.

Clinical Signs

The large colon rotates 180 degrees around the mesenteric attachment. The end result of this is that the colon becomes located between the cecum and body wall on the right. The horse may exhibit very mild to violent uncontrollable pain which is dependent upon the gas distention and tension on the mesentery. If the displacement causes an obstruction to the duodenum, gastric reflux is possible. The animal's heart rate, mucous membrane color, and hydration will all depend on the severity of the displacement and consequential gas accumulation. Rectal examination will reveal a transverse orientation across the pelvic inlet of the right colon. Edema may be palpable within the colonic walls and mesenteric lymph nodes and fat may also be present. The pelvic flexure will not be palpable because it has relocated into the cranial abdominal region due to the rotation of the colon.

Treatment

Right dorsal displacement requires surgical correction. The colon is exposed and replaced in its proper position. If the condition is diagnosed early, the prognosis is very good.

LEFT DORSAL DISPLACEMENT

Etiology

The cause of a left dorsal displacement of the colon is unknown. The left portion of the large colon relocates between the body wall and the left kidney. The pelvic flexure moves into the gastrosplenic space and becomes entrapped at the nephrosplenic notch. The nephrosplenic ligament supports the colon in its displaced position. Two possible mechanisms are thought to predispose this colon entrapment and are as follows. 1.) Migration of the pelvic flexure over the top of the nephrosplenic ligament is the first mechanism. 2.) A splenic contraction which allows the colon to migrate between the spleen and the body wall followed by a subsequent splenic expansion which traps the colon in this dorsal location.

Clinical Signs

The clinical signs of this displacement resemble those of an impaction within the colon. Mild to moderate pain is evident and dependent on how much obstruction is present due to the colon hanging over the nephrosplenic ligament. The heart rate, mucous membranes, and hydration levels are usually normal unless this condition has been present for a long period of time. A rectal exam will usually provide a diagnosis since it is normally possible to trace the colon over the nephrosplenic ligament. The spleen is usually rotated caudally away from the left abdominal wall due to the tension on its suspensory ligament.

Treatment

Surgical intervention is usually necessary to correct this displacement. Correction is provided in the surgical field by pushing the spleen medially and elevating the colon dorsal to the spleen. Once the colon is free from the nephrosplenic space, the pelvic flexure can be retrieved and replaced within its normal position.

It has been reported that 40% of the nephrosplenic entrapments can be corrected by rolling the horse. The animal is placed under general anesthesia on its right side. A rectal examination is then done to determine if the spleen will shift medially due to the weight of the colon. The anesthetized animal is then elevated by its rear legs vertically and let down slowly. Another rectal exam is done to see if the colon has pulled the spleen medially and ventrally. If this is accomplished, the horse is then elevated vertically again and rolled to the right. This should allow the colon to float to the top of the abdomen. This procedure should be done where economic considerations prevent a surgical option.

LARGE INTESTINAL DISORDERS RESULTING IN DIARRHEA

SALMONELLOSIS

Salmonella spp. are gram negative anaerobic bacteria which produce a potent endotoxin causing symptoms of colic and diarrhea in the horse. Many sterotypes of *Salmonella* are reported ubiquitous in equine population with those classified in group B as the most pathogenic. It has been shown that approximately 10 - 20% of the equine population are infected and actively shed *Salmonella*. These animals serve as a potential source of infection to all suseptible horses. Transmission of this disorder is by oral innoculation. Salmonellosis effects horses of all ages, but it is more common in younger animals. Stress such as training, transportation, surgery, dietary changes, or anesthesia predispose the horse to salmonellosis.

Clinical Signs

Animals that are infected with *Salmonella* can exhibit any one of four distinct clinical signs:
1.) An active carrier state in which the horse appears normal.
2.) The animal appears depressed, febrile, and anorexic with no apparent sign of any diarrhea.
3.) A severe case of enterocolitis with diarrhea.
4.) Septicemia.
Animals that are asymptomatic, in a carrier state, may clinically exhibit bone and joint infections,

Potomac Horse Fever

Artwork by S. Hakola / J. Dirig
Copyright Equistar Publications, Ltd.

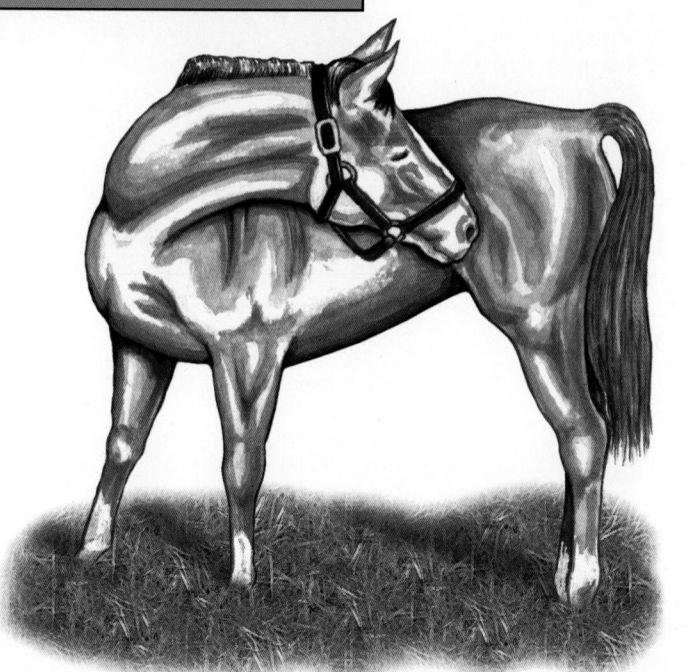

Horse looking at flank with painful colic.

Potomac Horse Fever

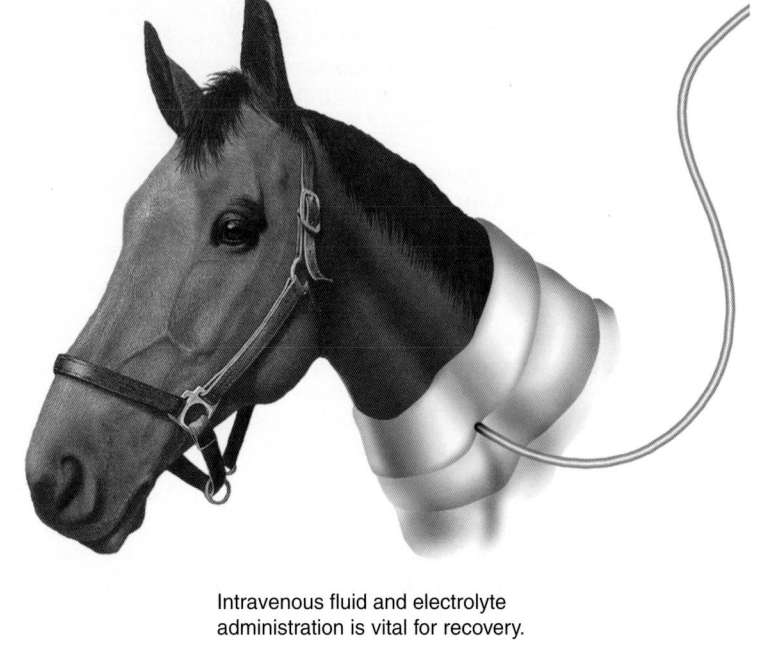

Intravenous fluid and electrolyte administration is vital for recovery.

Stage III - IV laminitis is a common sequel to Potomac horse fever.

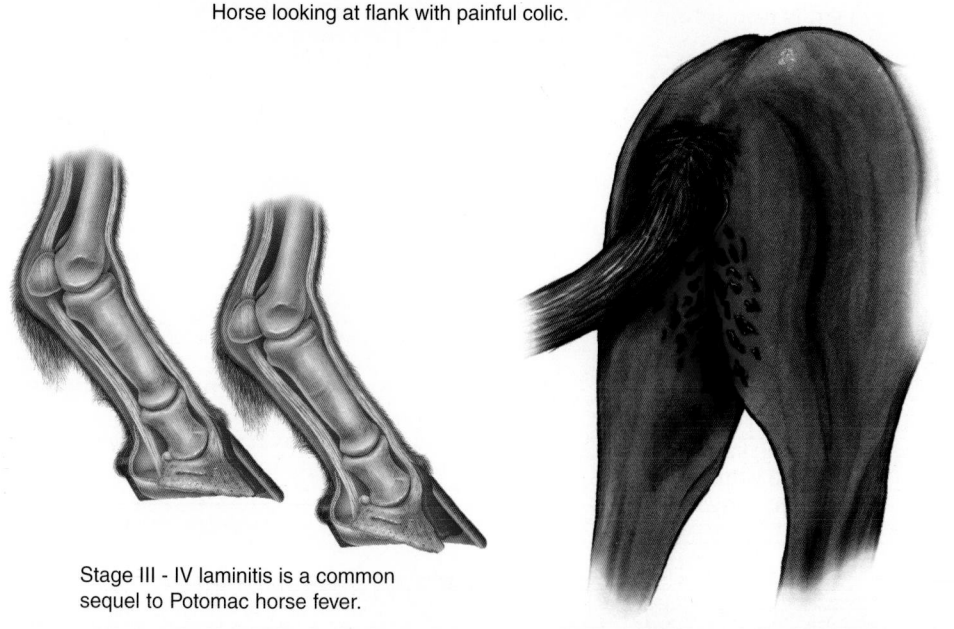

Diarrhea may be an important clinical sign.

Good cushioning pad and shoe may help in preventing laminitis.

subcutaneous abscess formation, and pneumonia. The diarrhea that is produced by these animals with enteric salmonellosis is profuse, foul smelling, and sometimes bloody. When the horse is in the nonacute state, it is possible that the stool has a characteristic "cow-patty" consistency. The animal is usually dehydrated depending on the severity of the diarrhea and fever. Auscultation of the abdomen reveals a hypermotile bowel that has the characteristic "tinkling" sounds. Blood work on these animals will usually reveal some degree of dehydration as well as a leukopenia (less than 3,000 WBC). Chemical profiles of the blood will also exhibit a hyponatremia, hypokalemia, and a hypochloremia.

Diagnosis

Fecal samples are submitted to the laboratory for the recovery of the *salmonella* organism. Samples should be taken for a culture on a daily basis for three to five days. Note that the *salmonella* organism may also be recovered from a fecal culture in association with other enteric diseases such as Potomac horse fever and proximal duodenitis.

Treatment

Treatment for salmonellosis requires fluid and electrolyte therapy, control of pain, control of the endotoxemia, and the reestablishment of normal flora within the bowel. Fluid therapy should be by both oral and parenteral administration. Dehydration, electrolyte imbalances, and acid-base abnormalities must be corrected through aggressive fluid therapy techniques.

Nonsteroidal antiinflammatory drugs should be administered in low doses on a regular basis to control inflammation. Sensitivity tests from the fecal culture should be consulted as to the proper antibiotic therapy for these cases. Tetracycline and oxytetracycline are contraindicated. Antidiarrheal medications are indicated because of their local antiinflammatory effect, thereby decreasing fluid secretion within the bowel. Medications such as bismuth subsalicylate, kaopectate, and activated charcoal can all be administered via a nasogastric tube.

In severe cases, plasma transfusions may have some value. The administration of 5 - 10 liters for a 450 - 500kg horse may help in the re-establishment of plasma protein values. Commercially available antiserum can be administered IV and may be useful in the treatment of horses with acute colitis. DMSO in a 10 - 20% solution administered IV may be useful as an antiinflammatory medication. Utilizing this treatment, there may also be some prophylactic benefit in the prevention of these horses from developing laminitis.

Prognosis

The prognosis is guarded for all cases of the salmonellosis. The use of antibiotics in the treatment of these cases should also be judicious since this organism readily develops bacterial resistance. Approximately 90% of those animals receiving proper treatment will survive the salmonellosis. However, unfortunately some of these horses will remain carriers of the organism and will serve as a source of infection to other animals.

POTOMAC HORSE FEVER

Etiology

Potomac horse fever is also referred to as equine monocytic ehrlichiosis and is caused by an infectious blood-born rickettsial organism. This organism, *Ehrlichia risticci* is not spread by contact or direct exposure from the environment. This organism requires blood transmission by an insect, arthropod, or even an avian intermediate host. This organism can infect horses of all ages; however, foals seem to be the least infected. In a geographical area where infection has occurred, infection rates are sporadic. Usually, only small groups of horses are infected. These animals are usually under areas of intense confinement such as that which occurs at a racetrack or a large training stable. Since its occurrence in 1982, twenty different states have reported this disease.

Clinical Signs

After the organism has infected the horse, clinical signs develop approximately 10 - 15 days later. Symptoms can range from very mild to severe and be complicated with a resulting case of laminitis. These horses are depressed, febrile, have mild to severe colic, diarrhea, and may in shock.

The diarrhea from these animals is usually not as foul smelling as that which occurs with salmonellosis. The mucous membranes may exhibit petechiation which is the formation of small areas of blood clots . Subcutaneous edema may occur along the ventral surface of the body and also throughout the limbs. Auscultation of the abdomen will reveal everything from no gut sounds to that of a hypermotile bowel. Laminitis is usually a sequela to this disorder and may be mild or severe and effect all four feet. Sinker syndrome or third phalanx displacement may also occur with these cases of laminitis.

Treatment

Treatment of these cases involves aggressive fluid and electrolyte replacement therapy, the administration of oxytetracycline, and the prevention of laminitis. Tetracyclines administered at a dose of 10 mg/kg intravenously twice a day can effectively stop this disease if given in the very early stages. Unfortunately, tetracycline may induce salmonellosis in these cases. Since approximately 25 - 30% of the Potomac horse fever cases exhibit laminitis, initial lateral radiographs of all four feet should be made for baseline reference. Frog pads should be applied and treatment with nonsteroidal antiinflammatory drugs should be initiated. There is a commercial vaccine available for this disorder; but vaccination in the face of a Potomac horse fever outbreak has little prophylactic value.

Intestinal clostridiosis causes extremely painful colic.

Intestinal Clostridiosis

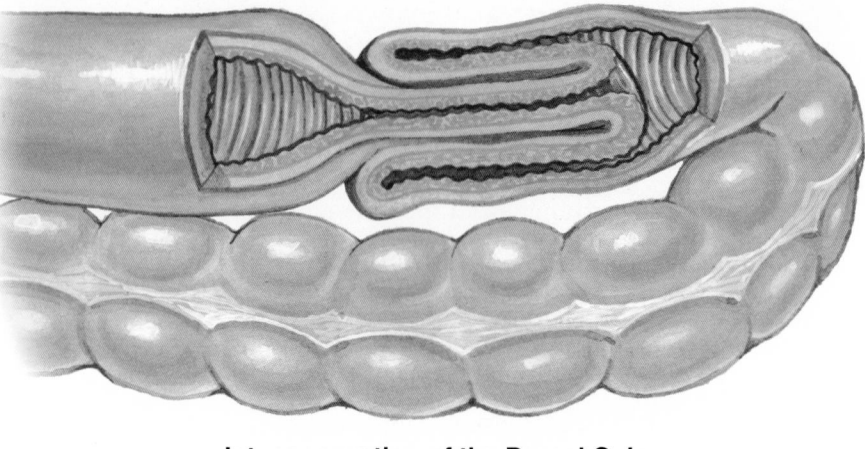

Swollen, inflammed mucous membranes and gingiva as seen in intestinal clostridiosis.

Intussusception of the Dorsal Colon

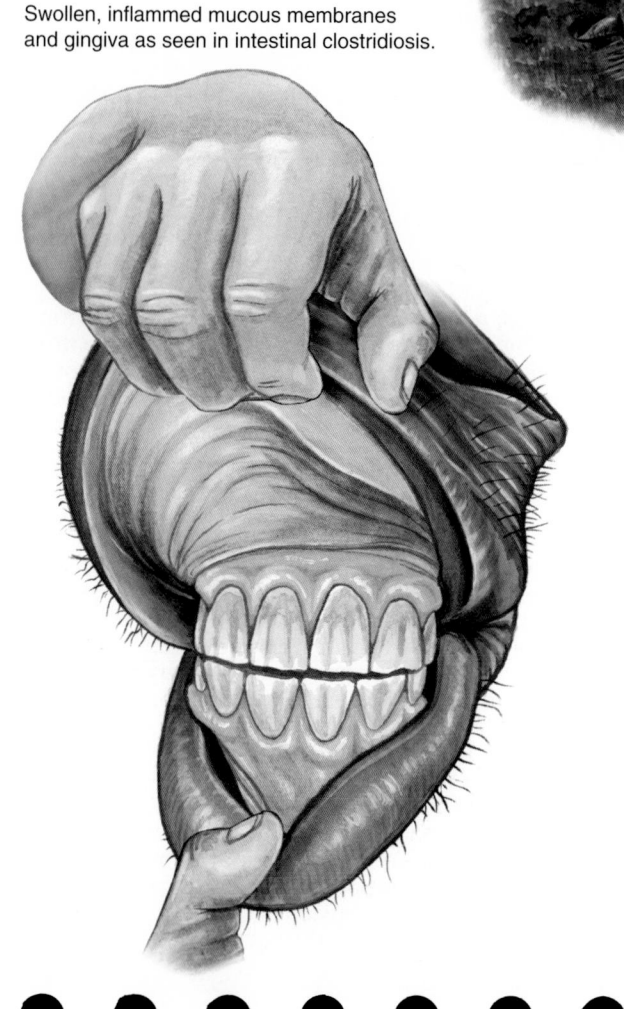

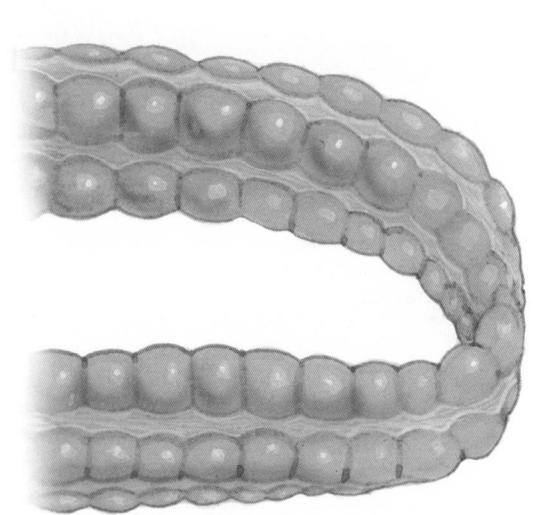

Nonstrangulated torsion at the sternal flexure

Torsional Colic

Strangulated 360 degree torsion of the diaphragmatic flexure

EQUINE INTESTINAL CLOSTRIDIOSIS

Etiology

Infection with *Clostridium perfringens* type A has been an important cause of enterocolitis within the foal. It is also the cause of acute colitis within adult horses. This disorder has also been referred to as "colitis X" and edematous bowel syndrome. The clinical severity of this disorder depends on the ability of the *Clostridium* organism to produce enterotoxins. *Clostridium* normally inhabits the gastrointestinal tract in low numbers but does not usually produce an enterotoxin; however, sometimes, these organisms do occassionally produce enterotoxins. These situations are not fully understood; but treatment with oxytetracycline has been shown to result in enterotoxin production.

Clinical Signs and Diagnosis

These animals are usually in extreme uncontrollable pain. They exhibit characteristic signs of toxemia which include fever, injected mucous membranes, and even tachycardia. Death may occur even before the onset of any diarrhea. Neutropenia, leukopenia, and hemoconcentration are common with this disorder. Diagnosis is based on the fecal culture of *Clostridium perfringens* type A.

Treatment

Aggressive oral and intravenous fluid administration to maintain hydration, electrolyte, and acid-base balance is important. The administration of nonsteroidal antiinflammatory drugs and plasma containing antibodies are also indicated to prevent the systemic effects of the endotoxins. Gastrointestinal protectants are beneficial in reducing inflammation and secretions within the bowel. Antibiotic therapy should include third generation cephalosporins.

INTUSSUSCEPTION

Etiology

When the bowel becomes hypermotile, it predisposes the animal's bowel to intussusception. This usually occurs in younger horses such as yearlings. Intussusception will usually occur at the pelvic flexure and left dorsal colon or at the apex of the cecum. Intussusception of the cecum has been associated with *Eimeria leukarti, Anoplocephala perfoliata,* and *Strongylus vulgaris* infections.

Clinical Signs and Diagnosis

The abdominal pain resulting from this condition may range from mild and intermittent to acute and severe. This pain may last a few hours to several days. If an obstruction results, there will be a gaseous distention of the bowel which results in more severe pain. Rectal palpation may reveal the vague clinical signs of gaseous distention in the bowel.

Treatment

Surgical intervention is the only treatment available for this disorder. The intussusception is reduced with a portion of the strangulated intestine resected. Supportive care and systemic treatment postoperatively are indicated since peritonitis usually results from this condition.

TORSION

Etiology

The cause of a colon torsion is unknown. Hypomotility with subsequent gas distention may allow the large ventral colon to float over the smaller dorsal colon along its entire length allowing displacement. This disorder usually effects only older horses. Brood mares just after parturition are especially susceptible.

Clinical Signs

These animals exhibit a very severe acute abdominal pain. The administration of analgesic agents does not control this pain. These horses soon go into shock, and their mucous membranes, which initially have a normal color, become pale pink to even gray in color.

The colon usually twists clockwise. The right dorsal colon moves laterally while rotating ventrally, and the right ventral colon moves medially while rotating dorsally. This rotation often continues past 180 degrees up to a possible 720 degrees. The cecum may or may not be involved with this twist. Rectal palpation will reveal a twist within the bowel and a thickened, edematous portion of the colon.

Treatment

Immediate surgical intervention is necessary to correct this condition. Since the bowel is twisted, the blood supply to this portion is severely compromised. Careful evaluation of the bowel during surgery is necessary to decide if correction of this torsion is even feasible. Prognosis for a torsion is very poor since irreversible circulatory damage occurs rapidly after the onset of this twist.

BLISTER BEETLES TOXICITY "CANTHARIDIN TOXICITY"

Beetles of the genus *Epicauta* are commonly referred to as blister beetles which contain the toxic principle cantharidin. *Epicauta* beetles are ingested by horses that eat contaminated hay. When they are ingested, the toxic principle is released from the tissues of the beetle and absorbed by the intestinal tract. The lethal dose of cantharidin is less than 1mg/kg. Depending on the species of beetle, ingestion of as many as 100 to as few as 6 to 8 can be lethal to the horse. Most of these cases occur in the states of Texas or Oklahoma. This toxin irritates the bowel which results in an enteritis and possible diarrhea.

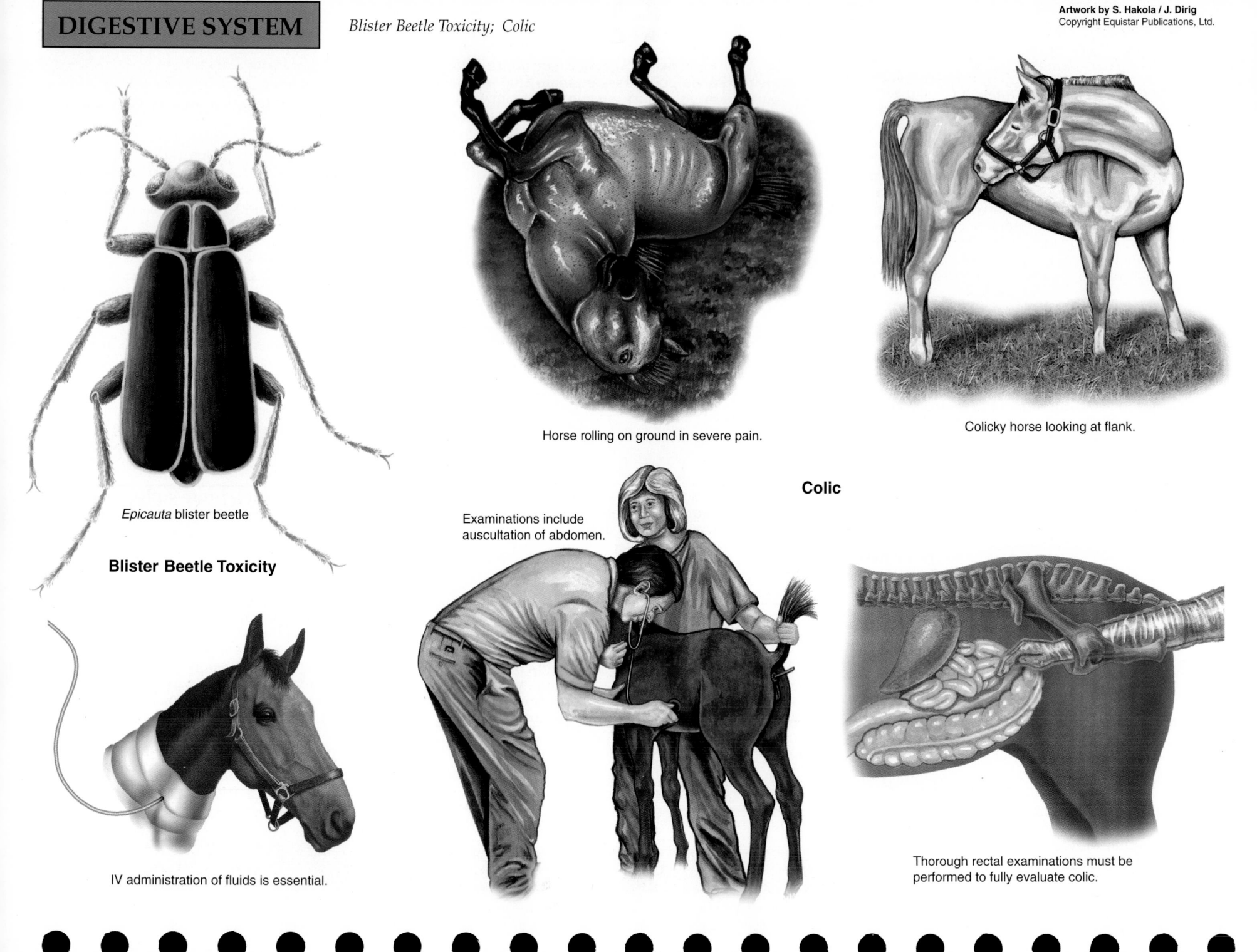

Artwork by S. Hakola / J. Dirig
Copyright Equistar Publications, Ltd.

Epicauta blister beetle

Horse rolling on ground in severe pain.

Colicky horse looking at flank.

Blister Beetle Toxicity

IV administration of fluids is essential.

Colic

Examinations include auscultation of abdomen.

Thorough rectal examinations must be performed to fully evaluate colic.

Clinical Signs

Blister beetle toxicity can cause a wide range of clinical signs. These vary from a mild depression and mild colic to severe toxemia and death. The clinical signs depend on the number and the type of beetles ingested. A mild depression and slight abdominal pain coupled with an elevated heart and respiratory rate will occur before the animal exhibits any sign of diarrhea. These animals frequently stand in a posture to urinate and will have a stilted gait when walked.

The diagnosis of blister beetle toxicosis is based on clinical signs and the finding of blister beetles within the hay. A definitive diagnosis can be reached with a measurement of cantharidin concentration within the urine.

Treatment

Supportive care comprised of oral and intravenous fluid therapy is the most important aspect in the treatment of blister beetle toxicosis. The administration of furosemide coupled with aggressive fluid therapy may help prevent any renal or urinary tract damage from this toxic agent. Nonsteroidal antiinflammatory medications may help control abdominal pain. The oral administration of mineral oil mixed with activated charcoal will help prevent further absorption of the toxin.

TREATMENT OF ABDOMINAL PAIN "COLIC"

Because there are over 75 causes of abdominal pain or colic in the horse, diagnosis of the disease or the disorder should be the goal of every examination. Careful consideration should be given to the history, clinical signs, physical examination, and all diagnostic tests to help define the diagnosis. All colic cases should be considered an emergency. Each case should be investigated on its own merits, but every minute of delay will reduce the prognosis and inevitably, the chance for survival.

Predisposing Factors to Colic

1. The horse is unable to vomit.
2. The left colon has a fixed position.
3. The cecum is a large unattached blind sac.
4. The length of the small intestine.
5. The upward movement of the ingesta at the pelvic flexure where there is a narrowing of the lumen.
6. Anatomically, the small colon narrows at the termination of the right dorsal colon.

Patient History

The questioning and gathering of a patient history is often difficult due to the gravity of the situation dictated by the amount of abdominal pain being experienced by the animal. An attempt should be made to obtain as much general and historical information as possible to help determine a final diagnosis and should include the following: the husbandry practices, the current feeding program, the use of the horse, the parasite control program, and the daily routine of the farm. The owner or trainer should also be able to supply the information as to when the animal was last fed, when did the abdominal pain first become evident, whether the animal is pregnant, any recent administration of medication, change of bedding, travel, or exercise schedule. While a physical exam is being undertaken, information such as the time of the last bowel movement and its consistency, signs of sweating, pawing, rolling, or staring at the flank can be gleaned.

Physical Exam

Initially, baseline data should be gathered which determines the animal's pulse, rectal temperature, and respiration rate. An assesment of pain should be made to include the type of pain, its intensity, and the duration can be noted. A general practice rule of thumb in the field is that any proximal lesion within the bowel associated with strangulation or fluid and gas accumulation will produce severe pain, whereas nonobstructive lesions without strangulation will produce mild or a moderate degree of pain. Acute uncontrollable

pain is typically the result of some spasmodic contraction of the intestinal wall in response to gas accumulation or fluid.

The mucous membranes of the animal are the barometer by which the circulatory status can be evaluated. Both the level of hydration and blood pressure can be determined from them. Digital pressure can be applied to these tissues and the capillary refill time can be measured. Normal refill time for the mucous membranes should be one to one and one-half seconds. The normal color of the mucous membranes is pink. As the level of hydration falls and the level of toxemia rises, these membranes will become a dark red with a dark ring appearing around the base of the teeth. If the animal develops severe shock from the endotoxemia, these membranes will become cyanotic and turn blue.

Auscultation of the Abdomen

Auscultation with a stethoscope should be accomplished over at least four sites along the upper and lower paralumbar regions. Normal sounds of "gurgling" and fluid mixing with gas should occur. Normal mixing sounds should occur at a rate of 2 - 4 per minute. Progressive motility sounds of the ingesta should be heard once every 2 to 4 minutes when the animal has not recently ingested any feed. Hyperperistalsis or a hypermotile bowel results when there are spasms within the musculature of the intestinal wall. Obstructions will generally cause a decrease in the motility. When an absence of motility is noted, there is an indication that the animal is in trouble, and the diagnosis should be reached with expedience. Gastrointestinal sounds should be auscultated several times during the treatment regime to constantly reassess the animal.

Rectal Examination

The rectal exam plays an important part in the determination of a diagnosis. This examination should be systematic and accomplished under adequate restraint. All organs should be palpated to determine their size, shape, and position in relation to the other organs contained within the abdomen.

Diagnosis and Management of Colic

Artwork by S. Hakola / J. Dirig
Copyright Equistar Publications, Ltd.

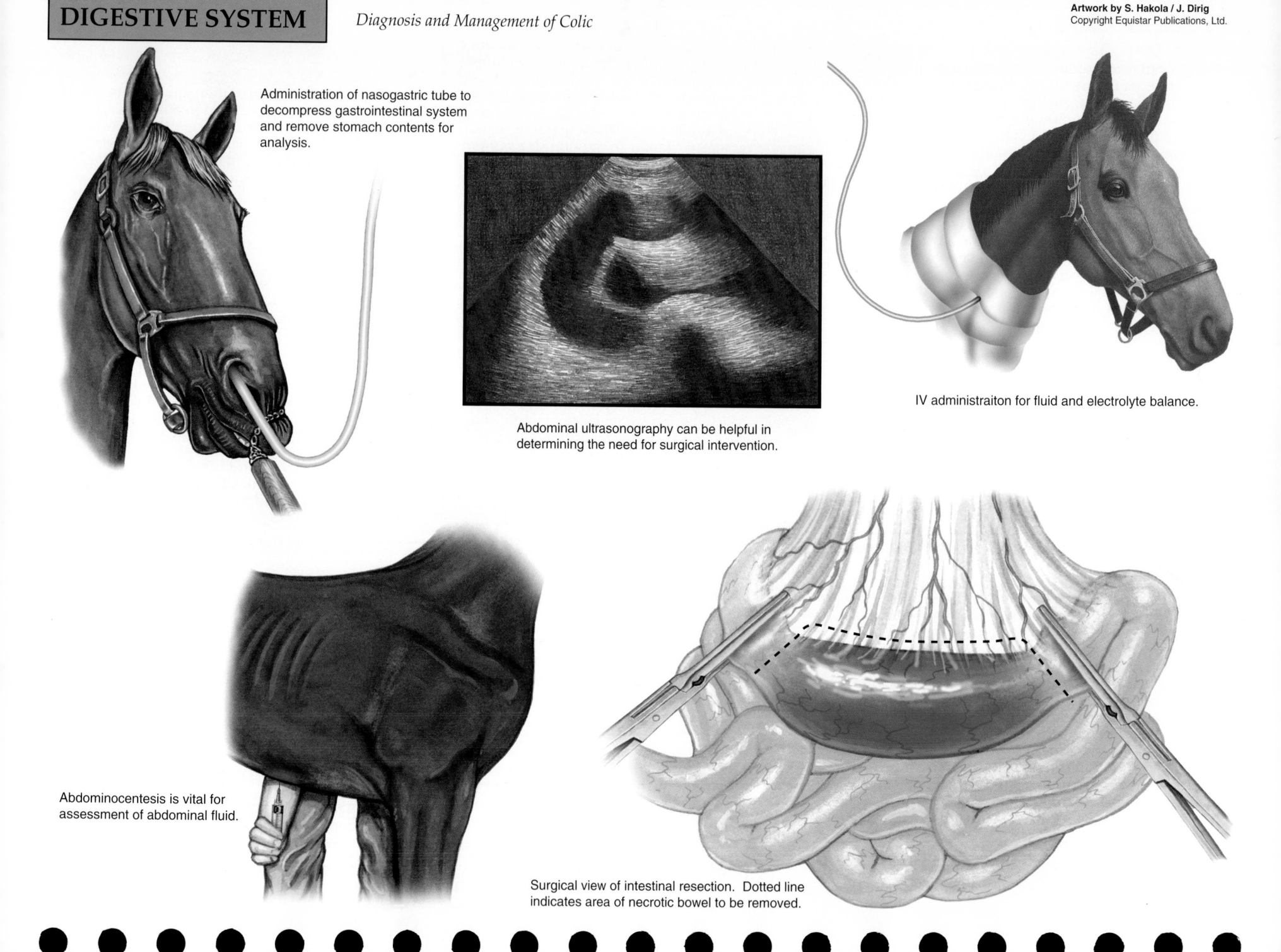

Administration of nasogastric tube to decompress gastrointestinal system and remove stomach contents for analysis.

Abdominal ultrasonography can be helpful in determining the need for surgical intervention.

IV administraiton for fluid and electrolyte balance.

Abdominocentesis is vital for assessment of abdominal fluid.

Surgical view of intestinal resection. Dotted line indicates area of necrotic bowel to be removed.

Diagnostic Aids

Nasogastric intubation allows a decompression of the stomach and the administration of oral fluids and protectant medications. Gastrc decompression of the stomach will prevent a possible stomach rupture and determine if there is any reflux of gas or fluid. In most cases, the tube is left in the animal by suturing it in place or merely taping it to the halter.

The condition of the abdominal contents can be assessed through the collection of fluid by abdominocentesis. After a surgical preparation, this procedure is accomplished using an 18 gauge 1 1/2 inch needle inserted at the most dependent point of the abdomen. This fluid can be examined grossly and will indicate the health of the bowel. Determination of blood cell count, electrolyte levels, and biochemical values will establish the level of hydration, toxemia, and the possible level of infection present within the animal. A complete blood count will indicate a leukocytosis as seen with duodenitis. A leukopenia would indicate a gram negative endotoxemia as that seen with salmonellosis, Potomac Horse Fever or a ruptured intestine. Electrolyte levels will not aid in making a diagnosis but provide information essential in the treatment of the animal.

Special techniques such as ultrasonography, radiography, and endoscopy may be useful in determining which horses require surgery and which do not. The stool sample should be examined for blood, foreign objects, and then submitted to a laboratory for bacterial culture.

Medical Management of Abdominal Pain

One of the most important facets in the medical management of abdominal pain is to provide analgesia to the patient. This can be accomplished by the administration of nonsteroidal anti-inflammatory drugs such as: flunixin meglumine, dipyrone, ketoprofen, and phenylbutazone. Xylazine and detomidine will provide analgesia in addition to muscle relaxation. Xylazine is a potent drug for abdominal pain and generally lasts 30 to 45 minutes in duration. Detomidine is more potent than xylazine and will provide analgesia and

sedation for up to 90 minutes. Narcotic analgesics such as morphine, oxymorphone, meperdine, and butorphanol provide analgesia but also reduce gastrointestinal motility.

Laxatives/ Lubrications

The administration of laxative or lubricating agents along with the oral administration of fluid therapy will provide lubrications of impactions and coat the bowel to protect it. The most commonly used lubrication is mineral oil. This facilitates the passage of ingesta through the lumen of the bowel and reduces intestinal water absorption. Psyllium hydrophilic mucilloid is administered orally to absorb water and act as a laxative to increase the water content and bulk to the stool. Psyllium can be administered several times during the day and is the agent of choice for the elimination of ingested sand. Dioctyl sodium sulfosuccinate is usually mixed with mineral oil and acts to decrease the surface tension which allows an increased penetration of water to facilitate breakdown of sand impactions. Agents that coat the bowel such as bismuth subsalicylate and kaopectate will have a local antiinflammatory affect and therefore decrease secretion.

Fluid Therapy

Those animals suffering from severe abdominal pain or any gastrointestinal disease that shows evidence of diminished cardiovascular function should receive large volumes of fluid therapy which can be administerd orally via a nasogastric tube on an hourly basis in the amount of 6 - 8 liters. It is not unusual to administer 25 - 50 liters of fluid IV within a 24 hour period. The most common fluid therapy provided in the field is Lactated Ringer's solution.

Surgical Intervention

There are numerous factors that must be considered before a decision is made to perform surgery for the treatment of abdominal pain. Indications for surgery are as follows:
    1. The animal is in uncontrollable or severe abdominal pain.

    2. Rectal exam reveals a distended small intestine, a distended or displaced large colon, or a palpable foreign object.
    3. Gastric reflux is evident through a nasogastric tube and there is no relief provided to the animal.
    4. Borborygmi are absent upon auscultation.
    5. There is an increased protein, RBC, and neutrophilic content of the abdominal fluid gathered through abdominocentesis.

Surgery is not indicated in animals where the pain is easily controlled, the rectal temperature is normal, and the CBC exhibits a neutropenia. The decision to refer or perform surgery on an animal with abdominal pain is a very difficult one. Even when a diagnosis is known, economic considerations and the quality of life after surgery should be given considersation.

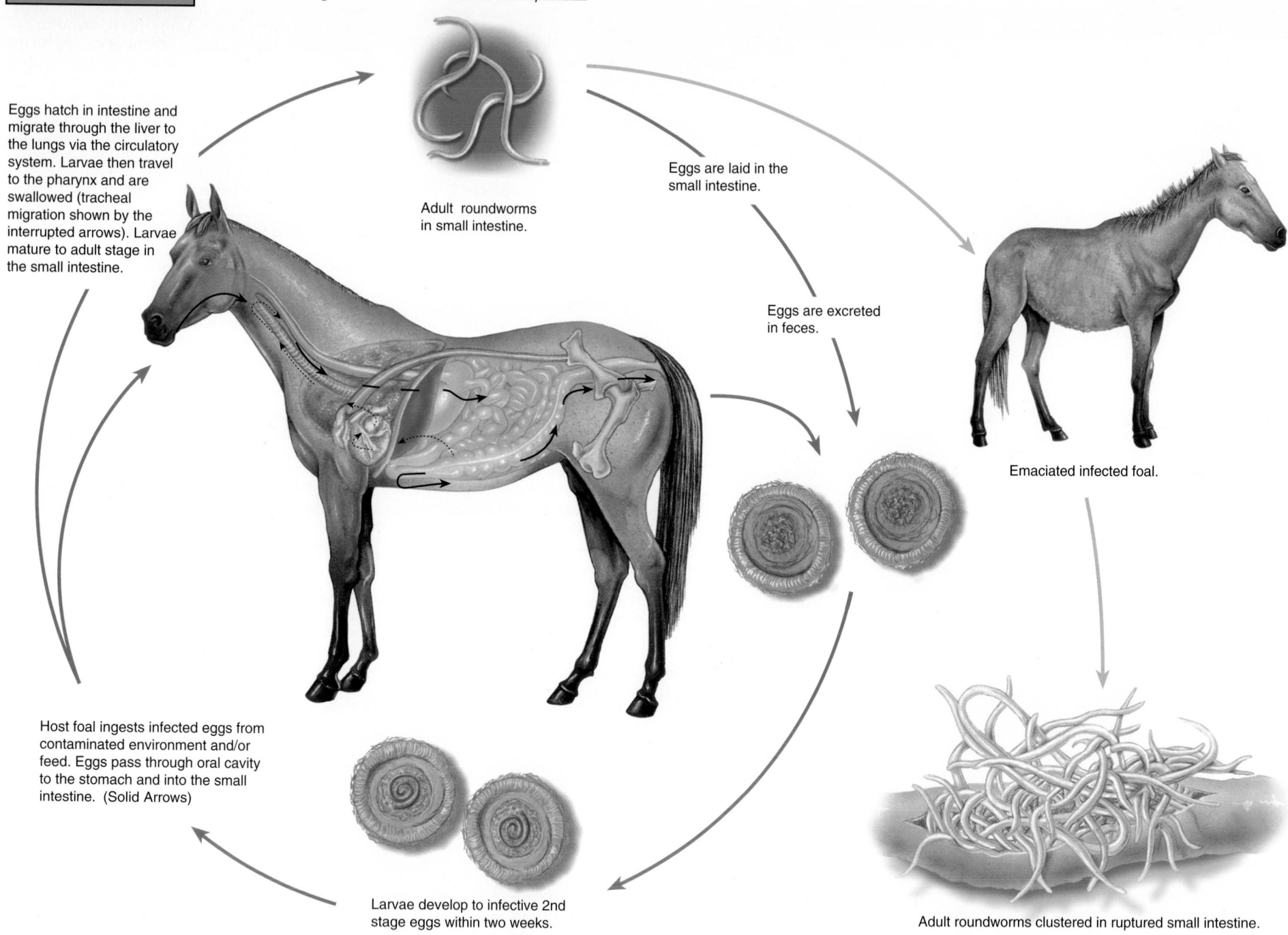

PARASITES

Ascarids: Large Roundworms (Parascaris equorum)

Eggs hatch in intestine and migrate through the liver to the lungs via the circulatory system. Larvae then travel to the pharynx and are swallowed (tracheal migration shown by the interrupted arrows). Larvae mature to adult stage in the small intestine.

Adult roundworms in small intestine.

Eggs are laid in the small intestine.

Eggs are excreted in feces.

Emaciated infected foal.

Host foal ingests infected eggs from contaminated environment and/or feed. Eggs pass through oral cavity to the stomach and into the small intestine. (Solid Arrows)

Larvae develop to infective 2nd stage eggs within two weeks.

Adult roundworms clustered in ruptured small intestine.

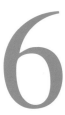

6

The Parasites

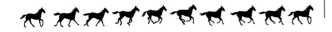

ASCARIDS

Infestation due to *Parascaris equorum* manifests itself in foals between 6 - 8 weeks and one year of age. Often, infestation of these roundworms results in symptoms closely resembling that of a respiratory disease. *Parascaris equorum* is found worldwide and becomes a problem where there is a high concentration of foals located where there is a heavy accumulation of eggs in the environment.

Life Cycle

Mature female worms within the bowel produce eggs that are passed in the feces. The structure of these eggs is such that their thick wall protects them from extreme environmental conditions. This allows them to remain dormant for up to five years. These eggs are also sticky on the surface and adhere easily to environmental surfaces, including the mare's udder. The mature female worms are extremely prolific, and it is possible for them to pass several million eggs on a daily basis from infected foals.

When proper environmental conditions exist, infected larvae will develop within these eggs within a 1 - 2 week period. The eggs containing the infective larvae are then ingested by the foal and subsequently hatch within the bowel. These larvae then migrate through the wall of the bowel, through the liver, and eventually through the lungs where they are brought up in respiratory secretions and then again swallowed. After these eggs are ingested, immature adults appear within the gastrointestinal tract in approximately 2 - 4 weeks. These immature adults reside within the duodenum and proximal jejunum. As the infestation increases, the adults may occupy the entire small intestinal tract. When these parasites reach maturity, they are quite large and average 2 1/2 to 14 centimeters in length.

Foals develop immunity to this parasite, and it is rare for a horse that is greater than two years of age to develop an infestation of this parasite with mature females actually shedding eggs. When older animals ingest infected larvae, they develop

an inflammatory reaction within the liver and lungs against this parasite which prevents the immature adult's migration to the intestinal tract.

Clinical Signs

Initially the clinical signs of *Parascaris equorum* can be easily confused with those clinical signs exhibited with a respiratory problem. Within a few weeks after parasitic infection, the foal may exhibit a cough and a mucopurlent discharge. As the infestation continues to grow, foals will exhibit a poor hair coat and be anorexic. They are unthrifty and have a slower growth pattern than expected. These foals may be permanently stunted in severe infections. As the infestation with mature worms becomes more severe, the foal may develop diarrhea and small bouts of colic. A heavily parasitised foal will be severely depressed, have poor muscle mass, a pendulous abdomen, and a poor appetite.

Diagnosis

The identification of the characteristic eggs on a fecal examination is diagnostic for an infestation of *Parascaris equorum*. It is not necessary to know the number of eggs per gram of feces since one female may lay thousands of eggs per day. Clinical signs associated with a heavily parasitised foal less than six months of age is diagnostic enough to warrant treatment. Adult *Parascaris equorum* are susceptible to a wide variety of anthelmintics. However, the migrating larvae from this parasite are difficult to control. Foals should be dewormed initially at four weeks of age and then at 4 - 6 week intervals until six months of age. Ivermectin at a dosage rate of 2 micrograms/kilogram has been proven to be effective against immature adults within the intestinal tract. Prevention of these immature adults' development into fertile adults therefore prevents the contamination of the environment with this parasite's eggs.

Treatment

Treatment of a foal with a suspected heavy infestation of *Parascaris equorum* should be carefully undertaken. Impaction of the bowel with adult ascarids may produce an obstruction that may

Ascarids

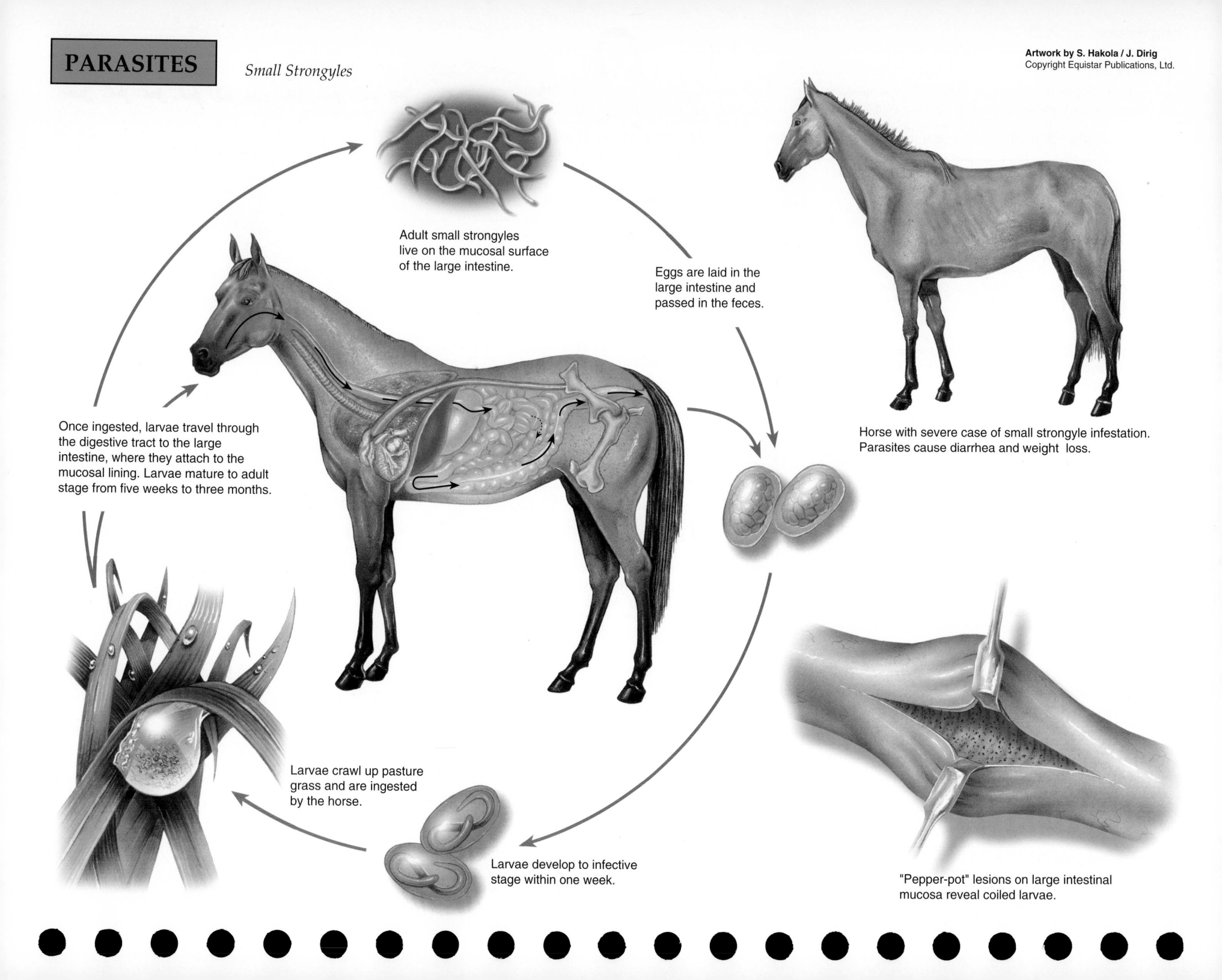

PARASITES

Small Strongyles

Artwork by S. Hakola / J. Dirig
Copyright Equistar Publications, Ltd.

Adult small strongyles live on the mucosal surface of the large intestine.

Eggs are laid in the large intestine and passed in the feces.

Once ingested, larvae travel through the digestive tract to the large intestine, where they attach to the mucosal lining. Larvae mature to adult stage from five weeks to three months.

Horse with severe case of small strongyle infestation. Parasites cause diarrhea and weight loss.

Larvae crawl up pasture grass and are ingested by the horse.

Larvae develop to infective stage within one week.

"Pepper-pot" lesions on large intestinal mucosa reveal coiled larvae.

even require surgery. An anthelmintic such as one of the benzimidaole products may be administered orally along with a dosage of mineral oil. Another approach to these heavily infested foals may be the administration of Pyrantel tartrate (Strongid C & C2x) administered as a daily dewormer. This will slowly rid the foal of the mature parasites.

SMALL STRONGYLES

Small strongyle infection is referred to as cyathostomiasis and is a cause of diarrhea and large intestinal disease within the horse. Chronic diarrhea, severe weight loss, and hypoalbuminemia characterize cyathostomiasis. There are about 40 species of cyathostomes that can infect the cecum and colon of the equine with the possibility of 20 different species present in one infective case.

Life cycle

Small strongyle infection begins with the ingestion of third stage larvae which hatch from eggs that are laid by the mature adults in the large intestine and passed in the feces. Migrating from the feces, these larvae are available for ingestion to the horse on the various forages within the pasture. These third stage larvae invade the mucosa and submucosa of the cecum and colon. A fibrous cyst forms around the parasite for 30 - 60 days. If the development is not terminated, fourth stage larvae emerge from these tissue cysts and develop into adults within the intestinal lumen. These fourth stage larvae can undergo arrested development termed hypobiosis within their respected mucosal cysts for up to 2 1/2 years. There is a poor understanding as to why this hypobiosis occurs and what eventually triggers the emergence of these arrested larval forms. When these larval forms do emerge from the mucosa, an intense inflammatory reaction within these tissues is initiated. This usually results in a severe diarrhea and edema within these tissues.

The prepatent period, that time period between the introduction of the parasite into the body and its appearance within the bowel, is only five to six weeks in the summer months. This is a much shorter time period than that of the large strongyle parasites.

Simplified Chart

Infection occurs from the ingestion of contaminated grass - - Larvae travel to the large bowel - - Larvae encyst into the bowel wall - - Encysted larvae emerge to become egg-laying adults attached to the bowel wall - - Eggs are produced and passed in the feces.

Clinical Signs

Cyathostomiasis is characterized in the early stages by a moderate weight loss, poor weight gain, and a poor hair coat. Upon emergence of the fourth stage larvae from their mucosal cysts, the horse may clinically develop ventral edema, fever, and mild colic. These clinical signs are more apparent in the spring. Some horses may have a ravenous appetite, but the appetite is usually normal, even though almost all cases exhibit diarrhea.

The clinical signs of cyathostomiasis may be from a mixed infection. There could be signs from the blood sucking adults that are within the lumen of the large intestine and/or the larvae that are in the lining. These parasites are termed "plug feeders" in that they tear away sections of the bowel wall to digest. This results in hemorrhage and sometimes bloody diarrhea. The emergence of the encysted larvae create signs that resemble an inflammatory reaction. Both of these symptoms can occur individually or simultaneously.

Diagnosis

Examination of fecal samples does not always reveal the small strongyle eggs. Clinical signs such as diarrhea may be apparent in the horse at a period of time in the life cycle where eggs are not being passed. Scrapings of the rectal mucosa may reveal cyathostome larvae. A definitive diagnosis may be made when a biopsy specimen of the

cecum or ascending colon is examined microscopically. A profound hypoalbuminemia is usually seen when the horse is chronically exhibiting ventral edema.

Control

Control of small strongyle infections is based on controlling the level of pasture contamination of the parasite's eggs. Animals should be treated and then placed on a clean pasture to break the life cycle of this parasite. In the spring, special consideration should be given to the emergence of the insistent larvae. During this time, a concentrated effort to treat these animals should be undertaken. If it is possible, fecal material should be removed from the pasture since harrowing or bush hogging may only lead to an increase in pasture contamination. Initiation of a proper worming program is essential in establishing control through pasture hygiene.

Treatment

While the administration of most readily available anthelmintics are effective against the mature adult stages of small strongyles, there are only three anthelmintics that have proven efficacy against the immature larvae. The administration of fenbendazole, at 50 mg/kg orally for five days, ivermectin at 200 mg/kg orally, and recently moxidectin are effective against encysted cyathostomes. The most important time to concentrate the worming program directed toward small strongyles is in the spring. It is at this time that the encysted and migrating larvae emerge to become egg laying adults. The daily administration of pyrantel tartrate will greatly aid in the control of pasture contamination of this parasite.

The treatment of a case of cyathostomiasis may not only require the administration of an anthelmintic, but may also require the administration of an anti-inflammatory medication and other supportive care. Nonsteroidal antiinflammatory drugs will reduce the inflammation in the colon and other affected tissues. Intravenous fluid administration and specialized nutritional support may be indicated to ensure a speedy recovery.

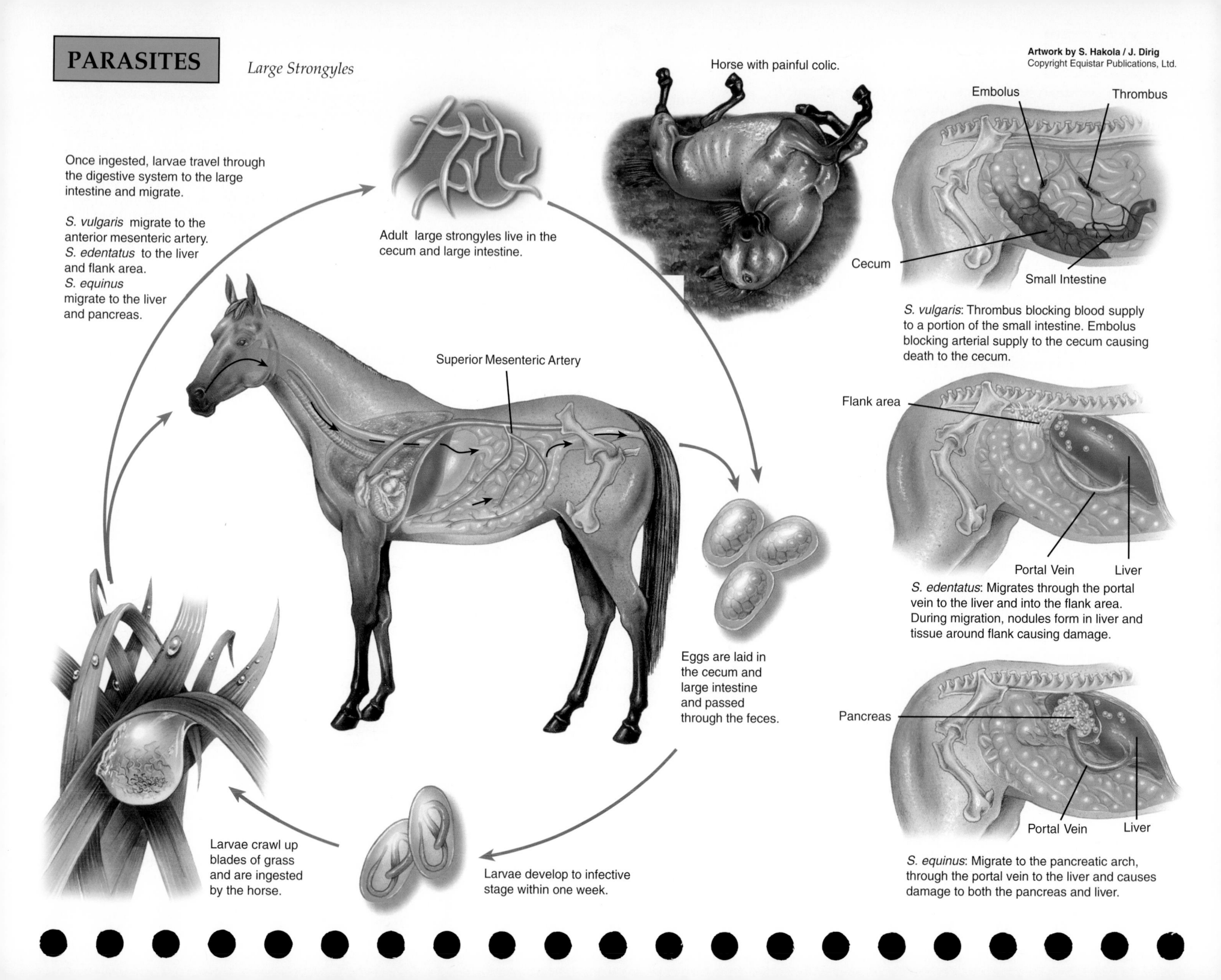

PARASITES

Large Strongyles

Artwork by S. Hakola / J. Dirig
Copyright Equistar Publications, Ltd.

Once ingested, larvae travel through the digestive system to the large intestine and migrate.

S. vulgaris migrate to the anterior mesenteric artery.
S. edentatus to the liver and flank area.
S. equinus migrate to the liver and pancreas.

Adult large strongyles live in the cecum and large intestine.

Horse with painful colic.

Superior Mesenteric Artery

Eggs are laid in the cecum and large intestine and passed through the feces.

Larvae crawl up blades of grass and are ingested by the horse.

Larvae develop to infective stage within one week.

Embolus

Thrombus

Cecum

Small Intestine

S. vulgaris: Thrombus blocking blood supply to a portion of the small intestine. Embolus blocking arterial supply to the cecum causing death to the cecum.

Flank area

Portal Vein

Liver

S. edentatus: Migrates through the portal vein to the liver and into the flank area. During migration, nodules form in liver and tissue around flank causing damage.

Pancreas

Portal Vein

Liver

S. equinus: Migrate to the pancreatic arch, through the portal vein to the liver and causes damage to both the pancreas and liver.

LARGE STRONGYLES

The large strongyles that are the most pathogenic in horses include the following: *Strongylus vulguris*, *Strongylus edentatus*, and *Strongylus equinus*. Of these large strongyles, *S. vulgaris* is the most important pathogenic parasitic infection in the horse. This is due mainly to the ability of *S. vulgaris* to migrate through the blood vessels which results in aneurysm formation within the vasculature. All of the large strongyles are commonly referred to as "blood worms." This term depicts the worm's color after it ingests blood from the host animal.

There are two forms of large strongyle infection in the horse: acute and chronic. There are a number of factors that determine which one of these two forms has manifested such as: the age of the horse, the resistance of the horse to the parasite, the number of larvae that are ingested, and the anatomical size and location of the arteries that are affected by the migrating larvae. Acute strongylosis is a result of a sudden ingestion of a large number of infective larvae. Chronic strongylosis is the ingestion of fewer infective larvae over a long period of time by a more resistant host. Colic is usually the result of acute strongylosis, whereas chronic strongylosis tends to result in debilitation, periodic colic, and diarrhea.

When one of the large strongyle larva migrate through the blood vessels, an aneurysm is usually formed which is the dilation of an arterial wall which weakens the structure. This weakened arterial wall may lead to a point of rupture within the artery or the formation of emboli that may eventually block the smaller arteries and therefore, stop blood from reaching other important tissues. This commonly occurs in the anterior mesenteric artery and is referred to as embolic colic which is very often terminal. As the result of a large strongyle migration, embolic colic usually leaves a lasting impression on both the owner and the attending veterinarian. Unfortunately, it is Mother Nature's cruel teaching tool reminding us to deal with the parasite management at this particular farm.

Life Cycle

Within the bowel, the adult females lay a large number of eggs which are passed out in the feces. Each one of these adults can produce as many as five thousand eggs per day. With ideal conditions, the first stage larvae can be hatched from each egg within 24 - 36 hours. Most larvae will hatch in one or two days after being passed. Almost all of them will be hatched within one week of deposition within the environment.

This larva then progresses to its second stage within the feces. The larva feeds on the bacteria in the fecal material. In one week, the third stage larvae develop which are now infective and are searching for a new host for food. The larvae actually migrate from the fecal material and contaminate soil and vegetation surrounding the fecal material from which they are passed as eggs. They will migrate up along the blades of grass to allow the new host to ingest them when the grass is eaten. Moisture is critical in providing the ideal conditions for these infective third stage larvae to develop and present themselves for ingestion. This can be in the form of rainfall within the environment or merely heavy dew in the morning.

Within a few days of ingestion, the infective larvae develop into a fourth stage after penetration of the bowel wall. The larvae of *S. vuglaris* enter nearby blood vessels and circulate within the arterial system for several weeks before they reach the anterior mesenteric artery. They can remain in this anterior mesenteric artery for as long as four months. It is here that they develop into immature adults and are now ready to return to the lumen of the large bowel. At this time, they can burrow completely through the blood vessels in order to reach the lumen of the large bowel to develop into mature egg-laying adults. This new generation of egg-laying adults will start producing eggs approximately 6 - 8 months from the time of initial infection.

S. equinus larvae migrate to the liver after developing into immature adults. They then travel via other abdominal organs before maturing into a new generation of egg-laying adults in the large bowel. This progression takes approximately nine months after the initial infection.

S. edentatus larvae migrate to the liver tissues before developing into their fourth stage larvae and are located in the tissues surrounding the liver, such as the peritoneum, for approximately nine weeks. These larvae are characteristic in that they form nodules in the large bowel wall before entering the lumen and maturing into egg-laying adults.

Clinical Signs

S. vulgaris clinically has a serious effect on the blood vessels through the formation of aneurysms; this results in embolic colic. Initially, these animals exhibit depression with moderate to severe incidences of colic. In almost all cases, this colic is accompanied by a fever. This acute strongylosis will not always cause an associated diarrhea.

Chronic infection with large strongyles produces weight loss or poor weight gain, poor appetite, frequent diarrhea, and intermittent bouts of colic. This typically occurs in young horses that are introduced into an infested environment over a long period of time. Rectal palpation will sometimes reveal a thickening within the cranial mesenteric artery. These chronically infected animals may also appear septic, endotoxemic, and have a profuse watery diarrhea.

Control and Treament

Controlling the environment through pasture hygiene and removal of fecal material aides in breaking the cycle of infection with large strongyles. It may be even necessary to plow the land in heavily infected areas. Routine fecal exams will monitor the progress of the worming program.

The treatment of an acute or chronic case of a large strongyle infection requires treatment of the migrating parasitic larvae and the lesions produced by this parasite. Anthelmintic administration of fenbendazole at 50 mg/kg orally every 24 hours for five days, ivermectin at 200 mg/kg orally once every seven days for 3 weeks, and moxidectin

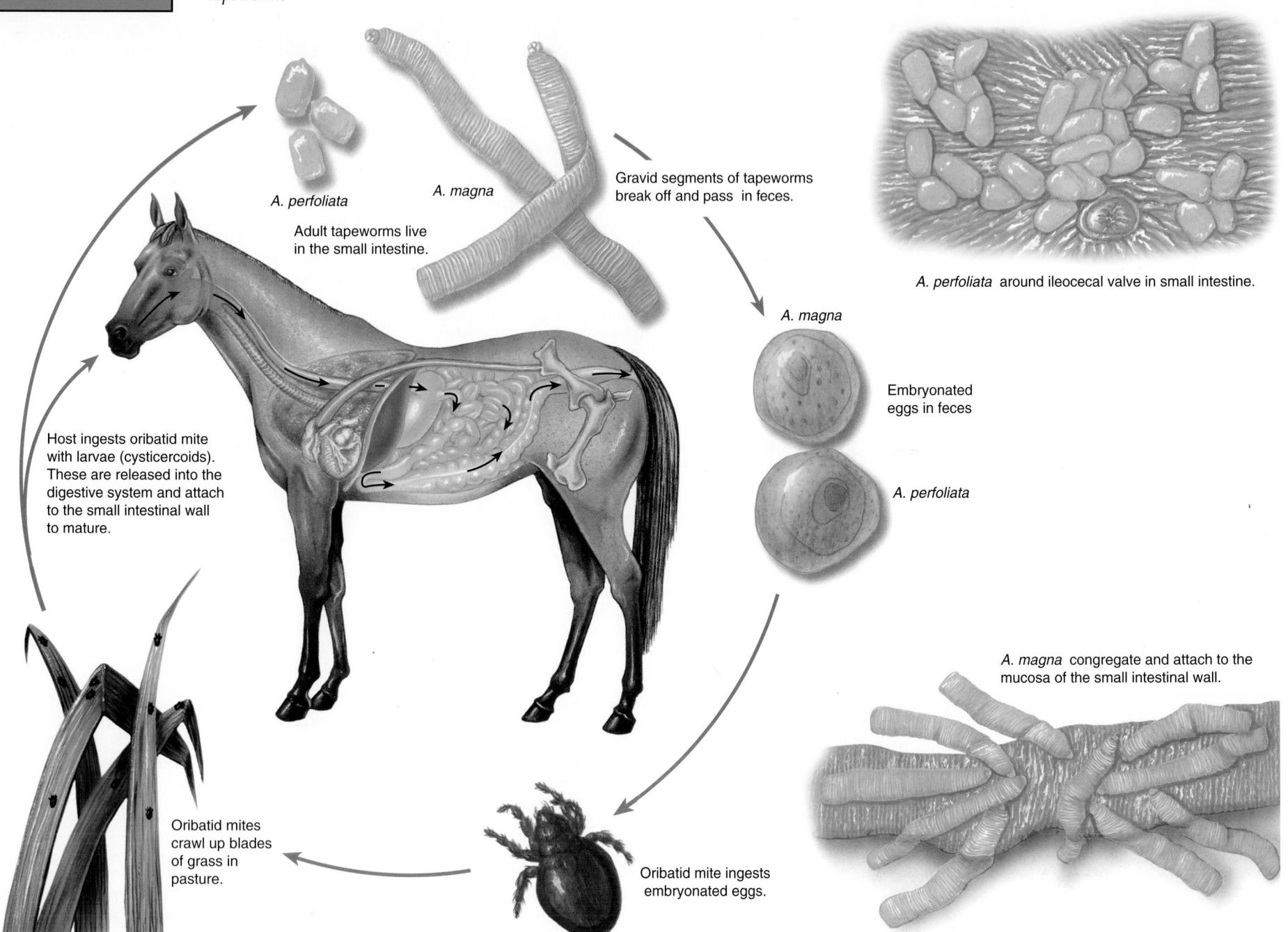

A. perfoliata

A. magna

Gravid segments of tapeworms break off and pass in feces.

Adult tapeworms live in the small intestine.

A. perfoliata around ileocecal valve in small intestine.

A. magna

Embryonated eggs in feces

A. perfoliata

Host ingests oribatid mite with larvae (cysticercoids). These are released into the digestive system and attach to the small intestinal wall to mature.

A. magna congregate and attach to the mucosa of the small intestinal wall.

Oribatid mites crawl up blades of grass in pasture.

Oribatid mite ingests embryonated eggs.

orally once a week for three weeks have been found to be effective in killing the fourth stage larvae. Daily administration of pyrantel tartrate will continuously eliminate the large strongyle adults. This in turn also prevents larval migration from occurring within the horse.

Unfortunately, the efficacy of any of the anthelmentics against the larvae within the thrombi is not known. Thrombolytic and antithrombic therapy should be administered to reduce the thrombi induced by the larvae. A dosage of aspirin and/or heparin has shown to be effective as an anticoagulant and inhibit the release of platelet products to prevent clot formation.

In both the chronic and acute cases, supportive care in the treatment of the diarrhea or colic is essential. Administer intravenous fluids, analgesic therapy, and antibiotics. One should always consider protection of the gastrointestinal tract with the oral administration of kaolin/pectin or bismuth subsalicylate. Management procedures are essential in preventing large strongyle infection. Overcrowding should be avoided, and the management of pastures is one of the keys to this managerial scheme. Proper deworming programs should be established and closely monitored with fecal egg counts to evaluate the efficacy of the parasite control programs that are in place.

TAPEWORMS

The three species of tapeworm, or cestodes, found in the horse are *Paranoplocephala mamillana*, *Anoplocephala magna,* and *Anoplocephala perfoliata*. *A. perfoliata* is the most common, and in some geographical areas it has been reported to infect 50% of the horses. Adult *A. magna* can reach as long as 80 cm. in length and be approximately 2 cm. wide. *A. perfoliata* are very short and are closely attached to each other. The anterior end or scolex is spherical, unarmed, and contains four structures called suckers. The bodies of tapeworms are divided up into segments called proglottids which are broad, thin, and immediately follow the scolex.

Paranoplocephala mamillana anatomically are found in the horse in the duodenum and proximal jejunum. *A. magna* is usually located in the distal portion of the small intestine. *A. perfoliata* will be found in large numbers clustered around sphincters or orifices such as the ileocecal junction. *A. perfoliata* can also be found in a distal jejunum and within the colon.

Life Cycle

The segments or proglottids at the distal end of the tapeworm become enlarged with eggs and are finally released to pass with the fecal material. The wall of this segment then decomposes which allows the eggs to be released and ingested by intermediate hosts. The oribatid mite is the intermediate host that ingests the tapeworm eggs and allows the larvae to develop within it. These larvae become infective within 2 - 4 months after ingestion.

The oribatid mite ascends vegetation and is eaten by grazing horses. This is how the infective tapeworm larvae are introduced into the gastrointestinal system of the horse, its final host. These larvae then develop to maturity within the lower small intestine, cecum, and colon in approximately 4 - 6 weeks. Once mature, these tapeworms then begin to produce eggs; therefore repeating the life cycle.

Clinical Signs

Tapeworms or cestodes do not in themselves cause clinical disease. However, when the tapeworm occurs in large numbers, it is not beneficial to its host. In an animal that is already on the verge of debilitation, the tapeworm will compete with the host for food and nutrients that the host has ingested. This will result in further stress and debilitation of the host. When the tapeworms occur in large numbers, intestinal irritation may result in thickening of the bowel wall, ulcer formation, and possible perforation. When *Anaplocephala perfoliata* occurs in large numbers around the sphincters such as the ileocecal junction, a blockage may result. This would then be revealed clinically as a loss of weight, colic, and even diarrhea.

Diagnosis

The diagnosis of a tapeworm infection is the result of the identification of the tapeworm eggs within the feces. Since the discharge of proglottids and eggs in a light infection are sporadic, a single fecal examination may not disclose a tapeworm infection. Therefore, a negative fecal result does not necessarily mean that there are no tapeworms found within the bowel.

Control and Treatment

Good pasture hygiene is essential for the control of tapeworms within the horse. Treatment with the proper anthelmintic drug is essential to rid the horse of the tapeworms within the bowel. Pasture management and the control of the oribitid mite will also result in limiting the possibility of infection by tapeworms.

The administration of double the normal dose of pyrantel pamoate is effective against equine tapeworms. Niclosamide administered orally at 100 mg/kg is also effective in the elimination of equine tapeworms. While not yet approved by the FDA at the time of this printing, current research indicates that daily administration of pyrantel tartrate may be efficacious in treating tapeworms.

Conclusion

Traditionally, tapeworms have always been thought incapable of causing serious disease within the horse. This has been repeatedly proven to be a false statement. In many instances, there are certain geographical areas where tapeworms are not given consideration because of the belief that the horses are not infected, yet 50% of the horses that are autopsied in Kentucky have shown to be infected by tapeworms. The time from ingestion to that point where the tapeworm is laying eggs is only a mere four to six weeks. Larvae become infective within the oribatid mite within 2 - 4 months. Numerous fecal examinations should be conducted in order to ensure that tapeworms are not a problem within your horse. If they are present, proper administration of pyrantel pamoate at double the dose should be used to effectively eliminate them.

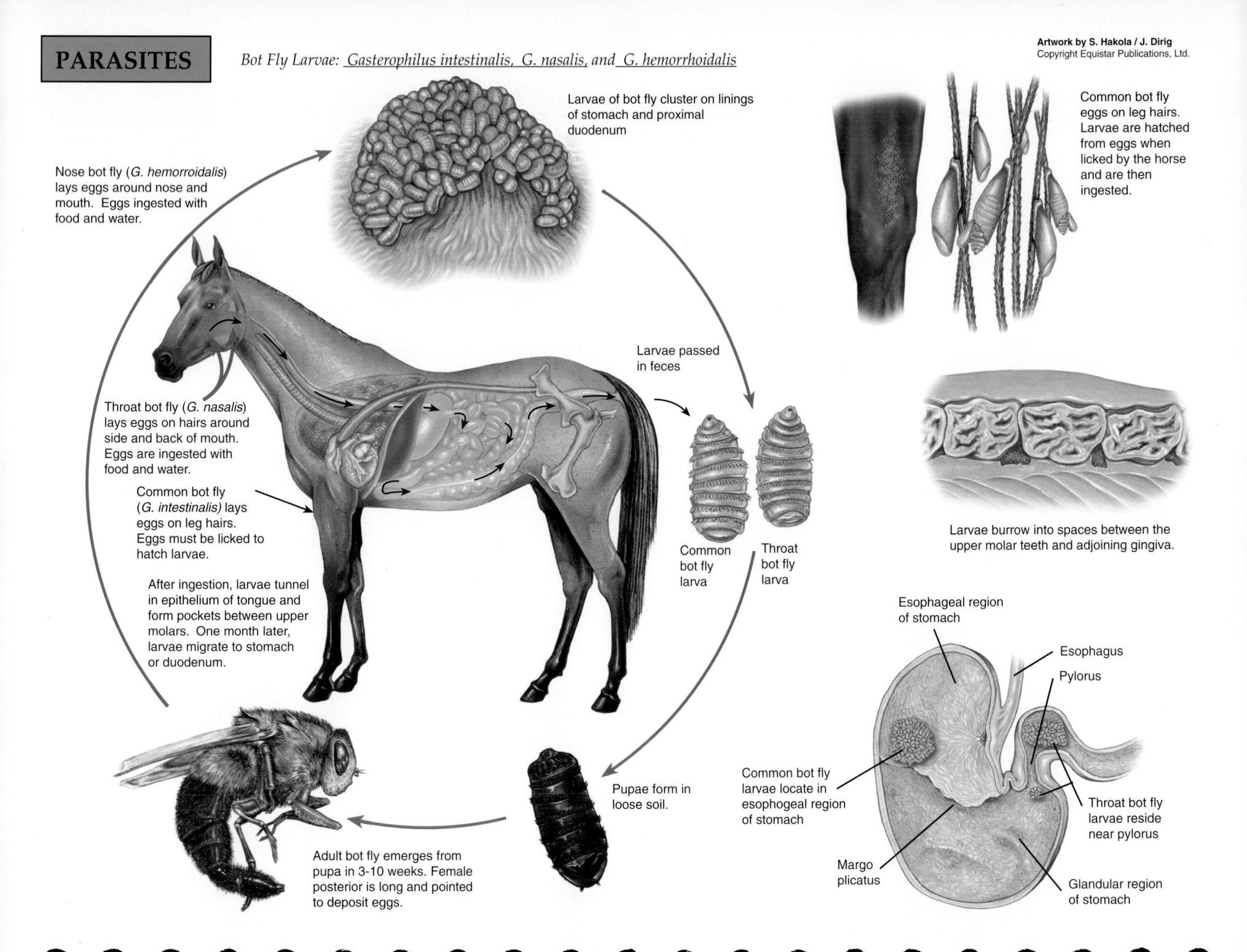

PARASITES

Bot Fly Larvae: <u>*Gasterophilus intestinalis,*</u> *G. nasalis,* and <u>*G. hemorrhoidalis*</u>

Larvae of bot fly cluster on linings of stomach and proximal duodenum

Common bot fly eggs on leg hairs. Larvae are hatched from eggs when licked by the horse and are then ingested.

Nose bot fly (*G. hemorroidalis*) lays eggs around nose and mouth. Eggs ingested with food and water.

Throat bot fly (*G. nasalis*) lays eggs on hairs around side and back of mouth. Eggs are ingested with food and water.

Common bot fly (*G. intestinalis*) lays eggs on leg hairs. Eggs must be licked to hatch larvae.

After ingestion, larvae tunnel in epithelium of tongue and form pockets between upper molars. One month later, larvae migrate to stomach or duodenum.

Larvae passed in feces

Common bot fly larva

Throat bot fly larva

Larvae burrow into spaces between the upper molar teeth and adjoining gingiva.

Pupae form in loose soil.

Adult bot fly emerges from pupa in 3-10 weeks. Female posterior is long and pointed to deposit eggs.

Esophageal region of stomach

Esophagus

Pylorus

Common bot fly larvae locate in esophogeal region of stomach

Throat bot fly larvae reside near pylorus

Margo plicatus

Glandular region of stomach

BOTS

Unless your horse is enclosed indoors in a fly-free environment year round or walks around under mosquito netting the entire summer, it will become infected with bots. It is possible to see foals that are less than 24 hours old already have botfly eggs deposited on the hairs of the abdomen and legs. This means that a seven day old foal can already have a bot infection. Unless the animal is on an extremely good worming program, it is very unusual to do a necropsy on a horse at any time of the year and not find bots within the stomach.

Three species of botflies are present within the United States and other temperate climates around the world. One research study has shown that 90% of the horses in the world have been infected with bots. *Gasterophilus intestinalis* and *Gasterophilus nasalis* are the two most common species of botflies and are present world wide. *Gasterophilus haemorrhoidalis* is present within the United States, but are not as common.

Life Cycle

During the summer, the adult botflies lay eggs on the hairs of the host animal. These eggs are yellow in color and occur in little patches or rows. They are very difficult to remove either with grooming equipment or one's fingers. Each botfly female can lay as many as 1,000 eggs.

G. intestinalis hatch under the influence of moisture usually provided by the horse licking its own hair coat. The *G. nasalis* eggs are deposited around the chin or throat and hatch in approximately one week regardless of the moisture content. *G. haemorrhoidalis* have black colored eggs which are deposited about the lips and mouth and hatch in 48 to 72 hours.

Once the *G. intestinalis* eggs hatch into larvae, these larvae remain in the mouth of the horse for approximately 2 - 3 weeks. When these larvae enter the host, the larvae are approximately 1 mm in length. The larvae burrow into the soft tissues of the mouth and grow until they are about 6 - 7 mm

long. At this point, they emerge from the soft tissue and attach to the base of the tongue. They are then swallowed and passed down the esophagus into the stomach. *G. nasalis* and *G. haemorrhoidalis* both burrow through the skin to gain entry into the host's mouth where they burrow into the soft tissues of the tongue and cheeks. Once the larvae migrate to the stomach, they usually spend up to a year here, especially during the winter months, before they are passed in the feces.

Once these larvae pass out through the feces, they leave the fecal material and enter the soil. It is here they pupate and take 3 - 10 weeks to develop into an adult fly. This adult fly then is capable of depositing eggs on the hairs of the horse, and the cycle repeats itself.

The adult flies are brown and almost have bee-like characteristics. They are approximately 18 mm long and have one pair of wings. The reddish brown larvae is approximately 2 cm long and 1 cm wide when it is present within the stomach of the horse. It is narrow anteriorly with a tapered end and a rounded body.

Diagnosis

Infection with bots cannot be diagnosed with a fecal floatation. The eggs are easily recognized on the body, limbs, and mane of the horses and can be distinquished from other foreign material by their resistance to removal by brushing. If the eggs have been present on the hair for at least one week in duration, this is enough evidence to indicate an internal infection.

Control and Treatment

Proper grooming of the horse and the removal of the bot eggs when they are present on the hair coat is essential. This can be accomplished using a special grooming tool or a strong brush combined with a strong arm. Providing the horse shelter from flies may help, but it is almost impossible to use this as the only management tool in controlling bot infection.

Traditionally, dichlorvos and trichlorfon have been the anthelmintics of choice to eliminate bots. These are strong chemicals and somewhat difficult to administer. Moxidectin and ivermectin are now the treatments of choice to eliminate bots from the horse. Ideally, the administration of either one of these anthelmintics should be done in the fall approximately 1 month after the first severe frost and then be given again in the early spring so that any larvae still remaining in the stomach are eliminated.

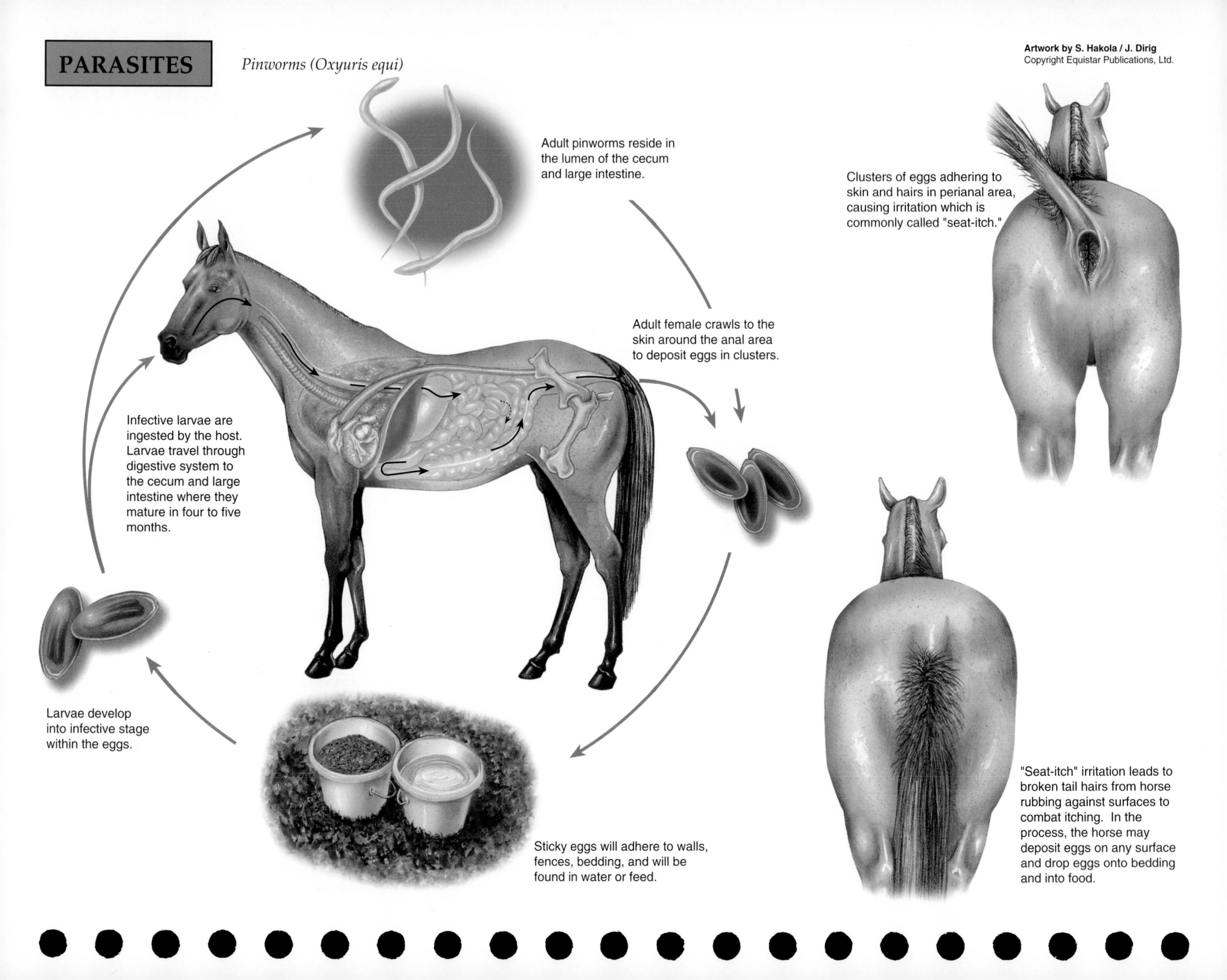

PARASITES

Pinworms (Oxyuris equi)

Adult pinworms reside in the lumen of the cecum and large intestine.

Clusters of eggs adhering to skin and hairs in perianal area, causing irritation which is commonly called "seat-itch."

Adult female crawls to the skin around the anal area to deposit eggs in clusters.

Infective larvae are ingested by the host. Larvae travel through digestive system to the cecum and large intestine where they mature in four to five months.

Larvae develop into infective stage within the eggs.

Sticky eggs will adhere to walls, fences, bedding, and will be found in water or feed.

"Seat-itch" irritation leads to broken tail hairs from horse rubbing against surfaces to combat itching. In the process, the horse may deposit eggs on any surface and drop eggs onto bedding and into food.

PINWORMS

Oxyuris equi is the pinworm of the horse. This parasite obtains its name from its pin-like tail. The male pinworms are usually only 10 - 12 millimeters in length, whereas the female pinworms are much larger and can be 10 centimeters or longer in length. Pinworm larvae are plug feeders; therefore, they can cause damage to the lumen of the bowel. Adult pinworms, however, feed only on intestinal contents.

Life Cycle

The female pinworm lays her eggs outside the anus on the skin of the perineum within a sticky fluid. It is possible for the female to lay 50,000 eggs, all of which can become infective in 3 - 5 days. These sticky eggs drop off into the environment where they contaminate the ground, the stalls, or the feed and water containers. This then provides the route where the horse can ingest the infective larvae from these surfaces. The animal may also become infected by directly biting at the local tissue irritations around the anus. The larvae then travel through the digestive system to the cecum and large intestine where they mature to adults in four to five months.

Clinical Signs

The most significant clinical sign of a pinworm infection is the horse rubbing his tail or rear quarters on any available surface. This constant rubbing gives the tail a characteristic "seat itch" or "rat-tailed" appearance. The pruritus is the result of the irritation caused by the females depositing eggs in the perineum. When the infestation is heavy, the scratching and local irritation can be profound. Pinworms, however, are not the only cause of the horse rubbing his tail. Tail rubbing can merely be a stable habit or can even be the result of a selenium toxicity.

Diagnosis

A small strip of transparent adhesive tape can be used to collect the eggs around the perineum. These eggs can then be identified under a microscope in the laboratory. The eggs are pale yellow to cream colored and contain fluid. Sometimes they can be visualized with a hand held lens.

Control

A clean environment is essential in the control of pinworms. As the horse rubs his tail on any available object, clumps of eggs may fall into water buckets, feed tubs, or bedding. Cleanliness of these containers is essential in limiting the ingestion of the larvae. Periodically, stalls can be steam-cleaned or thoroughly cleaned coupled with the application of hydrated lime. Early detection of the eggs on the perineum through daily grooming will allow early treatment and removal of this parasite.

Treatment

Most modern anthelmintics are effective against adult pinworms. Ivermectin and moxidectin have shown to be almost one hundred percent effective in the elimination of pinworms. All of the benzimidazoles and pyrantels are also effective in the elimination of pinworms. This in turn also prevents larval migration from occurring in the host. Early detection of pinworm infection through daily grooming is essential to the elimination of this problem. Once the pinworm has been eliminated through the treatment via an anthelmintic, good stable hygiene is essential to eliminate recontamination.

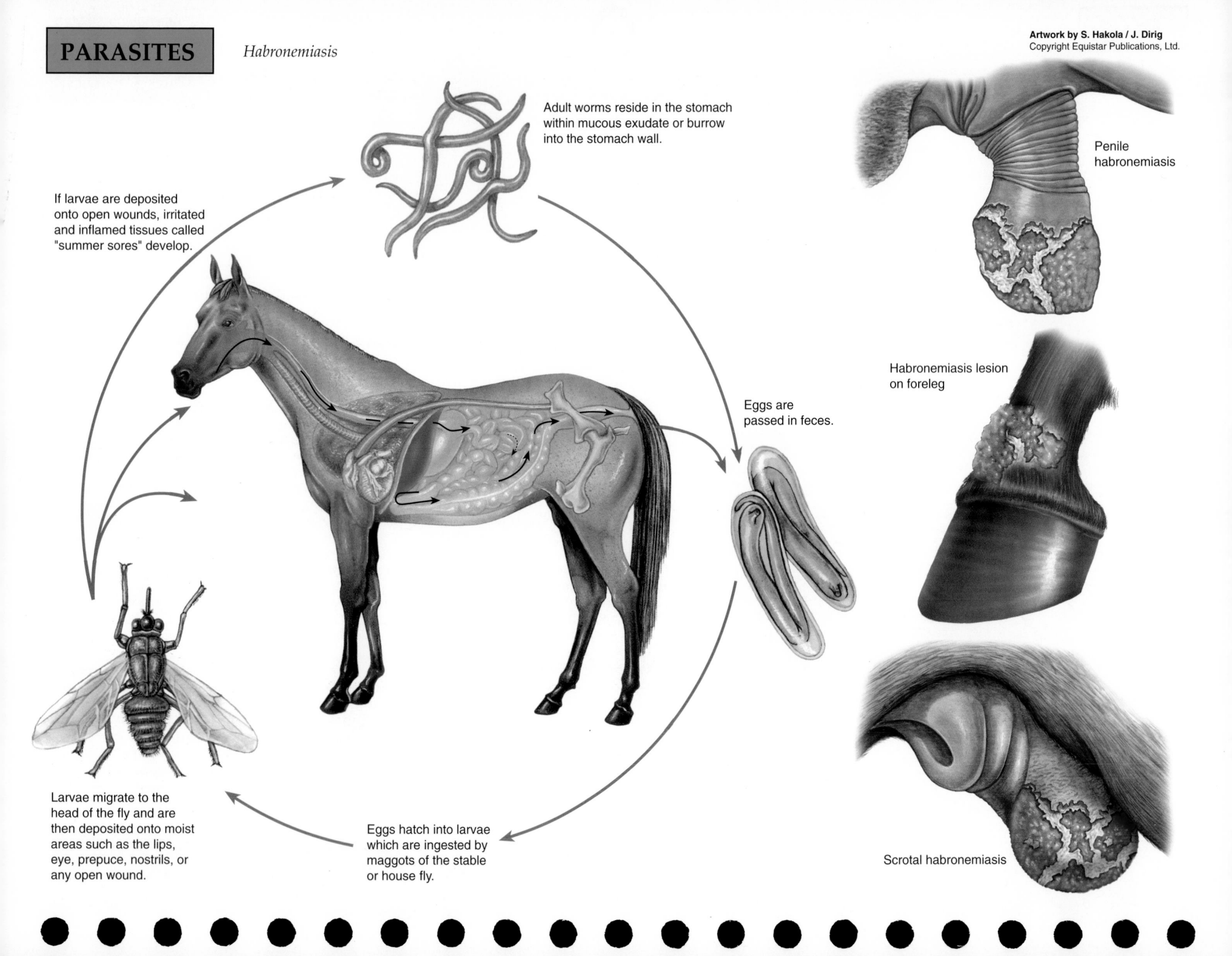

PARASITES *Habronemiasis*

Artwork by S. Hakola / J. Dirig
Copyright Equistar Publications, Ltd.

Adult worms reside in the stomach within mucous exudate or burrow into the stomach wall.

If larvae are deposited onto open wounds, irritated and inflamed tissues called "summer sores" develop.

Eggs are passed in feces.

Larvae migrate to the head of the fly and are then deposited onto moist areas such as the lips, eye, prepuce, nostrils, or any open wound.

Eggs hatch into larvae which are ingested by maggots of the stable or house fly.

Penile habronemiasis

Habronemiasis lesion on foreleg

Scrotal habronemiasis

HABRONEMIASIS

There are three species of stomach worms or spirurids that are found within the equine stomach: *Habronema muscae*, *Habronema majus* and *Draschia megastoma*. The adults of these stomach worms are usually white to cream colored and can measure from 1 cm to 3 1/2 cm in length. The females only lay a small number of eggs in comparison with the other internal parasites. The infective larvae of these species often invade skin wounds and result in a condition commonly referred to as "summer sores."

Life Cycle

The adults within the horse's stomach lay eggs that are passed in the feces and hatch into larvae very quickly after they are passed. The larvae are then ingested by housefly or stable fly maggots that develop in the manure. These larvae become infective within these maggots in about one week. This is approximately the same time the adult fly emerges from its pupae. These larvae migrate within the fly to its head where they are deposited on moist areas like the lips, nostrils, prepuce, or on open wounds on which the flies feed.

Once licked and swallowed, the larvae develop to maturity in the stomach. When the larvae are deposited by the flies onto an open wound or any area of broken skin, the larvae invade these skin wounds and cause an irritation termed summer sores. These larvae may also invade the eyes and the membranes surrounding the eyes causing a persistent case of conjunctivitis. If the larvae find their way through the nostrils into the pulmonary system and eventually the lungs, tiny abscesses develop around the larvae within the lung tissue. Once in the stomach, *Habronema spp.* become imbedded in the mucus exudate covering the glandular areas of the stomach, whereas *D. megastoma* produces abscesses within the stomach walls where the worms live in colonies. These worms then mature and begin to pass eggs which initiates the cycle again.

Clinical Signs

Any cut or open wound during the fly season that exhibits a rapid production of granulation tissue usually indicates stomach worm larvae within it. Some horses are hypersensitive to these larvae which results in edema around the wound and intense itching which may lead to further self-inflicted injury.

Wounds infected with these larvae typically refuse to heal. The larvae migrate and feed within the wound sometimes extending the size of the wound. The wound may appear to be healing during the winter months, but as soon as the fly season begins, the wound again becomes active.

When the larvae are deposited within the eye, wart-like lesions occur on the conjunctiva. The eyes are reddened and water profusely. Small ulcerated nodules also appear near the medial canthus of the eye.

Any area of the body that is moist will attract the flies and be more prone to infection with these larvae. Lesions may occur along the prepuce, urethral process, the ventral anatomical structures of the body, and around the heels and lower parts of the leg.

Within the lining of the stomach, the adult worms reside under thick plugs of mucus. *D. megastoma* actually forms nodules in the horse's stomach which develop into tumor-like growths. These can be visualized during a fiberoptic exam. Digestion is affected when the adult worms are present in large numbers. If a severe infection occurs, the passage of food through the stomach and into the small intestine may be blocked from passing.

Diagnosis

Fecal floatation may reveal embryonated eggs within the feces. Under microscopic examination, there is a characteristic diagonal line formed by the folded larvae within the egg. Skin scrapings of granulomatous wounds may expose the presence of larvae within these tissues.

Control and Treatment

Proper administration of anthelmintics will eliminate the adult worms from the stomach. Effective fly control within the stable environment will reduce the chances of infection. All wounds during the fly season should either be covered or treated with an appropriate fly repellent to help prevent larval infection.

The use of ivermectin and moxidectin on a weekly basis for 3 - 5 treatments orally will effectively kill the larvae within any open wounds. Both of these anthelmintics will also control the adult worms within the stomach. Normal wound hygiene processes should be initiated to prevent further larval contamination of the wounds. Any ocular lesions that occur may require surgery to remove them safely.

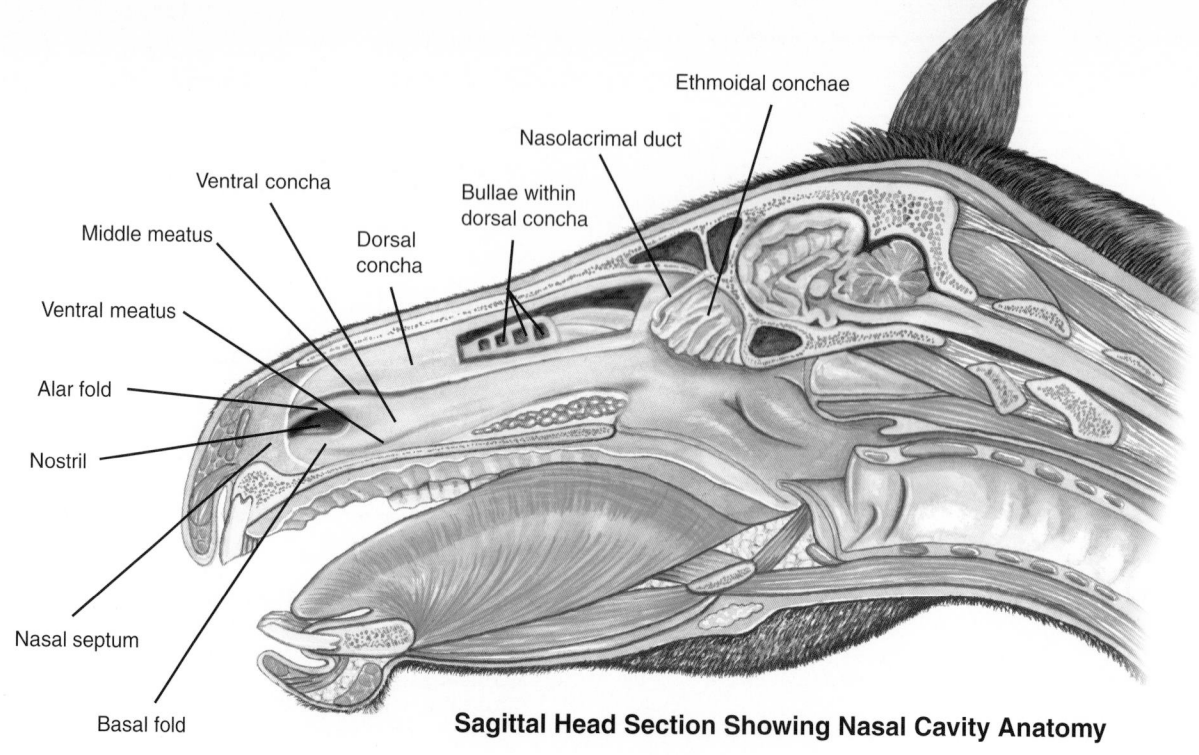

Ethmoidal conchae

Nasolacrimal duct

Ventral concha

Middle meatus

Dorsal concha

Bullae within dorsal concha

Ventral meatus

Alar fold

Nostril

Nasal septum

Basal fold

Sagittal Head Section Showing Nasal Cavity Anatomy

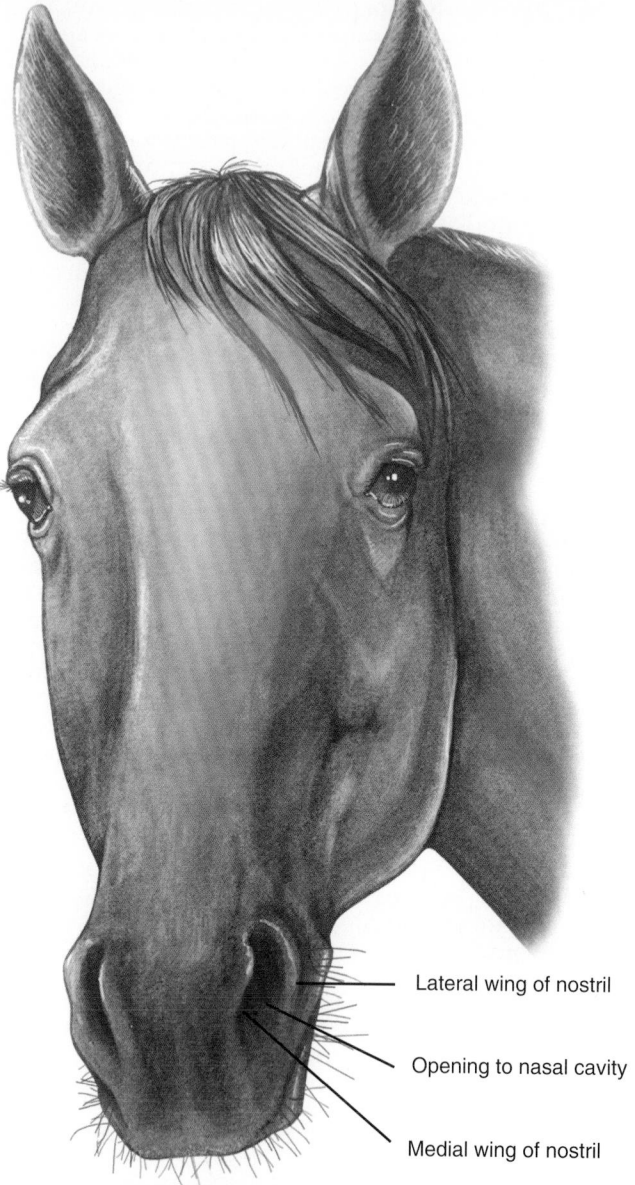

Lateral wing of nostril

Opening to nasal cavity

Medial wing of nostril

External Nasal Anatomy

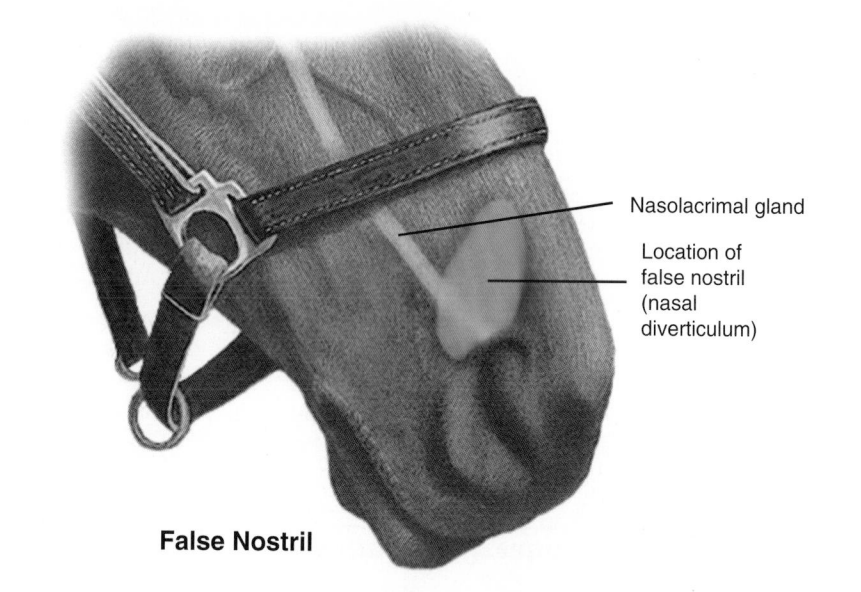

Nasolacrimal gland

Location of false nostril (nasal diverticulum)

False Nostril

7 The Respiratory System

ANATOMY OF THE RESPIRATORY SYSTEM

The respiratory system begins with the nostrils, includes the nasal cavity or passages, travels through the nasopharynx, the larynx, the trachea, down through the bronchi and bronchioles to conclude in the alveoli of the lungs where gas exchange occurs between the inspired air and the circulating blood. The respiratory system also includes structures such as the turbinate bones, the paranasal sinuses, and the guttural pouches. Externally, the nostrils are the first structures of the nasal cavity which allow communication from the external environment to the pharynx. The nasal cavity contains the olfactory apparatus which facilitates the sense of smell. The pharynx is the continuation of the horse's nasal passageway and the larynx. Since demarcation of this area is sometimes difficult, it is also referred to as the nasopharynx. In this anatomical area, there is a common passageway for both air and food. The larynx is that anatomical structure which regulates the volume of air that passes through the respiratory tract. The larynx is also the apparatus used by the horse to vocalize its sentiments. The trachea and bronchi are simply conducting tubes for the air to reach the alveoli of the lungs.

THE NASAL CAVITY

The Nostrils

The nostrils are the entrances to the nasal cavity. They are referred to as nares and are somewhat oval in shape, outlined with tissue, and placed obliquely. The rims of the nostrils are comprised of cartilage which prevents them from closing during inspiration. The nares are bounded on either side by two wings which meet above and below to form the commissures of the nostril. The lateral wing is concave in structure, whereas the medial one is convex above and concave below. The upper commissure forms a false nostril which is a pocket about 10 cm deep and is lined by a continuation of the skin. It is located on the upper inside of the nostril and functions to filter off dirt that enters the airway. This filtering can be visualized if one imagines this anatomical area on the second horse of a race immediately following the leader of that race. Dirt from the leader will be kicked back up into the second horse's face. The false nostril then filters out some of the dirt.

The nasal cavity can be entered by passing through the lower commissure of the nostril. Within this structure, the nasolacrimal duct opens about 5 cm from the external edge. Tears drain from the eye to the nose through this orifice. Just beyond the opening to this duct, the skin covering the nostrils becomes a pink mucous membrane which lines the rest of the nasal passages.

Blood supply to the nostrils is provided by the palatolabial, the superior labial, and the lateral nasal arteries. Venous drainage is provided by the corresponding veins. Both the facial and the infraorbital nerves innervate this area.

The Nasal Passages

The nasal passages are divided into two similar halves by a median nasal septum. These passages are further bounded on the roof by the nasal bones, laterally by the maxillary bones, and ventrally by the hard palate. Just before the entrance into the nasopharyngeal region, the ethmoturbinates form a caudal wall. There are two closely-rolled turbinate bones called chonchae on either side of the nasal septum. These dorsal and ventral chonchae appear as delicate scrolls that coil in opposite directions from their lateral attachments. Both these dorsal and ventral chonchae communicate with sinuses. The caudal portion of the dorsal choncha is occupied by a rostral extension of the frontal sinus. The caudal space within the ventral choncha communicates with the rostral maxillary sinus. Many small ethmoidal chonchae project into this area to extend the amount of surface membrane to which incoming air is exposed.

These major chonchae divide each nasal passage into three channels: the dorsal meatus, the middle meatus, and the ventral meatus. It has been presumed that the dorsal meatus allows air to flow to the olfactory mucosa. The middle meatus falls between the two turbinates with its posterior

Artwork by S. Hakola / J. Dirig
Copyright Equistar Publications, Ltd.

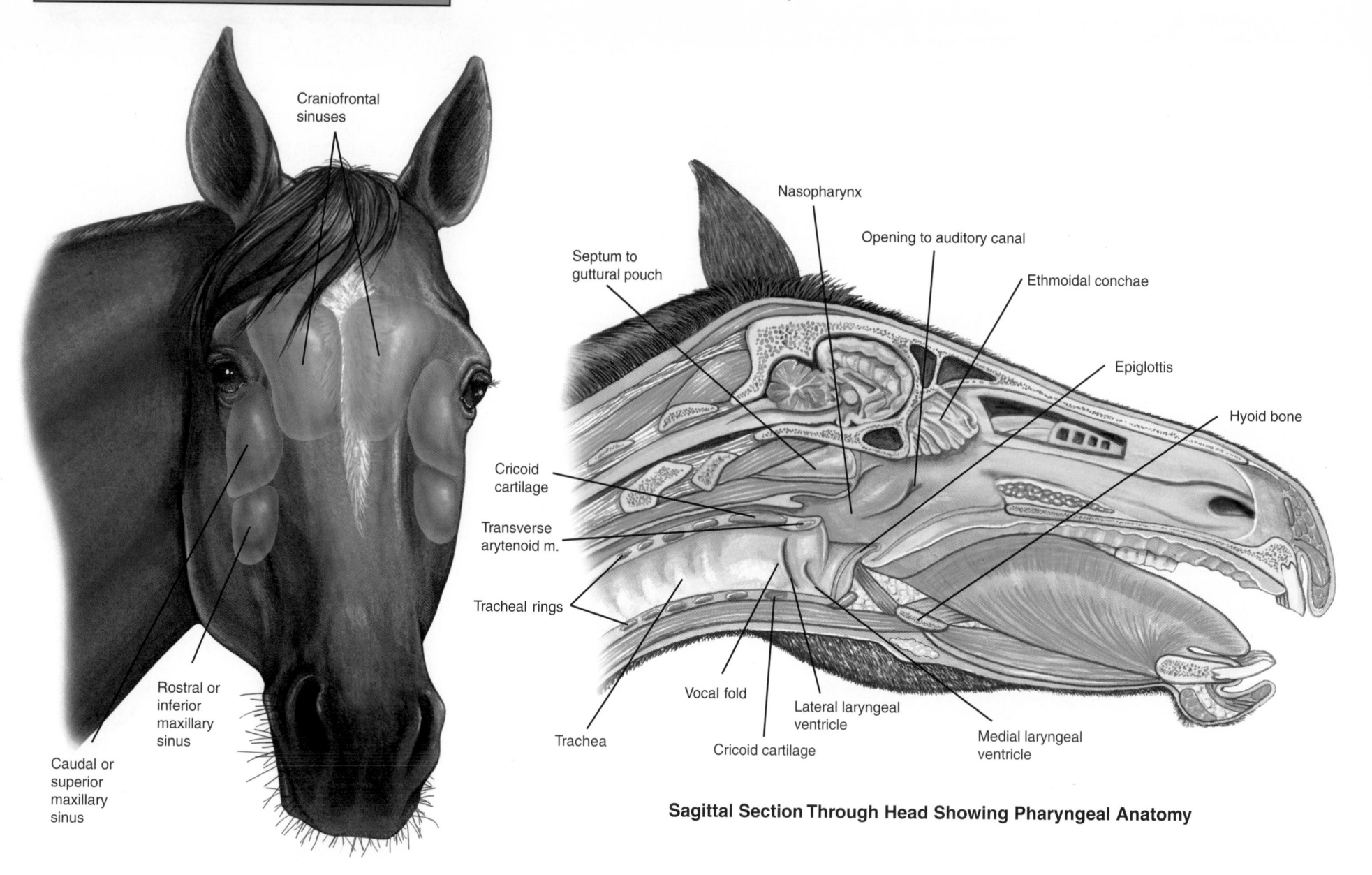

Craniofrontal sinuses

Rostral or inferior maxillary sinus

Caudal or superior maxillary sinus

Anatomy of the Sinuses

Nasopharynx

Opening to auditory canal

Ethmoidal conchae

Septum to guttural pouch

Epiglottis

Hyoid bone

Cricoid cartilage

Transverse arytenoid m.

Tracheal rings

Vocal fold

Lateral laryngeal ventricle

Cricoid cartilage

Medial laryngeal ventricle

Trachea

Sagittal Section Through Head Showing Pharyngeal Anatomy

end communicating with the maxillary sinus. The ventral meatus is the largest meatus and forms a direct channel between the nostrils and the pharynx. Stomach tubes and endoscopes are normally passed through this structure. The vascularity of the mucosa that covers this ventral area sometimes leads to hemorrhage produced by the passage of a stomach tube or an endoscope.

Arterial blood supply to this area is provided by branches of the ethmoidal, sphenopalatine, palatine, superior labial, and lateral nasal arteries. Innervation is provided by branches of the olfactory and trigeminal nerves.

The Paranasal Sinuses

Sinuses are air-filled cavities within the bone. Evolution has provided an extremely large skull for the horse. This accommodates the substantial eating apparatus that the horse needs to survive in nature. If this skull would have been achieved solely through extra bone, the weight of the horse's head would have been excessive. Therefore, sinuses evolved so that there could be an increase in area of the skull without any increase in weight.

On each side of the skull are frontal, caudal, and rostral maxillary sinuses, and sphenopalatine and ethmoidal spaces. These sinuses play no part in the horse's ability to smell. They are all lined by a continuous mucous membrane. The sinuses communicate with the air passing during expiration, so they are susceptible to infection which may be transmitted by this air and spread from the nose or from an abscess within the roots of the teeth.

The frontal sinus consists of two parts: the frontal and the turbinate portion. The frontal portion of the frontal sinus is bounded by the two plates of the frontal bone and ventrally by the lateral mass of the ethmoid. Medially, it is separated from the sinus on the opposite side of the skull by a complete septum. The turbinate portion of the frontal sinus is the posterior portion of the dorsal turbinate bone, and is bounded by the nasal and lacrimal bones. This turbinate portion extends forward and in a transverse plane between the anterior margin of the orbit and the infraorbital foramen. It communicates freely behind with the frontal part over the lateral mass of the ethmoid bone. This provides a frontomaxillary aperture which allows natural easy drainage with the caudal maxillary sinus. Direct drainage from this frontal sinus into the nasal cavity can be obtained by punching a hole in the thin wall of the conchal extension. Trephination in the roof of the sinus allows for irrigation of the sinus or facilitates the removal of a molar by repulsion.

The two maxillary sinuses occupy the upper jaw where they oppose the embedded portions of the caudal cheek teeth. These two sinuses share a communication termed the nasomaxillary opening with the middle meatus of the nasal cavity. An oblique septum divides this cavity into an anterior and a posterior portion.

The sphenopalatine space is comprised of two parts which communicate under the lateral mass of the ethmoid and with the maxillary sinus. The ethmoidal space communicates with the maxillary sinus through an opening in the lateral lamina. It is the cavity of the largest ethmoturbinate.

THE PHARYNX

The pharynx allows communication between the posterior nares and the larynx. In the adult horse, it is approximately 15 cm in length. On its long axis, it courses downward and backward. It lies beneath the skull and the rostral third of its roof is directly opposed. The communicating passageway can be divided into two parts by the soft palate and the palatopharyngeal arches which extend over the lateral walls to meet directly above the entrance to the esophagus. The upper compartment, which is sometimes termed the nasopharynx, contains flaps which guard the entrances to the auditory tubes. These flaps are about 3 cm long, directly oppose the pharyngeal wall, and can become stiffened by a flange of cartilage. The opening below the flap is normally held closed, but opens when the animal swallows. This opening allows an equalization of the pressure on both sides of the tympanic membrane. This flap can also be elevated manually to introduce an endoscope or a catheter within the guttural pouch.

Both the oropharynx and the laryngopharynx comprise the lower compartment of the pharynx. The oropharynx extends between the palatoglossal arches to the tongue and the epiglottis. All along the walls and floor of this area is diffuse tonsilar tissue. The long palatine tonsil is also located in this area. The projection of the larynx occupies the laryngopharynx which narrows as it approaches the origin of the esophagus.

Arterial blood supplying this area arises from the common carotid, the external carotid, and the external maxillary arteries. Innervation is supplied by the trigeminal, the glossopharyngeal, and the vagus nerves.

The Guttural Pouches

The guttural pouch is unique to the horse family. It is actually a dilation of the auditory or eustachian tube. Each guttural pouch has a capacity of 300 to 500 ml. The base of the skull and atlas lie dorsally, whereas the pharynx and origin of the esophagus lie ventrally. Lateral boundaries are provided by the pterygoid muscles and the parotid and mandibular glands. Medially, there is a thin septum ventrally. Along the dorsal portion, the two pouches are separated by the ventral striated muscles of the head. The floor of the guttural pouch opposes the pharynx, but it also involves the stylohyoid bone which produces a ridge that incompletely divides the medial and lateral compartments of the guttural pouch.

There are many other important structures that have a relationship with the guttural pouches. The facial, glossopharyngeal, vagus, excessory, and hypoglossal nerves directly oppose the guttural pouch as they pass from their foramina along the caudal portion of the skull. The internal carotid artery and branches of the sympathetic trunk are also found here.

The specific function of the guttural pouch is unknown, but it has been theorized that it is involved in the equalization of air pressure on either side of the tympanic membrane of the

THE RESPIRATORY SYSTEM

Anatomy of the Larynx

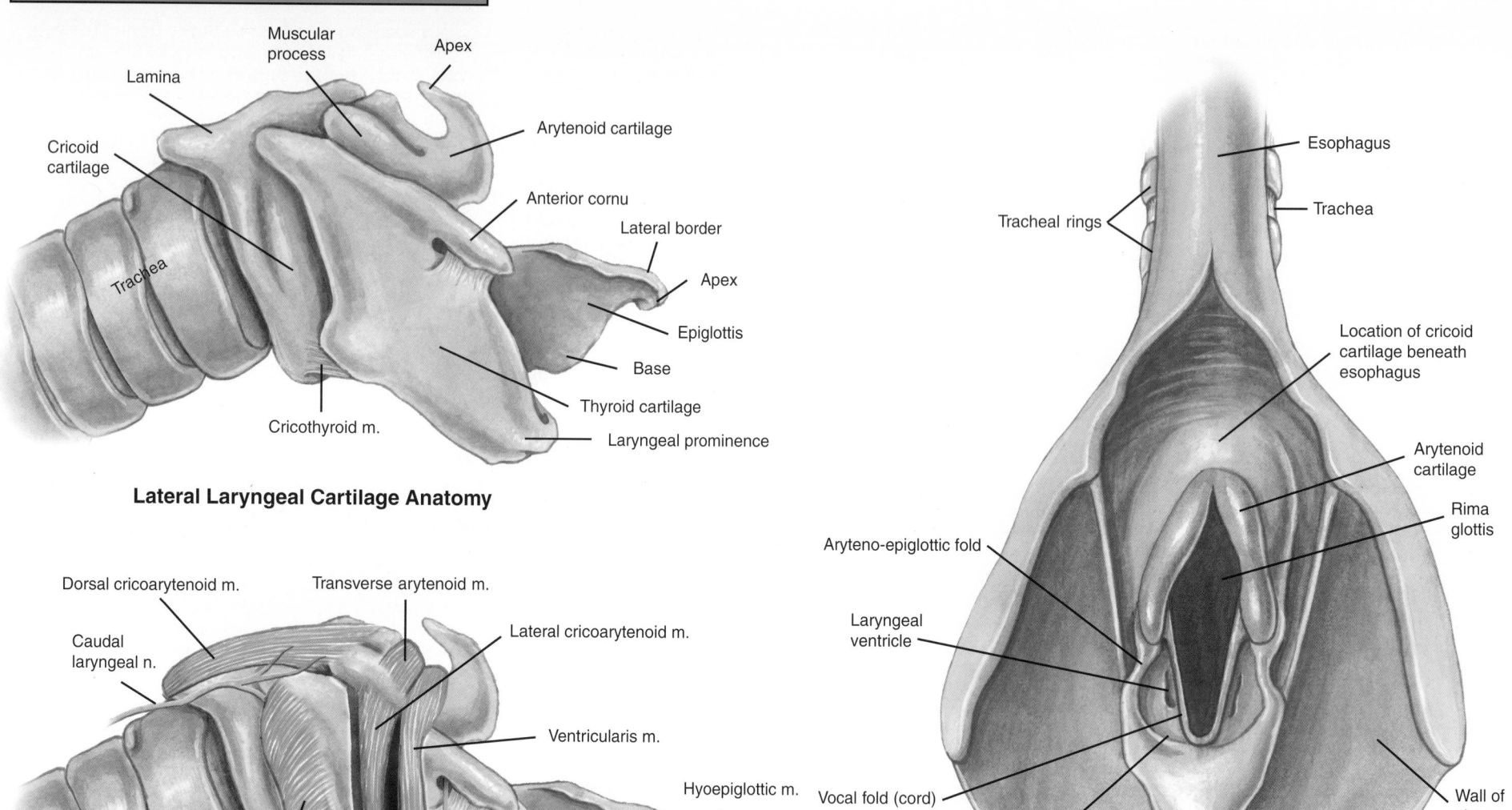

Lateral Laryngeal Cartilage Anatomy

Muscular process · Apex · Lamina · Arytenoid cartilage · Cricoid cartilage · Anterior cornu · Lateral border · Apex · Trachea · Epiglottis · Base · Thyroid cartilage · Cricothyroid m. · Laryngeal prominence

Lateral Laryngeal Muscular Anatomy

Dorsal cricoarytenoid m. · Transverse arytenoid m. · Lateral cricoarytenoid m. · Caudal laryngeal n. · Ventricularis m. · Hyoepiglottic m. · Cricothyroid m. · Cranial laryngeal n. · Thyrohyoid m. · Thyrohyoid bone

Dorsal View of Laryngeal Anatomy

Esophagus · Trachea · Tracheal rings · Location of cricoid cartilage beneath esophagus · Arytenoid cartilage · Rima glottis · Aryteno-epiglottic fold · Laryngeal ventricle · Vocal fold (cord) · Wall of pharynx · Vestibular fold · Epiglottis · Soft palate (cut)

middle ear. The guttural pouches fill with air during expiration or swallowing. When the horse swallows, the eustachian tubes on the roof of the pharynx open, and the soft palate contacts the pharyngeal roof behind them. This prevents the passage of any food material upward into the guttural pouches.

The lining of the guttural pouch normally produces a mucous secretion which drains into the pharynx when the head is lowered. If drainage is impeded or the mucus accumulates within the pouch, the pouch distends and produces a palpable, often visible swelling behind the jaw. This exudate may also become contaminated by bacteria or fungal organisms that spread from the neighboring retropharyngeal lymph nodes. This bacterial or fungal infection will involve structures that have a relationship with the guttural pouch and may produce an inflammation within the middle ear. The facial muscles may become paralyzed from involvement or irritation of the facial nerve. Difficulty in swallowing may arise from irritation of the glossopharyngeal and vagus nerves. Irritation to the vagus nerve may produce laryngeal hemiplegia. Congestion of the nasal passages may also result from these infections.

THE LARYNX

The larynx is a short tubular structure which connects the pharynx and the trachea. It is a very complex valvular apparatus which has three basic functions. It primarily regulates the volume of air during respiration. The larynx also prevents the aspiration of any foreign material such as food, and it is the chief organ for the horse's voice. When the head and neck are in the normal upright position, its long axis is horizontal. Dorsally, it is related to the pharynx and the origin of the esophagus. Skin, fascia, the sternohyoid, and the omohyoid muscle occur ventrally. Laterally, the larynx is related to the medial pterygoid, the occipitomandibularis, the digastricus, the stylohyoid, the pharyngeal constrictors, and the parotid muscles. The parotid and mandibular glands also occur laterally. There is an attachment to the body and thyroid cornu of the hyoid bone.

The larynx is made up of five cartilages that articulate together. The single cartilages are the cricoid, the thyroid, and the epiglottis. The arytenoid cartilages are paired. These cartilages serve as the attachments for the muscles which open and close the glottis (the opening into the larynx.) The epiglottis lies in the median plane and is the most anterior of the laryngocartilages. It projects in front of the glottis. The cricoid appears like a man's signet ring. Dorsally, it contains a broad thick quadrilateral plate called the lamina. Across this dorsal surface, a median ridge separates the cricoid into two shallow cavities and provides origin for the dorsal cricoarytenoid muscle. Two articular facets occur on either side of these depressions. The anterior facet articulates with the arytenoid cartilage, and the posterior facet articulates with the posterior cornu of the thyroid cartilage. The posterior border of this cricoid cartilage is attached to the first ring of the trachea by the cricotracheal membrane. Internally, this cartilage is lined by mucous membranes.

The thyroid cartilage is comprised of a thick median body and two lateral laminae. The body contains a prominence ventrally which can be palpated digitally on the horse. Dorsally, the body is related to the base of the epiglottis to which it is attached by an elastic ligament. On either side of the body, lamina arise to form the lateral wall of the larynx. Each lamina forms a slightly convex lateral surface where the thyrohyoid and thryo-pharyngeal muscles meet. Dorsally, the border is nearly straight and gives attachment to the pharyngeal fascia and the palatopharyngeus muscle. The interior cornu articulates with the cartilage of the thyroid cornu of the hyoid bone. The posterior cornu articulates with the cricoid cartilage.

The epiglottic cartilage, which is termed the epiglottis, is located above the body of the thyroid cartilage and curves toward the root of the tongue. When viewed through an endoscope, it is pointed much like a foliage leaf. It contains two surfaces, two borders, a base, and an apex. The oral or anterior surface is concave in its length and convex transversely. The pharyngeal surface is configured reversibly. The borders of the epiglottic cartilage are thin and somewhat inverted. The base of the

epiglottis is thick, and it is attached to the dorsal surface of the body of the thyroid cartilage through elastic tissue. The pointed apex curves ventrally.

The arytenoid cartilages are paired and occur on either side of and in front of the cricoid cartilage. These paired cartilages appear soft in form and contain three surfaces, three borders, a base, and an apex. The medial surface is covered by mucous membranes and is slightly curved and convex. The lateral surface is separated by the lamina of the thyroid cartilage, the cricoarytenoideus lateralis and vocalis muscles, and appears to be concave. The dorsal surface serves an attachment for the arytenoideus muscle and is also concave. The anterior and posterior borders are convex and converge ventrally to a wide angle. The vocal process serves as an attachment to the vocal ligament. The dorsal border forms a deep notch with the apex. The base of the arytenoid cartilage is concave and faces backward, whereas the apex curves upward and backward.

Blood supply to the larynx arises from the laryngeal and ascending pharyngeal arteries. Venous drainage corresponds to that of the arterial supply. Innervation arises from the vagus and recurrent laryngeal nerves, and the posterior laryngeal nerve which is the motor nerve to the muscles of the larynx with the exception of the cricothyroid. Sensory innervation to the crico-thyroid is provided by the anterior laryngeal nerve.

THE TRACHEA

The trachea is a tube that connects the larynx with the bronchi of the lungs. It is palpable on the lower surface of the neck where it lies just dorsal to two thin muscle layers. It is kept permanently open by a series of 50 - 60 incomplete cartilaginous rings that are imbedded in its wall. Each one of these rings measures between two and three centimeters from front to back and five to six centimeters in diameter. The average length of the trachea in the adult horse is usually 75 - 80 cm. The trachea can be divided into a cervical and a thoracic portion. The cervical portion of the trachea is related dorsally to the esophagus for a short distance but is mainly related to the longus colli muscles.

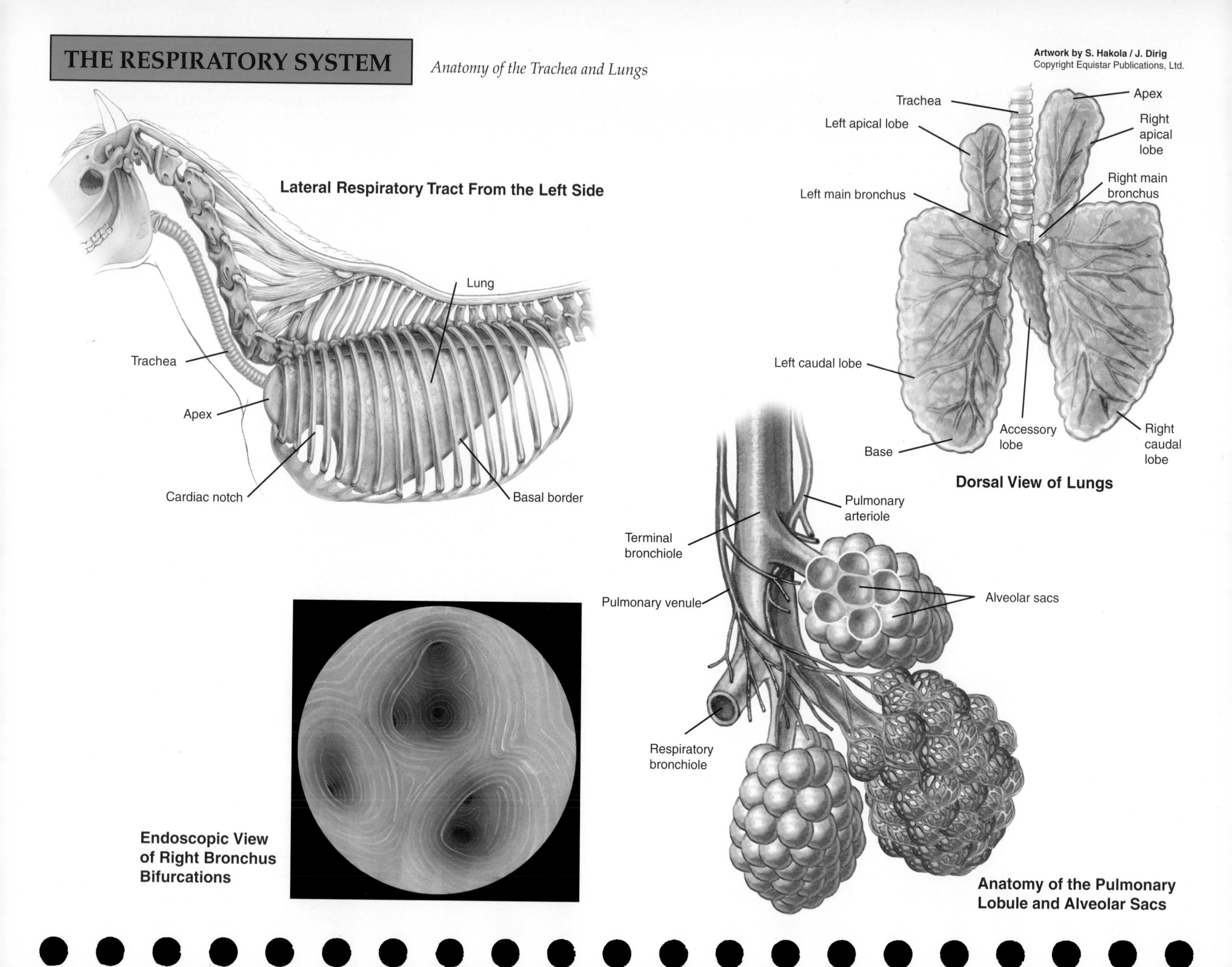

THE RESPIRATORY SYSTEM

Anatomy of the Trachea and Lungs

Artwork by S. Hakola / J. Dirig
Copyright Equistar Publications, Ltd.

Lateral Respiratory Tract From the Left Side

- Lung
- Trachea
- Apex
- Cardiac notch
- Basal border

Dorsal View of Lungs

- Trachea
- Apex
- Left apical lobe
- Right apical lobe
- Left main bronchus
- Right main bronchus
- Left caudal lobe
- Accessory lobe
- Base
- Right caudal lobe

Anatomy of the Pulmonary Lobule and Alveolar Sacs

- Terminal bronchiole
- Pulmonary arteriole
- Pulmonary venule
- Alveolar sacs
- Respiratory bronchiole

Endoscopic View of Right Bronchus Bifurcations

Laterally, it relates to the lateral lobes of the thyroid gland, the carotid artery, the jugular vein, the vagus, the sympathetic, and the recurrent laryngeal nerves, the tracheal lymph ducts, and the cervical lymph glands. The esophagus lies on its left surface from the third cervical vertebra backward. The thoracic portion of the trachea passes backward between the pleural sacs and divides into two bronchi over the left atrium of the heart. Dorsally, it is related to the longus colli for a short distance. Beyond this, the trachea is related to the esophagus. The aortic arch, the left brachial artery, and the thoracic duct cross its left face. On the right face, it is crossed by the right vagus nerve, the vena azygos, the dorsal cervical and the vertebral vessels. Ventrally, it is related to the anterior vena cava, the brachiocephalic vein, the common carotid trunks, the cardiac, and the left recurrent nerves.

Opposite the fifth rib and about four to five inches ventral to the sixth rib is the bifurcation of the trachea. The trachea is composed of a fibroelastic membrane which encloses the cartilaginous rings, a muscular layer, and a mucous membrane. The cartilaginous rings of the trachea are composed of hyaline cartilage. These rings resemble the letter "C" and are incomplete dorsally. In the cervical portion of the trachea, the free ends of the cartilaginous rings overlap, while in the thoracic portion, they do not meet. These rings are approximately 1.5 cm. wide ventrally, whereas dorsally they are wider and thinner. The first ring is attached by the cricotracheal membrane to the cricoid cartilage. A fibroelastic membrane encloses these rings and attaches to the perichondrium of the rings. Along the dorsal portion of the trachea, the trachealis muscle stretches. When this muscle contracts, the caliber of the trachea is lessened. The mucous membrane that lines the trachea is pale and contains numerous longitudinal folds comprised of bundles of elastic fibers.

Arterial supply to the trachea arises from the common carotid arteries and venous drainage is supplied by the jugular veins. Innervation arises from the vagus and the sympathetic nerves.

The Bronchi

The bifurcation of the trachea produces a right and left bronchus. These bronchi pass backward and outward to the hylus of the corresponding lung. The right bronchus is slightly larger and less oblique in direction than the left. Each bronchus divides into innumerable smaller bronchioles which gradually reduce in size as they approach the alveoli of the lungs. Bronchioles that are larger than one millimeter are usually supported by a cartilaginous framework that consists of plates rather than rings.

THE LUNGS

The right and left lungs are elongated, shallow, and occupy the greater portion of the thoracic cavity. The two lungs differ in both form and size. There is no external evidence of lobulation except for the accessory lobe at the base of the right lung which is considerably larger than the left lung, mostly in width. Both lungs are extensively joined by connective tissue caudal to the bifurcation of the trachea. The lung tissue itself is soft, spongy, and highly elastic. When the chest cavity is opened, the lung collapses to approximately 1/3 of its original size and loses its proper form. The lung tissue will vary in color according to the amount of blood that is contained within the lung. Normal color, however is pink. The form of the lung corresponds to the pleural cavity in which it is situated. There is a deep cardiac notch on the left lung which allows the pericardium extensive contact with the chest wall between the third and sixth ribs. The right lung also contains a notch, but it is much smaller and extends from the third rib to the fourth intercostal space. With moderate inspiration, the base of each lung reaches to a line passing through the upper part of the sixteenth rib, the middle of the eleventh rib, and the costochondral junction of the sixth rib.

The chief bronchus, the pulmonary vein and artery, the bronchial artery, the pulmonary nerves, and the pulmonary lymph vessels all form the root of the lung as they enter or leave the lung at the hilus on the mediastinal surface. At this root, the

bronchus is situated dorsally with the bronchial artery on its upper surface and the pulmonary artery immediately below it. The pulmonary veins lie chiefly below and behind the pulmonary artery.

As each bronchus enters the lung, it gives off branches both dorsally and ventrally. The structure of these large bronchial tubes is similar to that of the trachea, except their walls contain irregular plates of cartilage instead of rings. As these bronchial tubes diminish in size to approximately one millimeter in diameter, the cartilage component disappears. Interlobular bronchi are formed by repeated branching. From these, interlobular and lobular bronchioles arise. Once the lobular bronchioles enter a lobule and branch, a respiratory bronchiole is formed which then gives off alveolar ducts. The walls of these ducts are then pouched out to form hemispherical diverticula or alveoli. A lobular bronchiole with its branches, air cells, blood and lymph vessels, and nerves forms the basic unit of lung structure called the pulmonary lobule. Interlobular tissue forms the support framework for these units.

The blood supply to the lung is of major importance. Unoxygenated blood is carried to the lungs through branches of the pulmonary artery which accompany the bronchi and form rich capillary plexuses on the walls of the alveoli. It is within these plexuses where the blood is oxygenated and then returned to the heart via the pulmonary veins. Bronchiole arteries are small vessels which carry blood for the sole purpose of nutrition to the lung tissue. Branches of these bronchiole arteries travel as far as the alveolar ducts but do not extend to the alveoli themselves. Innervation to the lung arises from the vagus and the sympathetic nerves. These nerves enter the lung area at the hylus and supply branches to both the bronchiole arteries and the air tubes.

The Pleura

The pleura are two thin transparent serous membranes which enclose the pleural cavity and cover the tissues of the lungs themselves. A clear serous fluid is found within the pleural sacs formed by these membranes which lubricates these

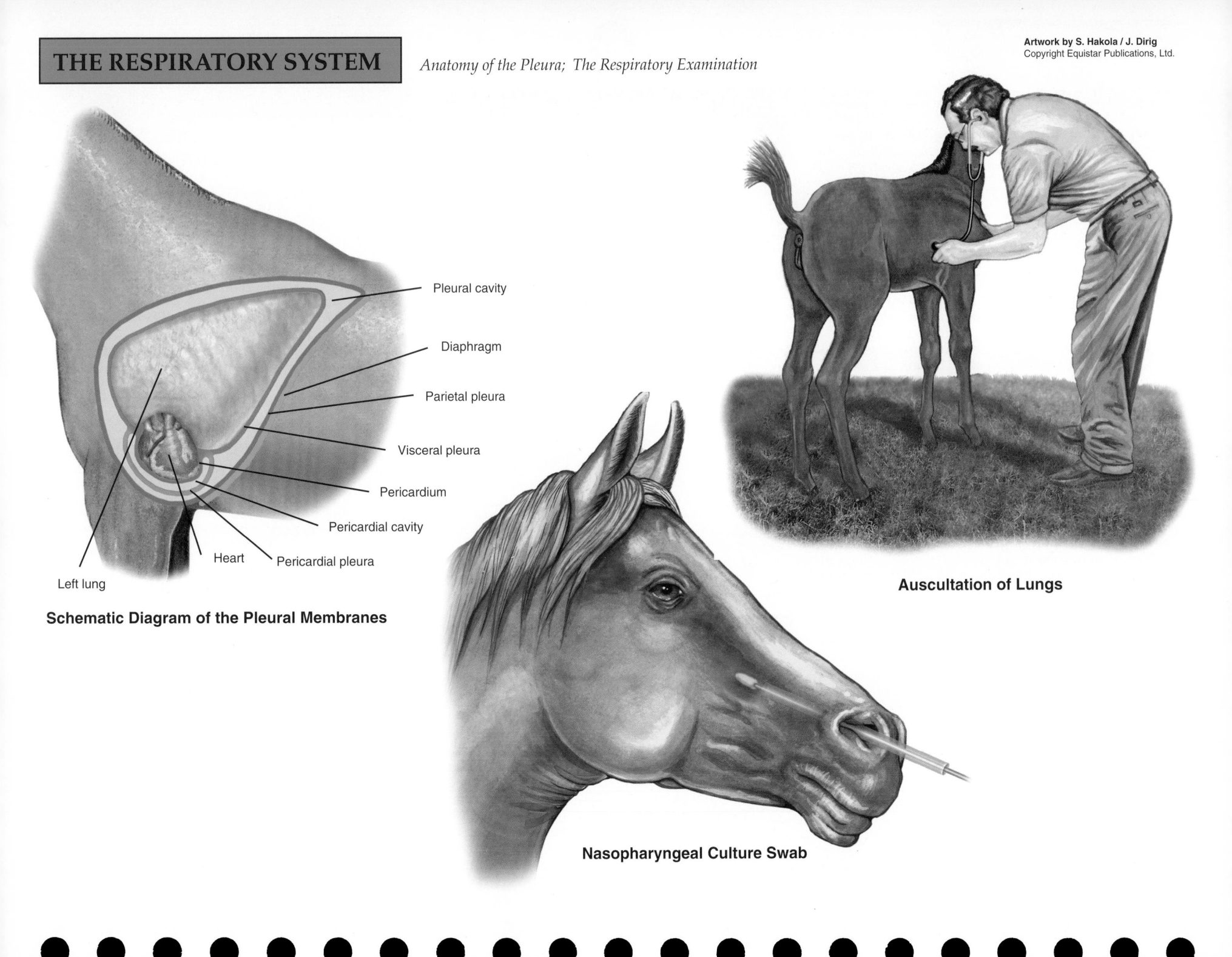

Pleural cavity

Diaphragm

Parietal pleura

Visceral pleura

Pericardium

Pericardial cavity

Pericardial pleura

Heart

Left lung

Schematic Diagram of the Pleural Membranes

Nasopharyngeal Culture Swab

Auscultation of Lungs

surfaces and facilitates the expansion and contraction of the lungs during breathing.

These pleural membranes can be divided up into three distinct parts: the parietal, the mediastinal, and the pulmonary or visceral portion of the pleura. The parietal pleura covers the lining of the chest wall and is attached by the endothoracic fascia. The portion of the parietal pleura that is adherent to the ribs and intercostal muscles is termed the costal pleura. That which is attached to the diaphragm is termed the diaphragmatic pleura. The mediastinal pleura covers the organs in the mediastinal space, part of which is adherent to the pericardium and is termed the pericardial pleura. Each pleura is reflected from the mediastinum upon its corresponding lung. This reflection of membranes occurs around and behind the hilus of each lung, and is termed the pulmonary or visceral pleura.

The Diaphragm

The posterior wall of the chest cavity is formed by the diaphragm. This thin, muscular structure separates the thoracic cavity from the abdominal cavity. It is extremely convex toward the thorax and concave toward the abdomen. It is muscular in composition and is a vital part of the respiratory system.

CLINICAL EXAMINATION OF THE RESPIRATORY SYSTEM

Disorders of the respiratory system frequently result in generalized systemic signs. It is, therefore, important to begin an examination of the respiratory tract in a systematic and routine manner. General assessments should be made concerning the animal's haircoat, rectal temperature, heart rate, and hydration status, all to be done while the animal is at rest. Each individual anatomical area, starting with the nostrils to the lung tissue, should then be evaluated and examined.

General Examination

Disorders within the respiratory system are the result of an obstruction, inflammation, septicemia, toxemia, neoplasia, or a reduced capacity to exchange oxygen and carbon dioxide within the alveoli. Initial impressions should be made of the respiratory rate, effort, pattern, and abnormal inspiratory or expiratory sounds. Flaring of the nostrils, shallow breaths, difficulty in breathing, or an increased expiratory effort by the abdominal musculature should be noted. Nasal discharge should be observed and evaluated as to its type (serous versus mucopurulent,) and whether it is unilateral or bilateral in nature. Any coughing should be determined, noting its frequency and character.

At rest, an adult horse usually takes 18 - 20 breaths per minute. Within the first hour or so after birth, a foal will take as many as 60 - 80 breaths per minute and then average approximately 30 breaths per minute when monitored at rest. When a horse inspires, it is an active process, whereas expiration is a passive act. Inspiration and expiration should be in a regular sequence with a pause between these two events. Descriptive terms such as dyspnea, hyperpnea, hyperventilation, and hypoventilation are used in the evaluation of the respiration rate and breathing.

It is normal for the nasal passages and nostrils of the horse to exhibit a thin transparent, glistening film of moisture. This is especially true in cold weather or after transport. Nasal discharges can be characterized as either a serous secretion or mucopurulent discharge. When blood is present the term "sanguineous" is used. When food, water, or saliva is noted within the nasal discharge, an obstruction of the pharynx or esophagus is usually the cause.

Nasal discharges may originate from anywhere in the respiratory tract. Collection of these discharges for diagnostic interpretation must be done with caution since these airways are not sterile. Collection of bacteria with corresponding sensitivity testing and identification of viruses may be helpful in determining a diagnosis. Nasopharyngeal swabbing with a guarded culture

device and nasal lavage procedures may be useful in collecting a nasal discharge for examination. Nasopharyngeal swabbing is accomplished through the passage of a guarded culture swab into the nasopharyngeal region through the ventral meatus of the nostril. The swab is extended through its protective covering allowing it to come into contact with the pharyngeal mucosa. This sample is then immediately placed in transport medium, cooled, and then rushed to the laboratory.

Nasal lavage requires the placement of a catheter within the nasopharynx, the administration of a phosphate-buffered saline solution, and its subsequent collection as it flows back through the nostrils by gravity. The horse is placed under appropriate restraint, and the catheter passed up through the nasal passage so that its tip is located in the caudal nasal cavity. Approximately 30 ml of phoshate-buffered saline solution is passed through the catheter. A collection device, such as a beaker, collects this fluid as it flows from the nose.

Examination of the Paranasal Sinuses

If the paranasal sinuses fill with fluid or mucopurulent material, they illicit a dull sound when auscultated. This anatomical area is percussed, tapped, and compared in tone to the same anatomical area bilaterally. If the problem is bilateral, these are difficult to detect since there is no contralateral side producing a normal sound.

External Examination of the Trachea and the Larynx

The trachea should be digitally palpated from its origin at the larynx to as far distally as possible. The trachea should be checked for sensitivity by squeezing. This sensitivity is often due to an inflammatory reaction from an infection. Digital palpation of the larynx should also include sensitivity testing since slight pressure will often cause the horse to cough. Laryngopalpation is facilitated if it is possible to rest the horse's head on one's shoulder to create a slight extension.

Artwork by S. Hakola / J. Dirig
Copyright Equistar Publications, Ltd.

Border Limits of Lung Auscultation

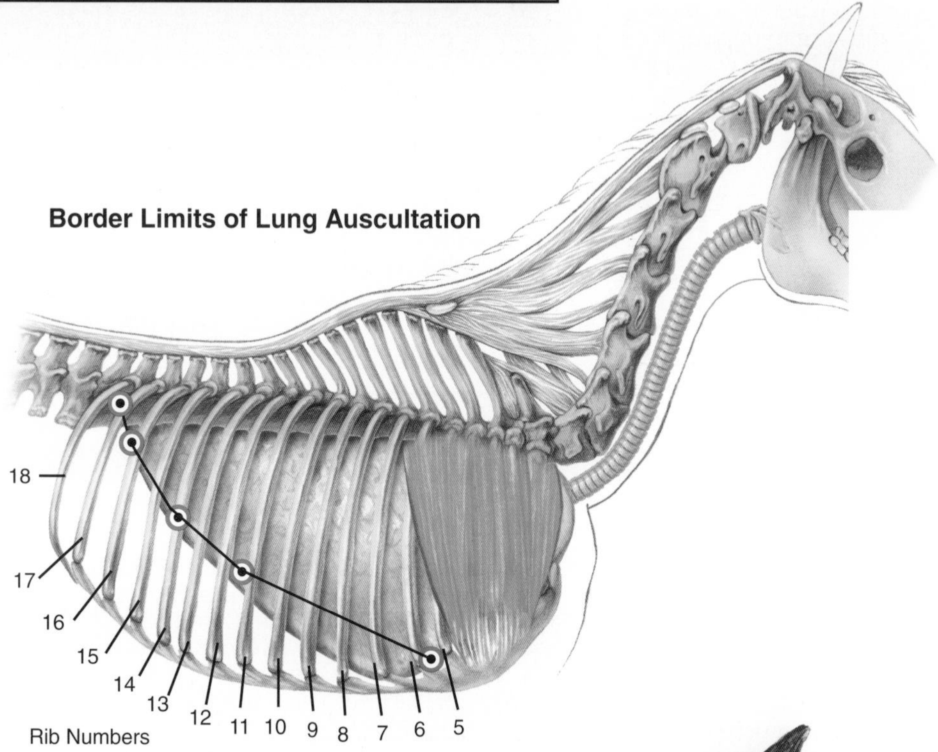

18
17
16
15
14
13 12 11 10 9 8 7 6 5

Rib Numbers

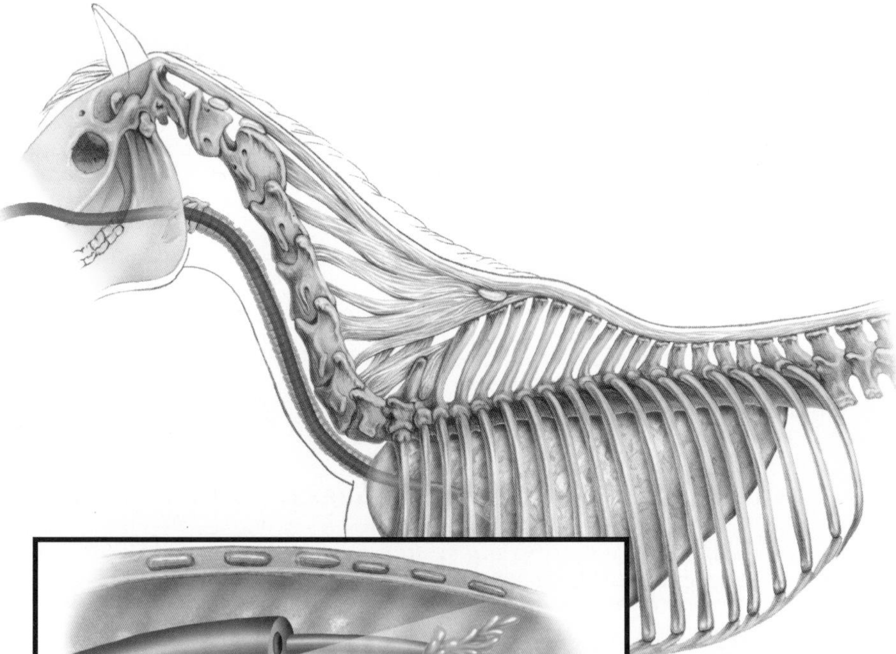

Endoscopic Examination of the Pharynx

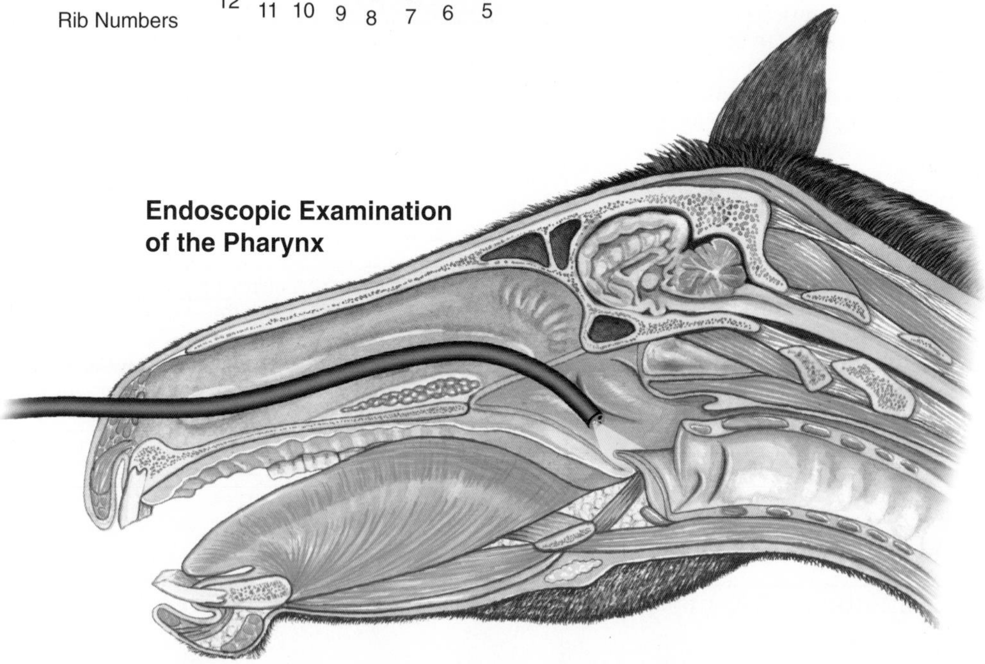

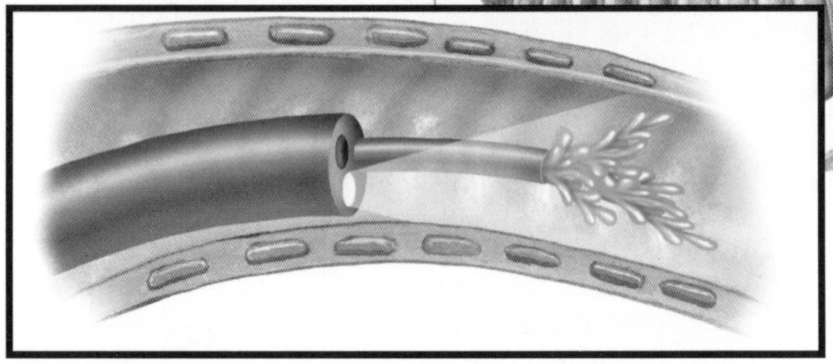

Insert shows end of endoscope injecting fluid for collection and aspiration of secretions.

Endoscopic Tracheal Wash

Auscultation of the Respiratory Tract

A systematic thorough examination of the respiratory tract through auscultation should be done in as quiet an environment as possible. Normal breath sounds that can be auscultated are produced by the flow of air in airways with diameters greater than two millimeters. These air sounds are largest over the trachea and extremely quiet over the caudal portion of the lungs. Normal lung sounds are called vesicular or broncho-vesicular and mimic the soft rustling sound of air. Crackles, wheezes, and sounds of friction are all abnormal sounds that can be heard. Crackles or sharp clicking sounds are produced by an equalization of pressures between different portions of the lung. Wheezes are produced by the vibration of material within the airways. Friction rubs are produced in cases of pleuritis where there is a less-than-normal lubrication between the pleura or pericardial surfaces. There are times when auscultation produces a total lack of any breath sounds as in a diaphragmatic hernia.

There are several methods to stimulate a horse to breathe deeper so that auscultation can be more accurate. The most common method utilized to stimulate breathing is to cover the nostrils with a plastic bag such as a rectal examination glove. This forces rebreathing of expired air and increases expiratory and inspiratory effort. The nostrils themselves can be squeezed closed manually to also facilitate an increased breathing rate. The last method of choice is the use of respiratory stimulants such as Doxaparm hydrochloride and Lobeline hydrochloride. These medications will produce hyperventilation for several minutes.

Careful auscultation of the chest should be performed in several areas. The external points of reference of the thoracic cavity are a point level with the tuber coxae at the eighteenth rib, mid-thorax at the thirteenth rib, the shoulder at the eleventh rib, with a marginal line that curves downward to the level of the elbow. Thoracic percussion is an examination technique that is used less frequently now than in years past. This has been due to the availability of ultrasonography. Direct thoracic percussion consists of directly striking a rib with either a finger or a percussion hammer. Indirect thoracic percussion involves a flat object, which is placed directly against the thoracic wall and then struck with a second instrument such as a finger or a hammer. The object of these percussion techniques is to detect abnormal sounds that would indicate the presence of fluid within the chest or consolidation near the lung surface.

ANCILLARY DIAGNOSTIC AIDS

Endoscopy

The respiratory tract can be examined with direct visualization through the use of a flexible endoscope. Endoscopes have an external diameter of 8 - 10 mm with a length of 60 cm to 3 m. The animal should be examined under sufficient restraint, but the use of chemical sedation should only be utilized when necessary, because it may influence the examination findings. In most cases, it is only necessary to apply a twitch to the animal.

Endoscopic examination should be done thoroughly and systematically. An endoscope is passed through the ventral nasal meatus into the nasal passages. Examination of this area should include the nasomaxillary ostium of the paranasal sinuses, the ethmoid region, the pharynx, the larynx, the openings to the guttural pouches, the internal lining of the pouches, the trachea, and some of the major bronchi. Endoscopy will reveal laryngeal hemiplegia, aryepiglottic entrapment, pharyngeal cysts, nasal tumors, lymph node hyperplasia, polyps, guttural pouch infections, purulent or bloody drainage, exercise induced pulmonary hemorrhage, or the accumulation of abnormal fluid, infection, debris, or hemorrhage within the trachea or bronchi.

Endoscopic examination of the larynx also allows for a system of grading laryngeal function. This examination is done in the resting horse but can be extrapolated to the horse during exercise. The grading system is as follows:
Grade One: Both the left and right arytenoid cartilages complete full asynchronous abduction and adduction movement. During exercise, full abduction occurs.
Grade Two: The left arytenoid cartilage exhibits asynchronous movement during any phase of breathing. Swallowing or nasal occlusion will allow full abduction of the left arytenoid cartilage. There is also full abduction of the left arytenoid cartilage during exercise.
Grade Three: There is an asynchronous movement within the left arytenoid cartilage during any phase of breathing. Full abduction cannot be induced by nasal occlusion. During exercise, most of these horses will have full abduction.
Grade Four: There is no significant movement of the left arytenoid cartilage during any phase of breathing. This produces a marked asymmetry between the right and left arytenoid cartilages with collapse of the arytenoid.

Transtracheal Wash

Transtracheal aspiration allows the sterile collection of fluids and secretions from the respiratory tract for cytological and microbiological examination. These samples can be collected using an endoscope or by inserting a catheter percutaneously.

Using an endoscope, it is possible to collect or wash secretions either from the trachea or the bronchi. Most endoscopes contain a biopsy channel into which a catheter can be placed. It is important to thoroughly clean or sterilize the endoscope before this procedure. The endoscope is passed into the trachea, and direct visualization of the area to be washed is found. Approximately 30 to 40 ml of sterile buffered saline is injected through the catheter onto the tracheal tissues where it forms a pool in the region of the thoracic inlet. The endoscope is then advanced until the tip is close to the fluid to be aspirated through the catheter and into a syringe. As much of the fluid as possible should be recovered to provide evaluation and bacteriological assessment. This same procedure can be accomplished even at the level of the bronchi. It is often advantageous at this bronchus level to infuse two or three aliquots of 30 - 40 ml of fluid with aspiration carried out after each infusion.

THE RESPIRATORY SYSTEM

Examination of the Respiratory Tract

Artwork by S. Hakola / J. Dirig
Copyright Equistar Publications, Ltd.

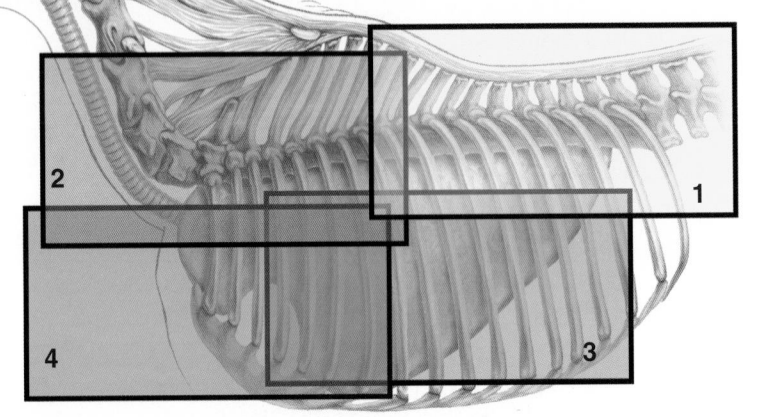

Each colored screen represents a region of lateral exposure for radiographs. Overlapping ensures coverage of entire lung field, distal trachea, bronchi, and cardiac areas.

Radiographic Examination

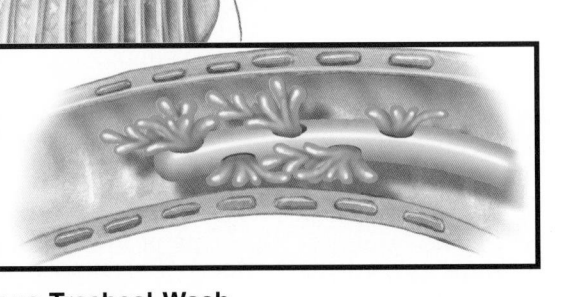

Insert shows end of multi-perforated catheter injecting fluid for aspiration of secretions.

Percutaneous Tracheal Wash

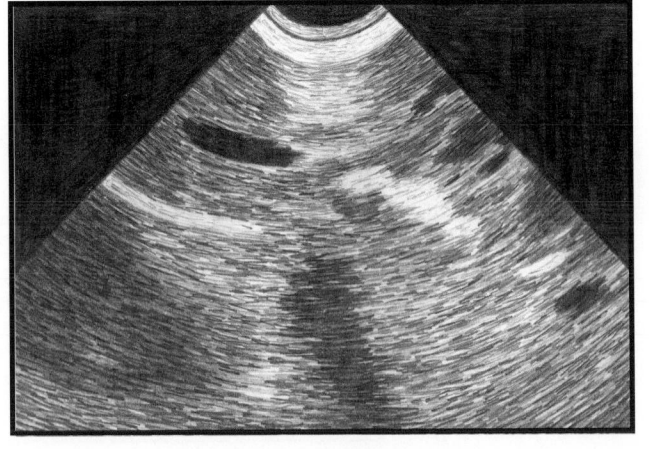

Ultrasonography is useful for detection of fluid and masses within the thorax.

Thoracic Ultrasound

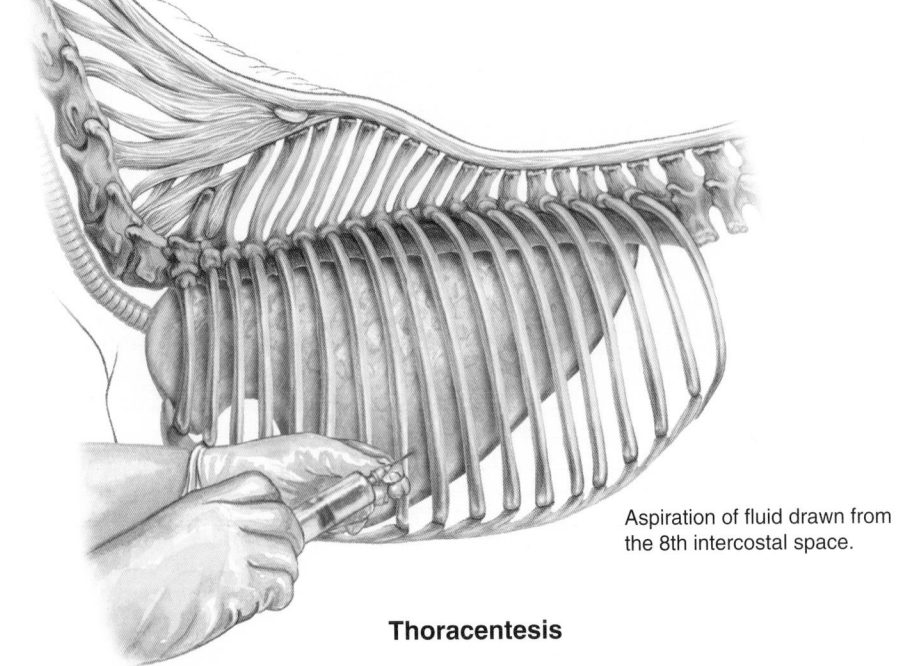

Aspiration of fluid drawn from the 8th intercostal space.

Thoracentesis

Percutaneous transtracheal washing and aspiration refers to the placement of a catheter within the trachea, infusion of a lavage fluid, and then collection by aspiration. This is accomplished by prepping an area over the middle third of the trachea with povodine-iodine, as if surgery is going to be performed. A pair of adjacent tracheal rings is chosen and a small amount of local anesthetic is injected subcutaneously. A stab incision is then made in the skin with a needle or trocar between the tracheal rings and directed down the trachea. A catheter is then inserted through the needle or trocar and then advanced. Sterile buffered saline is infused and immediately aspirated. This lavaged sample of secretions can then be submitted for cytological and bacterial examination.

Ultrasound Examination of the Chest

Ultrasonography is useful for the detection and characterization of fluids and masses within the thorax. A scanner with a frequency of 3.0 - 5.0 MHz is used. It is necessary to clip the hair over the region of the thorax that must be imaged, because intact hair traps air which interferes with the quality of the image. An acoustic coupling gel is then applied liberally before the scanner is put to the area for examination.

Lung tissue itself is poorly penetrated by sound waves. Normal pleural surfaces are smooth and highly echogenic. If these pleural surfaces are irregular, it is an indication that there is pneumonia or pleuritis present. Pulmonary abscesses and pulmonary consolidation are only visible when they are in direct contact with the thoracic wall. Adhesions between visceral and parietal pleura are often present.

Radiographic Examination of the Respiratory Tract

Radiographic techniques involving the respiratory tract will aid in the diagnosis of sinusitis, neoplasia, ethmoid hematomas, tooth root problems, guttural pouch disorders, tracheal stenosis, and the thoracic contents. Rare earth screens and high speed film have allowed diagnostic radiographic techniques to improve so

that even films of the adult thorax taken laterally can be diagnostic. Both lateral and ventrodorsal exposures are possible in the foal. When adult horses are involved, multiple lateral exposures should be made. It is often necessary to place the horse under anesthesia or heavy sedation to obtain high quality films. Lateral radiographs should be positioned so that there are four overlapping exposures which include: the caudodorsal area, the craniodorsal area, the caudoventral area, and the cranioventral area. These areas are termed one, two, three, and four respectively. If possible, these exposures should be taken during full inspiration.

Utilizing the overlapping technique, certain structures will be present on more than one radiograph. Field one will reveal a large portion of the caudal lung lobes, the pulmonary arteries and veins, the caudal vena cava, the diaphragm, the caudal thoracic vertebrae and ribs, and the distal most airways. Field two will reveal the dorsal portion of the heart, aorta, both the pulmonary arteries and veins, the trachea and tracheal bifurcation, a few thoracic vertebrae, the ribs, and possibly most importantly, the main bronchi. The caudal portion of the heart, the pulmonary vessels, the ribs, the ventral diaphragm, the trachea, and the tracheal bifurcation are visible in field three. Field four is a very difficult field to obtain. It usually involves the scapula, the humerus, and the overlying muscular structures. A major portion of the heart, the aorta, the trachea and the cranial portion of the mediastinum should also be visible.

Thoracentesis

When fluid is detected within the thorax either by auscultation, percussion, ultrasonography, or radiography, a procedure called thoracentesis is utilized to recover the fluid. This procedure should be done to prove if the fluid is present and to allow cytological and microbiological analysis.

It is important to carry out this procedure under extremely sanitary conditions. An area in the ventral third of the thorax over the sixth, seventh, and eight intercostal spaces approximately 10 cm above the level of the olecranon is clipped, shaved, and aseptically prepped with surgical scrub. This

area can be infiltrated with a local anesthetic to provide more comfort to the patient. The horse should be under sufficient restraint and may even be heavily sedated for this procedure. A large needle or cannula is inserted into the pleural space, and fluid is aspirated into a sterile syringe. A "popping" sensation is usually detected as the cannula or needle enters the pleural cavity. The samples are then processed by placing the fluid into Vacutainer(™) tubes and into transport media for microbiological evaluation.

RESPIRATORY TRACT DISORDERS

ATHEROMA (EPIDERMAL INCLUSION CYST)

An atheroma or epidermal inclusion cyst is a fluid-filled structure that creates a firm round swelling within the caudal aspect of the nasal diverticulum or false nostril. Microscopic examination reveals these cysts to be epidermal in origin and not sebaceous. The cause of these cysts is unknown, but since they occur mostly in younger horses, it is presumed that it is a congenital ectopic sequestration of epithelial tissue.

Clinical Signs

Most atheromas usually occur unilaterally in the false nostril. They can be palpated in the caudal space of the nasal diverticulum and rarely cause any obstruction with airflow. Therefore, they usually do not impair athletic performance. These cysts typically are painless in nature and enlarge very slowly. If a needle is inserted in them, fluid can usually be aspirated.

Differential Diagnosis

1.) Nasal Septum Deformation
2.) Abscesses
3.) Tumor

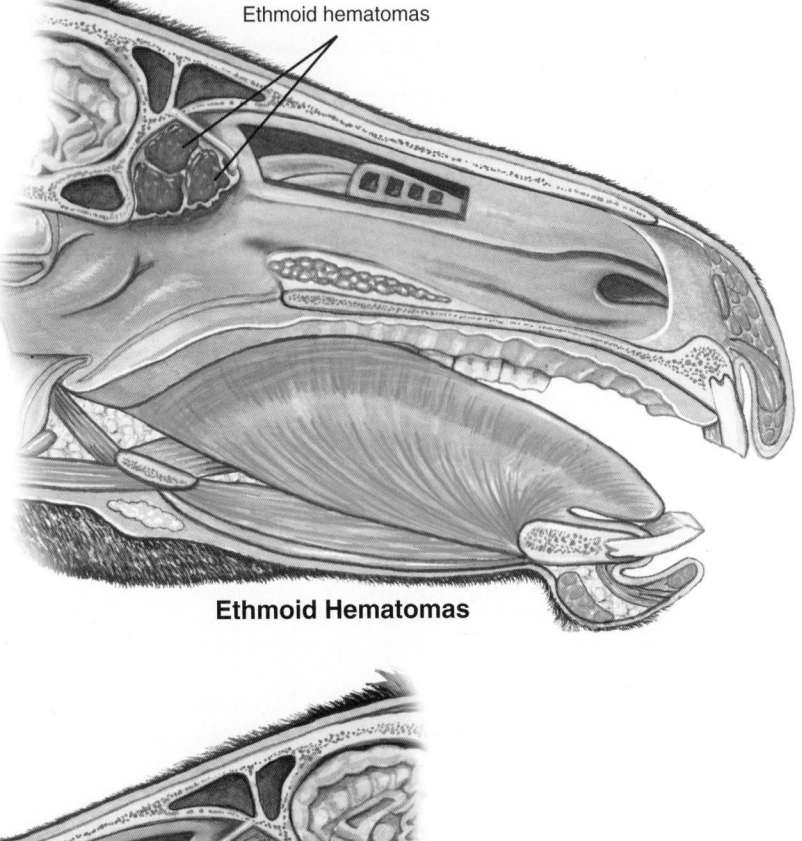

Ethmoid hematomas

Ethmoid Hematomas

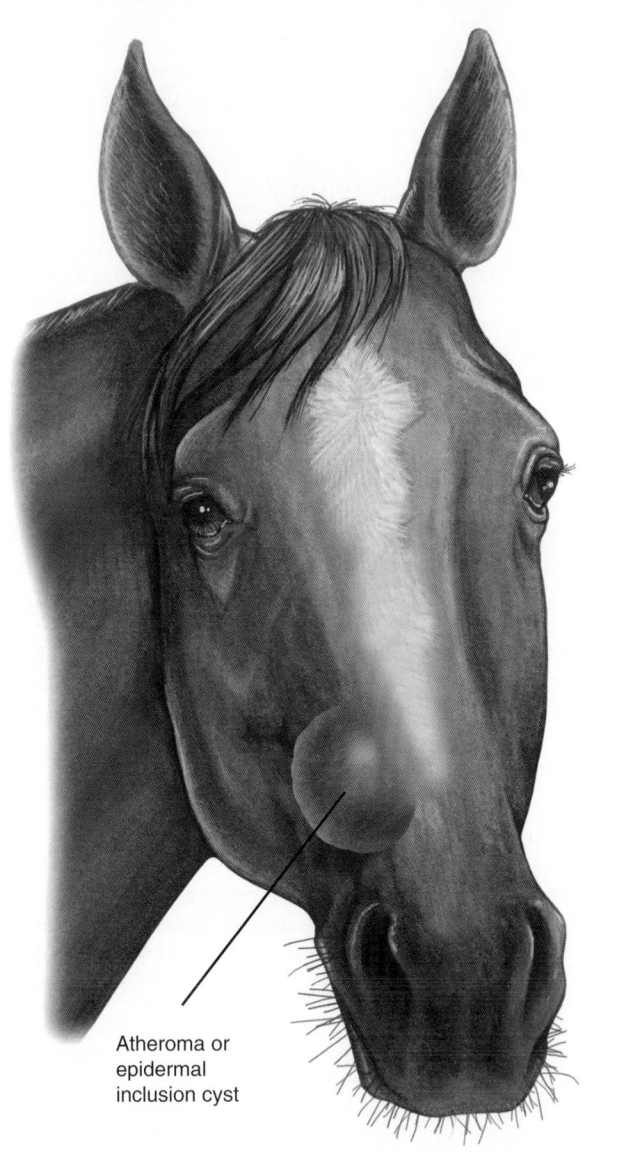

Atheroma or
epidermal
inclusion cyst

Atheroma

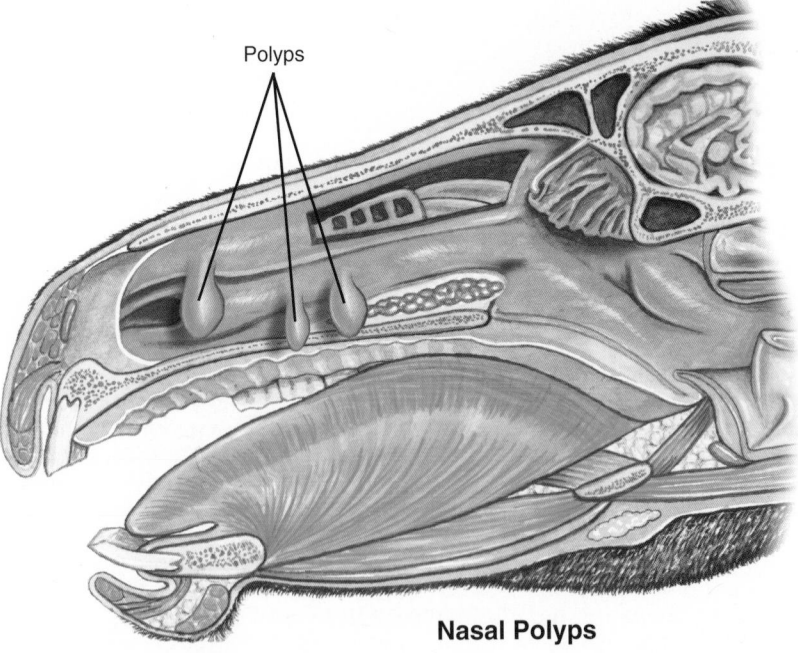

Polyps

Nasal Polyps

Treatment of Atheromas

These cysts can be drained or surgically removed. The animal is sedated and given a local infiltration of anesthetic which allows the cyst to be lanced through the nasal diverticulum. This incision then heals by second intention. If the cyst is large enough and needs to be removed for cosmetic purposes, a surgical approach can be gained dorsally. The cyst is then completely dissected away from the other tissues and the skin is closed in the normal manner.

ETHMOID HEMATOMA

An ethmoid hematoma is a hematoma that develops under the respiratory mucosa within the caudal cavity of the paranasal sinuses. There are three possible causes of this disorder, but the real pathogenesis of this problem is unknown. It has been theorized that it is a congenital weakened area that forms a hematoma from repetitive trauma, that it arises from neoplastic cells, and lastly, that its etiology is merely from chronic irritation and trauma.

Clinical Signs

These animals are presented with a small bloody nasal discharge usually arising from just one nostril. Blood may appear while the horse is at rest or after exercise. There may be some difficulty in breathing, because the hematoma may physically block a portion of the airway.

Differential Diagnosis

1.) Trauma
2.) Foreign Body
3.) Exercise-Induced Pulmonary Hemorrhage
4.) Fungal Infection
5.) Sinusitis

Diagnosis

In most cases, endoscopy will reveal a definitive diagnosis. A radiographic examination should also be conducted to define the limit of the mass and its extent within the tissues. The lesion itself occurs beneath the respiratory mucosa and appears greenish in coloration. Since it is located beneath the mucosa, the hematoma enlarges rostrally within the nasal cavity or caudally into the nasopharynx.

Treatment

Surgical removal of this mass is difficult, because it often requires access through the frontal bone and sinus. This area is highly vascular, and there will be a great deal of blood loss during this procedure. Cryosurgery techniques will freeze the mass and allow its removal while frozen, therefore decreasing the amount of hemorrhage during the procedure. Care must be taken during cryosurgery to minimize the amount of damage to surrounding local healthy tissue. It is often necessary to pack the nasal cavity postoperatively to reduce the amount the postoperative hemorrhage. If packing is necessary, a temporary tracheotomy may have to be performed. Follow-up endoscopic examinations on a periodic basis ensure the total removal of this hematoma and no recurrence.

NASAL POLYPS

Nasal polyps are slow-growing tumors that are comprised of connective tissue with an overlying layer of respiratory epithelium. They are usually pedunculated in shape and originate from the nasal mucosa, the septum, and even around the roots of the teeth. They are usually unilateral in nature but may occur bilaterally.

Clinical Signs

Initially, the animal will have an odorous nasal discharge that may be mucopurulent in nature. There will be intermittent bleeding from the nostril termed "epistaxis." This disorder can occur within horses of any age. In some cases, the polyp can be visualized by the owner or trainer. When these polyps grow in size, the animal will have difficulty breathing during exercise because the polyps will restrict the airflow through this area.

Differential Diagnosis

1.) Foreign body
2.) Neoplasia
3.) Infection

Diagnosis

Endoscopy will confirm the diagnosis of a nasal polyp. When visualized, these polyps appear white in color, are pedunculated, and have a smooth surface. There have been polyps that have been up to 30 cm in length that have even protruded out the nostril. Radiographic techniques will also define the margins of the mass and the tissues that they encompass.

Treatment

Surgical removal is the treatment of choice. The use of electrosurgical techniques is recommended because this technique facilitates hemostasis. Care must be taken to remove all abnormal tissue since regrowth of these polyps is possible.

STRANGLES (*STREPTOCOCCUS EQUI* INFECTION)

"Strangles" is the common name given to a horse that has a *Streptococcus equi* infection. This organism is highly contagious. Infection is spread by either inhalation or ingestion of this organism. The most common route of infection is the horse coming in contact with the nasal discharge of an infected animal through either grooming utensils, the water or feed sources, and humans. Strangles is a disorder that is predisposed to younger horses that are usually 6 months to five years old. Periodic outbreaks of strangles are common at boarding stables, stud farms, and training complexes.

Clinical Signs

The incubation period after exposure is usually 3 to 20 days. Most animals will exhibit clinical signs within 10 days of infection. These symptoms are variable depending on the horse's immune status

Artwork by S. Hakola / J. Dirig
Copyright Equistar Publications, Ltd.

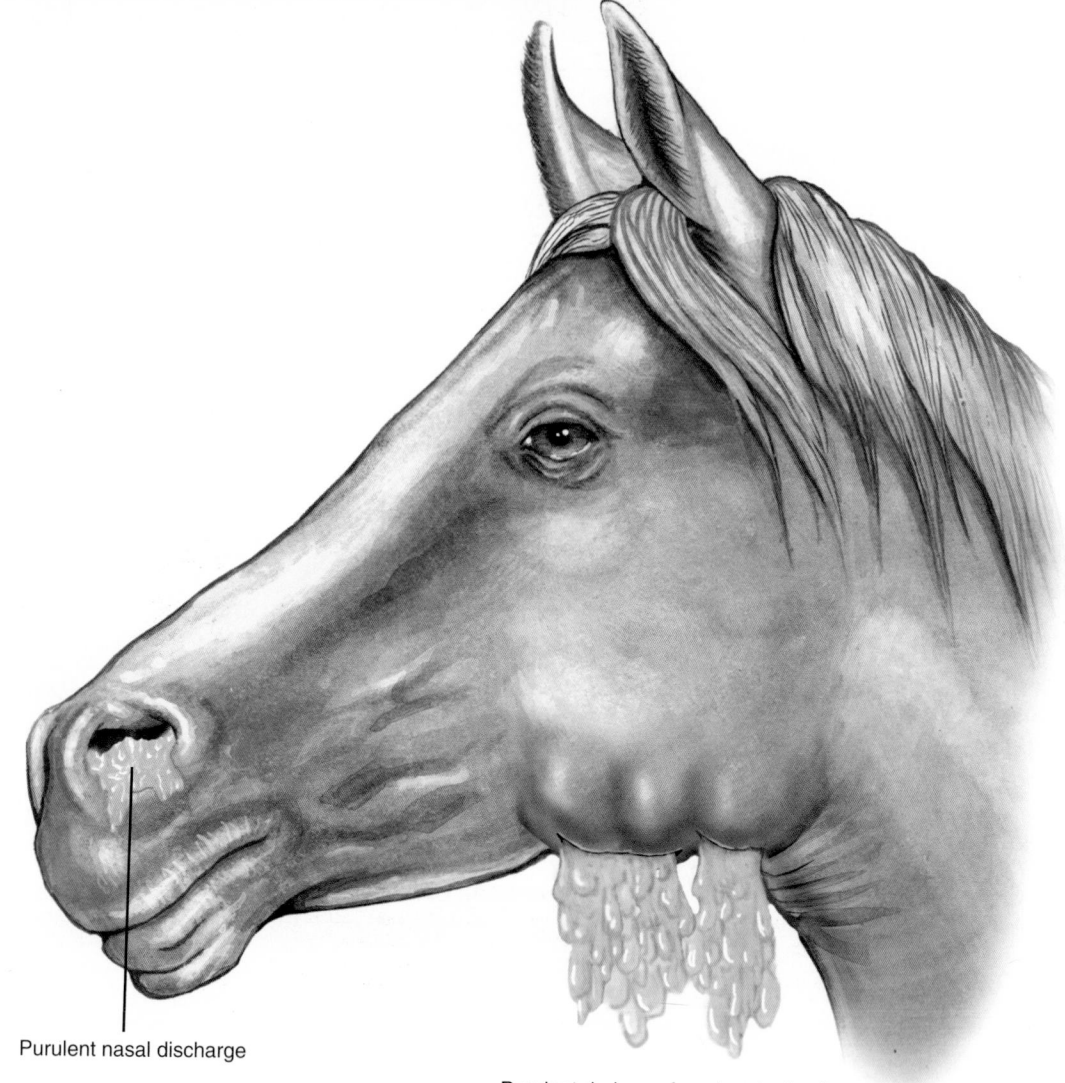

Purulent nasal discharge

Purulent drainage from lymph glands

Strangles (*Streptococcus equi* Infection)

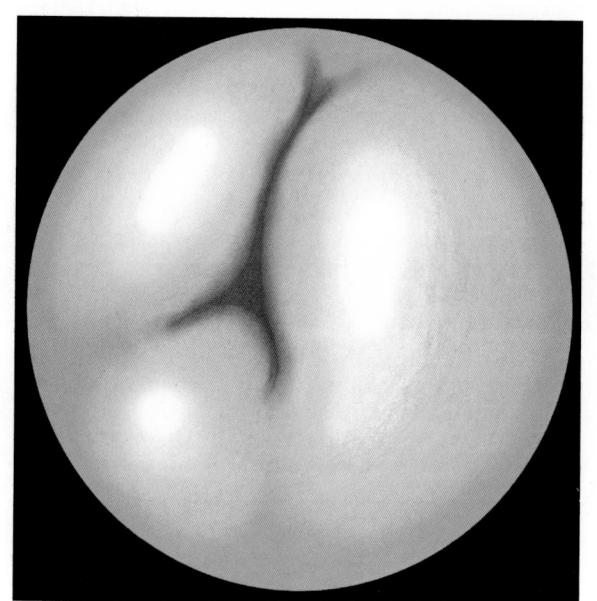

Maxillary Sinus Cyst as Seen Through an Endoscope with Protrusion of Sinus Walls into Pharynx

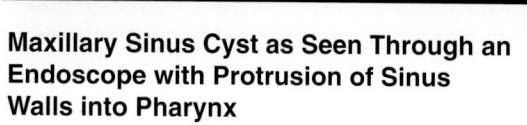

and the antibodies that the horse may have developed from an earlier exposure.

During the acute phase, the horse will exhibit depression, loss of appetite, fever, and a nasal discharge. As the disorder advances, it becomes localized within the submaxillary, mandibular, and retropharyngeal lymph nodes. The animal will experience pain from these swollen nodes, and this lymph node enlargement may obstruct respiration and affect swallowing. This is how "strangles" received its name.

Diagnosis

Diagnosis of *Streptococcus equi* is based on a culture of this organism. Nasal and pharyngeal cultures should be submitted to the lab for isolation of the *Streptococcus* organism. When these specimens are collected, a selective transport medium such as Strepswab (Medical Wire and Equipment Company, Cleveland, OH) should be used to reduce contamination with other organisms and improve the isolation of the causative organism.

Differential Diagnosis

1.) Bacterial Pneumonia
2.) Guttural Pouch Infections
3.) Viral Respiratory Disease

Treatment

Treatment should be initiated by placing all affected horses under quarantine and initiating personal hygiene restrictions for all those people handling these animals. These horses can spread the disease for 45 - 60 days after the disappearance of clinical signs. Animals should remain in isolation for at least four weeks after all clinical signs have disappeared. Ideally, repeated negative culture results should be obtained before they are allowed back into their normal environment.

In certain instances, the use of antibiotics depends on the severity of the symptoms. Mild infections that are localized to the lymph nodes or upper respiratory tract usually do not require systemic antibiotic treatment. Tradition has indicated that

the use of antibiotics in these cases predisposes these animals to "bastard strangles." The current literature states this is not true, and antibiotics should not be avoided because of this potential sequel to the disease. Pneumonia, pleuritis, sinusitis, synovitis, and guttural pouch infections are often complications of this disease and require rigorous effective antibiotic treatment. The drug of choice for this disorder is procaine penicillin. This antibiotic should be given at an appropriate dose (15,000 - 20,000 IU/kg) every twelve hours for at least 7 days. Regardless of which antibiotic is used, appropriate dosages and proper dose regime should be followed so as to not create a resistant strain of this bacteria which will be difficult to resolve.

Purpura hemorrhagica can be a complication from strangles. This will require long term antibiotic and antiinflammatory therapy.

Physical therapy techniques will help reduce the pain and swelling within the lymph nodes. Hot packs, or more ideally, warm moist heat should be applied twice daily to the swollen lymph nodes. This will help the mature to facilitate their drainage, and will also reduce the swelling in the area. This will in turn reduce the difficulty in breathing and swallowing for the animal. Even after the lymph nodes rupture and drain, continued applications of warm moist heat at least twice a day will greatly speed the healing process.

Prevention of strangles is an important aspect of this disorder. Stringent quarantine measures are an important way of preventing infection throughout the rest of the native horses at that location. Numerous commercial vaccines are available which reduce the morbidity and severity of the clinical signs of this disorder but do not prevent the disease. A new commercial intranasal vaccine is now available which shows promise in its route of administration and its effectiveness.

DISORDERS OF THE PARANASAL SINUSES

SINUS CYSTS

Fluid-filled cavities developing within the maxillary sinuses are referred to as sinus cysts. The etiology of these cysts is unknown with the only evidence of their origin lying in the fact that they all have an epithelial lining.

Clinical Signs

The initial clinical sign of these sinus cysts is that there is an increased degree of difficulty breathing for the horse. The animal will experience an intolerance to exercise. There may be some swelling that occurs along the facial tissue. There is a clear to mucoid nasal discharge that usually occurs unilaterally.

Differential Diagnosis

1.) Fibroma/Fibrosarcoma
2.) Bacterial Sinusitis
3.) Congenital Malformation of the Nasal Cavity
4.) Trauma
5.) Ethmoidal Hematoma

Diagnosis

Diagnosis of a cyst within the sinus consists of an endoscopic examination of the paranasal sinus and radiographic techniques. When one looks through an endoscope, the paranasal sinuses will appear to bulge into the airway. This is caused by an enlarged ventral concha. A radiographic exam will reveal fluid-filled cavities within the sinuses and may also reveal a sclerosis of the surrounding bone and displacement of the molar or premolar roots.

Treatment

Surgical removal of the sinus cysts and its lining is the treatment of choice. An appropriate incision is made and a bone flap technique is used to gain access to the appropriate sinus area. The cyst and

Empyema; Pharyngeal Cysts

Empyema

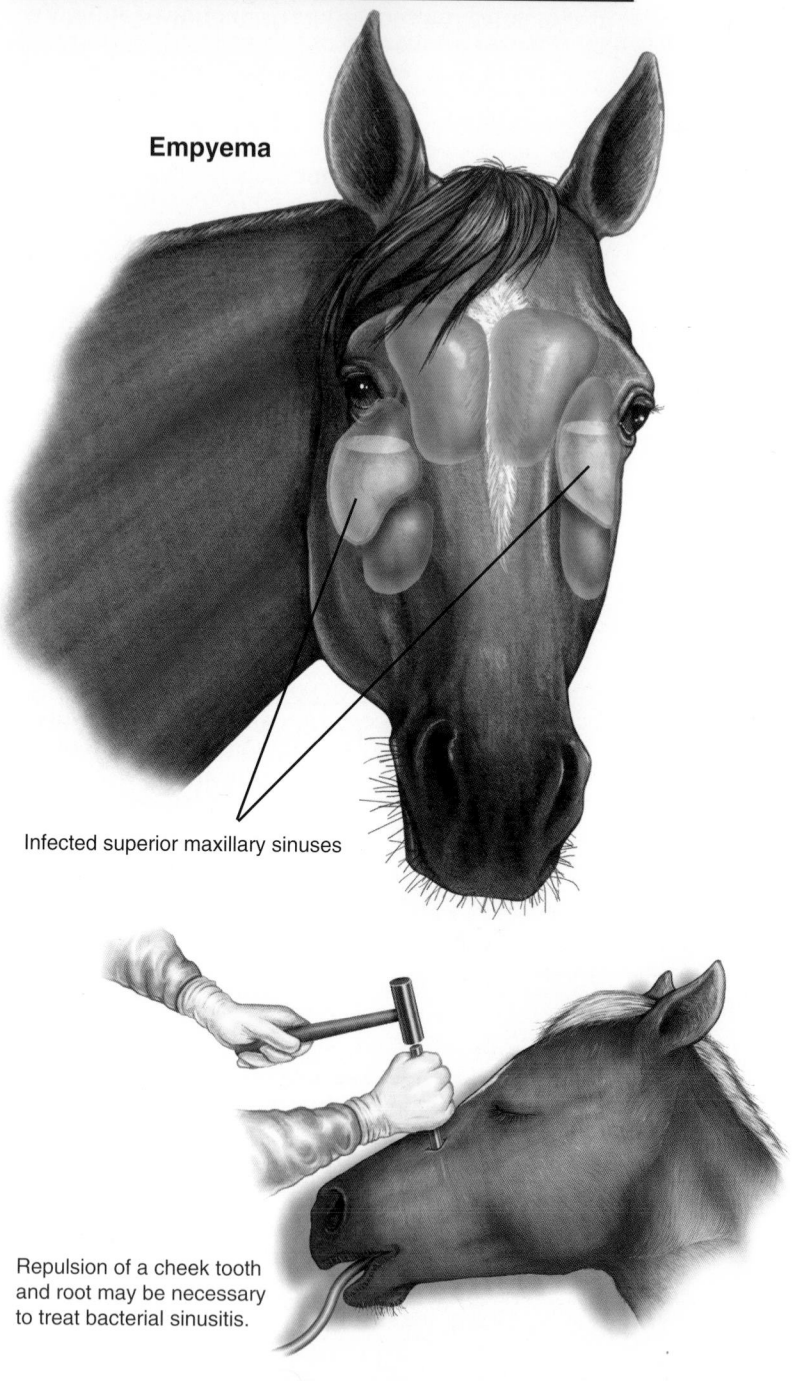

Infected superior maxillary sinuses

Repulsion of a cheek tooth
and root may be necessary
to treat bacterial sinusitis.

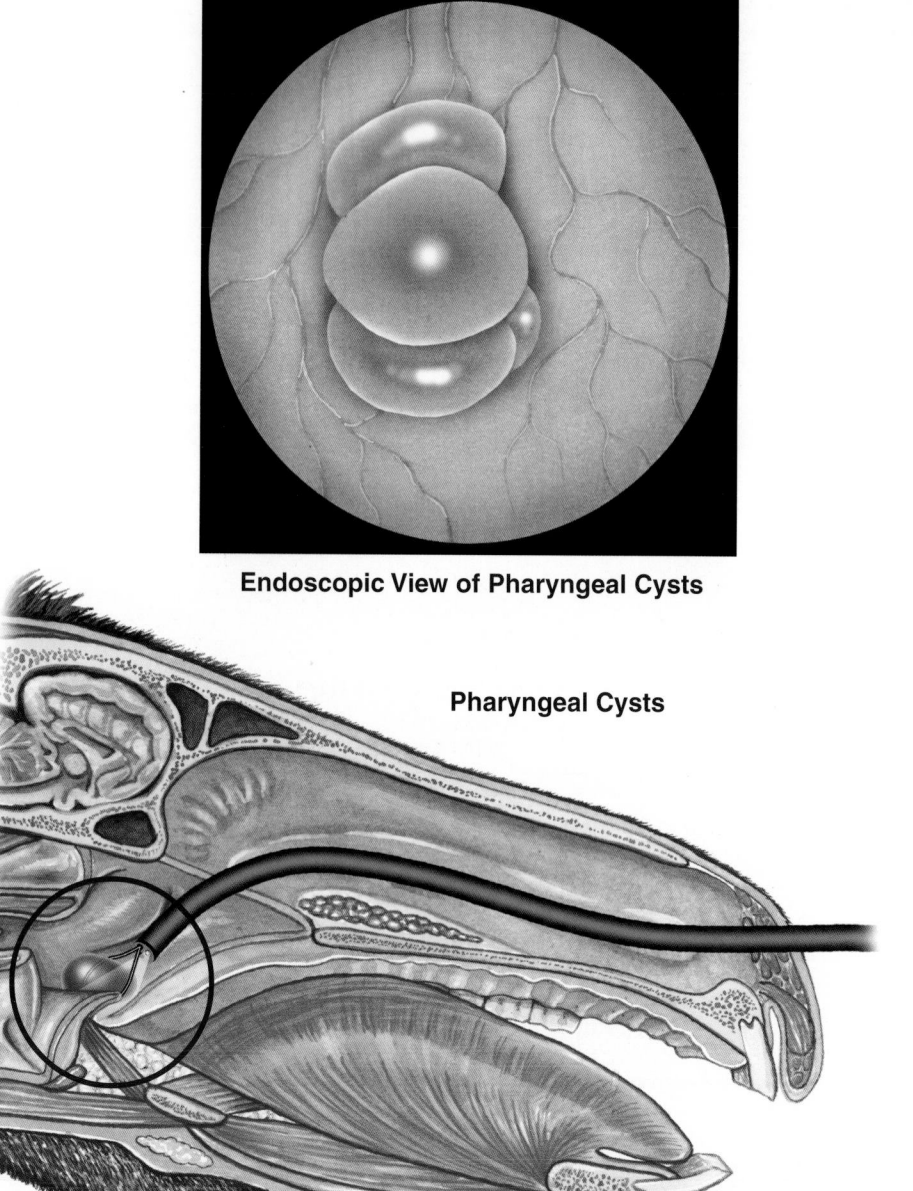

Endoscopic View of Pharyngeal Cysts

Pharyngeal Cysts

**Endoscopic Removal of Pharyngeal
Cyst Using a Wire Snare**

its lining are then excised from the surrounding sinus tissue. There will be considerable bleeding and care must be taken to control the hemorrhage. These cysts very rarely recur which allows for a favorable prognosis after this procedure.

BACTERIAL SINUSITIS (EMPYEMA)

Etiology

Bacterial infections of the frontal and maxillary sinuses can be either primary or secondary in nature. Primary bacterial sinusitis occurs because of the open communications between the nasal cavity and the sinuses. This allows upper respiratory tract infections to involve these paranasal sinuses. Secondary bacterial sinusitis occurs as an extension of the infections that involve the tooth roots. Respiratory infections such as those caused by *Streptococcus equi* and equine influenza virus readily involve the paranasal sinuses. Alveolar periostitis may also involve the paranasal sinuses.

Clinical Signs

These animals will usually exhibit pain over the affected sinus. Systemically, these animals will exhibit a fever, inappetence, difficulty in breathing, and exercise intolerance. In most cases, these horses will have a nasal discharge that is usually mucopurulent. In extreme cases, especially when the frontal sinuses are invloved, the horse may show signs of meningitis and other neurological dysfunctions.

Diagnosis

A definitive diagnosis can be reached with radiographic techniques. Fluid lines and radiographic signs of dental disease will be visualized on the films. Endoscopic examination will reveal a purulent drainage from the nasomaxillary opening. A sinuscentesis can be performed on the standing sedated patient and will produce samples of discharge that can be submitted for culture and sensitivity.

Treatment

Treatment of bacterial sinusitis that results from a dental problem focuses on alleviating that problem tooth. Removal of the tooth is often necessary since preservation of a diseased tooth usually allows recurrence of the sinus infection. After the tooth is removed, systemic treatment with antibiotics is necessary.

Lavage and drainage of the sinus in addition to antimicrobial therapy resolves most cases of sinusitis. A catheter or polyethylene tube is inserted into the sinus through a trephine hole. This catheter is then sutured in place so that it can be used repeatedly to flush and lavage the sinus. At least one to two liters of flushed solution should be infused once or several times a day through this catheter.

A maxillary bone flap technique can be used to gain access to the entire sinus. This surgical technique may be necessary to remove the chronic tissue or allow repulsion of an abnormal tooth.

Antimicrobial therapy should be considered on a case to case basis and be administered in a sufficient amount of time so as to prevent a recurrence. The selection of the antibiotic used should be based on culture and sensitivity results. In all cases this systemic antibiotic therapy should be coupled with a lavage and drainage technique.

PHARYNGEAL CYSTS

These cysts are sometimes referred to as subepiglottic cysts. They occur near the larynx, soft palate, and other sites within the pharynx.

Etiology

The origin of pharyngeal cysts is the result of a defect within the embryological development of these tissues. These cysts arise from remnants of the thyroglossal duct or form as an inclusion cyst within the fold of the aryepiglottic tissue or soft palate.

Clinical Signs

Pharyngeal cysts contain a thick yellow or tan mucoid material. Because of the frequency which standardbred and thoroughbred racehorses undergo endoscopic examination, these cysts are commonly found within the pharyngeal area. In most cases with these race horses, the endoscopic examination resulted from a reduced performance level or an intolerance to exercise. The animal may experience difficulty breathing or may have a chronic cough. When these animals perform, they may produce a respiratory noise during inspiration and expiration.

Differential Diagnosis

1.) Laryngeal Hemiplegia
2.) Guttural Pouch Infection
3.) Pharyngeal Lymphoid Hyperplasia
4.) Entrapment of the Epiglottis
5.) Nasal Polyp

Diagnosis

An endoscopic examination will allow an easy definitive diagnosis of pharyngeal cysts. When examining the pharyngeal area, some of these cysts may not be visible until the horse is made to swallow.

Treatment

Surgical removal of the offending cyst is the treatment of choice. An oral approach using a speculum or fiberoptic endoscope and wire snare is a popular technique that allows a rapid recovery time. If the cyst is large enough, it may require a surgical removal through a ventral midline pharyngotomy incision. This incision is allowed to heal by second intention and recovery is in terms of months instead of weeks.

Artwork by S. Hakola / J. Dirig
Copyright Equistar Publications, Ltd.

Dorsal Displacement of the Soft Palate

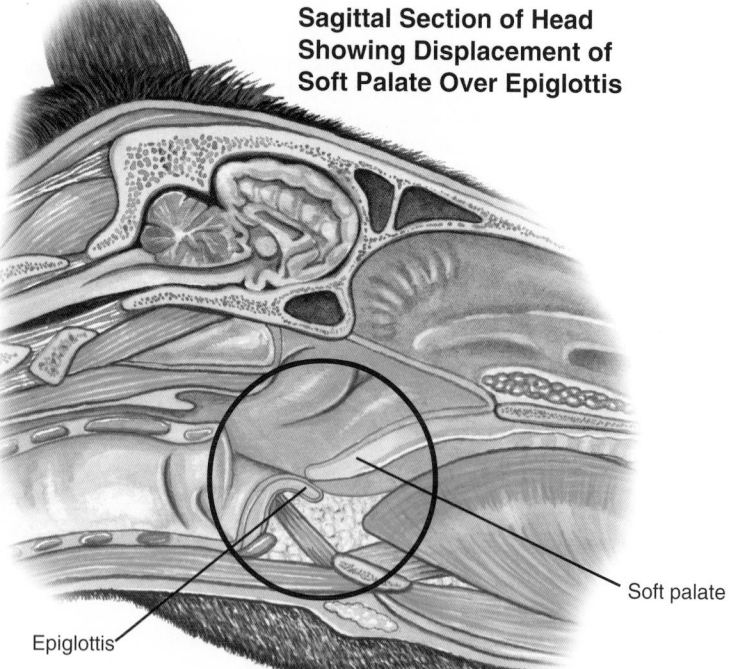

Endoscopic view of soft palate displacement

Sagittal Section of Head Showing Displacement of Soft Palate Over Epiglottis

Soft palate

Epiglottis

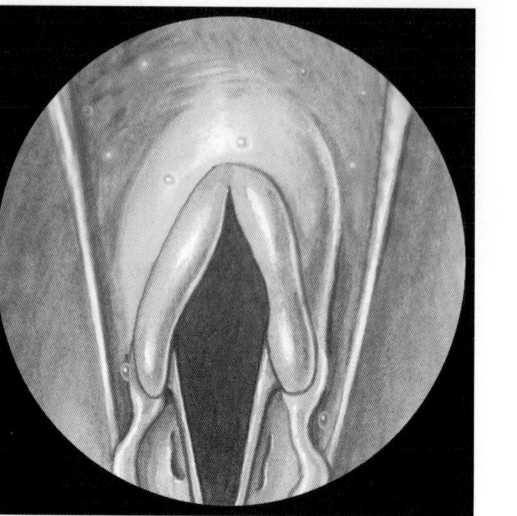

Stage 1

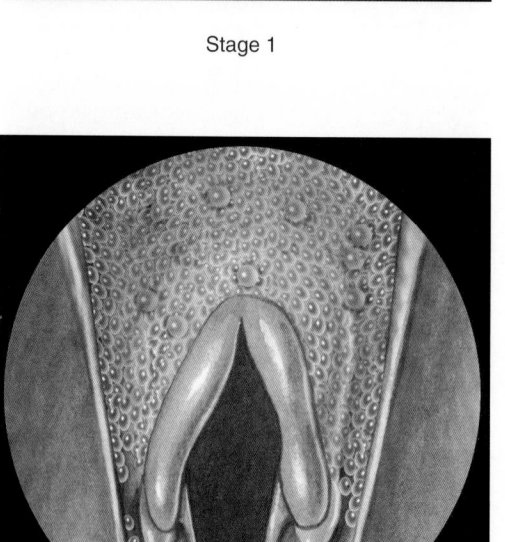

Stage 2

Stage 3

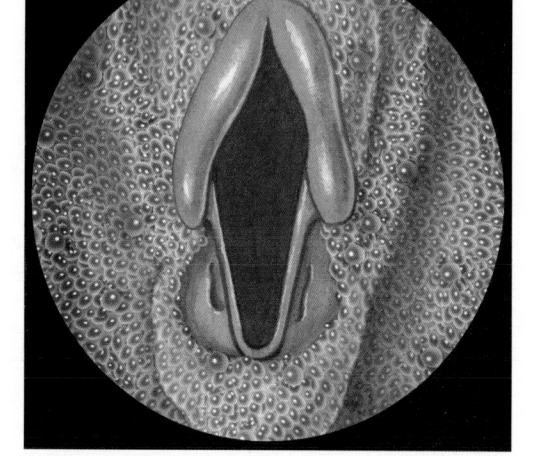

Stage 4

Pharyngeal Lymphoid Hyperplasia

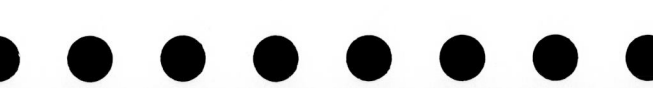

DORSAL DISPLACEMENT OF THE SOFT PALATE

During the act of swallowing, the soft palate displaces dorsally. If the external nares are occluded, the soft palate can be induced to displace dorsally. When there is a dorsal displacement of the soft palate, there is an obstruction to the airway. Therefore, if the soft palate is displaced dorsally, and the animal breathes over the free border of the soft palate which is obstructing the epiglottis, then there is a characteristic gurgling noise produced. If there is an obstruction of the airway over the opening of the larynx, there is a turbulent and reduced airflow in this area that results in a lack of athletic performance.

Etiology

Displacement of the soft palate dorsally may be in response to pain which might originate from a lameness disorder. During this displacement, there is a caudal retraction of the larynx and a dislocation of the larynx from the palatopharyngeal arch. This may be due to pharyngeal lymphoid hyperplasia, laryngeal and subepiglottic cysts, or chondritis. When evaluating a dorsal displacement of the soft palate, it is necessary to examine all the systems of the horse to eliminate possible causes.

Clinical Signs

Initially, the animal may swallow repeatedly. Swallowing will result in the replacement of the soft palate to its normal position. This disorder is usually seen in race horses. When they are exercised at high speeds, a gurgling noise can be heard. If the airway is severely obstructed, these animals may attempt to mouth breath and become weak and unstable.

Differential Diagnosis

1.) Sinus Cyst
2.) Guttural Pouch Infection
3.) Nasal Polyp
4.) Subepiglottic Cyst
5.) Laryngeal Hemiplegia

Diagnosis

A definitive diagnosis of a dorsal displacement of the soft palate is difficult. An endoscopic examination done when the animal is at rest usually results in no abnormalities found. An endoscopic examination immediately following a very strenuous exercise regime may reveal the soft palate dislocation. Therefore, a diagnosis is usually made when all other upper respiratory problems are eliminated as possibilities, and when the horse gurgles or chokes at the end of a race.

Treatment

The most conservative treatment is the use of a tongue tie. This limits a caudal retraction of the larynx. Surgical intervention involves trimming the soft palate and the excision of the ventral neck muscles that cause a caudal retraction of the larynx. Portions of the sternothyrohyoideus and omohyoideus muscles can be removed. This myectomy can be performed while the horse is in a standing position. Training of these animals is usually resumed within two weeks. Approximately 50% of the animals will show improvement after this myectomy procedure. Since 10 - 12 cm sections of these muscles should be removed, postoperative care should include applications of warm moist heat, massage, and the systemic administration of antibiotics.

PHARYNGEAL LYMPHOID HYPERPLASIA

Pharyngeal lymphoid hyperplasia is commonly seen in young race horses during training. The ability to perform endoscopic examinations has greatly increased the awareness of this disorder. Some horses with a mild to moderate degree of lymphoid hyperplasia perform poorly, while others with a similar degree enter the winner's circle. Therefore, there is some controversy as to the significance of these lesions.

Etiology

Causes of pharyngeal lymphoid hyperplasia could be from viruses that damage the upper respiratory tract, air pollution, inhaled irritants (such as dust from the race track,) or from a low grade bacterial infection. Any factor that induces the hyperplasia of these lymphoid follicles within the pharynx results in this disorder.

Clinical Signs

These animals all exhibit a chronic shallow cough. Finding hyperplasia of these pharyngeal lymphoid follicles is usually concurrent with poor performance on the track.

Grades of Pharyngeal Lymphoid Hyperplasia

Grade 1: This is a normal finding upon endoscopic examination. There are very few small inactive follicles present within the pharyngeal tissues.
Grade 2: This grade is differentiated in that there are more follicles present, some of the follicles appear swollen, and are seen both on the dorsal and lateral surfaces of the pharynx.
Grade 3: This is the grade where there is a corresponding lack of performance and the initial signs of a chronic cough. The pharyngeal tonsilar tissues are hyperplastic and the follicles appear large and pink to red in color.
Grade 4: Most of the follicles at this level appear swollen and are spread over the dorsal and lateral pharyngeal walls, soft palate, and the epiglottis. These follicles resemble the appearance of a polyp.

Differential Diagnosis

1.) Laryngeal Hemiplegia
2.) Dorsal Displacement of the Soft Palate
3.) Viral Upper Respiratory Disease
4.) Subepiglottic Cysts

Diagnosis

Diagnosis of pharyngeal lymphoid hyperplasia is based on an endoscopic exam of the lymphoid tissues within the pharynx. Care must be taken during this endoscopic examination to eliminate other possible upper respiratory disorders that may be causing an effect on the airflow.

Artwork by S. Hakola / J. Dirig
Copyright Equistar Publications, Ltd.

Endoscopic Examination of the Guttural Pouch

A - Hyovertebrotomy incision

B - Viborg's triangle incision

C - Modified Whitehouse incision

D - Whitehouse incision

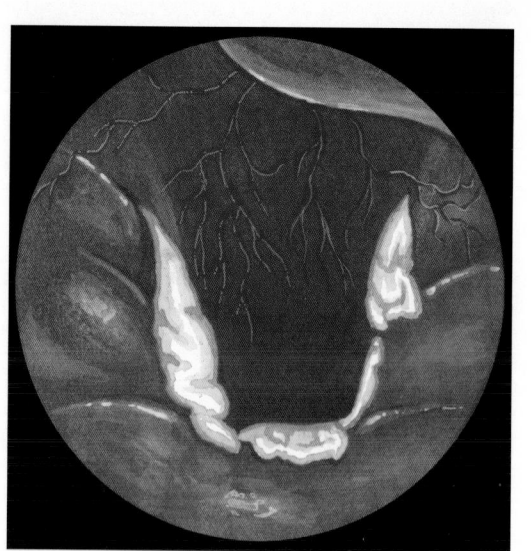

Endoscopic View of Guttural Pouch Empyema

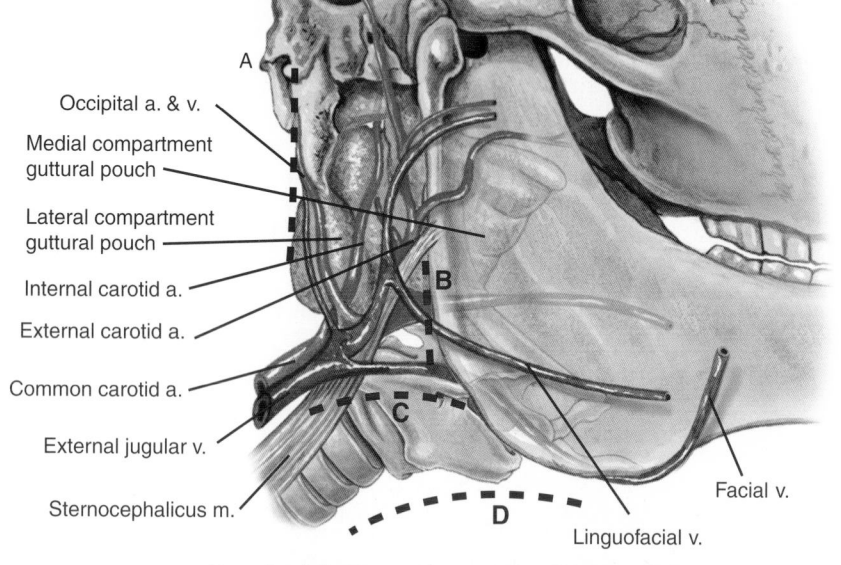

Occipital a. & v.

Medial compartment guttural pouch

Lateral compartment guttural pouch

Internal carotid a.

External carotid a.

Common carotid a.

External jugular v.

Sternocephalicus m.

Facial v.

Linguofacial v.

Surgical Approaches to the Guttural Pouch

Treatment of Pharyngeal Lymphoid Hyperplasia

There have been a wide variety of treatments proposed for this disorder which include a rest period for 8 - 12 weeks, cryosurgery, chemical cautery, electrocautery, and nebulization with anti-inflammatory drugs in combination with antibiotics.

GUTTURAL POUCH DISORDERS

There are three significant disorders involving the guttural pouch: guttural pouch tympany, mycosis, and empyema. The guttural pouches communicate through the epipharyngeal orifices with the pharynx. The location of these pouches on the lateral walls of the pharynx coupled with the fact that they open during swallowing predisposes this anatomical area to infections. Any infection within the guttural pouch will limit the performance level of the horse.

EMPYEMA OF THE GUTTURAL POUCH

The term "guttural empyema" means the accumulation of any exudate, such as pus, within the guttural pouch. This disorder is the most common guttural pouch problem. It may occur in horses of any age, but it is more common in those that are young. Guttural pouch empyema occurs secondarily to upper respiratory tract infections. In particular, it results from a *Streptococcus equi* infection (strangles) because of abscess formation in the lymph nodes around the adjacent anatomical areas.

Clinical Signs

There is a thick purulent discharge from the nostrils. It can be unilateral in nature or bilateral with unequal amounts of discharge from both nostrils. If the animal has its head in a lowered position and pressure is applied to the guttural pouch, an increased amount of discharge may be exhibited. Externally, enlargement of the guttural pouch region may not be noticeable. This is the

result of the structure of the guttural pouch which allows it to expand a great deal internally before an external enlargement is seen.

Differential Diagnosis

1.) Guttural Pouch Mycosis
2.) Sinusitis
3.) Foreign Body
4.) Ethmoidal Hematoma
5.) Trauma

Diagnosis

Endoscopic examination of this area will reveal a mucopurulent discharge from the guttural pouch opening. It may be necessary to pass the endoscope through the epipharyngeal orifice to confirm the diagnosis. Radiographs of this area will indicate a presence of fluid or accumulated material within the guttural pouches. A catheter can be placed within the guttural pouch to obtain a culture. This will confirm the specific positive agent, and sensitivity testing will lead to efficient treatment regimes.

Treatment

Systemic antibiotic treatment for at least 5 - 7 days will usually resolve the infection. A more aggressive and thorough treatment is obtained if this systemic antibiotic treatment is also coupled with a daily lavage of the guttural pouches. This lavage technique is ideally performed 2 - 3 times per day utilizing 500 ml of fluid. Isotonic polyionic solutions that are warmed to body temperature and contain antibiotics are used for this technique. Irritating solutions should not be used since they may lead to neurological damage.

If the guttural pouch discharge persists for several days after systemic antibiotic therapy and lavage of the pouches, than surgical drainage may be indicated. Due to the number of anatomical structures within the guttural pouch region, caution should be exercised in taking any approach to the guttural pouch. The approach through Viborg's triangle is one of the most common, and it is formed by the tendinous insertion of the

sternocephalicus muscle dorsally, the linguofacial vein ventrally, and the vertical ramus of the mandible rostrally. Dorsal to the linguofacial vein, a 6 - 8 cm skin incision is made vertically. Care must be taken to avoid the parotid salivary gland and the salivary duct. Dissection is continued ventral to the external carotid artery until the guttural pouch is reached. An incision is made into the pouch and all exudate within the pouch is removed. After surgery, the incision is left to heal as an open wound and to provide drainage to the area. This pouch should then be lavaged several times a day utilizing a catheter that is placed either through the surgical site itself or into the guttural pouch via the pharyngeal opening through the epipharyngeal orifice.

Other surgical approaches can be used. A lateral approach can be used to gain access to the guttural pouch. This approach falls cranial to the wing of the atlas and ventral to the base of the ear. This area however contains numerous vascular structures, and the drainage from the guttural pouch is not in its most ventral position. A modified Whitehouse approach utilizes a ventral paramedian incision that is ventral to the linguofacial vein and lies between the sternothyro-hyoideus and the omohyoideus muscles. This modified Whitehouse approach provides the best ventral drainage but has a disadvantage because of the numerous neurological structures that can be damaged during the surgical procedure.

MYCOSIS OF THE GUTTURAL POUCH

Fungal infections of the guttural pouch wall often involve damage to underlying neurovascular structures. These fungal infections occur more commonly in the Northern Hemispheres than the Southern Hemispheres. There is no breed or sex predisposition; however, it does seem to affect younger horses more commonly than older ones.

Etiology

Aspergillus nidulans is the most common fungal agent resulting in guttural pouch infection which usually occurs unilaterally. The actual

Artwork by S. Hakola / J. Dirig
Copyright Equistar Publications, Ltd.

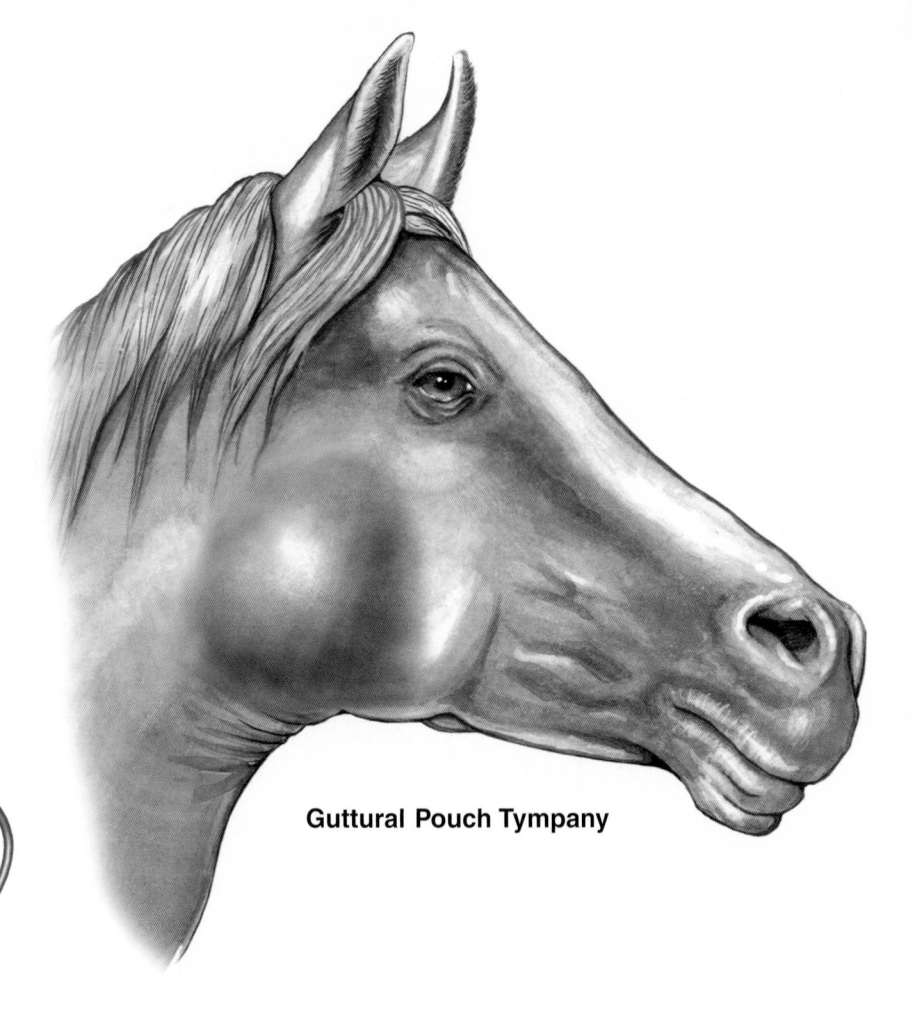

Endoscopic view of mycosis or fungal infection

Guttural Pouch Mycosis

Nebulization of antifungal medications in the treatment of mycosis

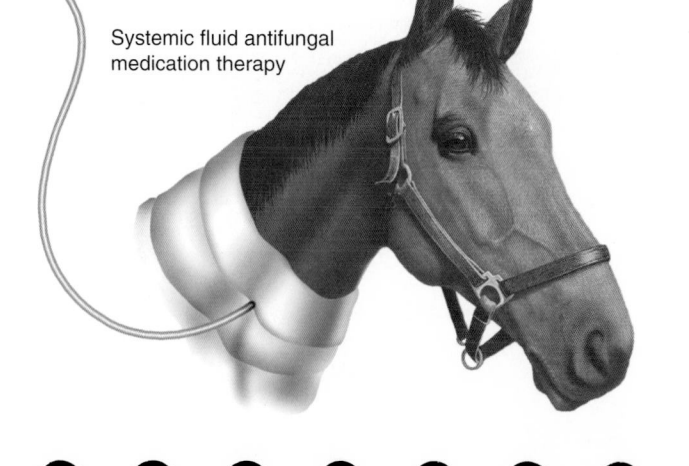

Systemic fluid antifungal medication therapy

Guttural Pouch Tympany

pathogenesis of this condition is unclear, but infection with this organism is opportunistic and requires appropriate environmental conditions or predisposing factors for its development. It has been theorized that there is a higher incidence with horses that are kept indoors in dusty environments. Horses that race or train on dusty surfaces may also be predisposed to these guttural pouch mycoses.

Clinical Signs

Guttural pouch mycosis may be completely asymptomatic. When the condition is symptomatic, the most common clinical sign is epistaxis. Even though the infection is usually unilateral, blood is typically seen exiting both nostrils. This blood may range from a few trickles to severe bleeding and is usually bright red in color which suggests an arterial origin.

The animal will also have difficulty swallowing, which is termed "dysphagia." This is usually the result of the fungal organism causing a loss of function within the pharyngeal branches of the vagus and the glossopharyngeal nerves. The animal may merely hold its head in an abnormal posture, and there may be parotid pain upon digital palpation.

Initially, the animal may merely exhibit a sudden predisposition to head shyness. The horse may present an abnormal respiratory noise or break out in a sweat for no reason. As the fungal infection becomes more advanced, the animal may exhibit signs of Horner's syndrome and may even show paralysis of the facial nerves.

Differential Diagnosis

1.) Guttural Pouch Empyema
2.) Sinusitis
3.) Ethmoidal Hematoma
4.) Trauma

Diagnosis

Endoscopic examination will confirm guttural pouch mycosis and will probably also reveal laryngeal hemiplegia, dorsal displacement of the soft palate, or hemorrhage through the pharyngeal openings.

Treatment

Guttural pouch mycosis usually involves the internal carotid artery, the glossopharyngeal, and the vagus nerves. The wall of the internal carotid artery is invaded by the fungus which results in the hemorrhages that are noted on the clinical signs. Therefore, the treatment of guttural pouch mycosis should involve stabilization of the patient and cessation of the hemorrhage. If blood loss has been severe, systemic fluid therapy may be indicated. The administration of systemic antibiotics may be necessary if there is a secondary bacterial infection to the fungus. Nebulization with antifungal medications will provide topical contact with the fungal organisms. Antifungal agents such as amphotericin B and ketoconazole are effective against *Aspergillus* but are relatively toxic to the animal. Griseofulvin is absorbed from the GI tract and is usually not effective against *Aspergillus*.

Placement of a catheter within the guttural pouch to allow lavage and drainage of this area may be an effective treatment. Lavage fluid should be warm sterile solutions that also contain antifungal agents.

Surgical intervention may be the only option in a chronic case of guttural pouch mycosis. This surgery will be quite challenging due to the location of the lesion adjacent to the internal carotid artery and the underlying nerves. Surgical removal of the mycotic mass may result in rupture of the internal carotid artery. To prevent hemorrhage, the internal carotid artery may have to be ligated before the lesion is removed. This ligation may have to be done both proximally and distally to the lesion to prevent hemorrhage in the area. If nerve function is severely compromised, humane destruction may be a consideration.

TYMPANY OF THE GUTTURAL POUCH

This disorder can be congenital or acquired. It is manifested by the accumulation of a large volume of air within the guttural pouch. Tympany usually occurs unilaterally but can occur bilaterally.

Etiology

The cause of guttural pouch tympany is unknown. This occurs due to a malformation of the pharyngeal orifice of the eustachian tube which acts as a one-way valve to allow air into the guttural pouch but not to leave. There may be a congenital abnormality to this valve, or it may be due to a secondary infection which has produced scarring of the orifice or thickening of the mucous membrane.

Clinical Signs

There is a nonpainful elastic swelling in the parotid region. Percussion over the swollen area will reveal an air-filled pocket. This can occur in foals shortly after birth, and these foals will exhibit a "snoring" sound when suckling. When the enlargement is significant, there may be an obstruction of air flow which produces dyspnea.

Differential Diagnosis

1.) Congenital Malformation
2.) Guttural Pouch Empyema

Diagnosis

A diagnosis is usually based on the clinical signs. An endoscopic examination will typically reveal normal pharyngeal openings. Radiographs will determine whether the condition is unilateral or bilateral in nature.

Artwork by S. Hakola / J. Dirig
Copyright Equistar Publications, Ltd.

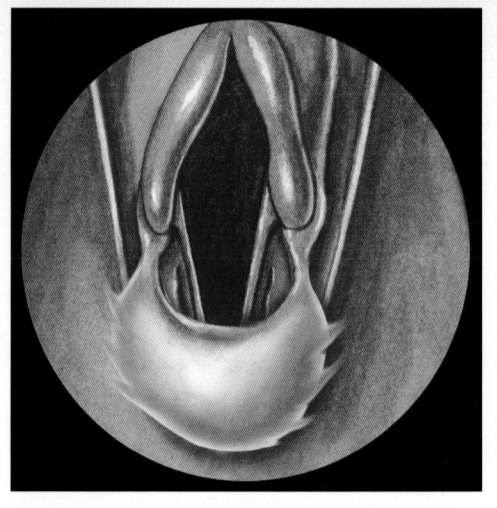

Endoscopic view of epiglottis ensnared by the aryepiglottic membrane.

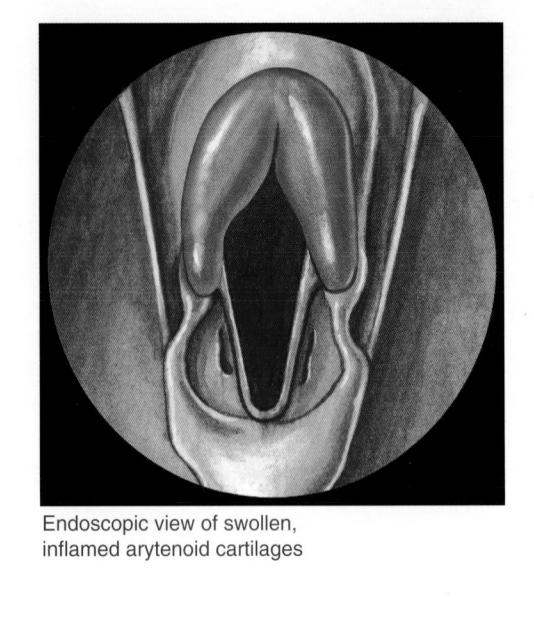

Endoscopic view of swollen, inflamed arytenoid cartilages

Epiglottic Entrapment

Transendoscopic laser division of the aryepiglottic membrane.

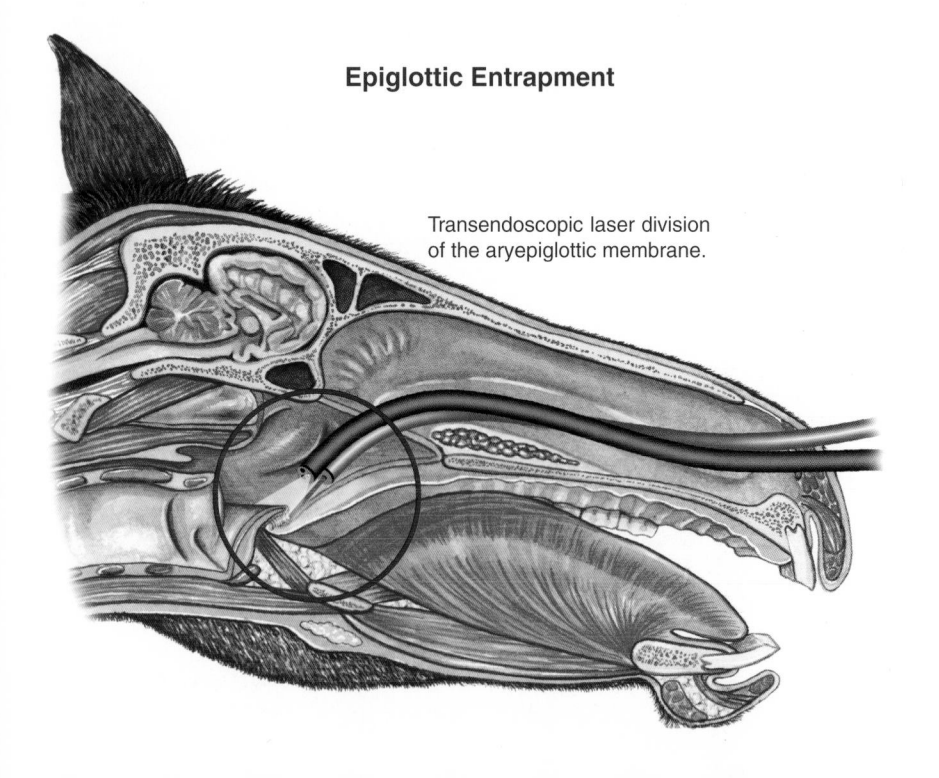

Arytenoid Chondritis

Surgical Views of Arytenoid Chondroplasty

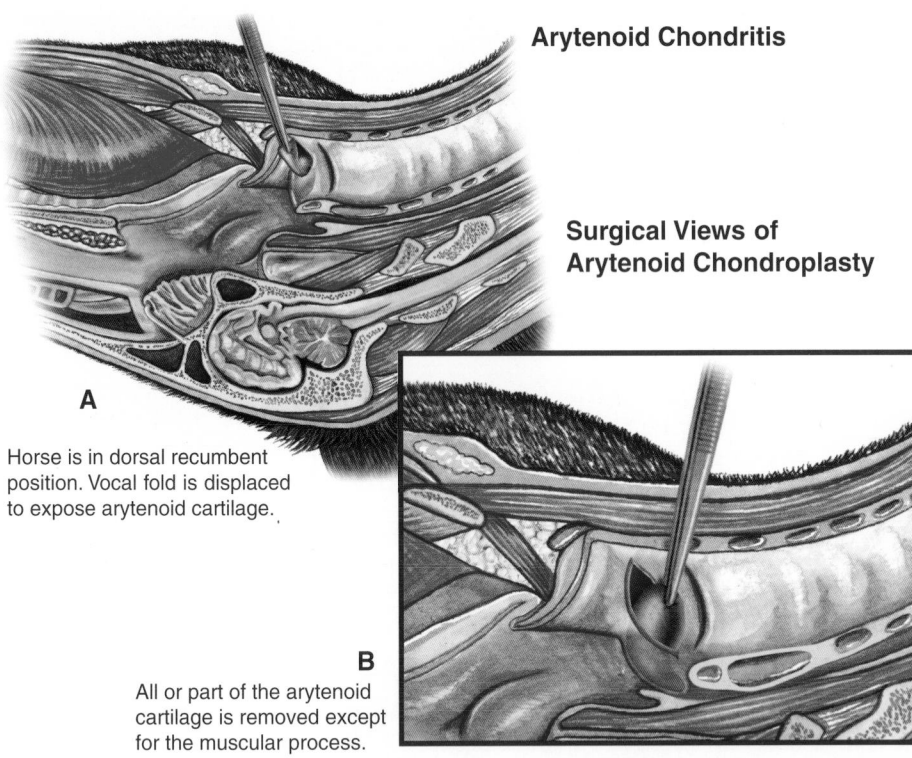

A

Horse is in dorsal recumbent position. Vocal fold is displaced to expose arytenoid cartilage.

B

All or part of the arytenoid cartilage is removed except for the muscular process.

Treatment of Guttural Pouch Tympany

Temporary relief to the accumulation of air can be accomplished through the placement of a catheter into the guttural pouch via the nasopharynx. Simple digital pressure on the pouch may also temporarily relieve the condition.

Surgical enlargement of the pharyngeal openings to both guttural pouches will provide a more definitive treatment. Access to the guttural pouch is gained through Viborg's triangle. The medial lamina of the eustachian tube and its mucosal fold is excised within the guttural pouch orifice to create a larger opening to the pharynx. The medial septum is then incised to remove a 2 cm segment which allows trapped air from the tympanic pouch to exit through to the normal side. Provided there are no secondary complications such as pneumonia or guttural pouch empyema, the prognosis for complete recovery is very good.

EPIGLOTTIC ENTRAPMENT

Etiology

Epiglottic entrapment occurs when the aryepiglottic folds envelope the epiglottis. These folds are the thick bands of mucous membrane that attach to the ventral surface of the epiglottis and extend caudally and dorsally to communicate with the mucous membranes that join the corniculate processes. Subepiglottic epithelium is loose and allows for the elevation of the epiglottis during swallowing. Entrapment occurs when this loose tissue surrounds the apex and lateral aspects of the epiglottis.

Clinical Signs

There is an abnormal respiratory noise that occurs during exercise, particularly in thoroughbred and standardbred race horses. The animals initially exhibit a decrease in athletic performance before the respiratory noise can be heard. The trainer or owner may complain that the animal has a chronic cough or has signs of nasal discharge.

Differential Diagnosis

1.) Left Laryngeal Hemiplegia
2.) Laryngeal Chondritis
3.) Soft Palate Displacement
4.) Ethmoid Hematoma

Diagnosis

Endoscopic examination will reveal a definitive diagnosis. The epiglottis will still be visibly positioned above the soft palate. It will be covered with a folded mucosa which will obscure the serrated margins of the epiglottis and the dorsal epiglottic vasculature. If the animal is induced into swallowing, the entrapped membranes may be intermittently relieved.

Treatment

Correction of epiglottic entrapment involves a surgical division of the aryepiglottic membrane. This can be accomplished using a transendoscopic contact laser, a transnasal or transoral division of this membrane utilizing a curved bistoury, or a surgical incision through a laryngotomy or pharyngotomy.

ARYTENOID CHONDRITIS

This is a chronic inflammatory disease of adult horses that leads to laryngeal obstruction.

Clinical Signs

These animals exhibit coughing, have difficulty breathing, and exhibit a respiratory noise whether at rest or at exercise.

Differential Diagnosis

1.) Laryngeal Hemiplegia
2.) Sinusitis
3.) Trauma
4.) Guttural Pouch Empyema

Diagnosis

Endoscopic examination of the laryngeal area will provide a definitive diagnosis of arytenoid chondritis. The arytenoid will be swollen and displaced medially with no movement being noted during respiration. It is sometimes difficult to differentiate arytenoid chondritis from that of laryngeal hemiplegia. Mucosal projections and distortion of arytenoid cartilages are only present during arytenoid chondritis.

Digital compression of the larynx may produce a difficulty in breathing and result in an abnormal respiratory noise while the animal is at rest. The larynx may be firmer than normal when palpated. Radiographs may reveal a calcification of the area over the dorsum of the larynx and the arytenoid cartilages.

Treatment

There are two treatments of choice for arytenoid chondritis. Consideration should be given to the actual obstruction of the airway and the future use of the horse when a treatment regime is considered. The more conservative treatment regime involves an excision of projecting lesions on the arytenoid cartilages, curettage of sinus tracts within the cartilage, and ventriculectomy. This conservative approach should be considered when these animals are only exhibiting dyspnea during exercise.

The surgical procedure is accomplished through a ventral laryngotomy incision made through the cricothyroid ligament to expose the arytenoid cartilage. This cartilage is then removed through dissection to the level below the mucosal surface. The sinus tracts are examined and curetted with a small bone curette, and all surrounding granulation tissue is removed. A ventriculectomy is then performed on the affected side. The incision is not closed but allowed to heal as an open wound. Daily cleansing of this wound along with the administration of systemic antibiotics and antiinflammatory agents are administered.

A more aggressive surgical treatment for arytenoid chondritis is a partial arytenoidectomy. In this

Laryngeal Hemiplegia, "Roaring"

Laryngeal Hemiplegia

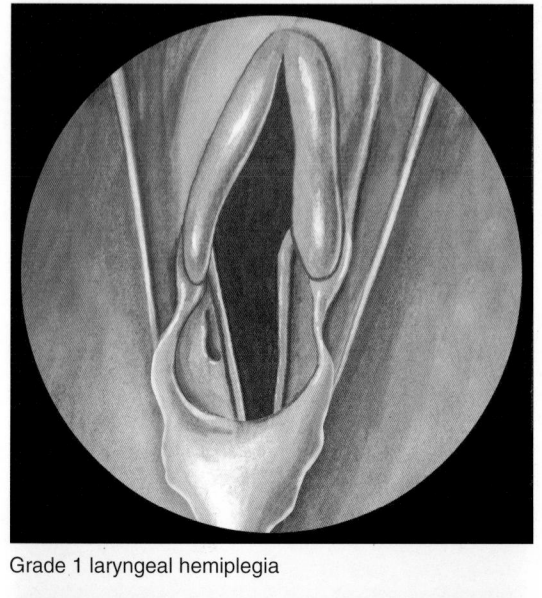

Grade 1 laryngeal hemiplegia

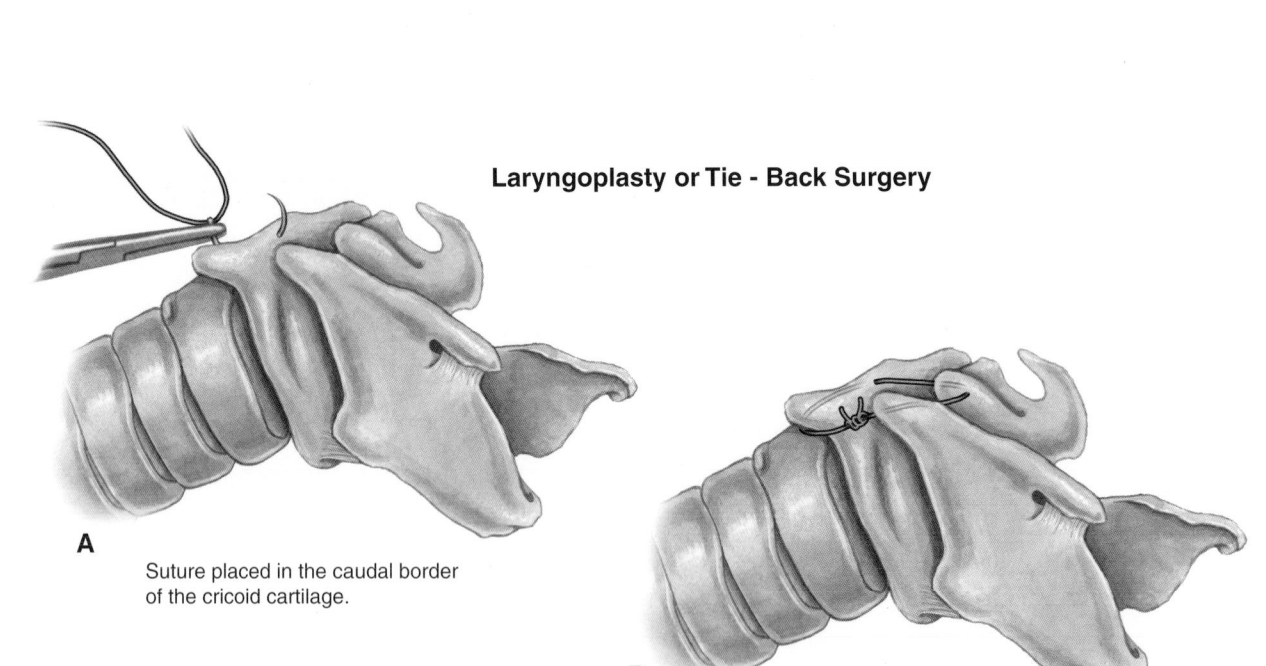

Stage 1   Stage 2   Stage 3

Roaring : Progressive Closure of Laryngeal Opening

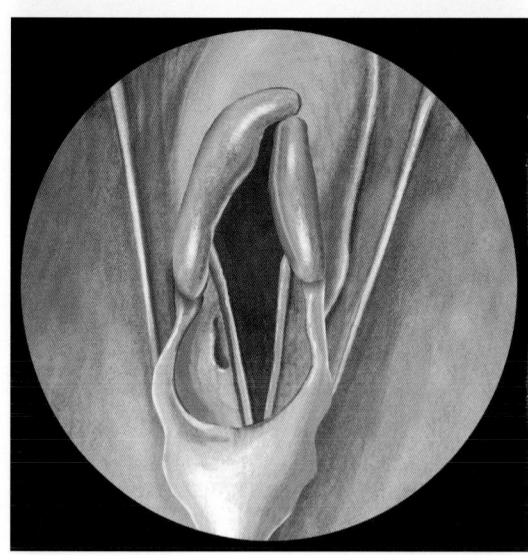

Grade 4 laryngeal hemiplegia: displacement of the left arytenoid cartilage toward the midline and shortening of the vocal cord.

Laryngoplasty or Tie - Back Surgery

A

Suture placed in the caudal border of the cricoid cartilage.

B

Completed suture pass through the muscular process and the cricoid cartilage prevents the arytenoid cartilage and vocal folds to intrude into the laryngeal lumen.

procedure, all of the cartilage is resected except for the muscular process. Postoperative coughing and difficulty in swallowing are expected. Care must be taken to monitor the horse for aspiration pneumonia. This procedure should be reserved for those animals that have difficulty breathing at rest and drastic treatment is required to provide some relief to the animal.

LARYNGEAL HEMIPLEGIA

Etiology

The cause of laryngeal hemiplegia is damage or irritation to the left recurrent laryngeal nerve. This results in denervation of the muscles of the larynx, in particular the cricoarytenoideus dorsalis, which is an abductor, and the cricoarytenoideus lateralis, which is an adductor muscle. The underlying cause to the irritation of the left recurrent laryngeal nerve may be from trauma, guttural pouch mycosis, neoplasia, organophosphate intoxication, lead poisoning, or poisoning from toxic plants. In some cases, there is also involvement of the right recurrent laryngeal nerve.

Clinical Signs

Laryngeal hemiplegia is referred to as "roaring" in performance horses. Initially, these animals will have a reduced capacity to perform, and then they develop a "whistling" noise during exercise. As the condition progresses, this whistling noise progresses to that of a roar. During the more progressive phases, the animal may exhibit a cough, signs of choking, or even gasping after light exercise. When the horse attempts to neigh, there is an impaired vocal ability with this condition.

Differential Diagnosis

1.) Epiglottic Entrapment
2.) Soft Palate Displacement
3.) Subepiglottic Cysts
4.) Laryngeal Chondritis

Diagnosis

Endoscopy is the most useful diagnostic tool in confirming laryngeal hemiplegia. There is the classic displacement of the arytenoid cartilage toward the midline and a shortening of the vocal fold. One will see a kink in the aryepiglottic fold and a failure by the left arytenoid cartilage to abduct. During the endoscopic examination, a slap test can be performed which will allow direct observation of the adductor function. The left thorax is slapped gently with the open hand which should result in the right muscular process adducting. When the right thorax is slapped gently, the muscular process of the left arytenoid cartilage should have the same motion. If the response is reduced or does not occur at all, it is a positive test for laryngeal hemiplegia.

Treatment

Surgical treatment should have the goal to create a larynx with minimal airflow turbulence and resistance. A combination of a laryngoplasty (tie back surgery) and a ventriculectomy will yield the best results. The goal of this is to prevent intrusion of the arytenoid cartilage and the vocal fold into the laryngeal lumen during exercise.

The animal is placed under general anesthesia, on its right side with its neck extended. The anatomical area over the left side of the larynx is surgically prepped. A 10 cm incision is made starting approximately 1 cm ventral to the linguofacial vein immediately cranial to its junction with the jugular vein. Utilizing blunt dissection and digital manipulation, the caudal border of the cricoid lamina is exposed which contains a prominence approximately 2 cm from the midline. These tissues are dissected free so that the cricoid arch and cartilage can be rotated outward. Sutures are then inserted behind the caudal border of the cricoid cartilage and advanced under the medial surface of this cartilage. Care should be taken to avoid penetration of the laryngeal lumen. Perforation of the lamina of the cartilage at least 2 cm rostral to its caudal margin is then accomplished. A flat instrument should be placed above the dorsal cricoarytenoid muscle which overlies the cricoid cartilage before the suture

needle penetrates this structure. This acts as a guard against possible penetration of the carotid artery or esophagus. A second suture is then placed in the cricoid cartilage. An incision is made with scissors between the thyropharyngeal and cricopharyngeal muscles to allow exposure to the muscular process of the arytenoid. This process is then dissected away from its surrounding fascia. A curved forceps is then passed close to the muscular process and caudally over the surface of the cricoid lamina. Both ends of the placed sutures are inserted within the jaws of this forceps and then retrieved. This procedure is repeated for the suture that was placed secondly. Using a 16 gauge hypodermic needle, a hole is drilled transversely through the muscular process. A length of twisted wire is then passed through the lumen of the needle. The sutures are placed through the end of the twisted wire, pulled through the muscular process, and retracted in a medial to lateral direction. Tension is then applied to these sutures, and they are then tied off.

The animal is repositioned in dorsal recumbency with its neck outstretched. The skin is surgically prepared so that an 8 cm incision can be made in the midline caudally from the caudal border of the mandible. The muscle tissues are divided on the midline and retracted. The triangular cricothyroid membrane is identified through palpation. An incision is made through this membrane and laryngeal mucosa. The left vocal fold is then identified. A Blattenburg bur is inserted into the left ventricle, then rotated and twisted in a rostromedial direction. Traction is applied until all the mucosa is removed from the ventricle. This entire incision is left to heal as an open wound.

Systemic antibiotics are administered before surgery and at least 5 - 7 days postoperatively. The incisions are cleaned several times a day and dressed with topical antibiotic ointment. Stall rest is recommended for at least four weeks. Periodic endoscopic examinations should be done before training is resumed.

Bacterial Pleuropneumonia

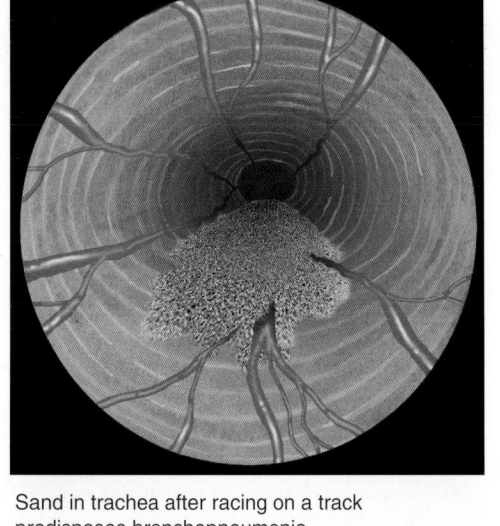

Sand in trachea after racing on a track
predisposes bronchopneumonia.

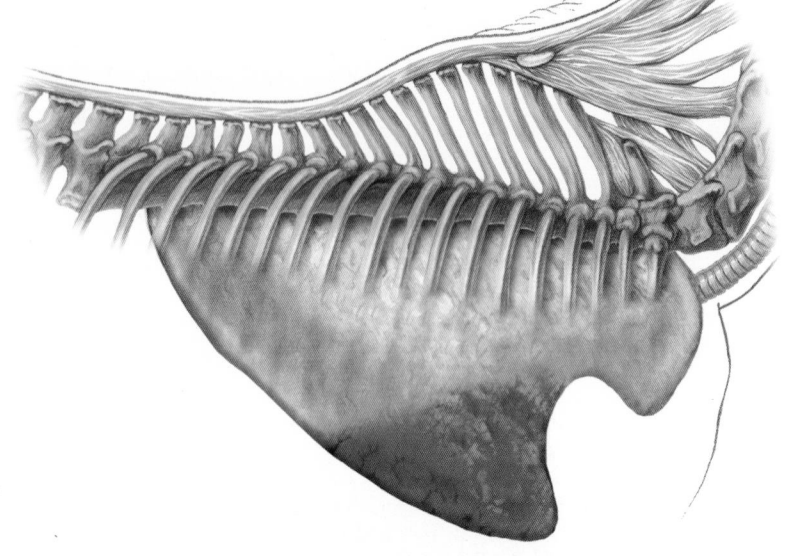

Consolidation of the ventral lung

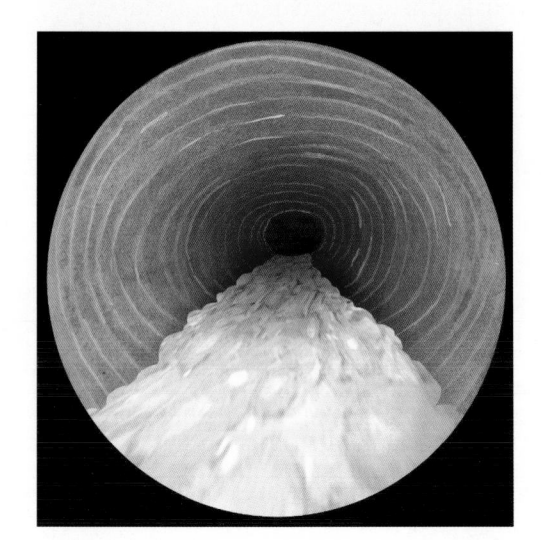

Purulent drainage in the trachea.

Transtracheal wash is utilized
to obtain secretions for culture.

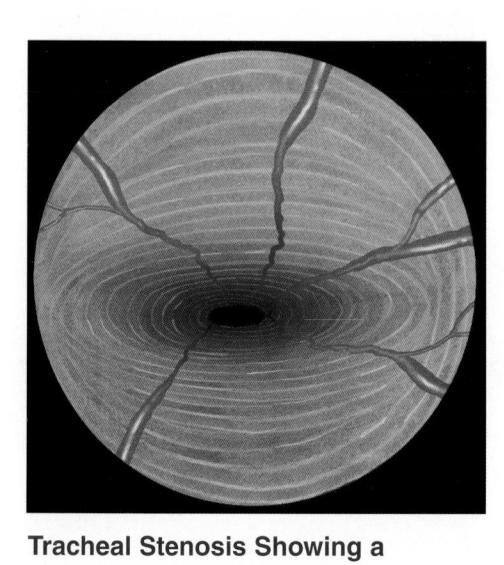

**Tracheal Stenosis Showing a
Narrowed Lumen as Seen in
an Endoscopic Examination**

TRACHEAL STENOSIS

Any narrowing or stricture of the tracheal lumen is referred to as tracheal stenosis.

Etiology

Severe mucosal hemorrhage results from prolonged endotracheal intubation during surgery. The cuff on the endotracheal tube may have provided pressure on these tissues which resulted in the formation of a stricture. *Streptococcus equi* abscesses on the lymph nodes may result in a narrow stricture formation within the trachea. Tumors such as lipomas are very rare, but could possibly result in the narrowing of the trachea.

Clinical Signs

In most cases, tracheal stenosis is an incidental finding. Coughing after exercise is the most common complaint for this disorder. The animal may perform poorly and have difficulty breathing in relation to exercise.

Differential Diagnosis

1.) Chronic Obstructive Pulmonary Disease
2.) Pneumonia
3.) Retropharyngeal Abscesses

Diagnosis

Palpation of the trachea may reveal a flattened area. Endoscopic examination of the trachea will exhibit a narrowed area, and lateral radiographs will show an area of stenosis.

Treatment

Treatment of tracheal stenosis is very difficult. Numerous surgical techniques have been proposed for treatment, but they involve many complications. Unless the animal is required to perform a considerable number of athletic endeavors, treatment should not be considered.

BACTERIAL PLEUROPNEUMONIA

Etiology

Bacterial pleuropneumonia is the result of bacterial organisms infecting and reproducing within the lung tissues which results in pneumonia, pulmonary abscesses, and pleural effusion (pleuritis). Bacterial pleuropneumonia is usually the sequelae of an immunocompromised event. This depressed defense mechanism is the result of stress or is secondary to a viral respiratory disease. Stress can include strenuous exercise, long-distance transport, poor ventilation, and aspiration of dust or dirt while racing.

There are four species of streptococci bacteria which result in infection of the lungs: *Streptococcus zooepidemicus*, *S. equi*, *S. suis*, and *S. pneumoniae*. *Rhodococcus equi* infection is the primary cause of pulmonary abscesses in foals 2 - 4 months of age. Numerous other bacterial organisms have been isolated and found to produce bacterial pleuropneumonia in both foals and young horses.

Clinical Signs

Clinical signs that are exhibited by these animals inflicted with bacterial pleuropneumonia are functions of the causative organisms of the infection. Initially, these animals will be intolerant to exercise, exhibit a weight loss, and have a cough. Fever, lethargy, and a nasal discharge will soon follow. As this condition progresses, the animals will start breathing with flared nostrils and show signs of sternal edema.

Differential Diagnosis

1. Viral Respiratory Infections
2. Chronic Obstructive Pulmonary Disease

Diagnosis

Initial auscultation of these animals will reveal "wheezes" and "gurgling" respiratory sounds. There may be areas that are absent of all lung sounds, because pleural effusion may be present that is obscuring these sounds. Percussion techniques will usually reveal a horizontal line on the thorax where resonant sounds are in evidence dorsally and dull sounds ventrally.

Ultrasonic examination of the thorax will show localization of the pleural effusion, fibrin, consolidation, and abscess formation. Linear array scanners should be utilized with a 3.5 - 5.0 MHz transducer. Radiographic studies will indicate the extent of the infection within the tissues. Radiograph films can often be misleading when pleural effusion is present, therefore obscuring many of the lesions.

Specimens should be collected and submitted to the laboratory for aerobic and anaerobic sensitivity testing. Transtracheal washing is the preferred method, because contamination by upper respiratory bacteria is eliminated. Pleural fluid samples can be collected utilizing a thoracentesis technique. These samples should also be submitted to the lab for culture and antibiotic sensitivity testing.

Treatment

Treatment should include aggressive systemic antibiotic therapy, the administration of bronchodilators and nonsteroidal anti-inflammatory drugs. Supportive care such as fluid therapy and the administration of vitamins may also be indicated. Initial systemic antibiotic treatment can be based on results of gram stains of the specimens gathered through transtracheal aspiration. Initial antimicrobial therapy may include penicillin, cephalosporins, and aminoglycocides. This antimicrobial therapy may be altered once bacterial culture and sensitivity results return from the laboratory.

An effective bronchodilator will reduce the respiratory effort required by these animals infected with acute bacterial pleuropneumonia.

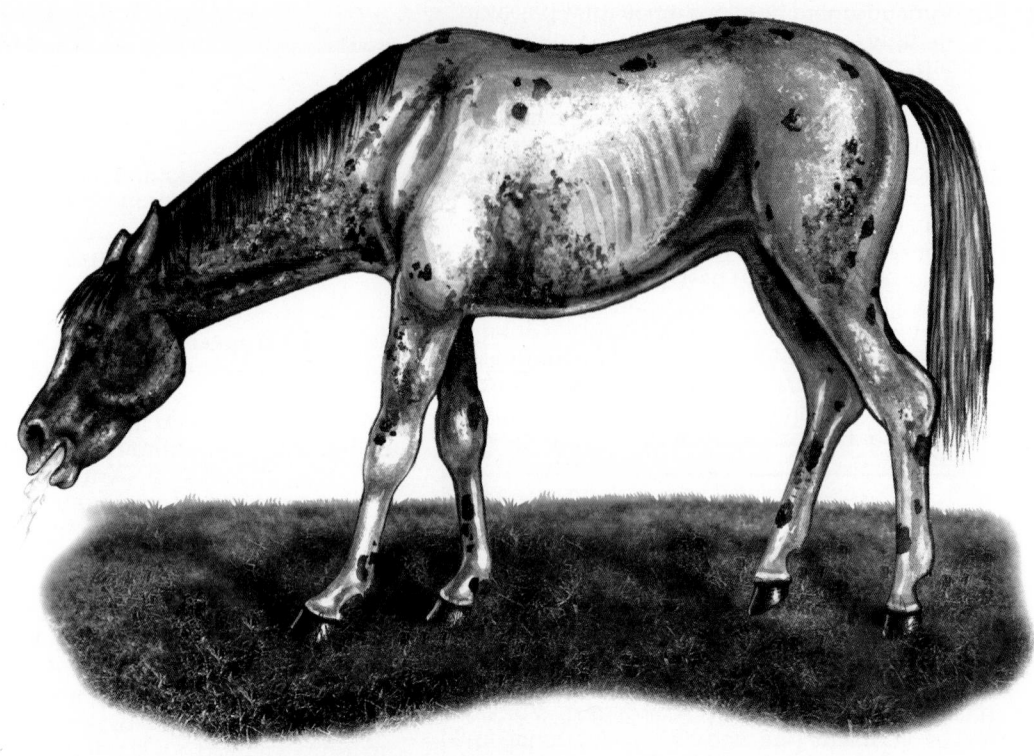

A depressed and coughing horse is a classic sign of viral pneumonia.

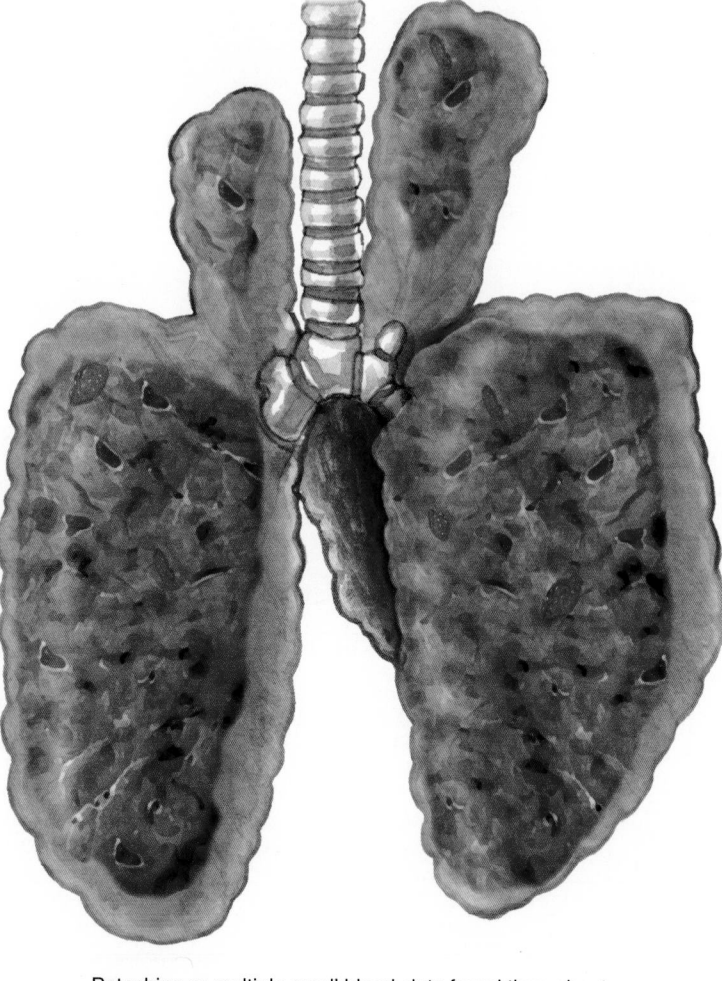

Petechiae or multiple small blood clots found throughout the lung parenchyma in viral pneumonia.

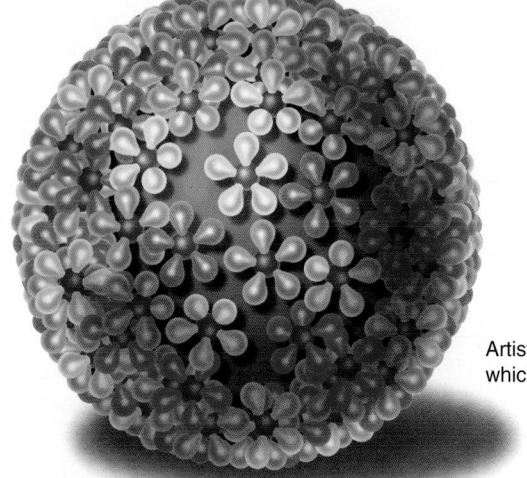

Artist's rendition of a virus particle which could cause a viral pneumonia.

The administration of bronchodilators will improve the clearance of the mucopurulent secretions from the lower airways. Administration of these bronchodilators, such as clenbuterol HCl, will also relieve bronchospasms that arise during the inflammatory reaction generated by the bacteria.

The administration of nonsteroidal anti-inflammatory drugs will allow the animal to be more comfortable and possibly increase its interest in the resumption of food and water intake. Care must be taken however, to not administer these medications in a way that would mask a fever generated by a failing antimicrobial regime. Nursing and supportive care should always be a component for horses with bacterial pleuropneumonia. High quality palatable food stuffs should be provided to encourage these animals to eat. Fresh water must be available at all times. The fluid and electrolyte needs of these horses may have to be supplemented intravenously.

VIRAL RESPIRATORY DISORDERS

Disorders of the respiratory system caused by viruses affect the equine industry worldwide. One cannot be a horse owner or trainer for a very long time without being confronted with a viral respiratory disorder.

Etiology

Numerous viral agents attack and result in respiratory disease and include: equine herpesviruses (of which there are five distinct types), influenza (A/equine I and II), rhinovirus, and equine arteritis virus. In most cases, these viral infections and resulting outbreaks among animals that are stabled together spread as a result of direct contact, aerosol, fomites, and even venereal pathways as in equine viral arteritis.

There are five types of equine herpesviruses. Equine herpesvirus type 1 (EHV-1) primarily attacks the respiratory system, but is also associated with abortion and sometimes

neurological disorders. Equine herpesvirus type 2 (EHV-2) can be found in most of the horse population but has never been linked to any particular disorder. Equine herpesvirus type 5 (EHV-5) can also be isolated from the majority of the horse population but has yet to be established as a causative agent for a disorder. Equine herpesvirus type 3 (EHV-3) results in coital exanthema and is transmitted venereally. The major cause of viral respiratory disorders is equine herpesvirus type 4 (EHV-4). EHV-4 is also associated with sporadic outbreaks of abortions.

Equine influenza is caused by two types of influenza A virus. These are designated A/equine 1 and A/equine 2. Influenza is a major viral disease of the horse. When any immunologically depressed animal is exposed to this virus, it usually manifests itself as a disease.

Equine rhinoviruses are very similar to the human rhinoviruses that result in the common cold. This has been identified as equine rhinovirus type 1 which is spread by direct contact and aerosol exposure.

Equine arteritis virus can be spread by the respiratory route, although venereal transmission is usually the route of contamination.

Clinical Signs

Viral respiratory disorders result in a variety of clinical signs dependent upon the type of virus involved, the age of the animal, and the level of the animal's immune system. Initially, these animals will be depressed, show no interest in food, and have a fever. As the virus progresses, they will develop a nasal discharge and a cough.

Clinical signs exhibited by EHV-1 and EHV-4 are usually characterized by a fever, inappetence, and depression. There is an initial serous nasal discharge that becomes mucopurulent as the virus progresses. Submandibular and retropharyngeal lymph nodes become enlarged. These animals may cough occasionally, but coughing is usually not a manifestation of this virus. Unfortunately, infections with EHV-1 or EHV-4 can be further complicated by neurological disorders and

abortions. The neurological manifestations may be only a mild incoordination, but can progress to hind limb ataxia and bladder incontinence.

The incubation time for equine influenza is very short. The onset of this virus is very sudden, characterized by a rapid elevation in body temperature and the development of a dry hacking cough. These animals immediately go off feed, become severely depressed, and exhibit severe muscle soreness. Secondary bacterial infections are very common resulting in bacterial pneumonia.

Equine rhinovirus infection is characterized by pyrexia, pharyngitis, and nasal discharge. The infection may be mild enough that the only symptom may be a diminished performance.

Equine viral arteritis may exhibit mild subclinical signs or range to severe symptoms. Abortion in these animals occurs mid-to-late gestation with these horses showing no other clinical abnormalities. Respiratory characteristics may include a nasal discharge, coughing, and/or respiratory distress.

Diagnosis

In most cases, identification of a specific virus is not performed because of the self-limiting nature of these agents. However, in the face of an outbreak, a specific diagnosis may be beneficial. Numerous serological testing techniques can be utilized to isolate and identify the causative agent. Compliment fixation tests and serum neutralization tests are utilized in the identification process.

Treatment

Treatment of these animals involves providing supportive and nursing care, and reducing the stress to the animal. An effort to minimize potential secondary problems should be the goal in handling these viral respiratory disorders. Infected horses should be isolated with sanitation procedures initiated to help stem the spread of the virus. Systemic antibiotics need to be given in the acute stage of this disorder to prevent

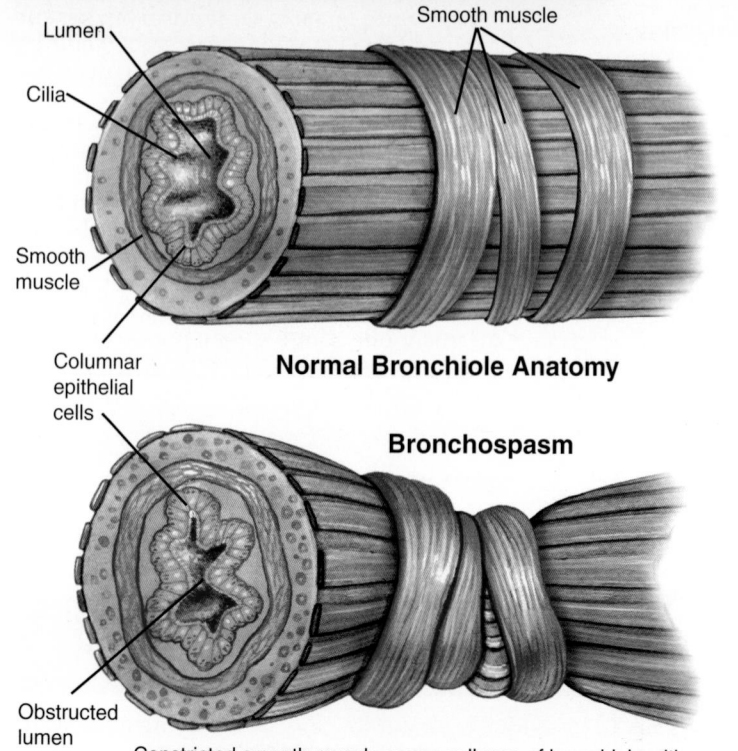

Lumen

Cilia

Smooth muscle

Smooth muscle

Normal Bronchiole Anatomy

Columnar epithelial cells

Bronchospasm

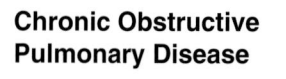

Obstructed lumen

Constricted smooth muscle cause collapse of bronchiole with subsequent partial-to-complete obstruction of the lumen.

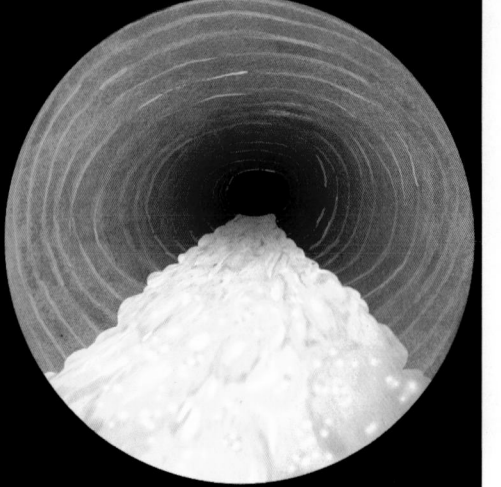

Endoscopic view of mucous secretions in trachea as seen in COPD

Chronic Obstructive Pulmonary Disease

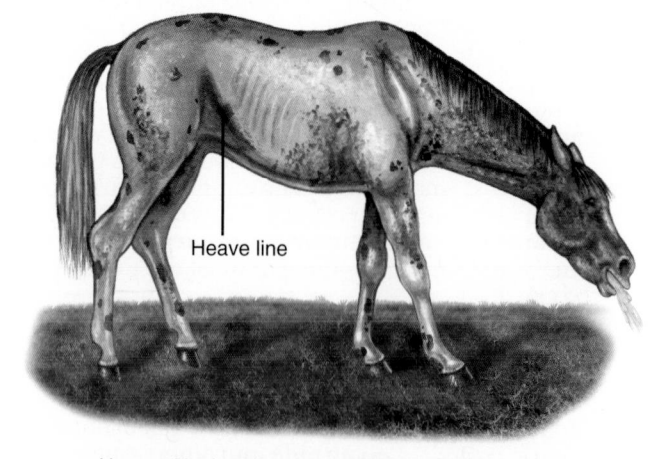

Heave line

Horse with chronic cough and "heave line" caused by hypertrophy of the external abdominal oblique muscles.

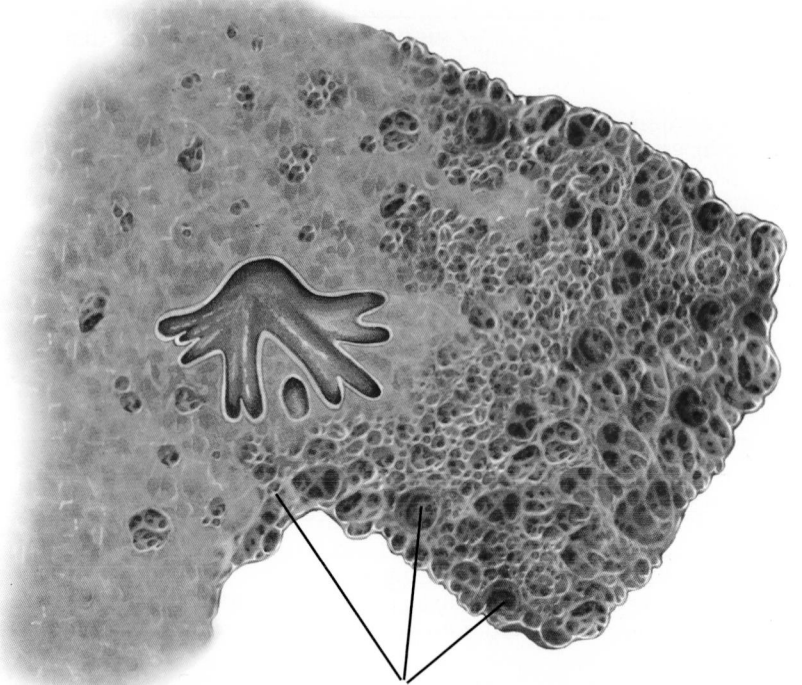

Saccular lesions in apex of lung tissue contribute to decreased lung expansion during inspiration.

secondary bacterial infections. Nonsteroidal anti-inflammatory drugs should be utilized in those animals that have a fever. Bronchodilator drugs such as clenbuterol have therapeutic considerations that may be beneficial. In all cases, supportive therapy such as fluid and electrolyte replacement should be considered to hasten the recovery and reduce the stress on these animals.

Prophylaxis

Vaccines have been developed for EHV-1, EHV-4, equine influenza A/1 and 2, and equine viral arteritis. Vaccination of pregnant mares with EHV-1 at 5, 7, and 9 months of gestation reduces the incidence of abortions due to infections with this virus. Other vaccinations are effective in reducing the severity of signs, the degree of viral shedding, and the extent of the spread of the disease. Overvaccination however, has not been proven to be beneficial in totally preventing these viral disorders. Reducing the stress to these animals and providing a clean well-ventilated environment is probably the best mechanism for reducing the incidence and severity of viral respiratory problems.

CHRONIC OBSTRUCTIVE PULMONARY DISEASE

Chronic obstructive pulmonary disease, or "COPD," is a condition that is referred to commonly as heaves, broken wind, emphysema, chronic bronchitis, and recurrent airway obstruction. This disorder is found mainly in older horses that are kept in the colder climates. The reason behind the predisposition for colder climates is that these horses are usually kept in a stall for some part of the year which allows exposure to more dust, hay, and straw.

Etiology

The etiology of COPD is unknown. It is an inflammatory condition of the lower airways that also includes bronchospasms and changes within the bronchiolar walls which results in terminal airway obstruction. It is theorized that this is caused by a hypersensitivity reaction to specific antigens, a nonspecific hyper-reactivity reaction, or is merely an inflammatory reaction that is induced by dust. Some infectious disease may predispose the hypersensitivity and hyper-reactivity reactions by damaging the tissues within the airways and altering the immune responses. Viral respiratory infections oftentimes have the development of COPD as a complication.

Clinical Signs

The first complaint that will be heard is that the animal is becoming exercise intolerant. As the condition progresses, occasional coughing at the onset of exercise or while eating will be present. Further progression of this condition will lead to an increased respiratory effort and dyspnea. The nostrils will flare and a double expiratory effort will become evident. When the condition becomes chronic, the animal will loose weight, and a "heave line" will develop caused by the hypertrophy of the external abdominal oblique muscles.

Differential Diagnosis

1.) Bacterial Pleuropneumonia
2.) Viral Respiratory Disease
3.) Laryngeal Hemiplegia

Diagnosis

In the early stages when the animal is auscultated, normal sounds within the thorax will be heard. When the animal is forced to breathe deeply, wheezes and expiratory crackles can be heard along the periphery of the lungs. As the disease progresses, wheezing can be heard in the trachea and throughout the entire lung field. Endoscopic examination of the respiratory tract will reveal a large amount of mucus in the trachea. Examination of the lower airways will reveal hyperemic and edematous tissues throughout. A bronchoalveolar lavage should be conducted to obtain fluid for cytological evaluation which will confirm the presence of lower airway inflammation. This sample should also be examined for the presence of bacteria since these animals are predisposed to infection. There will be a neutrophilia within this lavage sample.

Treatment

There are three goals to treating COPD: 1.) to eliminate all dust from the animal's environment; 2.) to provide antiinflammatory medications for the treatment of the tissues of the lower airways; and 3.) to provide immediate symptomatic relief.

Any effort to prevent further exposure to dust should be undertaken. Hay can be replaced with pelleted hay or hay silage. If this is not possible, the hay should be soaked in water for at least a half an hour before feeding. This is often a difficult managerial procedure, but in some cases, it will induce clinical remission of the disorder. Straw can be replaced with wood shavings, shredded paper, or peat moss. If possible, it is important to move the horse out of a stall where hay stored overhead or a very dusty ceiling. The ventilation to the entire barn should be examined and improvements made when possible.

The administration of antiinflammatory drugs will decrease the inflammation within the lower airways. Nonsteroidal antiinflammatory drugs may be used, but unfortunately they are not as effective as the corticosteroids. Dexamethasone and prednisone are the usual drugs of choice in the treatment of this inflammatory condition. Care must be taken to use the minimum effective dose. Prolonged administration of these drugs should be avoided.

Inhalation therapy may be beneficial in the treatment of COPD. Corticosteroids and other medications such as expectorants and mucolytic agents can be administered through this means. Aggressive inhalation therapy should be undertaken for at least four days before determining that it is providing relief, or a decision is made to discontinue it. This type of therapy can also be used if there is an acute episode of inflammation within the horse to help bring it under control.

The administration of bronchodilators should be combined with environmental dust control and antiinflammatory therapy. Bronchodilators will aid in giving immediate relief in some of the clinical signs because of their rapid onset of action.

THE RESPIRATORY SYSTEM

Exercise - Induced Pulmonary Hemorrhage

Progressive Stages of Exercise-Induced Pulmonary Hemorrhage as seen on Endoscopic Examination

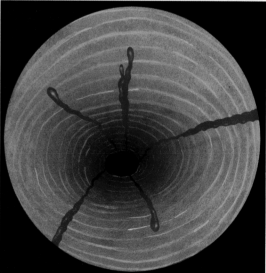

Stage 1: Small trickles of active bleeding.

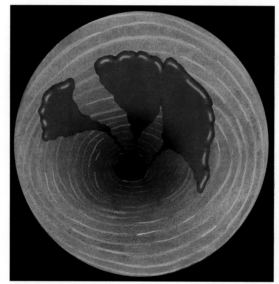

Stage 2: Heavier flow of blood accumulating in tracheal and bronchiole pasages.

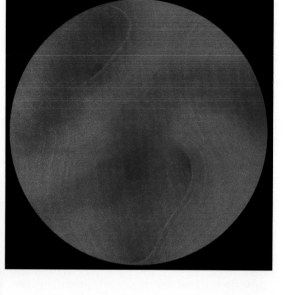

Stage 3: Massive hemorrhage obliterating visual field during endoscopy.

Dorsal view of lungs shows areas most commonly affected with EIPH

Epistaxis or bleeding from the nostrils may be the only noticeable symptom.

Clenbuterol is a bronchodilator that increases mucociliary transport, increases mucous secretions, and relieves bronchospasms.

The administration of expectorants increases pulmonary secretions, whereas mucolytic agents loosen the secretions. Any agent that increases the clearance of respiratory tract secretions is termed mucokinetic. Clenbuterol has both bronchodilator and mucokinetic properties allowing it to aid in the clearance of mucus from the airways. Potassium iodide will improve the clearance of bronchial secretions, but is also irritating to the respiratory tract and can induce bronchospasms. Antitussive agents should not be administered because the animal's ability to cough is its own mechanism for clearing the respiratory tract of secretions.

EXERCISE-INDUCED PULMONARY HEMORRHAGE

Exercised-induced pulmonary hemorrhage (EIPH) is a common disorder among performance horses and is characterized by the presence of blood in the airways after exercise. The more intense the exercise performed by the animal, the higher the incidence of EIPH. Thoroughbreds and quarter horses have an incidence between 50 and 75%. Standardbreds have an incidence of 40 - 60%. This also occurs in jumpers, polo ponies, ropers, and even in the draft horses that compete in pulling competitions. The hemorrhage that is present within the airways originates in the lung tissue.

Etiology

There are several hypotheses that have been suggested as to the cause of EIPH. One of the most believable explanations suggests that there is small airway disease present which predisposes the animal to EIPH. Airway obstruction from this small airway disease would result in forces on the lung tissue that are subtended by these airways. Therefore, the blood vessels within these lung segments would be subjected to an increase in the local paravascular blood pressure. This increased pressure is sufficient during exercise to produce vessel rupture and subsequent hemorrhage.

Clinical Signs

Since EIPH is a hemorrhage from the lungs as a consequence of exercise, epistaxis (bleeding from the nostrils), is the most evident clinical sign. Unfortunately about 5% of the affected horses exhibit epistaxis either during or at the end of their event. Other than this epistaxis, the animal usually exhibits no other clinical signs of lung disease.

Differential Diagnosis

1.) Viral Respiratory Disease
2.) Chronic Obstructive Pulmonary Disease
3.) All other disorders that produce exercise
    intolerance

Diagnosis

Endoscopic examination of the airway provides a definitive diagnosis of EIPH. This endoscopic exam should be done within thirty minutes after exercise. It is often necessary to endoscopically examine far down into the bronchial tree to see evidence of EIPH in the early stages. If an endoscope is unavailable, a transtracheal lavage or a bronchoalveolar lavage will demonstrate blood cells in the aspirated fluid.

Treatment

There are a number of management and therapeutic approaches that are undertaken to reduce or prevent EIPH. Unfortunately, few of these procedures or regimes have scientific justification for their efficacy.

The classic treatment for prevention of EIPH is furosemide. This medication is given prerace at the rate of 250 - 500 mg intravenously 1 - 4 hours before the event. Furosemide attenuates pulmonary capillary pressure. If the increased stress and pressure on the pulmonary capillaries predisposes the animal to EIPH, then a reduction in this pulmonary capillary pressure should reduce EIPH. Unfortunately, furosemide does not prevent EIPH in more than 50% of the horses to which it is administered. This medication's effect on racing times is still a matter of controversy.

There have been a number of other medications that have been suggested for the treatment of EIPH. These include bronchodilators, estrogen, coagulants, and even feed additives such as hesperidine.

Low level light therapy is currently being investigated as a possible treatment for EIPH. The preliminary results seem very encouraging, and its efficacy for this disorder appears to be quite high. If this modality is as successful in EIPH as it is in treatment of wounds and other soft tissue injuries, there may finally be an available modality that can manage this disorder.

THE NERVOUS SYSTEM

Anatomy of the Brain

Artwork by S. Hakola / J. Dirig
Copyright Equistar Publications, Ltd.

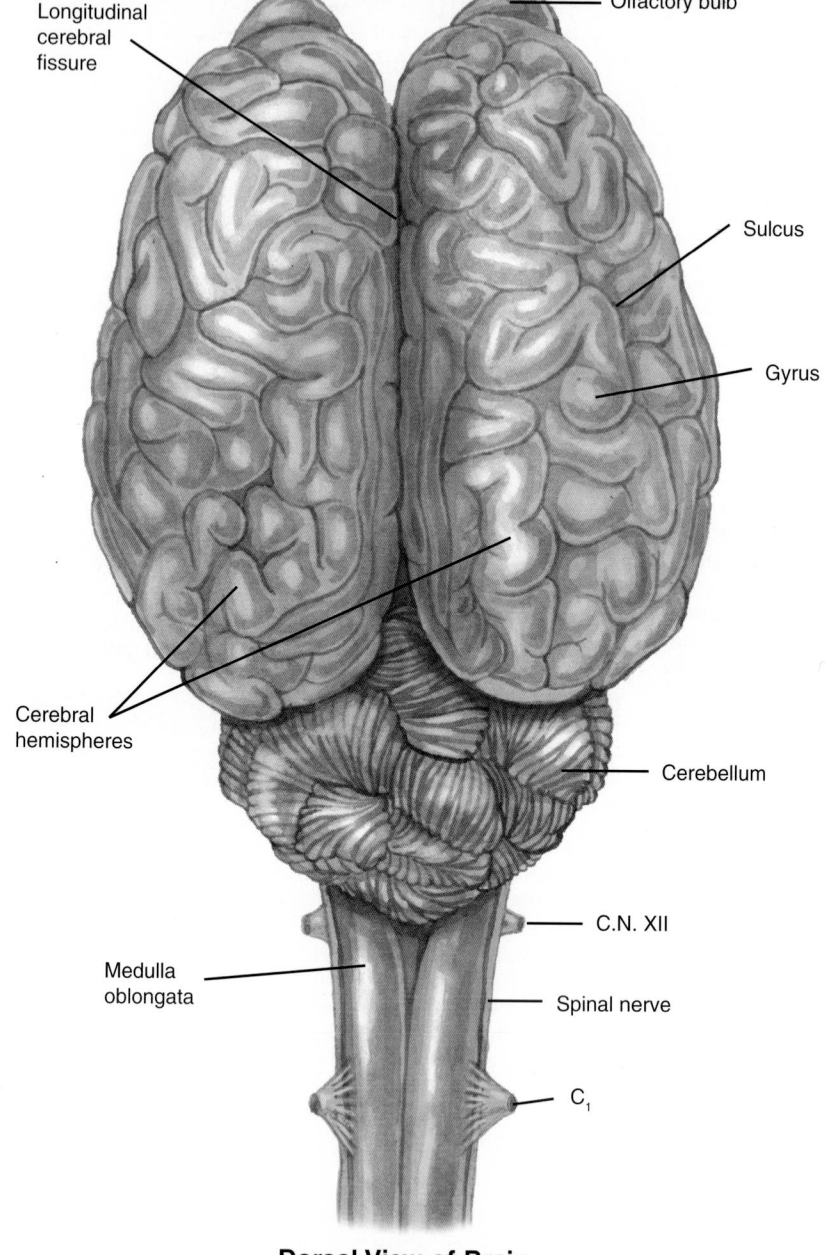

Longitudinal cerebral fissure

Olfactory bulb

Sulcus

Gyrus

Cerebral hemispheres

Cerebellum

C.N. XII

Medulla oblongata

Spinal nerve

C₁

Dorsal View of Brain

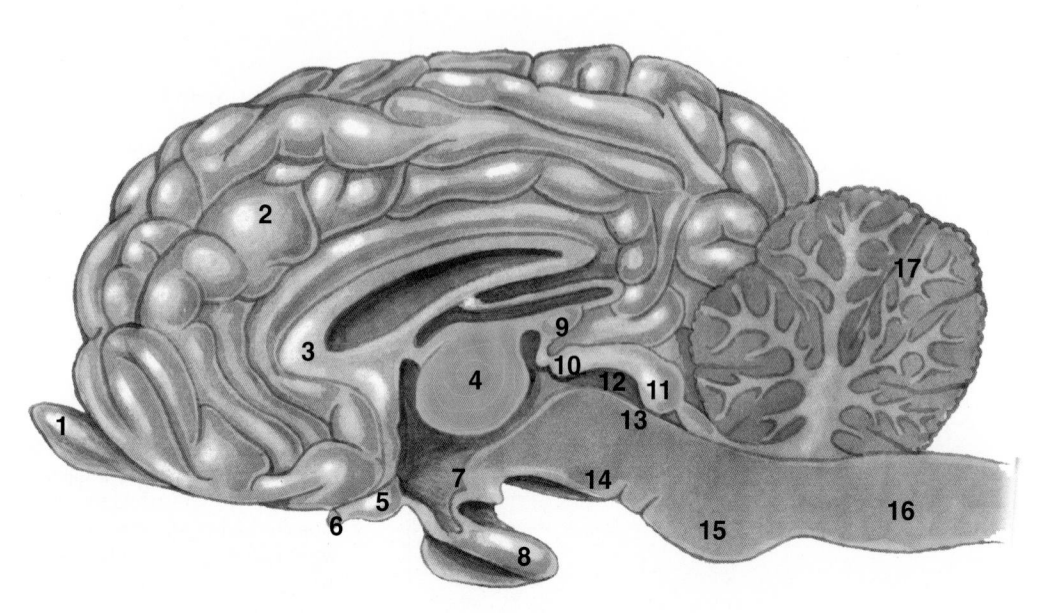

Median Section Showing Right Half of Brain

1. Olfactory bulb
2. Right cerebral hemisphere ⎤
3. Corpus callosum ⎦ Telencephalon

4. Thalamus
5. Optic chiasm
6. Optic nerve (C.N.II)
7. Hypothalamus
8. Pituitary gland ⎦ Diencephalon
9. Pineal gland

10. Rostral colliculus ⎤
11. Caudal colliculus ⎦ Tectum
12. Aqueduct
13. Tegmentum
14. Crus cerebri
15. Pons ⎦ Mesencephalon
16. Medulla oblongata ⎦ Rhombencephalon
17. Cerebellum

8 The Nervous System

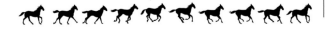

The nervous system is the most complicated system of the body. It functions as a complex mechanism that allows the organism to functionally relate to its environment. It is divided into two primary parts: the central and peripheral nervous systems. The brain and spinal cord comprise the central nervous system, whereas the peripheral nervous system is composed of the cranial and spinal nerves, their ganglia, and the autonomic nervous system.

THE CENTRAL NERVOUS SYSTEM

The Brain

The brain is that part of the central nervous system that is located within the cranial cavity and anatomically conforms to the cavity's size and shape. The brain of the horse weighs between 400 and 700 grams. This represents a ratio of 1:800 when compared to total body weight. The ratio in the dog is about 1:100. Therefore, when comparing body weight, the horse has a relatively small brain.

The brain of the horse can be divided into four parts: the rhombencephalon, the mesencephalon, the diencephalon, and the telencephalon.
The dorsal part or hindbrain is termed the rhombencephalon. This structure is comprised of the medulla oblongata, the pons, and the cerebellum. The medulla oblongata and pons form successive portions of the brain stem. Many of the cranial nerves originate on the ventral surface of the medulla oblongata. The trigeminal, the abducent, the facial, the vestibulocochlear, the glossopharyngeal, the vagus, the accessory, and the hypoglossal nerves all arise from this ventral surface. The pons is that part of the brain stem which is separated from the medulla and cerebral peduncles by the anterior and posterior grooves. The cerebellum is located in the posterior fossa of the cranium and is separated from the cerebral hemispheres by a transverse fissure and the tentorium cerebelli. The fourth ventricle is the

cavity of the rhombencephalon which communicates with the central canal of the spinal cord behind and through the cerebral aqueduct with the third ventricle in front.

The mesencephalon is often referred to as the midbrain. It connects the rhombencephalon with the forebrain. Ventrally, the midbrain exhibits the divergent crura cerebri, the interpeduncular fossa, and the origin of the oculomotor nerves. Dorsally, it is in direct opposition with the cerebral hemispheres and the cerebellum. It contains a lumen called the aqueduct which allows communication between the third and fourth ventricles. The tectum lies just dorsal to the aqueduct and is featured with four rounded surface swellings. The paired caudal swellings are referred to as the caudal colliculi. The paired rostral colliculi are closer together. The core of the midbrain is continuous with the corresponding stratum of the metencephalon and is comprised of tegmentum.

The most rostral part of the brain stem is termed the diencephalon. Dorsally, this structure connects with the large cerebral hemispheres through fibrous tracts. The most ventral portion of this division is the hypothalamus which is divided into three parts: the epithalamus, the thalamus, and the hypothalamus. The thalamus is the largest portion of the diencephalon. It is composed of a large number of nuclei that have specific functions and together form the most important relay and integration center of the brain stem. The epithalamus is the most dorsal portion of the diencephalon and includes the pineal gland which is a small, ovoid, red-brown mass that is believed to function as the center for sexual development and behavior. The hypothalamus forms the lower portion of the lateral walls of the third ventricle. It contains a number of nuclei associated with the visceral nervous system and hormonal regulation.

The largest part of the brain is the telencephalon. It is comprised mostly of the cerebral hemispheres. The surface of this structure is fissured by a large number of alternating ridges, called gyri, and grooves, which are called sulci. The olfactory bulbs are rostral to the cerebral hemispheres. The olfactory peduncles give rise to the olfactory bulbs

Ventral Anatomy of the Brain: The Cranial Nerves and the Cranial Vessels

Artwork by S. Hakola / J. Dirig
Copyright Equistar Publications, Ltd.

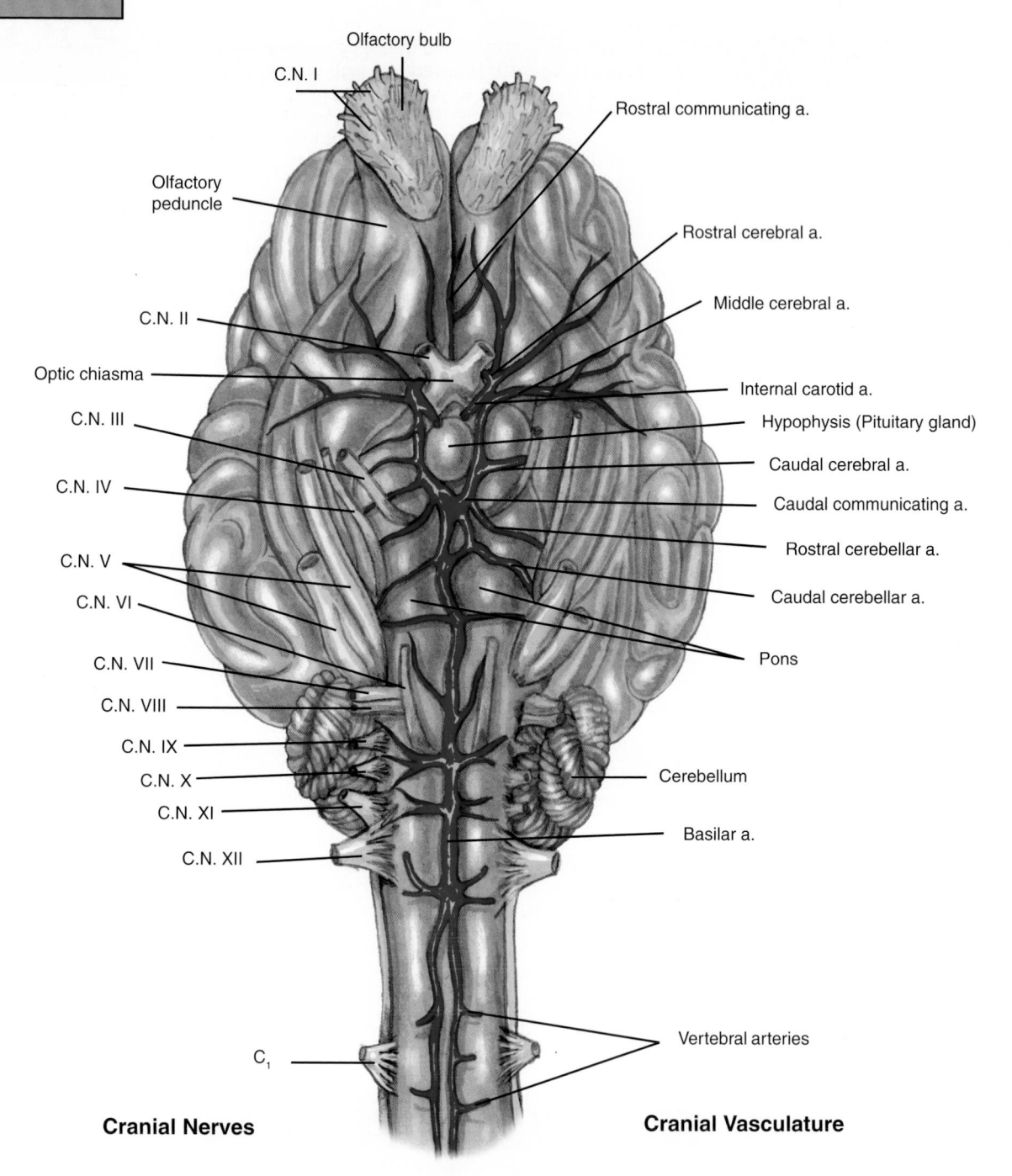

Olfactory bulb

C.N. I

Olfactory peduncle

C.N. II

Optic chiasma

C.N. III

C.N. IV

C.N. V

C.N. VI

C.N. VII

C.N. VIII

C.N. IX

C.N. X

C.N. XI

C.N. XII

C_1

Rostral communicating a.

Rostral cerebral a.

Middle cerebral a.

Internal carotid a.

Hypophysis (Pituitary gland)

Caudal cerebral a.

Caudal communicating a.

Rostral cerebellar a.

Caudal cerebellar a.

Pons

Cerebellum

Basilar a.

Vertebral arteries

Cranial Nerves

Cranial Vasculature

which give rise to the bundles of olfactory fibers.

There is a lumen or ventricular system to the brain. It extends from the interior of the olfactory bulbs through an array of ventricles and interconnecting ducts to the spinal cord. The largest invagination of this system is the fourth ventricle. This is located ventral to the cerebellum. The third ventricle lies rostral to the pineal gland, and two lateral ventricles send extensions into the olfactory bulbs.

The blood supply to the brain arises from the ventral surface. The arteries of the brain are derived chiefly from the internal carotid and occipital arteries. The basilar artery is formed by the union of the right and left cerebral branches of the occipital artery. This enters the cranial cavity through the foramen magnum. This basilar artery then divides at the interpeduncular fossa into the two posterior cerebral arteries. These cerebral arteries combine with branches of the internal carotid arteries to form an arterial circle on the base of the cerebrum. These basilar arteries then ascend from the circle to supply the general brain stem and basal ganglia. Cortical arteries run superficially and supply the cortical and medullary substances. Venous drainage enters sinuses of the dura mater which communicate with the ophthalmic, the dorsal and ventral cerebral, and the spinal veins.

The Cranial Nerves

There are twelve pairs of cranial nerves that are sequentially numbered cranially to caudally. The cranial nerves, listed by number, name, and functional characteristics are as follows:

I.	The olfactory nerve	sensory
II.	The optic nerve	sensory
III.	The oculomotor nerve	motor
IV.	The trochlear nerve	motor
V.	The trigeminal nerve	mixed
VI.	The abducent nerve	motor
VII.	The facial nerve	mixed
VIII.	The vestibulocochlear nerve	sensory
IX.	The glossopharyngeal nerve	mixed
X.	The vagus nerve	mixed
XI.	The spinal accessory nerve	motor
XII.	The hypoglossal nerve	motor

The **olfactory nerve (C.N. I)** is unique in that the fibers that comprise it do not form a trunk. These fibers ascend as central processes of the olfactory cells in the nasal mucosa. They are then collected into bundles that separately traverse the cribiform plate to join the adjacent surface of the olfactory bulb. These bundles or filaments are surrounded by sheaths that enclose the extensions of the subarachnoid space. These sheaths unfortunately provide a route of infection directly from the nasal cavities to that of the cranial cavities.

The **optic nerve (C.N. II)** is responsible for the transportation of stimuli from the retina to the diencephalon. Fibers from the retina converge within the eye to form the optic papillae where they collect into a round trunk referred to as the optic nerve. This emerges from the eye and passes backward and medially through the optic foramen. After passage through the optic foramen, it joins with its pair from the opposite side to form the optic chiasma.

The **oculomotor nerve (C.N. III)** arises from the basal surface of the cerebral peduncle. It contains somatic efferent fibers from the motor nucleus and visceral efferent fibers from the parasympathetic nucleus. These fibers supply the rectus dorsalis, the rectus medialis, the rectus ventralis, the levator palpebrae superioris, and the ventral oblique muscles.

The smallest of the cranial nerves is the **trochlear nerve (C.N. IV)**. It is a small motor nerve that supplies the dorsal oblique muscle. It arises from the anterior cerebellar peduncle and curves outward and forward through the cranium via a small foramen immediately above the orbital foramen.

The largest of the cranial nerves is the **trigeminal nerve (C.N. V)**. This nerve contains a large sensory portion and a smaller motor portion. The sensory portion supplies sensations to the skin and deeper tissues of the face, whereas the motor portion supplies the muscles of the first mandibular arch. The trigeminal nerve divides into three branches: the ophthalmic nerve, the maxillary nerve, and the mandibular nerve.

The opthalmic nerve is the smallest of the three branches of the trigeminal nerve. It is purely sensory in function. It has three branches itself, which are the lacrimal nerve, the frontal nerve, and the nasociliary nerve.

The maxillary nerve is larger than the ophthalmic and is purely sensory in function. It divides into the following branches: the zygomatic nerve, the sphenopalatine nerve, and the infraorbital nerve. These branches supply sensory innervation to the lower eyelid, the skin, the nasal cavity, the maxillary sinuses, and the palate.

The mandibular nerve is the result of the union of two roots. The large sensory root arises from the semilunar ganglion and the small motor root is the pars minor of the trigeminal nerve. It gives off the following branches: the massenteric nerve, the deep temporal nerves, the buccinator nerve, the pterygoid nerve, the superficial temporal nerve, the mandibular alveolar nerve, and the lingual nerve.

The fibers of the **abducent nerve (C.N. VI)** originate within the caudal brain stem, pass forward across the pons, and emerge through the orbital foramen. This nerve provides innervation to the rectus lateralis and retractor muscles of the eyeball. When there is damage to this nerve, the animal has the inability to deviate the eyeball laterally.

The **facial nerve (C.N. VII)** arises superficially immediately behind the pons. It divides into numerous branches which provides sensory and motor innervation to the facial region. The following collateral branches arise from the facial nerve: the greater petrosal nerve which has parasympathetic and sympathetic fibers, the stapedial nerve which supplies the stapedius muscle of the middle ear, the chorda tympani which mediates the sense of taste, the posterior auricular nerve which supplies the auricular muscles and skin of the external ear, the internal auricular nerve which supplies the skin of the concave surface of the ear, the digastric branch (the auriculopalpebral) which supplies the anatomical area of the eye, the cervical branch which receives cutaneous branches from the second to the sixth

THE NERVOUS SYSTEM

Anatomy of the Spinal Cord

Artwork by S. Hakola / J. Dirig
Copyright Equistar Publications, Ltd.

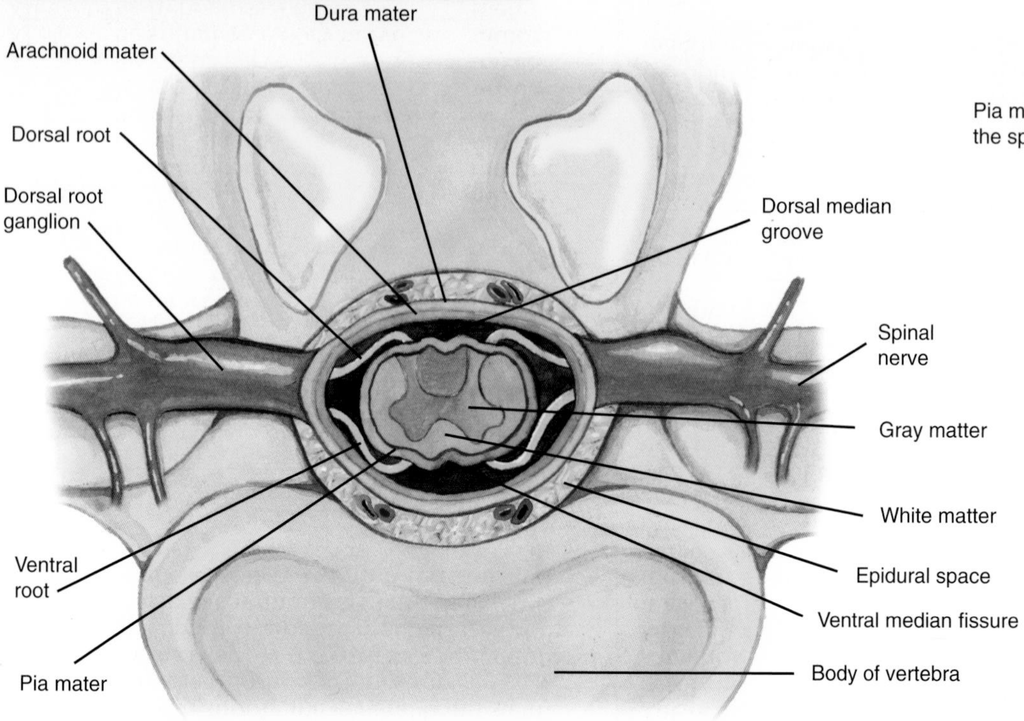

Cross Section of Spinal Cord Through Vertebra

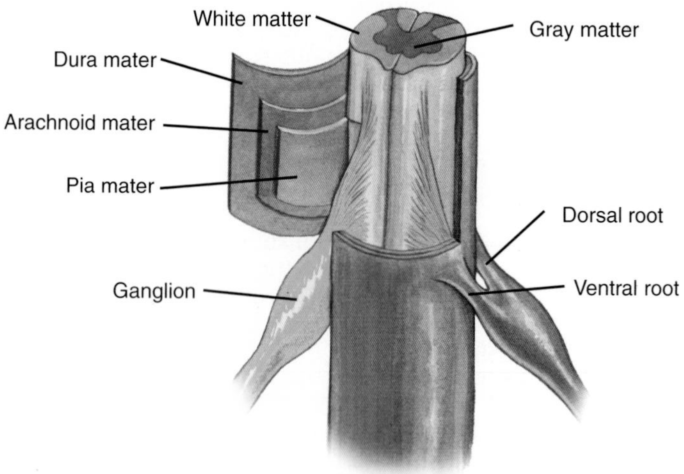

- Dura mater
- Arachnoid mater
- Dorsal root
- Dorsal root ganglion
- Dorsal median groove
- Spinal nerve
- Gray matter
- White matter
- Epidural space
- Ventral median fissure
- Body of vertebra
- Ventral root
- Pia mater

Meninges Covering the Spinal Cord

- White matter
- Gray matter
- Dura mater
- Arachnoid mater
- Pia mater
- Ganglion
- Dorsal root
- Ventral root

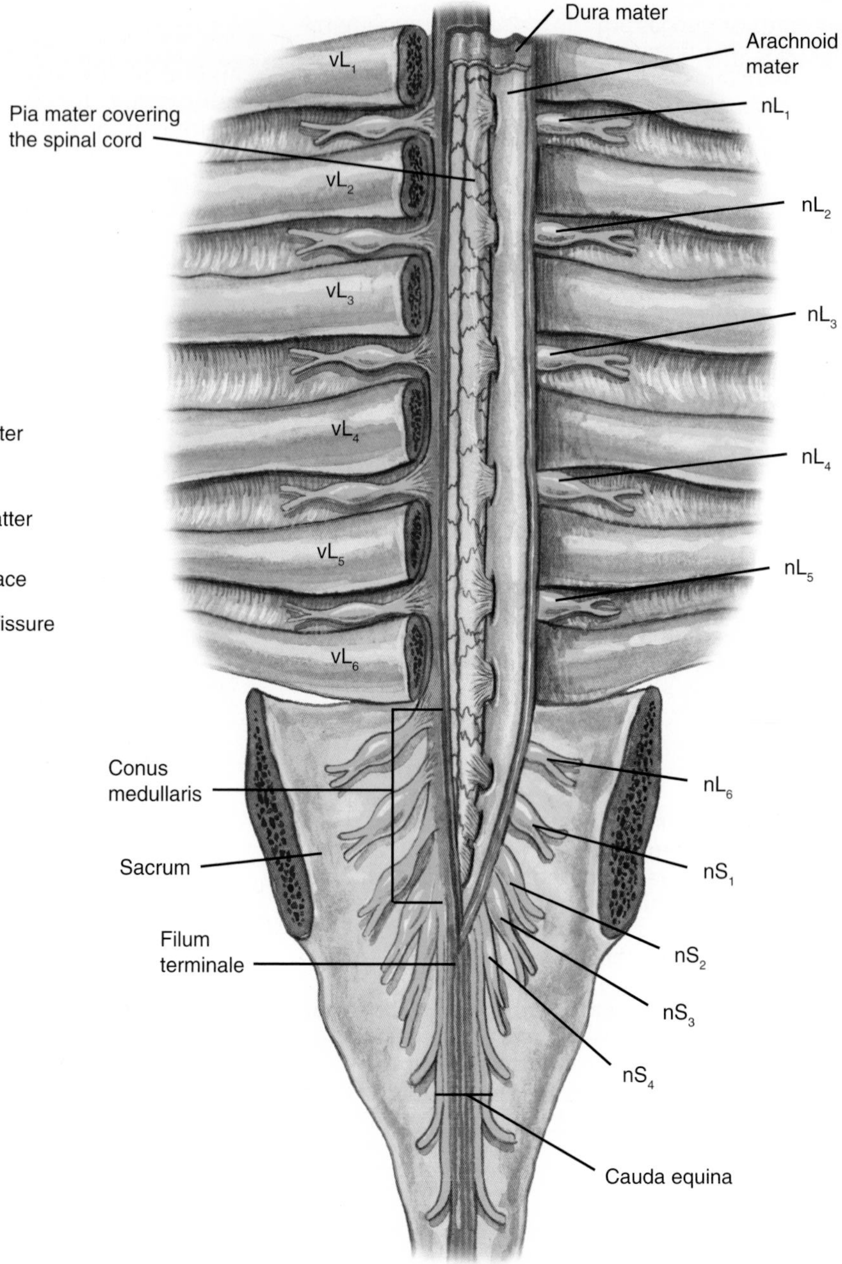

Dorsal View of Lumbosacral Nerves, Conus Medullaris, and Cauda Equina

- Dura mater
- Arachnoid mater
- Pia mater covering the spinal cord
- vL_1
- vL_2
- vL_3
- vL_4
- vL_5
- vL_6
- nL_1
- nL_2
- nL_3
- nL_4
- nL_5
- Conus medullaris
- Sacrum
- Filum terminale
- nL_6
- nS_1
- nS_2
- nS_3
- nS_4
- Cauda equina

cervical nerves, and the dorsal buccal and the ventral buccal nerves which supply innervation to the upper and lower lip and nostrils.

The **vestibulocochlear nerve (C.N. VIII)** originates from the lateral aspect of the medulla just behind and lateral to the facial nerve. Branches of this vestibulocochlear nerve help mediate the sense of balance and the ability to hear.

The **glossopharyngeal nerve (C.N. IX)** rises from the ventrolateral aspect of the medulla oblongata. It divides into the following branches: the tympanic nerve which forms a plexus with the facial and internal carotid nerves to supply the otic ganglion and the parotid gland, the carotid sinus branch which terminates in baroreceptors within the sinus walls and a chemoreceptor of the carotid body, the pharyngeal branch which supplies the pharyngeal musculature, and the linguinal branch, which provides sensory innervation to the mucosa at the root of the tongue. Damage to this nerve, especially to the linguinal branch due to inflammation within the guttural pouch, will lead to difficulties in swallowing.

The longest and most widely distributed of the cranial nerves is the **vagus nerve (C.N. X)**. It contains the parasympathetic fibers that innervate the cervical, thoracic, and abdominal viscera. The vagus branches into: the pharyngeal branch, the anterior or cranial laryngeal nerve, the recurrent laryngeal nerve, the cardiac branches, the tracheal and esophageal branches, and the bronchial branches.

The functions of the **spinal accessory nerve (C.N. XI)** are purely motor. The dorsal branch supplies innervation to the splenius, serratus ventralis, brachiocephalicus, omotransversarius, and trapezius muscles. The ventral branch supplies only one muscle, the sternocephalicus.

The **hypoglossal nerve (C.N. XII)** is also purely motor in function, since it innervates both the intrinsic and extrinsic muscles of the tongue. Any irritation or damage to this nerve usually results in paralysis of some of these muscles, which results in a deviation of the tongue toward the normal side.

The Spinal Cord

The vertebral canal contains that part of the central nervous system which is referred to as the spinal cord. This section of nervous tissue is approximately 75 - 80 inches in length and extends from the foramen magnum to the sacrum. At the initiation of the spinal cord, there is no specific line of demarcation between it and the medulla oblongata. Therefore, it is referred to as the spinal cord at the plane of the foramen magnum. It is surrounded and protected by meninges, appears somewhat cylindrical in shape, but is flattened on the dorsal and ventral surfaces. The end of the cord extends to approximately the first sacral vertebra. It is continued by the filum terminale (a tapered end) until the cord reaches approximately the fourth sacral segment. The filum terminale and the spinal nerves form a structure called the cauda equina in adult horses which begins at the lumbosacral junction.

There are divisions which divide the cord into two similar halves on the ventral and dorsal surfaces of the spinal cord. Dorsally, one finds a median groove. Ventrally, there is a median fissure. These anatomical demarcations divide the cord into bilateral symmetrical structures. The ventral median fissure penetrates nearly to the middle of the dorsoventral diameter of the cord. This fissure is occupied by a fold of pia mater. A dorsal median septum is a partition of the cord that descends from the dorsal median groove to about the middle of the cord. The two symmetrical halves of the spinal cord are connected by commissures of both gray and white substance. The gray commissure consists of a transverse band of gray substance at the ventral end of the dorsal septum. This band traverses medially through the central canal of the cord. The white commissure is a branch of white substance which connects the ventral columns of the cord over the dorsal end of the ventral median fissure and constitutes a conducting path from one side to the other.

When visualizing a transverse section of the spinal cord, the central canal is a dorsoventrally flattened oval. In the sacral segment of the cord, it is slightly flattened from side to side, whereas in the caudal

end of the cord, the canal is slightly expanded and communicates dorsally with the subarachnoid space. The anterior end of the central canal communicates with the posterior portion of the fourth ventricle of the brain. This canal is lined by epithelium and is surrounded by a layer of modified neuroglia.

A cross section of the spinal cord will reveal the gray substance roughly resembling the capital letter "**H**". The cross bar of this letter is formed by the gray commissure, whereas each lateral portion consists of the dorsal and ventral gray columns. The dorsal gray columns become elongated and taper to a point which extends almost to the surface of the cord at the attachment of the dorsal root fibers of the spinal nerves. The ventral column is short, thick, and rounded and is separated from the surface of the spinal cord by a thick layer of white substance through which the fibers of the ventral roots of the spinal nerves pass.

The white substance of the spinal cord can be divided into three pairs of columns: the dorsal, the ventral, and the lateral columns. The dorsal columns lie on either side of the dorsal median septum. The ventral columns are situated on either side between the median fissure and the ventral gray column. These ventral columns are connected above the fissure above the white commissure. Lateral to the gray columns on either side are the lateral columns of white substance.

Throughout the vertebral canal, the spinal cord is fairly uniform in size except for two areas of enlargement. Both of these enlarged regions involve segments with which the nerves of the limbs are connected. The cervical enlargement is initiated at the area of the fifth cervical vertebra and subsides in the area of the second thoracic vertebra. The lumbar enlargement begins at the fourth or fifth lumbar vertebra and terminates where the cord begins to taper to form the conus medullaris.

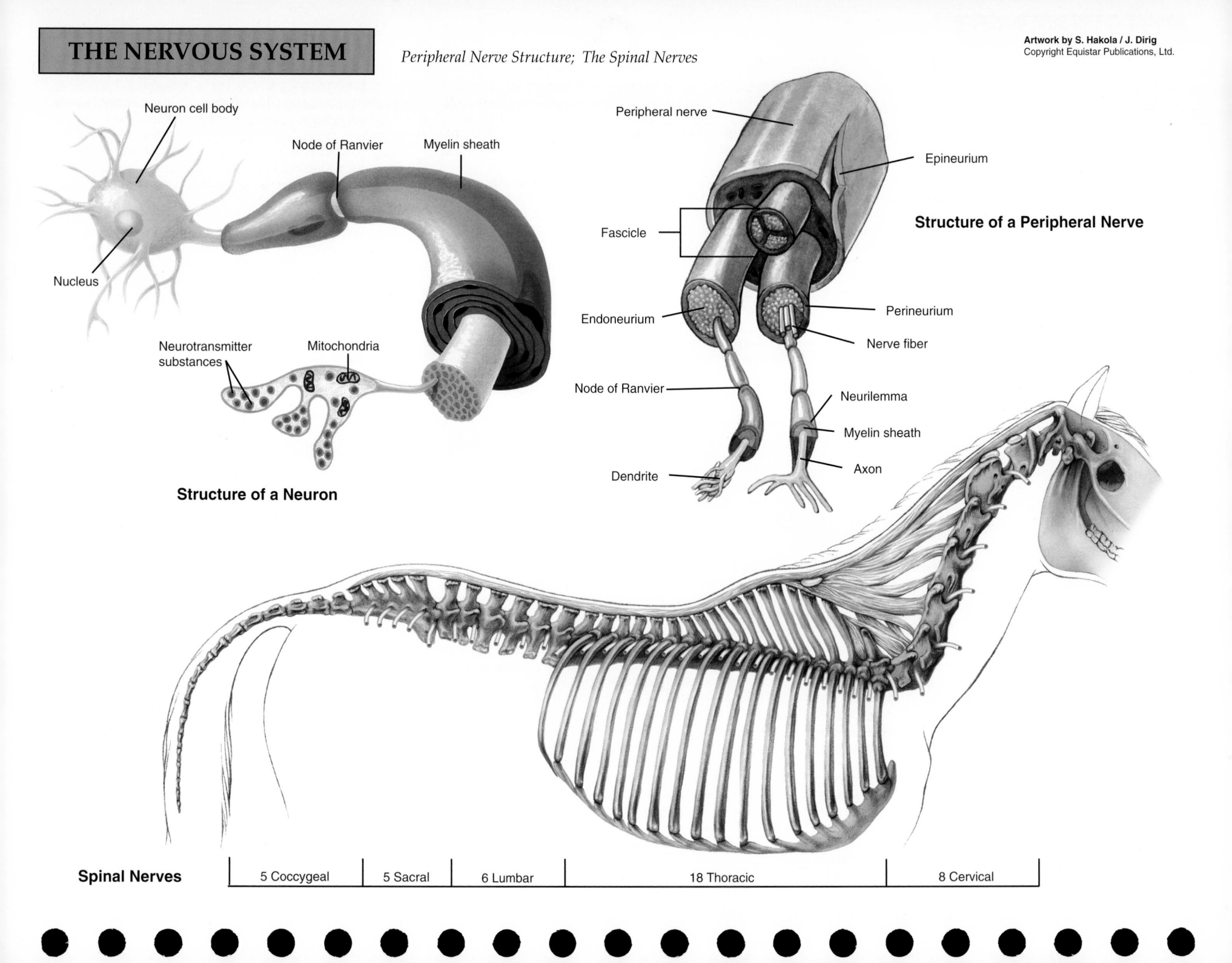

THE NERVOUS SYSTEM

Peripheral Nerve Structure; The Spinal Nerves

Neuron cell body

Node of Ranvier

Myelin sheath

Nucleus

Neurotransmitter substances

Mitochondria

Structure of a Neuron

Peripheral nerve

Epineurium

Fascicle

Structure of a Peripheral Nerve

Endoneurium

Perineurium

Nerve fiber

Node of Ranvier

Neurilemma

Myelin sheath

Axon

Dendrite

Spinal Nerves

| 5 Coccygeal | 5 Sacral | 6 Lumbar | 18 Thoracic | 8 Cervical |

STRUCTURE OF A NERVE

Nerves can be classified according to their central connections. Therefore, they are termed cranial, cerebral, spinal, or sympathetic nerves. These structures are composed of bundles of parallel nerve fibers which connect the structures of the body and allow the animal to be aware of and interact with its environment.

Neurons vary considerably in size and shape but they all are comprised of a cell body and tubular processes that contain cytoplasm and conduct nerve impulses to and from the cell body. The cell body contains the various organelles that are common to all cells: mitochondria, lysosomes etc. Two different fibers extend from the cell body of most neurons. These are the dendrites and the axons. The dendrites are short, highly branched structures that are the main receptive surfaces of the neuron to which processes from other neurons communicate. The axon is a slender smooth-surfaced structure that functions to conduct nerve impulses away from the cell body.

The epineurium is the outermost layer of connective tissue that covers the nerve fiber. Each bundle of nerve fibers is individually termed a fascicle and is covered by connective tissue called the perineurium. Each individual nerve fiber is surrounded by a small amount of loose connective tissue that is termed the endoneurium.

In general, nerves that conduct impulses into the brain or spinal cord are called sensory nerves, and those that carry impulses away from the central nervous system to muscles or glands are termed motor nerves. Most nerves contain mixed fibers that include both motor and sensory functions. Efferent fibers carry motor impulses outward from the brain or spinal cord, whereas afferent fibers carry sensory impulses into the brain or spinal cord. Therefore, nerve fibers can be divided into four groups as follows:
1. General somatic efferent fibers which carry motor impulses outward from the brain and spinal cord to the skeletal muscles.
2. General visceral efferent fibers which carry motor impulses to the various smooth muscles and glands associated with the internal organs.
3. General somatic afferent fibers which carry sensory impulses from the skeletal muscles to the brain and spinal cord.
4. General visceral afferent fibers which carry sensory impulses to the central nervous system from the blood vessels and internal organs.

An unconscious response to a stimulus by the body is called a reflex. A simple reflex pathway does not have a connection with any ascending or descending pathways within the central nervous system. An example of this would be a stimulus upon a tendon. There would be a stimulation to the receptor in the tendon, an impulse that travels to the sensory neuronal cell body in the dorsal root ganglion, which in turn stimulates an internuncial neuron that effects contraction of the limb muscle via a lower motor neuron which has its cell body within the ventral gray matter of the spinal cord.

THE PERIPHERAL NERVOUS SYSTEM

The Spinal Nerves

The spinal nerves are arranged in pairs and are identified according to the relationship which they have with the cervical, thoracic, lumbar, sacral, and coccygeal vertebrae. In the horse, there are usually 42 pairs of spinal nerves. Each one of these spinal nerves is connected with the spinal cord by dorsal and ventral roots. There are 8 cervical, 18 thoracic, 6 lumbar, 5 sacral, and 5 coccygeal pairs of spinal nerves.

Of the dorsal and ventral connecting roots, the dorsal root is the larger of the two. This dorsal root connects with the cord along the dorsal lateral groove. Fibers from this root form a compact bundle on which there is a gray nodular enlargement called the spinal ganglion. Distal to this ganglion, the dorsal root joins the ventral root to constitute the nerve. These spinal ganglia are located in the intervertebral foramina, except in the sacral and coccygeal areas. In these two regions, the ganglia reside within the vertebral canal. Except for the first cervical spinal nerve, the ventral root is smaller than the dorsal root. These ventral roots arise from the ventral surface of the spinal cord over an area of 3 - 5 mm in width. There are no ganglia on the ventral root.

There are eight pairs of cervical spinal nerves. The first cervical nerve emerges through the intervertebral foramen of the atlas and the eighth emerges between the last cervical and first thoracic vertebrae. The dorsal branches from these cervical nerves innervate the dorsal lateral muscles and the skin of the neck. The ventral branches of these cervical nerves are smaller than the dorsal ones and increase in size from the first to the last. The first five ventral branches of the cervical nerves supply the muscles and skin over the lateral and ventral aspects of the vertebrae. The last three ventral branches enter into the formation of the brachial plexus. The two or three branches proceeding the last provide roots to the phrenic nerve.

The Phrenic Nerve

The motor nerve that innervates the diaphragm is called the phrenic nerve. This nerve is formed from the ventral branches of the sixth and seventh cervical nerves with a small number of branches coming from the fifth cervical nerve. Some fibers from the seventh cervical spinal nerve also aid in the formation of the phrenic nerve, but these fibers join after passage through the brachial plexus.

Artwork by S. Hakola / J. Dirig
Copyright Equistar Publications, Ltd.

The Brachial Plexus

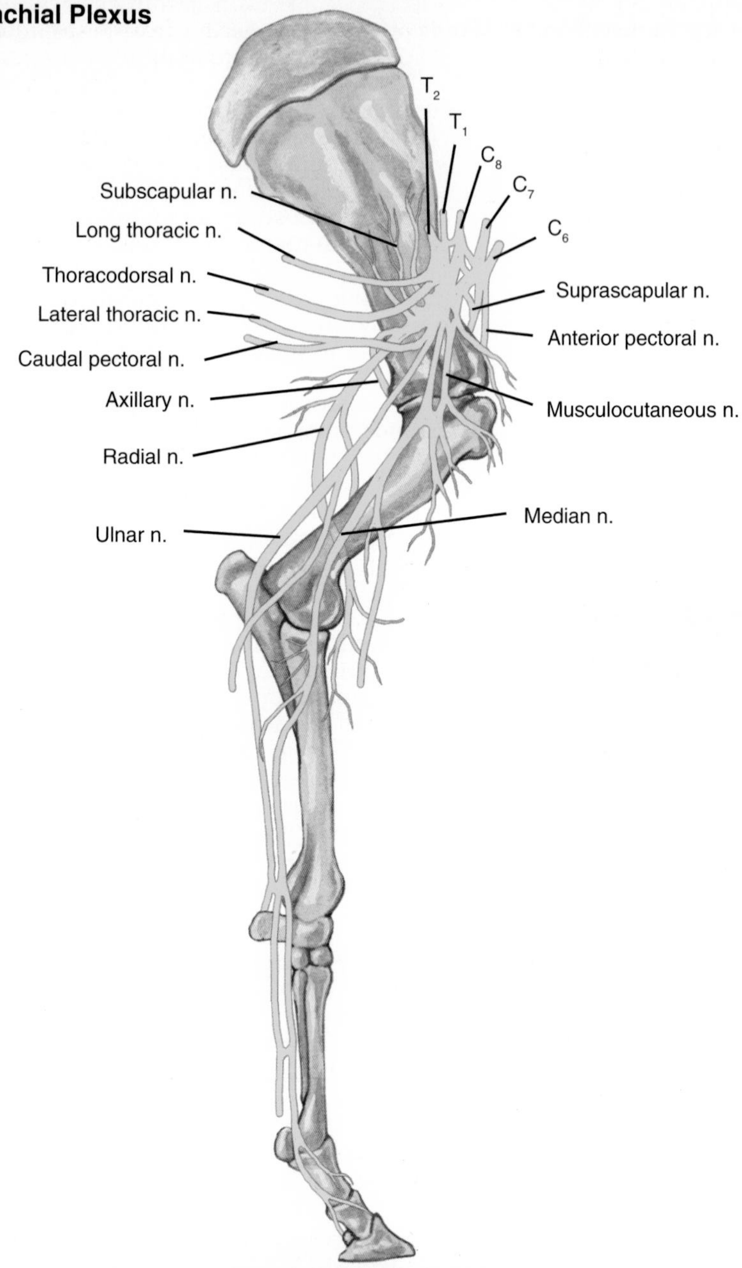

T_2
T_1
C_8
C_7
C_6

Subscapular n.
Long thoracic n.
Thoracodorsal n.
Lateral thoracic n.
Caudal pectoral n.
Axillary n.
Radial n.
Ulnar n.

Suprascapular n.
Anterior pectoral n.
Musculocutaneous n.
Median n.

Medial Left Forelimb

The Lumbosacral Plexus

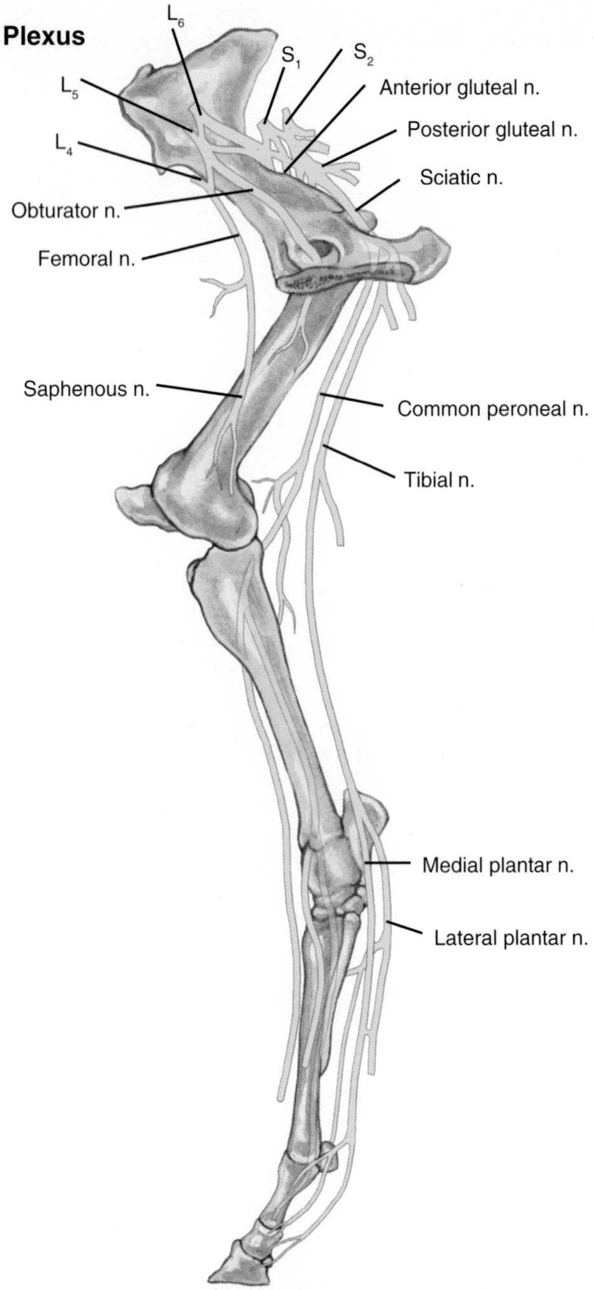

L_6
S_1
S_2
L_5
L_4

Anterior gluteal n.
Posterior gluteal n.
Sciatic n.

Obturator n.
Femoral n.

Saphenous n.

Common peroneal n.
Tibial n.

Medial plantar n.
Lateral plantar n.

Medial Right Hindlimb

The Brachial Plexus

Ventral branches arising from the last three cervical and first two thoracic spinal nerves anastomose to form the brachial plexus. This plexus is located between the two portions of the scalenus muscle and lies deep to the anterior deep pectoral and subscapularis muscles.

The brachial plexus gives rise to eleven different branches. These branches supply the thoracic limb and innervate portions of the chest wall. They are as follows:
1.) The *suprascapular nerve* provides innervation to the supraspinatus and infraspinatus muscles. This nerve is directly related to the bone and is vulnerable to injury. When this nerve becomes injured, it is referred to as "sweeny."
2.) The *subscapular nerve* divides into several branches which enter and supply the subscapularis muscle.
3.) Branches of the *anterior pectoral nerve* supply the deep pectoral, the superficial pectoral, the brachiocephalicus, and the posterior deep muscles.
4.) The *musculocutaneous nerve* supplies branches to the pectoral muscles.
5.) The *median nerve* is the largest branch of the brachial plexus. It arises with the ulnar from the posterior part of the plexus and forms a loop with the musculocutaneous nerve.
6.) The *ulnar nerve* arises with the median nerve through a short common trunk.
7.) The *radial nerve* arises from the posterior portion of the brachial plexus and descends with the ulnar nerve over the medial surface of the origin of the subscapular artery.
8.) The *axillary nerve* arises from the brachial plexus behind the musculocutaneous nerve.
9.) The *long thoracic nerve* arises along the anterior edge of the brachial plexus and divides into three branches.
10.) The *thoracodorsal nerve* arises medial to the axillary nerve and passes through the subscapularis muscle to innervate the latissimus dorsi muscle.
11.) The *external thoracic nerve* arises through a common trunk with the ulnar nerve and mainly functions to innervate the cutaneous muscles and skin of the abdominal wall as far back as the flank. Branches from this nerve also supply the deep pectoral muscles and form branches with the intercostal nerves.

The Thoracic Spinal Nerves

There are 18 pairs of thoracic nerves and each nerve divides into a dorsal and ventral branch. The dorsal branches divide again to form a medial and lateral branch. The medial branches supply the dorsal spinal muscles, whereas the lateral branches supply the longissimus dorsi, the serratus dorsalis, and the rhomboideus muscles. Still other small fibers from these lateral branches supply the skin over the ligamentum nuchae and the trapezius muscle. The ventral branches of the thoracic nerves are much larger than their dorsal counterparts and are sometimes referred to as the intercostal nerves. As their name indicates, these nerves supply the intercostal muscles, the abdominal muscles, and the skin in this region.

The Lumbar Spinal Nerves

There are six pairs of lumbar nerves, and the last pair emerges between the last lumbar vertebra and the sacrum. The dorsal branches of these nerves are much smaller than the ventral branches which are connected with the sympathetic nervous system and innervate the sublumbar muscles.

The iliohypogastric nerve is formed by the ventral branch of the first lumbar nerve. This nerve then forms superficial and deep branches. The second lumbar nerve gives rise to a ventral branch which is connected to that of the ventral branch of the third lumbar nerve. This then branches off to innervate the psoas major muscle and continues on as the ilioinguinal nerve and also divides into superficial and deep branches.

The third lumbar nerve gives rise to a ventral branch which anastomoses with a branch from the second lumbar nerve to provide a root to the lumbosacral plexus. This third lumbar nerve branches off to the psoas muscles and forms the external spermatic and lateral cutaneous nerves. The fourth, fifth, and sixth lumbar vertebrae give rise to ventral branches which anastomose to form the lumbosacral plexus.

The Lumbosacral Plexus

The ventral branches of the last three lumbar and first two sacral nerves form the lumbosacral plexus. The anterior portion of this plexus lies superficial to the internal iliac artery between the lumbar transverse processes and the psoas minor muscle. This plexus serves as the origin to the nerves of the pelvic limb.

The Nerves of the Pelvic Limb

There are nine main nerves of the pelvic limb and they are described as follows:
1.) The *femoral nerve* arises from the third, fourth, and fifth lumbar nerves and sometimes receives fibers from the sixth. It arises from the anterior portion of the lumbosacral plexus and gives rise to the saphenous nerve.
2.) The *saphenous nerve* branches off from the femoral nerve along the terminal portion of the iliopsoas muscle.
3.) The *obturator nerve* arises chiefly from the ventral branches of the fourth and fifth lumbar nerves but also receives some fibers from the third or sixth lumbar nerves.
4.) The *anterior gluteal nerve* arises from the fifth and sixth lumbar ventral roots and the first sacral ventral root. This root then divides into numerous branches to supply the musculature of this area.
5.) The *posterior gluteal nerve* is derived mainly from the sacral roots of the lumbosacral plexus, then divides into two trunks which emerge above the sciatic nerve.
6.) The *sciatic nerve* is the largest nerve in the body and arises from the sixth lumbar and first sacral roots of the lumbosacral plexus. Some animals also receive fibers from both the fifth lumbar and second sacral nerves to form the sciatic nerve which gives rise to numerous muscular and cutaneous branches.
7.) The *common peroneal nerve* arises from the sciatic nerve after it emerges from the pelvic cavity.
8.) The *tibial nerve* is a direct continuation of the sciatic nerve as it passes between the two heads of the gastrocnemius muscles.
9.) The *plantar nerves* are medial and lateral branches that result from the bifurcation of the tibial nerves on the distal portion of the limb.

Artwork by S. Hakola / J. Dirig
Copyright Equistar Publications, Ltd.

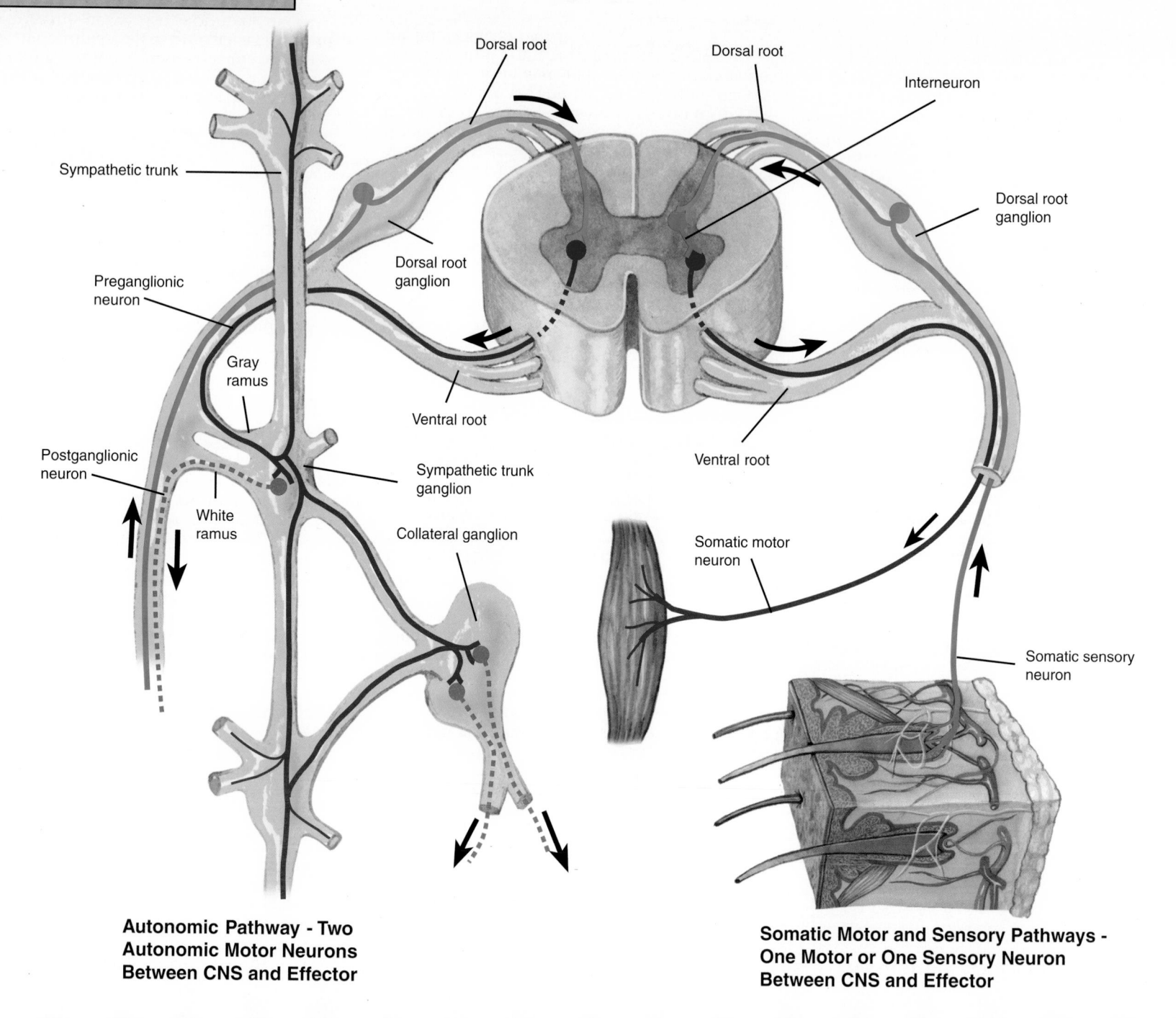

Dorsal root

Dorsal root

Interneuron

Sympathetic trunk

Dorsal root ganglion

Preganglionic neuron

Dorsal root ganglion

Gray ramus

Ventral root

Ventral root

Postganglionic neuron

Sympathetic trunk ganglion

White ramus

Collateral ganglion

Somatic motor neuron

Somatic sensory neuron

Autonomic Pathway - Two Autonomic Motor Neurons Between CNS and Effector

Somatic Motor and Sensory Pathways - One Motor or One Sensory Neuron Between CNS and Effector

The Sacral Spinal Nerves

There are five pairs of sacral nerves. Dorsal branches emerge from these sacral spinal nerves and pass through the dorsal sacral foramen and the space between the sacrum and the first coccygeal vertebra. Ventral branches of the sacral spinal nerves leave the ventral canal through the ventral sacral foramina and that space between the sacrum and the first coccygeal vertebra.

The Coccygeal Spinal Nerves

There are usually five pairs of coccygeal spinal nerves. Both their ventral and dorsal branches anastomose to form trunks which innervate the muscles and skin of the tail.

THE AUTONOMIC NERVOUS SYSTEM

An afferent pathway is when an impulse travels toward the spinal cord or a particular brain area. When an impulse is conveyed away from the spinal cord or the brain, it is termed an efferent pathway.

The autonomic nervous system is concerned with the regulation of various visceral functions. It can be divided into a peripheral autonomic nervous system and a central autonomic nervous system. The peripheral autonomic nervous system is that motor system which controls the activity of smooth muscle, cardiac muscle, and glandular functions. Afferent fibers from visceral structures are associated with reflex mechanisms utilizing discharges in nerve fibers of the autonomic nervous system. These afferent fibers are termed visceral afferents.

The autonomic nervous system can be subdivided into sympathetic thoracolumbar and parasympathetic craniosacral portions. These two systems differ in their origin, the relationship of the location of their peripheral ganglia with respect to the target organs which their fibers innervate, in transmitter substance secretion, and their actions

on the target organ which are often opposed. Generally, the sympathetic nervous system mediates visceral activities that would resemble a response observed in an animal behaving in the "flight" manner. For example, when a horse is "spooked," there is a general sympathetic discharge. This results in acceleration of the heart, elevation of blood pressure, and dilation of the pupils. Conversely, the parasympathetic system mediates many of the more placid functions of the viscera. An example of parasympathetic activity would involve the processes of slowing the heart and pupillary constriction. Parasympathetic activity is also associated with digestion of food, secretion of various digestive glands, and contractions of the intestine directed toward movement of food along the digestive system.

Information that is carried by the sympathetic nervous system to peripheral effector organs such as smooth muscle of the gut or cardiac muscle travels along a two-neuron path. The synapse between the two neurons occurs within the sympathetic ganglia. The cell bodies of the sympathetic preganglionic neurons are located within the spinal cord. These cell bodies are found at the levels between the upper thoracic segments and the lower lumbar segments of the cord.

There are two widely separated portions of the parasympathetic nervous system. The cranial portion is associated with several of the cranial nerves, whereas the lower portion originates from the sacral spinal cord around the level of the second, third, and fourth sacral vertebrae. In general, the cranial sympathetic nervous system supplies structures of the head, neck, thorax, and part of the abdomen, while the sacral parasympathetic nervous system innervates the remainder of the abdomen and the pelvis. In contrast to the sympathetic nervous system where the postganglionic fibers are of considerable length, the parasympathetic nervous system is organized in such a way that its ganglia are adjacent to the organs innervated, and the postganglionic fibers are relatively short.

EXAMINATION OF THE NERVOUS SYSTEM

The purpose of a neurological exam is to first determine whether or not there is a neurological disorder present. If a disorder is present, attempts should be made to localize the problem as to its anatomical location.

This examination should be undertaken in a cranial to caudal progression. A general clinical exam should be done initially to detect the presence of any other disorders within other body systems. By starting with the head and working toward the tail of the horse, one can also determine if a neurological problem is within the central nervous system or the peripheral nervous system. Examination progression should be done in the following order: cerebrum, brain stem, cerebellum, spinal cord, peripheral nerves, then musculature.

Evaluation of the Head

Variations in behavior should be examined. Behaviorial malfunctions usually an indicate an abnormal process within the cerebral cortex. A judgment should be made as to the animal's reaction and interaction to people and other horses. Is the animal developing aggressive behavior? Is the horse able to relax, or does it seem discontented when left undisturbed? Does the animal lie down normally or seem uncomfortable when lying down? These questions should be evaluated and answered.

An animal's state of awareness or mental status is an excellent indicator of brain stem and cerebral cortical function. Stimuli cause a response through input from the visual, auditory, olfactory, tactile, and gustatory systems. Normal mental state is manifested by normal responses to these stimuli. Abnormal mental status is evident when the animal exhibits depression, somnolence, lethargy, and eventually coma. When the horse is in a comatose state, there is no response at all to normal stimuli.

Artwork by S. Hakola / J. Dirig
Copyright Equistar Publications, Ltd.

Symptoms of Various Cranial Nerve Dysfunctions

Head Tilt

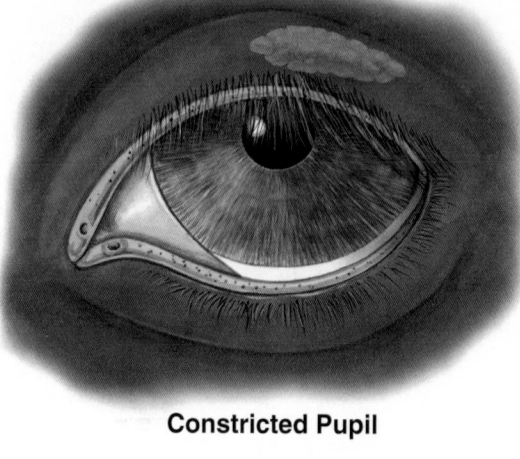

Head tilt positions may be a result of problems found in the cerebrum, the cerebellum, or the vestibular system.

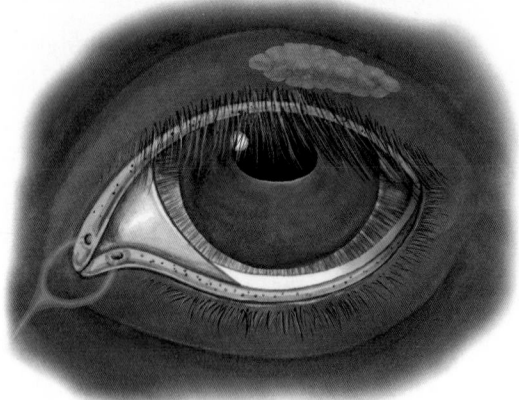

Constricted Pupil

Dilated Pupil

Abnormal pupil constriction may result from injuries affecting both the optic and/or oculomotor nerves.

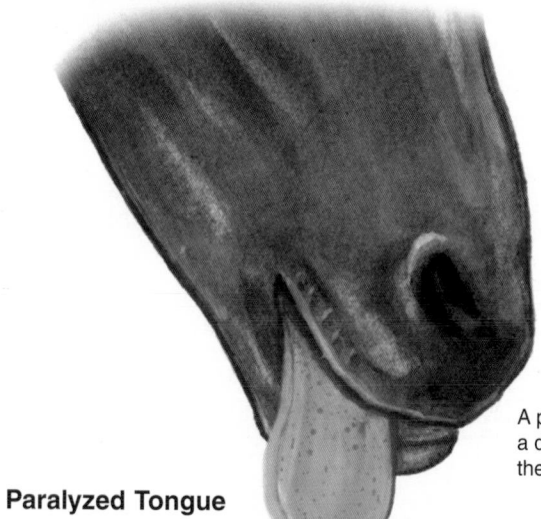

Paralyzed Tongue

A paralyzed tongue reflects a disorder which involves the hypoglossal nerve.

Facial Nerve Paralysis

Facial nerve paralysis results in drooping of the eyelids, ears, lips, and nostrils.

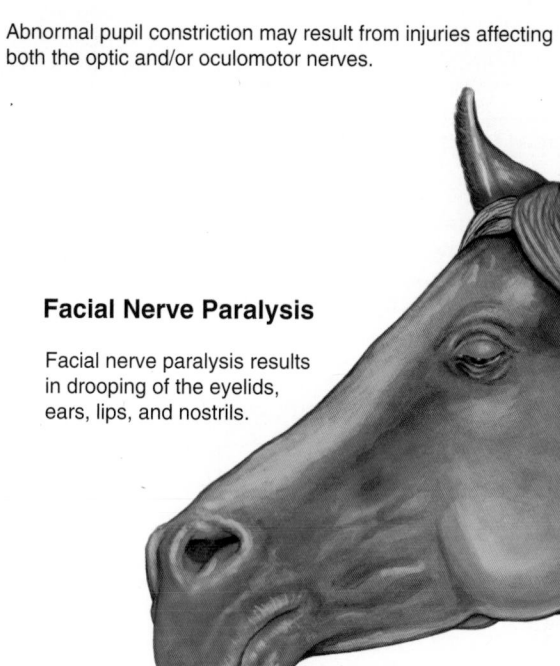

The cerebrum, the cerebellum, and the vestibular system control the movements of the head. Normal head motions involve flexion, extension, or rotation of the atlanto-occipital joint. An animal that presents with an abnormal head position could have a disorder which is the result of:

1.) A fracture or infection resulting in pain within the atlanto-occipital joint.

2.) A lesion within the vestibular system that results in a head tilt.

3.) A lesion within the cerebrum which would be manifested by a deviation of the head and neck toward the side of the lesion. (This would also cause the horse to circle.)

4.) Cerebellar lesions which would result in abnormal coordination and fine tremors within the musculature.

Coordination and posture of the head can be determined by an easy test. A treat or food is held beside the shoulder on either side of the horse. The horse should readily flex its head, reach for the treat, and attempt to eat it. The animal's motion, posture, and coordination can then be evaluated during this activity.

Cranial Nerve Evaluation

Examination of the cranial nerves should be done in a cranial to caudal procedure. The following is a list of the cranial nerves and their evaluation techniques:

C.N. I. Olfactory nerve: An evaluation should be made to determine the animal's ability to smell. This can be accomplished by placing food, a hand, or even a hand soaked in urine in front of the horse and noting the animal's nasal reaction to it.

C.N. II. Optic nerve: An evaluation can be made of the horse's abiltiy to see by conducting a menace reflex test. A threatening gesture is made in the vacinity of the eye which should result in a closure of the eye and a withdrawl of the animal's head. A strange object, such as a pen light, is moved slowly through the field of vision while observing the movement of the eye. The pupillary light reflex test depicts the functions of the optic and oculomotor nerves simultaneously. The size of the animal's pupil will depend on the balance between the constrictor muscles which are innervated by the parasympathetic fibers within the oculomotor nerves, and the dilator muscles which are innervated by sympathetic fibers from the cranial cervical ganglion.

C. N. III. Oculomotor nerve: A lesion within this nerve will result in the inability of the animal to respond to the pupillary light reflex which is indicated by a dilated pupil when a light is directed at the eye.

C. N. IV. Trochlear nerve: This nerve innervates the extraocular muscles which are responsible for the positioning of the eye within the orbit and for normal eye movement. The movement of the eye can be evaluated while the animal is at rest when the head is manually manipulated. Position of the eye is not just determined by the trochlear nerve, but may be the result of lesions within the oculomotor and the abducent nerves.

C.N. V. Trigeminal nerve: A lesion within this nerve causes the inability of the animal to close its jaw. Any damage to this nerve will result in an ineffective chewing capability.

C.N. VI. Abducent nerve: Lesions within this nerve are responsible for the dysfunction of the extraocular and retractor bulbi muscles. This results in an abnormal eye position at rest.

C.N. VII. Facial nerve: The functions of this nerve are tested by manually stimulating several areas around the eyelids, ears, and lips. Any lesions within this nerve will result in a drooping of the ear, the eyelid, lip, or nostrils on the affected side. Muscle tone within these areas should also be evaluated.

C.N. VIII. Vestibulocochlear nerve: Hearing loss is difficult to determine in the horse; however, the vestibular branch of this nerve involves the animal's sense of balance. Any lesions within this vestibular branch will result in a head tilt and nystagmus when the head is manipulated. It may be necessary to blindfold the horse to assess the early stages of lesions within the vestibular branch.

C.N. IX. Glossopharyngeal nerve/ C.N. X. Vagus nerve/ C.N. XI. Spinal accessory nerve: Evaluation of pharyngeal and laryngeal functions will allow a determination of their respective sensory and motor functions. An assessment can be made through observations of normal breathing, swallowing, and through an endoscopic examination of the pharynx and larynx. A slap test called the laryngeal adduction test will assess the function of the vagus nerve. A manual slap on the withers will produce a reflex response of adduction of the contralateral arytenoid cartilage. This can be visualized directly through the use of endoscopy.

C.N. XII. Hypoglossal nerve: Motor function to the tongue is provided by this nerve and its function can easily be evaluated through examination of these tissues.

Evaluation of the Horse's Gait

An evaluation of the animal's gait will determine whether an abnormality exists and its location within the spinal cord, the peripheral nervous system, the musculoskeletal system, or the brain stem. An exam should be made while the horse is observed at a walk, at a trot in straight lines, and turning in circles in both directions. The animal should also be evaluated walking over small obstacles and up and down an incline.

Gait abnormalities can be evaluated and assigned a grade as to the deficits that are being exhibited:

Grade 0: There are no deficits and the animal is normal.

Grade 1: This deficit is barely detectable when the horse is traveling normally. The deficit can be exaggerated however, by forcing the horse to back, turn, sway from side to side, or extend the neck.

Grade 2: When the animal is traveling at a walk or trot, deficits are present within the gait. When the horse is forced to back or turn, the deficit is greatly exaggerated.

Grade 3: Gait deficits are very obvious and the animal will stumble when provoked by any stress.

Grade 4: The deficits will be severe enough in this gait that it will cause the animal to fall or stumble when the horse is forced to move.

Grade 5: These horses are recumbent.

Artwork by S. Hakola / J. Dirig
Copyright Equistar Publications, Ltd.

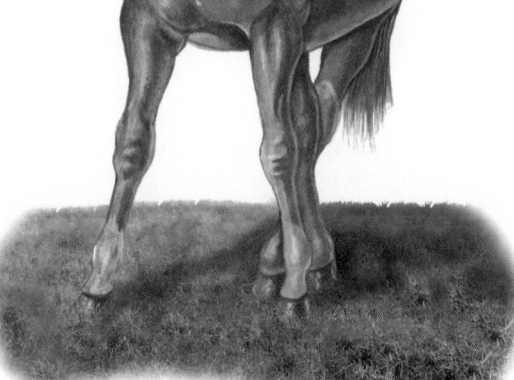

Ataxia, or loss of proprioception, is evidenced here by crossing of hind limbs, and abnormal positioning of the forelimbs and the head.

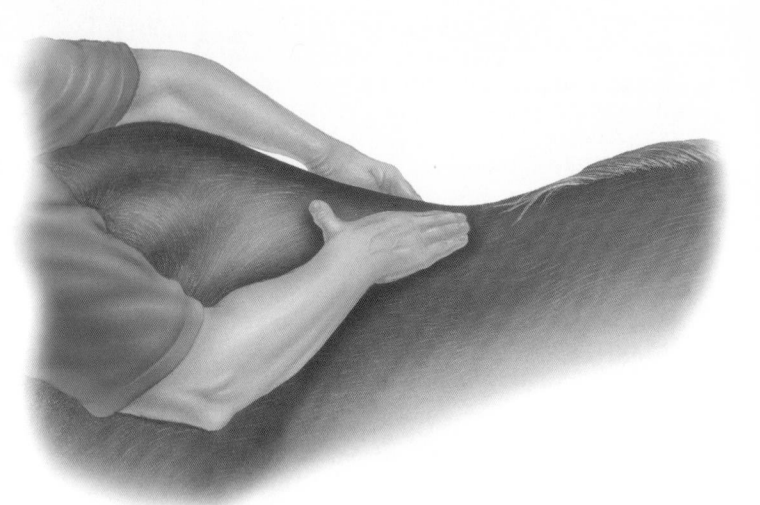

Palpation of the spine and lumbar musculature to check for asymmetry, localized sweating, atrophy, or pain response.

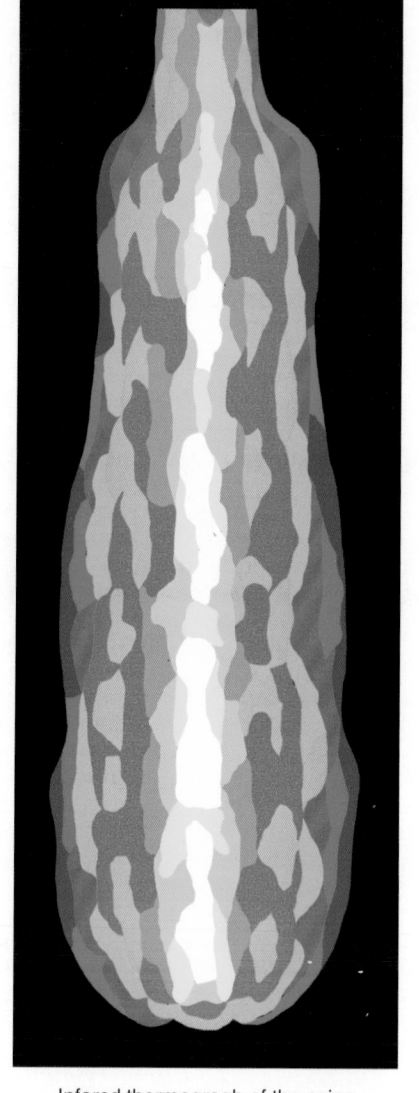

Infared thermogragh of the spine shows "hot spots" of increased thermal gradients along the spine.

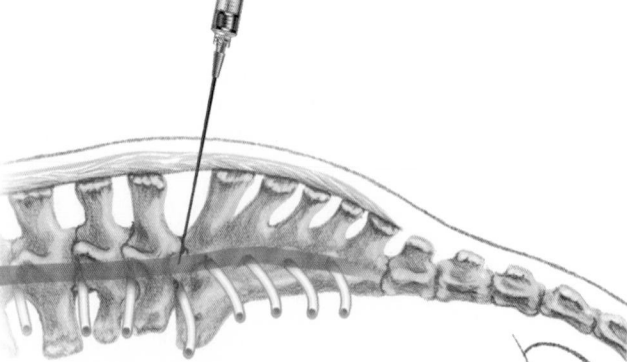

Collection of cerebrospional fluid via a lumbar puncture for evaluation may indicate an infection, the presence of toxins, or evidence of trauma.

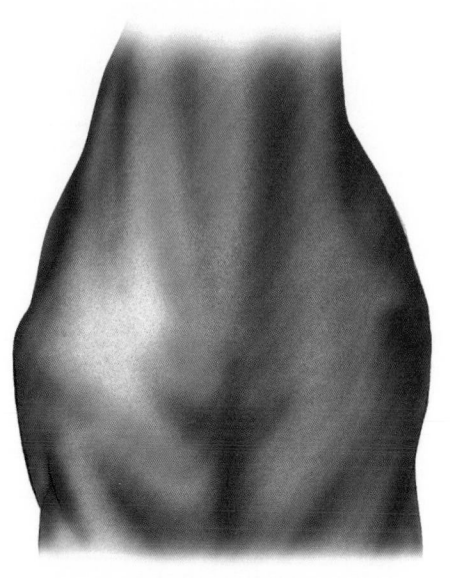

Atrophy of the supraspinatus muscle as seen in sweeny is the result of an injury to the suprascapular nerve.

Examination, Palpation, and Reflexes Utilized in the Neurological Exam

Initially, the animal should be evaluated while at rest from a distance to note any abnormality within the animal's posture. The horse's limbs should be positioned squarely beneath the body, although it is possible for the animal to be resting a limb while relaxed. An evaluation should be made to determine proprioception which is the ability of the animal to know the location of the limbs when displaced in an abnormal position.

A gait evaluation should be conducted while the animal is walking, trotting, moving in small circles in both directions, and backing. If possible, the animal should be asked to negotiate an obstacle course. This is easily accomplished by using the cross rails from jumps. The horse should also be asked to ascend and descend an incline when available. Any abnormalities within the gait should be evaluated and graded.

Evidence of weakness, ataxia, spasticity, or dysmetria should be noted. Weakness (paresis) is manifested by noting increased wear on the toe or cranial surface of the hoof. Ataxia is a loss of proprioception and is the inability to identify space between the limbs. Clinical signs of this will include swaying movements, crossing of the limbs when walking, and asymmetric placement of the feet on the ground. Spasticity is manifested by stiff movements with a decreased range of motion within the joints. A loss of control over the direction and range of motion of the limb such as over-reaching is described as dysmetria.

The neck and forelimbs should be carefully examined, palpated, and tested for reflexes. Palpation of the neck and shoulder area should detect any asymmetry, muscle atrophy, and localized sweating. The neck should be manually manipulated to evaluate reluctance to move the head and neck in any direction which would indicate pain in that anatomical region.

Stimulation should be performed with a blunt pin or the tip of a ball point pen. When performed on the skin over the cervical region, contraction of the cutaneous muscle results in twitching of the skin.

A sway reaction test can be made while the horse is standing still or walking. This test evaluates the animal's resistance to being pushed or pulled in a lateral direction and is a test to depict any weakness or ataxia present. Downward pressure on the withers will normally cause the horse to arch his back. When the animal is weak or ataxic, this downward pressure can result in a collapse. Testing of postural reactions through manipulations of the forelimbs may reveal subtle neurological deficits. Making the horse hop sideways by lifting each forelimb in turn may result in a manifestation of weakness or ataxia. The forelimb should then be placed in an abnormal position, to force the horse to return the limb to its normal position. This test evaluates proprioception.

The body of the horse and its hindlimbs should be examined and palpated. Any abnormalities such as asymmetry, muscle atrophy, and localized sweating should be noted. When there is damage to spinal sympathetic tracts or peripheral fibers, localized sweating will be produced. Stimulation should be applied to the skin using a blunt needle or instrument. Notation should be made of any areas of decreased sensation. Pressure should be applied to the pelvis or by pulling the tail from one side to the other. This will evaluate the sway reaction and therefore, allow detection of any evidence of weakness or ataxia within the animal. The tone of the anus and tail should be evaluated. Any lesions within the sacrococcygeal section of the cord will result in an absence of muscle tone or weakness within these areas. The perineal reflex, which is done by gently stimulating the skin of the perineum with a sharp object, will allow evaluation of the both the sensory and motor components of the cord.

Special Neurological Examination Procedures

Collection of cerebrospinal fluid, radiographic techniques, thermography, and electromyography will allow further assessment of the neurological system.

Cerebrospinal fluid (CSF) can be collected from either the atlanto-occipital or lumbosacral sites. Cerebrospinal fluid that is collected from the atlanto-occipital site is utilized to evaluate intracranial lesions, whereas CSF from the lumbosacral site is utilized for the evaluation of more distal lesions. Unfortunately, collection of cerebrospinal fluid from the atlanto-occipital space is done while the horse is under general anesthesia and in lateral recumbency. Lumbosacral site collection can be done while the horse is in a standing position and carries a lesser risk to the patient when done properly.

Collection of cerebrospinal fluid from the lumbosacral site is usually done while the animal is restrained by a twitch and stocks. Generalized sedation is only recommended when it is absolutely necessary, since sedation will usually cause the horse to stand asymmetrically. The site for collection is determined by using the caudal borders of each tuber coxae, the caudal edge of the spine at L6, the cranial edge of the spine of the second sacral vertebra, and the cranial edge of each tuber sacrum. This site is then clipped and surgically scrubbed. A local anesthetic solution is administered to this area and the area is again rescrubbed. A 15 cm spinal needle with a stilette is then advanced vertically until the resistance of the interarcuate ligament is felt. Penetration is made through this ligament, the dura mater, and the arachnoid. The stilette is then removed and the cerebrospinal fluid is collected.

The cerebrospinal fluid should be examined and evaluated as soon as possible after collection. The fluid may indicate the prescence of infectious diseases, trauma, or damage from toxins.

Radiological evaluation of the nervous system can be a very useful tool to localize and characterize trauma, infection, and malformations within the spine. A high output x-ray machine utilizing high speed film and rare earth screens is necessary to obtain diagnostic radiographs.

Infrared thermography can be utilized to obtain the precise temperature of the skin surface. This is a noninvasive technique that detects changes in skin temperature resulting from inflammation, atrophy,

Artwork by S. Hakola / J. Dirig
Copyright Equistar Publications, Ltd.

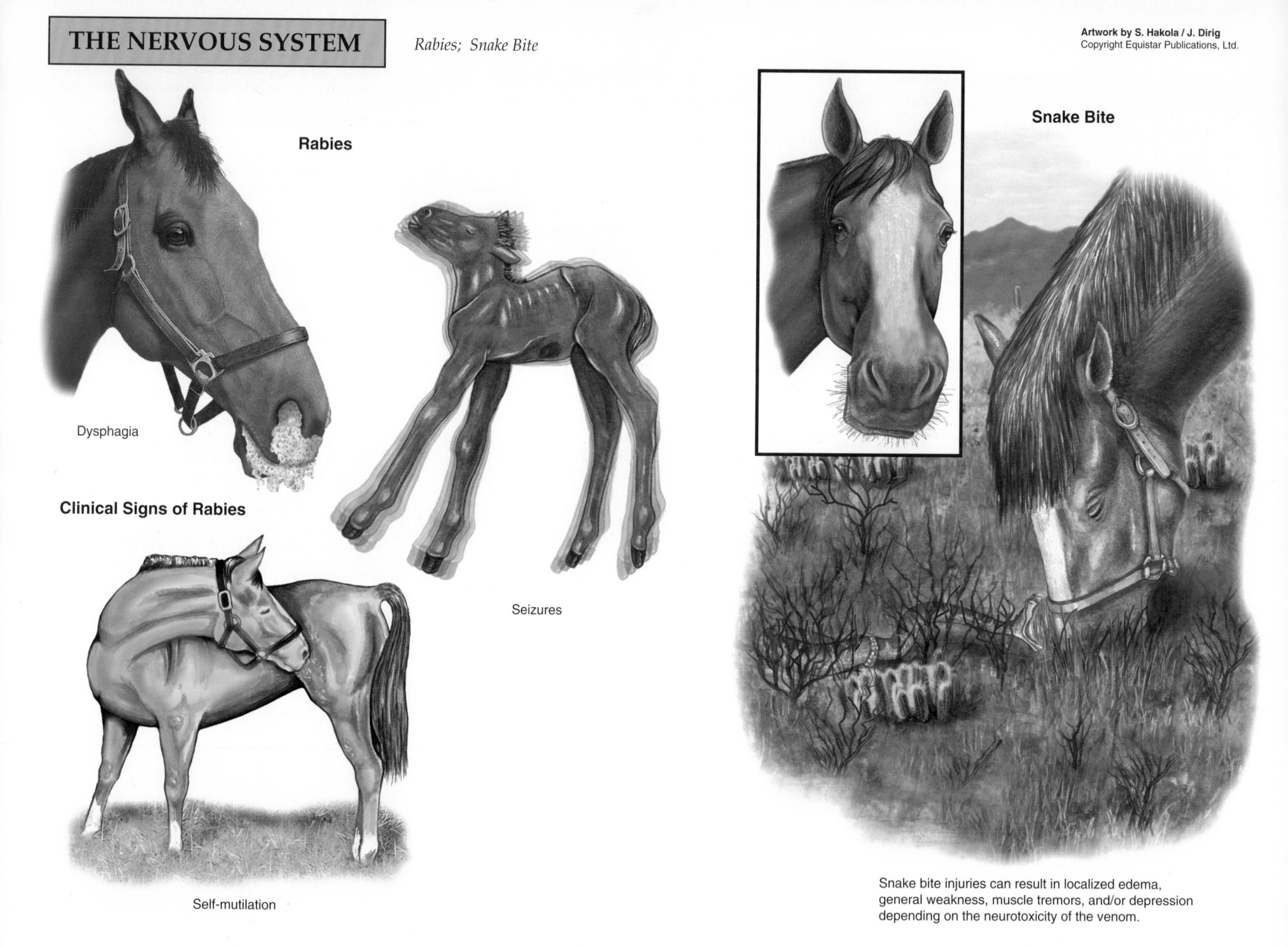

Rabies

Dysphagia

Clinical Signs of Rabies

Seizures

Self-mutilation

Snake Bite

Snake bite injuries can result in localized edema, general weakness, muscle tremors, and/or depression depending on the neurotoxicity of the venom.

neoplasias, and neurological lesions. These lesions can cause nerve irritation which result in deficits within the thermogradients found throughout the horse's limbs.

Electromyography is an evaluation of the electrical activity of the muscles. Needle electrodes are inserted into a muscle to measure the electrical current within this tissue due to a response from nerve stimulation.

COMMON DISORDERS OF THE NEUROLOGICAL SYSTEM

RABIES

Rabies is a viral disease that can occur in all warm-blooded domestic species and humans. The rabies virus is normally spread by bites from infected wildlife, particularly raccoons, skunks, foxes, and bats. The incidence in horses in endemic areas coincides with the number of reservoirs in that area. This virus effects all ages and all breeds.

Clinical Signs

There are three forms or manifestations of infection with the rabies virus: the cerebral form, which is referred to as a "furious" form of rabies, a "dumb" form where the brain stem is involved, and a paralytic form where the virus attacks the spinal cord. After the initial contact with the wild host, the incubation time for the horse ranges from two weeks to several months. The virus is a rhabdovirus. It travels from the site of inoculation, up the peripheral nerves, to the central nervous system. It then spreads centrifugally to all body organs that are highly innervated.

Clinical signs to this disorder can vary according to the site and dose of inoculation, and the pathogenicity of the specific rabies virus strain. Initially, the animal will exhibit an ascending ataxia and paresis. The horse may appear lame or have intermittent bouts of colic. It may exhibit signs of dysphagia, self-mutilation, salivation, hyperesthesia, or photophobia. Terminally, these

animals may become blind, suffer from seizures, and become aggressive. Any animal that is a rabies suspect should be handled with extreme caution because of the ability of this virus to spread to humans.

Differential Diagnosis

1.) Trauma
2.) Encephalitis
3.) Equine Protozoal Myeloencephalopathy
4.) Botulism
5.) Bacterial Meningitis
6.) Equine Cervical Vertebral Malformation
7.) Ingestion of Toxins

Diagnosis

Diagnosis is based mainly on history and clinical signs. The most reliable tests for rabies are unfortunately those that are performed on brain or spinal cord tissue on a postmortem examination. As required by most laboratories, the whole head is shipped in a sealed, cooled container to the appropriate state public health laboratory for histopathologic and fluorescent antibody testing. The standard diagnostic test is the use of the fluorescent antibody test for viral antigen within the brain tissue.

Treatment

There is no successful treatment for rabies and the administration of antiinflammatory medications will merely prolong the course of the disease.

Prevention

Vaccination with killed virus vaccines should be included in the annual preventive medicine regime. If rabies is suspected, the animal should be in quarantine and contact with human beings should be restricted. Prophylactic antirabies immunization for anyone in contact with this animal should be considered.

SNAKE BITE

Snake bites within the United States usually involve water moccasins, rattlesnakes, or copperheads. The venom from these snakes cause an intense localized reaction but seldom result in neurological symptoms. Venom from snakes such as cobras, mambas, and coral snakes of India, Africa, Asia, Central and South America however, are neurotoxic. Animals that are bitten by these snakes initially exhibit excitement and hyperesthesia. As the venom from these snakes spreads, it produces a generalized weakness, depression, dysphasia, and muscle tremors.

There is a marked local edema at the site of the bite. The rattlesnake, copperhead, and water moccasin bite has an insufficient amount of toxin to cause the death of a large horse. Infection at the site of the bite can produce a bacterial toxemia which is usually of more concern than the snake venom itself.

Broad spectrum antimicrobials and antihistamines should be administered to these animals. Since the antivenoms for the rattlesnake, copperhead, and water moccasin are all of equine origin, they should be utilized in treatment with great care. Corticosteroids are contraindicated in the treatment of snake bite.

Tetanus

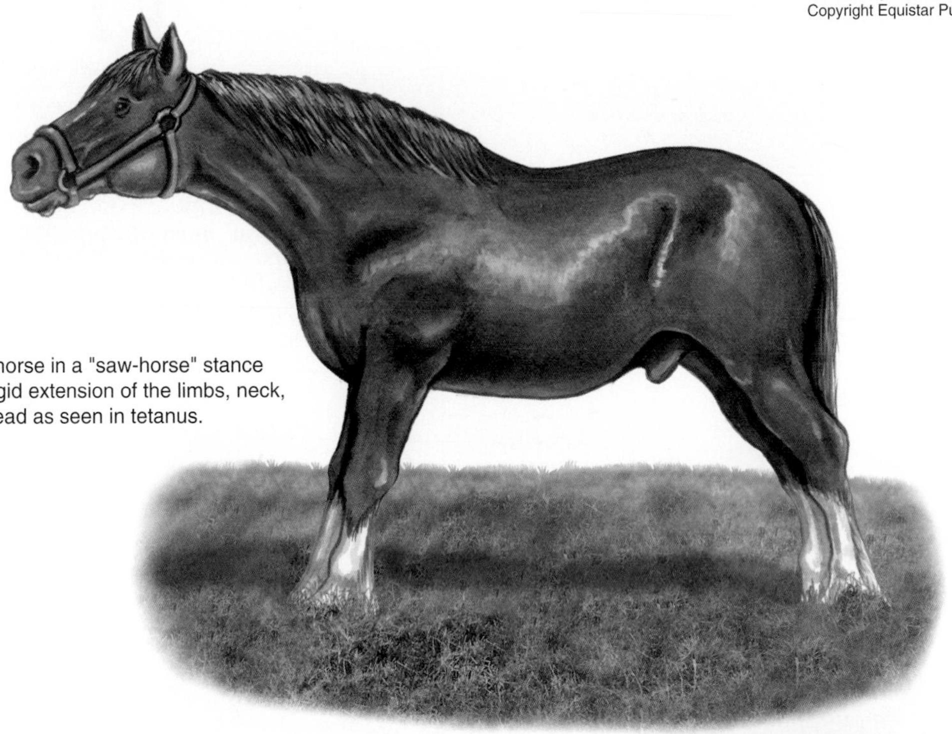

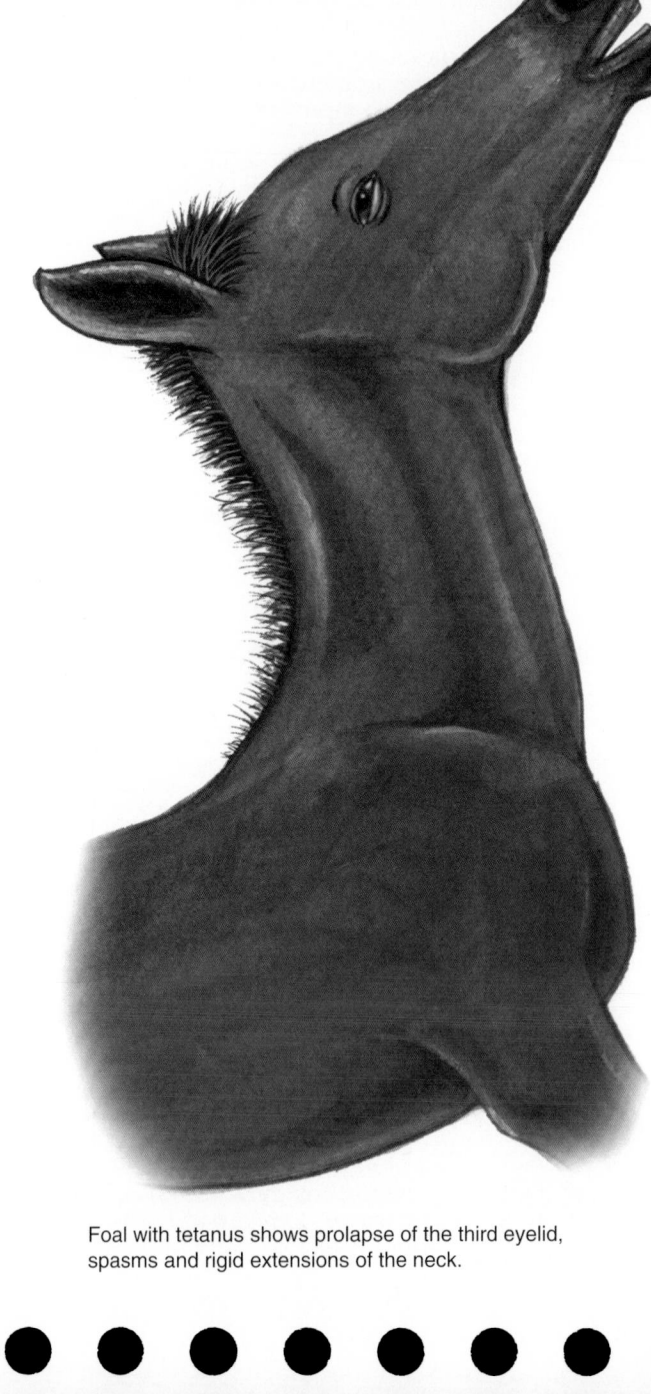

Adult horse in a "saw-horse" stance with rigid extension of the limbs, neck, and head as seen in tetanus.

Foal with tetanus shows prolapse of the third eyelid, spasms and rigid extensions of the neck.

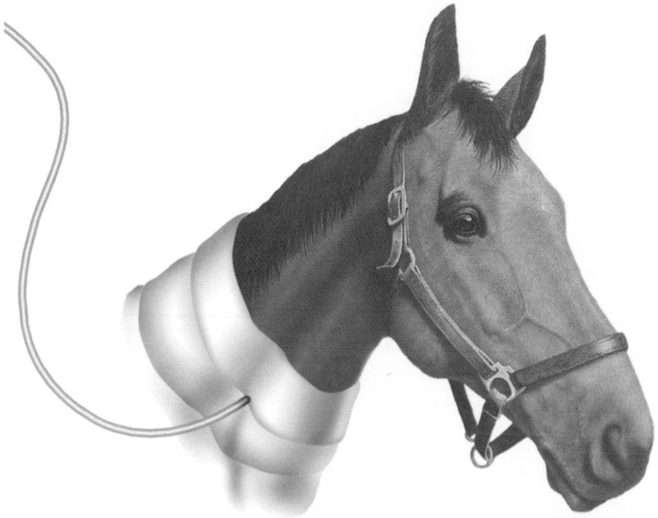

Systemic fluid and electrolyte therapy is essential in addition to supportive nursing care.

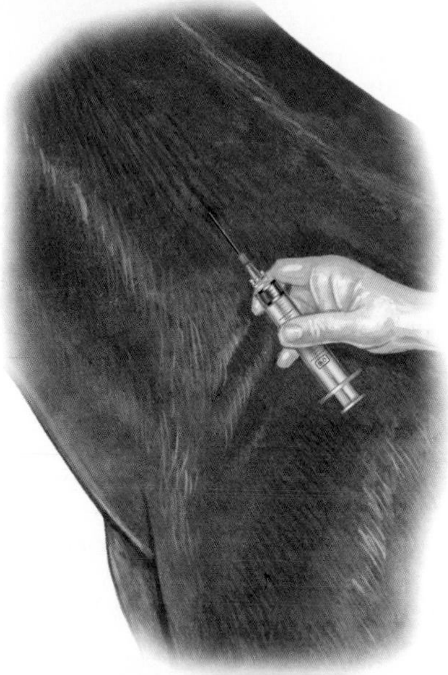

Intramuscular injections of tetanus antitoxin, penicillin and/or tetracycline.

TETANUS

Tetanus is commonly referred to as "lock jaw." It is a highly fatal infectious disease that is caused by toxins liberated from the bacterium *Clostridium tetani* which forms a spore and is capable of existing in the soil for many years. Therefore, horses are frequently exposed to the infective form of this bacteria. This can occur when these spores are deposited deep within the tissues as is caused by a penetrating wound that is contaminated. *Clostridium tetani* needs an anaerobic environment which is provided deep within the tissues of this type of wound. Deep puncture wounds are especially dangerous, but this organism may find ideal growth conditions in any break in the skin or mucous membranes. Suseptibility to *Clostridium tetani* includes wounds from castration procedures, metritis, injuries following a dystocia, or a retained placenta. Infection through the umbilicus is possible in the newborn foal. The incubation period of this organism may range from several days to several months, but usually occurs within one to three weeks.

After the organism gains suitable entry into the tissues, it releases exotoxins which enter the nervous system via peripheral nerve roots. The exotoxin itself is called tetanospasmin and is a water soluble protein that attacks the central nervous system. This exotoxin blocks inhibitory neurotransmitters within the descending motor tracks which results in abnormal contractions of muscles from reflex reactions after normal sensory stimulation.

Clinical Signs

The clinical signs of tetanus vary depending on the amount of toxin, the size of the horse, the age, and the immune status of the affected animal. Initially, these animals may appear to have a slight deficit in their gait or even be lame. This is the result of specific groups of muscles being first affected by the toxin. Some horses are initially reluctant to feed off the ground due to spasms within the cervical muscles.

As the disease progresses, there is a restriction of jaw movement and a prolapse of the third eyelid. The animal's tail may be held out stiffly, especially when the horse is asked to move backward.

The animals may initially exhibit signs of colic or constipation as these horses cannot posture in the correct position to void feces. Further progression of the disease includes over-reaction to normal external stimuli. The spasms of the muscles may initially occur while the animal is eating, but as the disease progresses, a simple tap on the forehead will provoke spasms of the facial, masseter, and extraocular muscles. A sawhorse stance may eventually occur as other striated muscles are affected. The limbs, neck, and tail will appear as if in rigid extension. Eventually, the animal will fall and generally, it is unable to regain its feet because its distress will cause further muscle spasms and further distress. Death is usually the result of asphyxia due to the spastic paralysis of the respiratory muscles, laryngospasms, or aspiration pneumonia. This usually occurs 5 - 7 days after the initial onset of clinical symptoms.

Differential Diagnosis

1.) Exertional Rhabdomyolysis
2.) Laminitis
3.) Heat Stroke

Diagnosis

The diagnosis of tetanus is usually based on history, clinical signs, and a lack of vaccination. The site of infection is often extremely difficult to determine since it may be a former wound that has healed completely. Isolation of this organism is very difficult.

Treatment

Treatment of tetanus can be approached in three parts. The main objective is to eliminate the causative organism *Clostridium tetani*. Secondly, there should be a neutralization of any residual toxins. Finally, the animal needs to be systemically treated to control any neuromuscular spasms and provide nutritional support.

Elimination of the *Clostridium tetani* organisms and neutralization of the toxins involves the administration of large doses of tetanus antitoxin, penicillin, or tetracycline administration and the thorough cleaning of any apparent wounds. Dosages of antitoxin administration have ranged up to 220 IU/kg of body weight every 12 hours. Intravenous administration of 5,000 - 10,000 IU is probably adequate since circulating toxin levels are usually very low. Dosages of 200,000 IU/kg of body weight of potassium penicillin per day divided into four equal doses should destroy any *Clostridium tetani* organisms deep within the tissues. If an infected wound is found, it should be immediately debrided and irrigated with disinfectant solutions.

Supportive nursing care is essential in the treatment of tetanus. This is accomplished through the use of systemic tranquilizers, antiinflammatory drugs, muscle relaxant agents, and fluid therapy. The animal should be kept in a dark stall with a minimum amount of external stimuli. Careful attention should be paid to the hydration and electrolyte status of these animals. Systemic fluid administrations via the intravenous and oral route may be required to correct these deficits. It may even be necessary to catheterize the urinary system and manually remove the fecal material from the rectum due to the effect that the exotoxins have on the excretory muscles.

Prognosis

The prognosis for any horse with tetanus is severely guarded and grave. Complications include laminitis, aspiration pneumonia, and pleuropneumonia. Each of these cases should be evaluated and treatment options should be considered carefully.

Prophylaxis

Any unvaccinated horse should have a prophylactic dose of 1,500 IU of tetanus antitoxin given subcutaneously after any injury. These injured horses should also receive a dose of tetanus toxoid. All mares should receive tetanus immunization in the last 30 days of gestation. Any foals that are born and have not acquired sufficient

Botulism

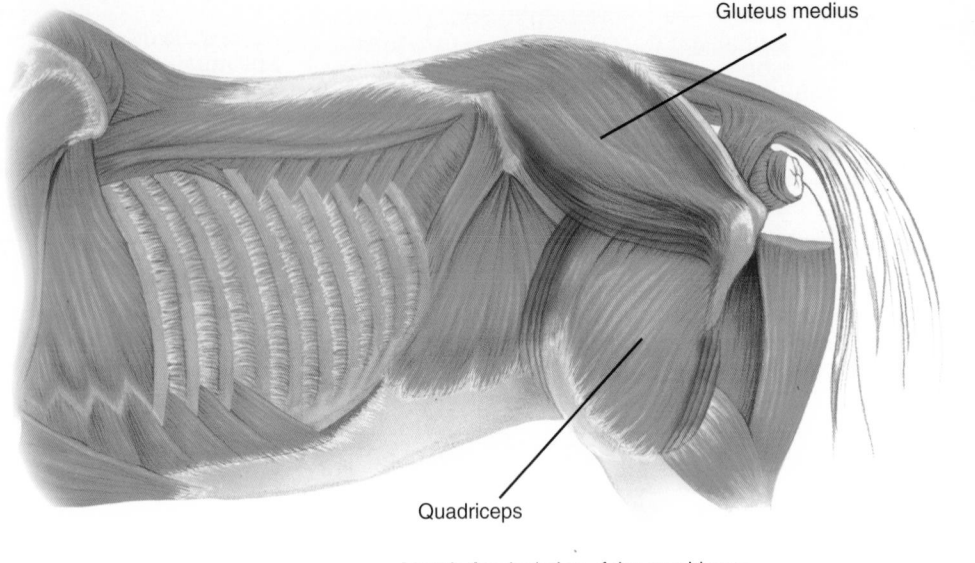

Gluteus medius

Quadriceps

Muscle fasciculation of the quadriceps
and gluteal muscles.

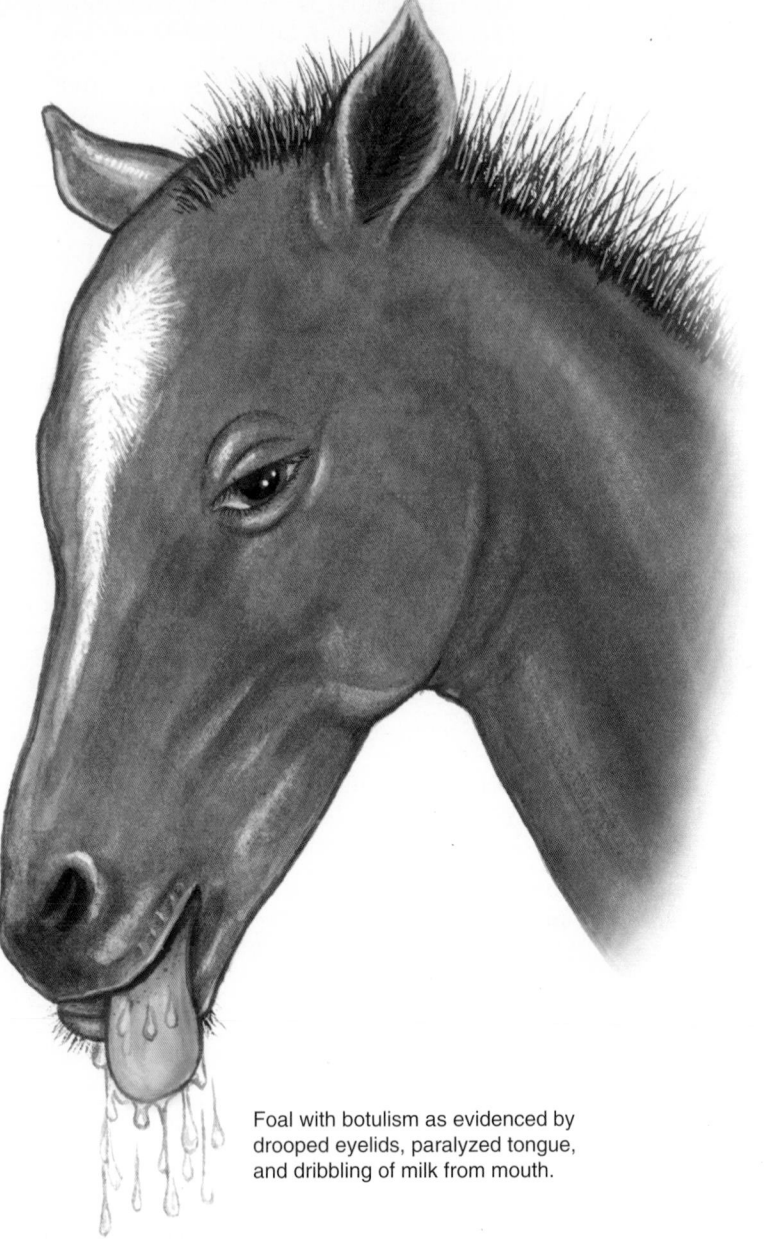

Foal with botulism as evidenced by
drooped eyelids, paralyzed tongue,
and dribbling of milk from mouth.

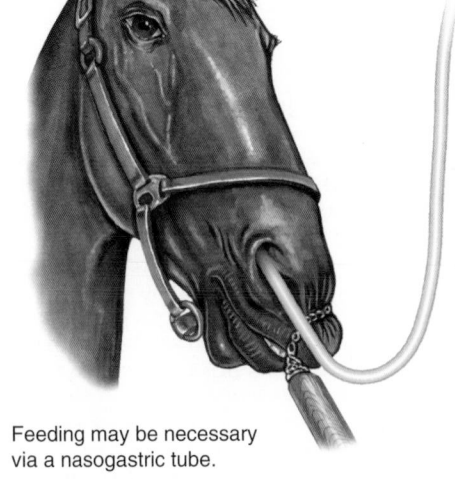

Feeding may be necessary
via a nasogastric tube.

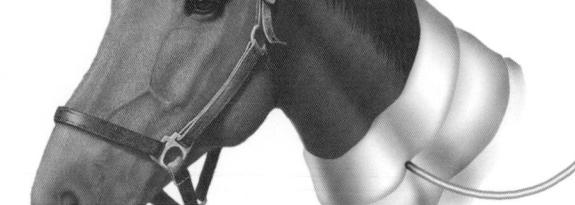

Intravenous fluid and electrolyte therapy.

passive antibodies from colostrum should receive 1,500 IU of tetanus antitoxin. Tetanus toxoid administration should begin at 3 - 4 months of age, boostered again at 6 months of age, and then be administered on an annual basis as part of the preventive health regime.

BOTULISM

Botulism is caused by the exotoxin of the gram-positive bacterium *Clostridium botulinum*. This disease has the ability to affect both foals and adult horses. It is commonly referred to in foals as "shaker foal syndrome." In adults, it is commonly referred to as forage poisoning. *Clostridium botulinum* is an organism that is found in the soil. When this organism multiplies and grows in an anaerobic environment, it produces a toxin. Contaminated feed or the ingestion of stagnant water is usually the source of an outbreak.

Etiology

There are three types of botulism that can occur. Forage poisoning is the ingestion of an already formed toxin. This usually occurs in adult horses and is caused by *C. botulinum* type B or C. The second type of botulism disease that occurs is when the toxin itself is produced within the gastrointestinal tract. This occurs in foals and is commonly referred to as shaker foal syndrome. This is thought to be caused by the type B toxin. An extremely rare form of botulism occurs when the organism grows and liberates its toxin from within a wound. This is commonly referred to as wound botulism. Botulism causes a progressive flaccid neuromuscular paralysis. This toxin blocks acetylcholine release at the sight of the neuromuscular junctions.

Clinical Signs

Clinical signs of botulism may vary from mild to severe. This is dependent upon the amount of toxin that is ingested or being produced within the tissues of the body. Botulism does not affect the central nervous system; therefore, these animals are usually bright and alert but suffer from some degree of paralysis.

Foals can exhibit clinical signs to this disease as early as two weeks of age. Initially, these animals will exhibit muscle weakness and spend a large amount of time lying down. As the effects of the paralysis progress, the animal will begin to dribble milk from both the nostrils and the mouth. Further progression will be evident by muscle tremors, and the foal will be distressed when it cannot keep up with the mare. These muscle tremors are what give the disease its name of shaker foal syndrome. Eventually, the horses will suffer from severe muscle weakness and have difficulty swallowing. The last stages are marked by respiratory distress and recumbency. Death of these animals is eventually due to respiratory paralysis.

The clinical signs in the adult are also toxin dose dependent. Initially, these animals will lose tone in their tail and eyelids. If an endoscopic exam is performed, there will be a slight paralysis of the pharyngeal musculature. Other signs at this stage will include difficulty swallowing, excessive salivation, and dropping of food from the mouth. If the tongue is manually removed from the mouth, the animal may just leave it hang outside and find it difficult to retract the tongue back into the mouth. Initial weakness within these animals will exhibit itself as a stiff short-strided gait. When the horse is exercised, small muscle fasciculations and tremors may be evident. The animal will also develop an intolerance to excercise. In the advanced stages, the weakness becomes more exaggerated, and the respiratory effort becomes increased. Death in the adult horse occurs from respiratory failure. The clinical signs of wound botulism closely resemble those of the adult horse forage poisoning.

Differential Diagnosis

In the foal:
1.) Septicemia
2.) Trauma

In the adult horse:
1.) Trauma
2.) Choke
3.) Equine Protozoal Encephalomyelitis
4.) Hyperkalemic Periodic Paralysis

Diagnosis

Botulism is diagnosed from the clinical signs it exhibits and a lack of any vaccination history. In foals, failure of passive transfer is another source of immune deficiency to be considered. Since the botulism toxin does not affect the central nervous system, the animals are usually bright and alert. This helps in the differentiation of botulism from other neurological disorders.

Treatment

The administration of polyvalent botulism antitoxin is the treatment of choice and should be given as early as possible after a diagnosis is made. It will absorb any free toxin within the system, but is not able to absorb toxin that is already bound to receptors. The recommended dose for treatment of the adult horse is 400 ml, whereas for the foal it is 200 ml.

Nursing care and nutritional support should be given consideration once the antitoxin has been administered. These animals may have to be fed via a nasogastric tube and be given fluid therapy intravenously. All complications involved with this infection should also be treated with either systemic antibiotics or antiinflammatory medications.

Prevention

Vaccination with *C. botulinum* has been very effective in preventing this disease. Brood mares should be vaccinated with three doses of this toxin with one month between vaccinations. The last vaccine should be given within thirty days of parturition. After this initial vaccination procedure, mares should then receive a yearly booster vaccination during their last month of gestation. All other animals should receive an initial three dose series and then be boostered yearly. Vaccination is usually not necessary where this disease is not prevelant.

Artwork by S. Hakola / J. Dirig
Copyright Equistar Publications, Ltd.

Equine Togaviral Encephalomyelitis

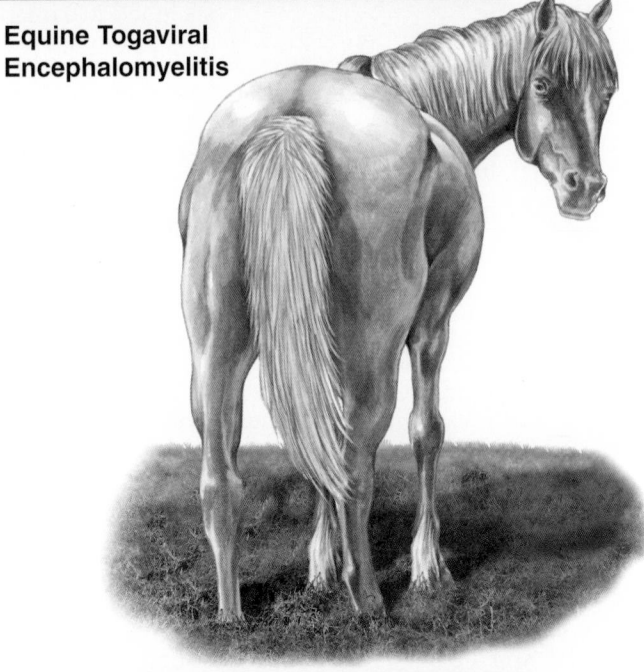

Circling, head pressing, and somnolence are symptoms of equine togaviral encephalomyelitis.

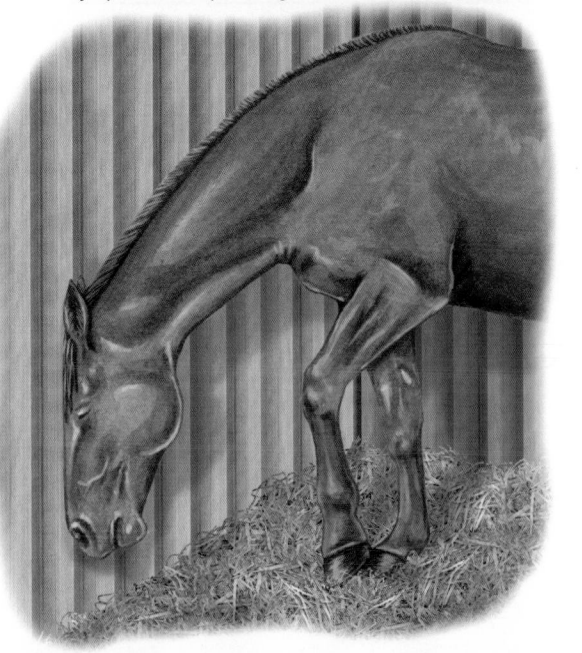

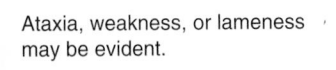

Ataxia, weakness, or lameness may be evident.

Equine Herpesvirus Myeloencephalopathy

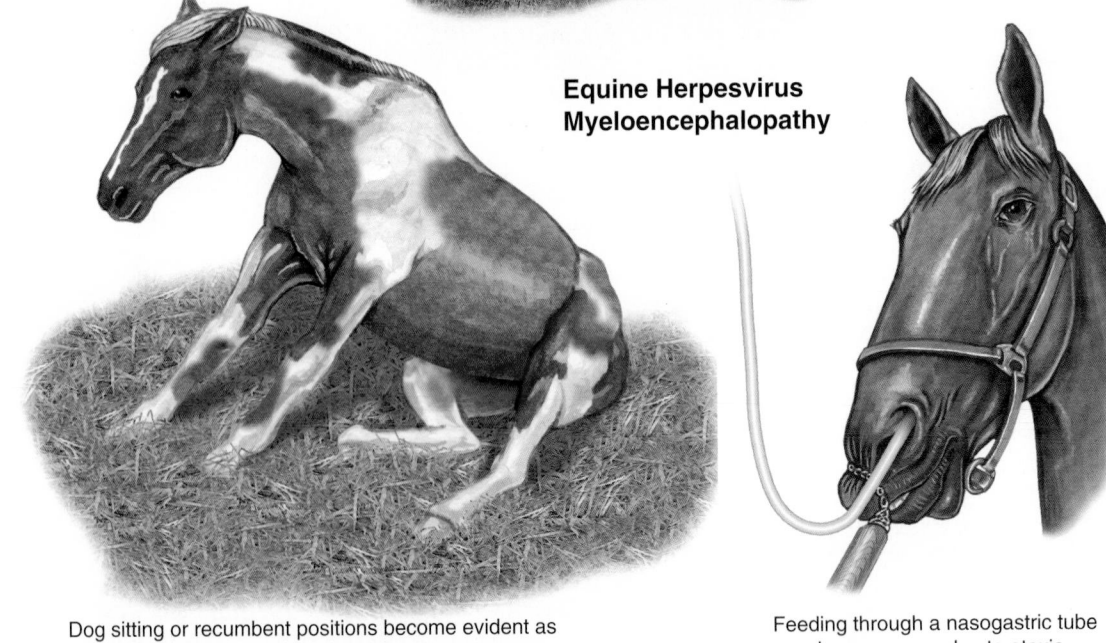

Dog sitting or recumbent positions become evident as equine herpesvirus myeloencephalopathy progresses.

Feeding through a nasogastric tube may be necessary due to ataxia.

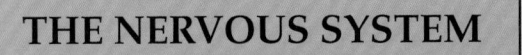

EQUINE TOGAVIRAL ENCEPHALOMYELITIS

Alphaviral encephalomyelitis includes Eastern (EEE), Western (WEE), and Venezuelan (VEE) equine encephalomyelitis. These viruses exist in a host population of birds. Mosquitoes are then responsible for spreading this virus to horses. These viruses affect all ages of horses, but it is rare to find an infection within a foal. Due to climatic conditions, these viruses can occur year round in the Southeastern part of the United States. During the summer and early fall when mosquitoes are present, these viruses can occur in the Northeast. As the name implies, WEE occurs in the West, Midwest and Southern United States, whereas EEE is usually found only in the East. All three viral encephalitis types occur in Mexico and throughout South America.

Clinical Signs

The initial clinical sign for viral encephalitis may be a subtle change in behavior. Normal docile animals may become aggressive or fail to respond to their owners at all. Within a short period of time, these animals will refuse to eat or drink. The horses will always have a fever and act depressed as the condition progresses. As the virus multiplies and the inflammatory response within the animal increases, the horse will exhibit head pressing, circling, blindness, seizures, and eventually end in a comatose state.

Differential Diagnosis

1.) Trauma
2.) Rabies
3.) Equine Protozoal Myeloencephalopathy
4.) Bacterial Meningitis

Diagnosis

Diagnosis of these alphaviruses is based upon clinical signs and the animal being in a geographic area where these diseases are prevalent during mosquito season. Clinical pathology tests on cerebrospinal fluids will usually indicate an increased total protein and a leukocytosis. Compared serum samples may be useful in assisting in the diagnosis. Titers will indicate a four fold increase between the acute phase and those samples collected 10 - 14 days later. Unfortunately, a definitive diagnosis can only be made on a postmortem evaluation of the central nervous system tissues.

Treatment

Currently, there is a lack of any specific treatment for viral encephalitis. Treatment consists of providing good supportive and nursing care. The systemic administration of nonsteroidal anti-inflammatory medications is indicated. If seizures occur, the administration of either diazepam or phenobarbital is often useful. Hydration and nutritional status should be maintained through the administration of IV fluid therapy coupled with feeding through a nasogastric tube. Prevention of viral encephalitis is accomplished through vaccination programs and insect control.

EQUINE HERPESVIRUS MYELOENCEPHALOPATHY

Where there is a large concentration of horses such as at a racetrack, a breeding farm, or a boarding stable, there is a higher incidence of viral infection. Equine herpesvirus type 4 (EHV-4) is a major cause of respiratory tract disease in horses, whereas EHV-1 is responsible for myeloencephalopathy. Equine herpesvirus type 1 can occur in horses of all ages. Depending on the immune status of a specific population of horses, it may affect a single horse, or a generalized outbreak may occur. The incubation time for this virus is approximately 7 days after initial exposure.

Clinical Signs

These animals initially develop a fever and have evidence of a mild respiratory tract disorder. This respiratory clinical sign may just be a cough or a slight nasal discharge. Pregnant mares may abort immediately before or during the development of any neurological clinical signs. Initially, the horse may be presented for a lameness disorder resulting from the abnormalities noticed in the gait. As the virus progresses, the animal may appear stiff and show signs of weakness and ataxia within the limbs. Eventually, these animals will assume the "dog sitting position" or be recumbent. Other neurological clinical signs will include urinary incontinence, penile prolapse, fecal retention, and hypalgesia in the tail and perineal regions.

Differential Diagnosis

1.) Trauma
2.) Rabies
3.) Equine Protozoal Myeloencephalopathy
4.) Viral Encephalititis
5.) Equine Cervical Vertebral Malformation

Diagnosis

Initially a diagnosis of EHV-1 myeloencephalitis can be made upon the characteristic clinical signs. Virus isolation can be done from a nasopharyngeal swab or from the buffy coat within a blood sample. Paired serum samples should reveal a four fold rise in titer with samples taken 7 - 10 days apart. Measuring titers however, may reveal a false negative result since some subtypes are not tested.

Treatment

There is no specific treatment for a viral infection. Supportive and nursing care are critical in the recovery of these affected animals. Systemic fluid therapy may be necessary to maintain hydration to these febrile patients. Animals that are suffering from severe ataxia may require nasogastric tube feedings. Antiinflammatory therapy is essential in allowing the horse to recover more quickly. The passage of urine and stool must be monitered carefully, and urinary catheterization and bowel evacuation may be required.

Prevention

Prevention of this disorder is available through commercial vaccines containing modified live and inactivated adjuvant-containing EHV-1. These vaccines should not be used in any animals showing clinical signs.

Artwork by S. Hakola / J. Dirig
Copyright Equistar Publications, Ltd.

Hyperkalemic Periodic Paralysis

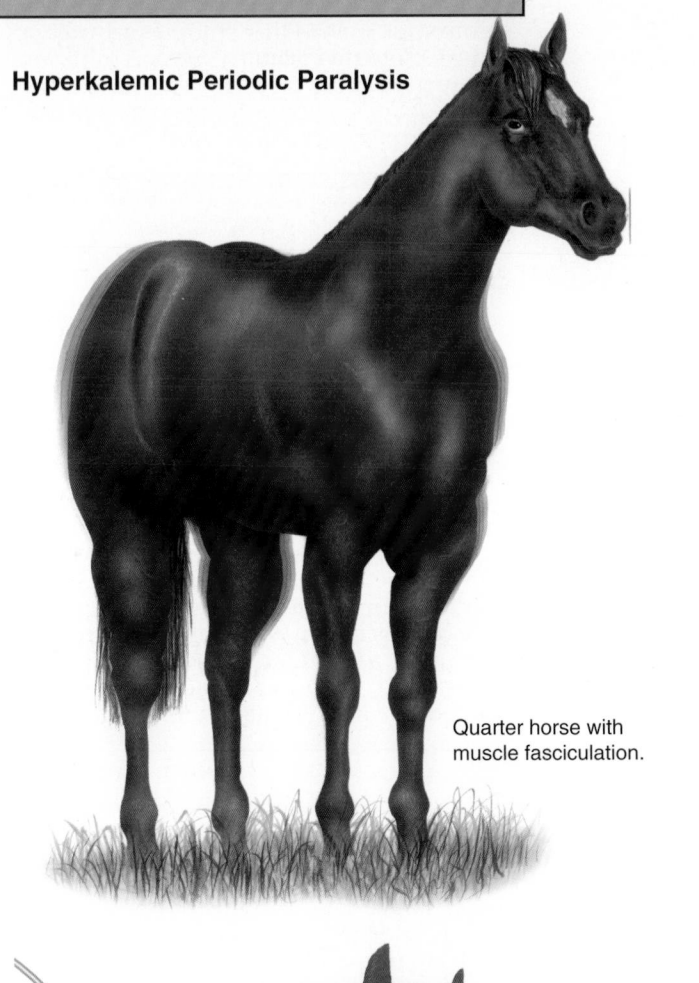

Quarter horse with muscle fasciculation.

Intravenous administration of dextrose with sodium bicarbonate, potassium-free fluids, insulin, and/or calcium gluconate.

Equine Protozoal Myeloencephalitis

EPM horse with severe muscle atrophy

As EPM progresses, abnormal gaits, weakness, or ataxia may become present.

HYPERKALEMIC PERIODIC PARALYSIS (HYPP)

This disorder involves the peripheral nerves and musculature. It is a familial disorder that affects pure and part quarter horses in North America. HYPP is similar to hyperkalemic periodic paralysis in people in that these animals undergo episodes of muscular weakness. It is more common in colts than in fillies, and it usually affects horses that are less than 4 years old.

Clinical Signs

These animals are extremely well muscled and appear absolutely normal between episodes of weakness. Any stressful stimuli such as exercise, high environmental temperatures, or transport may precipitate a clinical manifestation of this disorder. Episodes of hyperkalemic periodic paralysis, however, may be totally unpredictable and occur at random. Initially, the animal will appear still and will have a prolapse of the third eyelid. The horse will begin to sweat, and muscle fasciculation will occur. As the episode progresses, these animals become recumbent and the muscles develop flaccidity. The horse's respiratory and heart rates are usually elevated. The animal will be alert and able to respond to noise and visual stimuli. These episodes usually last between 15 and 16 minutes.

Differential Diagnosis

1.) Exertional Rhabdomyolysis
2.) Colic
3.) Seizures

Diagnosis

A diagnosis can be made when there is an episode of weakness in a relatively young quarter horse that is heavily muscled. These animals have a familial predisposition. This fact should be gathered when a history is taken. Before the episode occurs, serum potassium concentration is within the normal range of 3 - 5 mEq/L. This concentration rises to 7 - 9 mEq/L during the weakness episode and returns to normal following the episode.

A potassium chloride provocation test can be used to identify those animals that are predisposed to these episodes of weakness. This test has some risk involved and should be used with caution. Potassium chloride at a concentration of .088 g/kg is dissolved in 150 ml of water and is administered via a nasogastric tube following an overnight fast. This will usually produce clinical manifestations within affected animals. Blood testing will also indicate the genetic predisposition to this disorder.

Treatment

Intravenous administration of sodium bicarbonate, dextrose, potassium free isotonic fluids, and insulin are of benefit in the treatment of hyperkalemic periodic paralysis. The administration of calcium gluconate at a level of 40 - 90 mg/kg IV diluted in a dextrose solution usually results in a rapid remission of the clinical signs.

Dietary management should be directed at decreasing the potassium intake in the diet. Alfalfa and brome grass hays, which are high in potassium, should be removed from the diet and replaced with oat or grass hay. Oats should be fed 2 - 3 times a day, and any rapid changes in the diet should be avoided.

Acetazolamide has been utilized to successfully reduce the incidence of weakness episodes in those horses that do not respond to dietary management. This medication is administered orally at the level of 2 - 4 mg/kg.

Animals can also be blood tested for this disorder. Any horses with familial predispostion for HYPP should be strongly discouraged from breeding.

EQUINE PROTOZOAL MYELOENCEPHALITIS

Equine protozoal myeloencephalitis is a debilitating disease of horses that results in asymmetric incoordination, weakness, spasticity, and may be potentially fatal. This disorder is caused by the protozoan *Sarcocytis falcatula*. This organism can affect horses of all ages but is more commonly diagnosed in horses less than four years of age.

Etiology

Infection of the horse occurs after ingestion of *S. falcatula* sporocysts. The protozoal organism *Sarcocytis falcatula* has a unique two host species lifecycle. It has a natural intermediate host of passeroid, psittacorid, or columborid bird and a definitive host in the opossum. The intermediate host bird becomes infected when it ingests sporocysts that contaminate its feed or water. These sporocysts give rise to sporozoites which penetrate the intestinal tract of the bird and develop into merozoites within the muscle tissue of the bird. When this avian muscle tissue is eaten by the opossum, the organism undergoes sexual reproduction in the intestinal epithelium of the opossum. An oocyst is formed which contains infected sporocysts. These oocysts are disrupted when the opossum passes feces. Infected sporocysts are then passed in the stool which contaminate feed that is later ingested by the horse.

In reveiw of this lifecycle, horses are then aberrant intermediate hosts of *Sarcocyst falcatula*. Infective sporocysts are ingested and give rise to sporozoites which enter the tissues of the horse. These sporozoites develop into tachyzoites which migrate to the central nervous system where they continue to undergo asexual reproduction. Unique to the horse, these merozoites never form tissue cysts which is why a horse cannot transmit *S. falcatula* to other animals. After the ingestion of infective sporocysts, it takes a minimum of 4 weeks for clinical signs to develop or may even require years to develop and only be manifested when the animal is under stress.

Equine Protozoal Myeloencephalitis (EPM) Life Cycle

The *Sarcocystis* parasite undergoes asexual reproduction in the avian intermediate host.

An opossum feeds on contaminated avian muscle tissue and becomes a definitve host because the *Sarcocystis falcatula* parasite undergoes sexual reproduction in the intestinal tract of the opossum.

After ingestion of feed contaminated with sporocysts, sporozoites are formed in the intestinal tract of the bird which then migrate and develop into merozoites in the muscles.

Oocysts containing infective sporocysts are then passed in the feces which in turn contaminate the horse's feed.

The horse becomes an aberrant intermediate host after ingesting contaminated feed, particularly hay that has been lying on the ground. The sporocysts develop into sporozoites, then mature into merozoites which then migrate into the central nervous system.

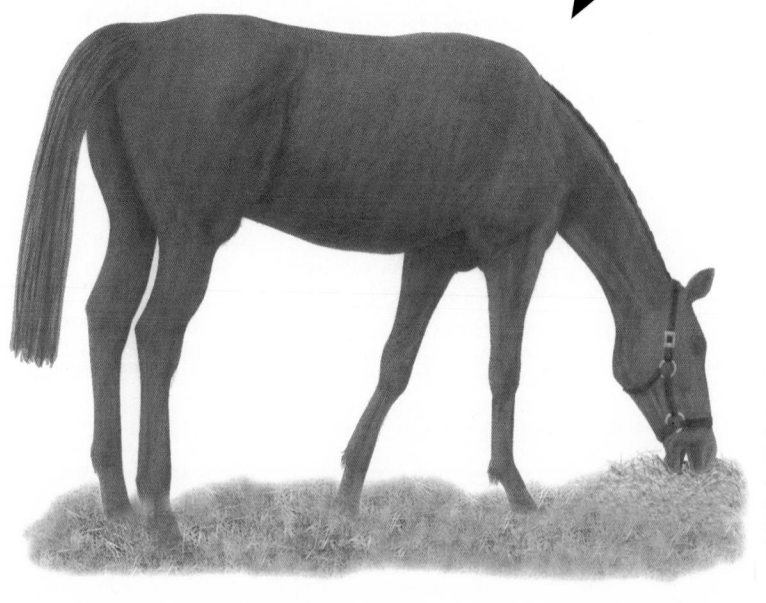

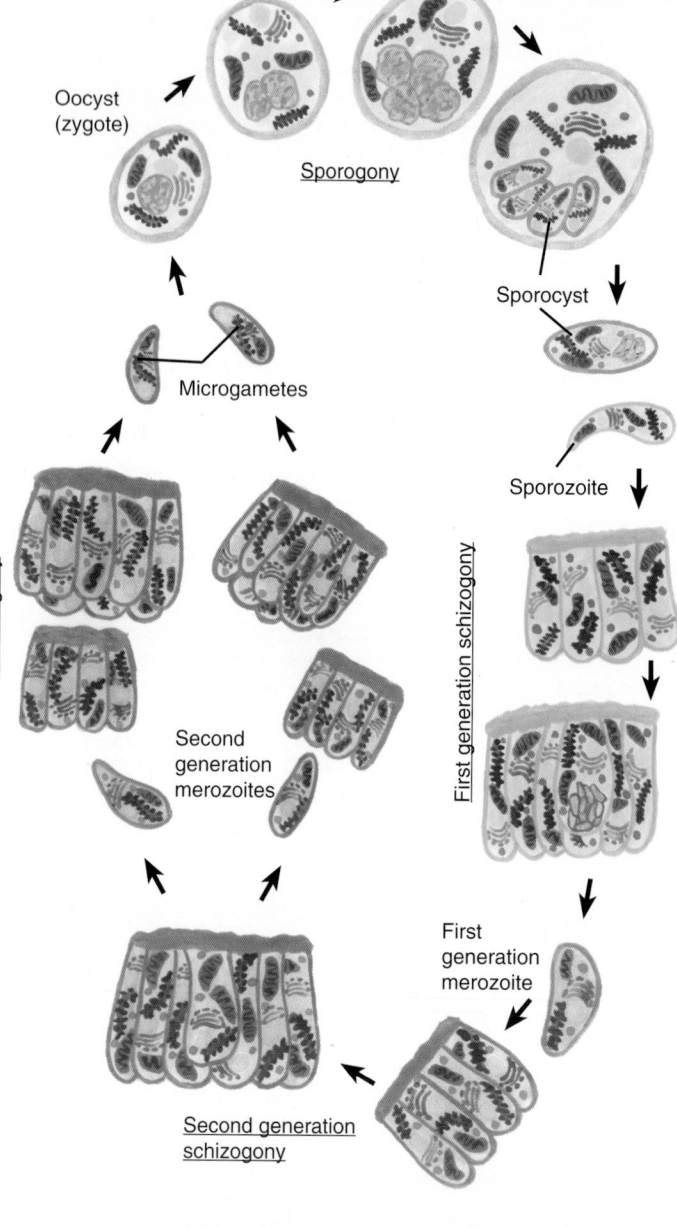

Oocysts with developing sporocysts

Oocyst (zygote)

Sporogony

Sporocyst

Sporozoite

Microgametes

Gametogony

First generation schizogony

Second generation merozoites

First generation merozoite

Second generation schizogony

Sarcocystis falcatula **Life Cycle**

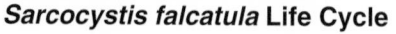

Clinical Signs

Clinical signs of horses suffering from EPM can vary from mild to severe. Initially, these animals may be presented with a lameness complaint since, in the early stages, it may be manifested as an abnormal gait. As the disorder progresses, ataxia, weakness, muscle atrophy, and occasionally behavioral changes will occur. The clinical signs that are evident are a function of the areas of the spinal cord or brain stem that are involved. Classical neurological clinical signs include an asymmetrical ataxia and atrophy of the muscle tissues.

Differential Diagnosis

1.) Rabies
2.) Viral Encephalitis
3.) Equine Herpesvirus Myeloencephalopathy
4.) Trauma
5.) Equine Cervical Vertebral Malformation

Diagnosis

The diagnosis of equine protozoal myeloencephalitis can be based on the exhibited clinical signs, the analysis of cerebrospinal fluid for the presence of anti-*S. falcatula* antibodies, and the response to treatment. If the animal exhibits clinical signs of asymmetrical ataxia and muscle atrophy, a diagnosis of EPM moves far up the differential diagnostic list. Diagnosis can also be based on a trial and error method for EPM by noting any response in the first 10 - 14 days of treatment. If the animal fails to respond within this two week period, additional diagnostic tests should be utilized.

Cerbrospinal fluid analysis is utilized to diagnose most cases of EPM. A sample taken from the lumbosacral space should reveal inflammation, high creatinine kinase activity, and anti-*S. falcatula* antibodies. Anti-*Sarcocystis* antibodies in the cerebrospinal fluid are detected using western blotting or immunoblotting techniques. These tests use the *S. falcatula* organism. Initial screening of serum from a blood sample can also be tested for antisarcistosis, but this test is unreliable.

Treatment

Treatment of equine protozoal myeloencephalitis has the goals of eliminating the parasite, reducing the inflammation within the nervous tissue, and treating any secondary complications. Current antiprotozoal treatment includes:
1.) pyrimethamine at 1.0 mg/kg orally, once daily.
2.) trimethoprim sulfathoxazole or sulfadiazine at 15 - 30 mg/kg in a combined dose orally, twice daily.

Both of these medications should be administered orally with a dose syringe making sure that the animal receives all of the medication. Attempts to treat these animals by adding the drugs to the feedstuffs has failed to achieve a high enough drug level within the body. Treatment with this regime should last a minimum of four months.

There are two other alternative treatments for EPM. Diclazuril, given at a dose of 5 mg/kg orally every 24 hours, has been reported to be efficacious. Toltrazuril is currently being examined as a possible treatment, and the early data is encouraging, but not definitive until all the studies have been completed.

Antiinflammatory therapy should accompany initial treatment with the antiprotozoal drugs. Nonsteroidal antiinflammatory drugs such as phenylbutazone and flunixin meglumine should be utilized. Acute cases of EPM may require additional treatment of diamethyl sulfoxide at a rate of 1g/kg in a 10% solution intravenously.

Diarrhea, colitis, and anemia are common complications involved in the antibiotic and antiprotozoal doses used in the treatment of EPM. Each of these complications should be handled on an individual basis, and the animal must be monitored continually. The anemia is produced by the interference of these drugs on folic acid metabolism by the horse. Therefore, it may be important to supplement folic acid to these animals throughout their treatment regime.

Prognosis

When EPM is diagnosed in early stages, recovery to normal usually occurs in 50 - 70% of the cases. Response to the treatment within the first 10 - 14 days of the treatment regime is a good indicator in the prognosis of recovery. There are always exceptions to this rule, but those horses that are diagnosed early and are mildly affected are more likely to return to normal.

Prevention

Prevention is centered on not allowing any of the feed ingested by the horses to become contaminated. The stable area and feed rooms should be kept clean, and the management practice of feeding grain swept up from the floor should be discontinued. Opossums can usually be trapped and relocated to a new location in an attempt to eliminate them from the horse's environment. Hay storage facilities should be built like a poured concrete bunker silo to eliminate access around the base to opossums and other rodents.

THE EYE AND ADNEXA

Anatomy of the External Eye and Nasolacrimal Duct

Artwork by S. Hakola / J. Dirig
Copyright Equistar Publications, Ltd.

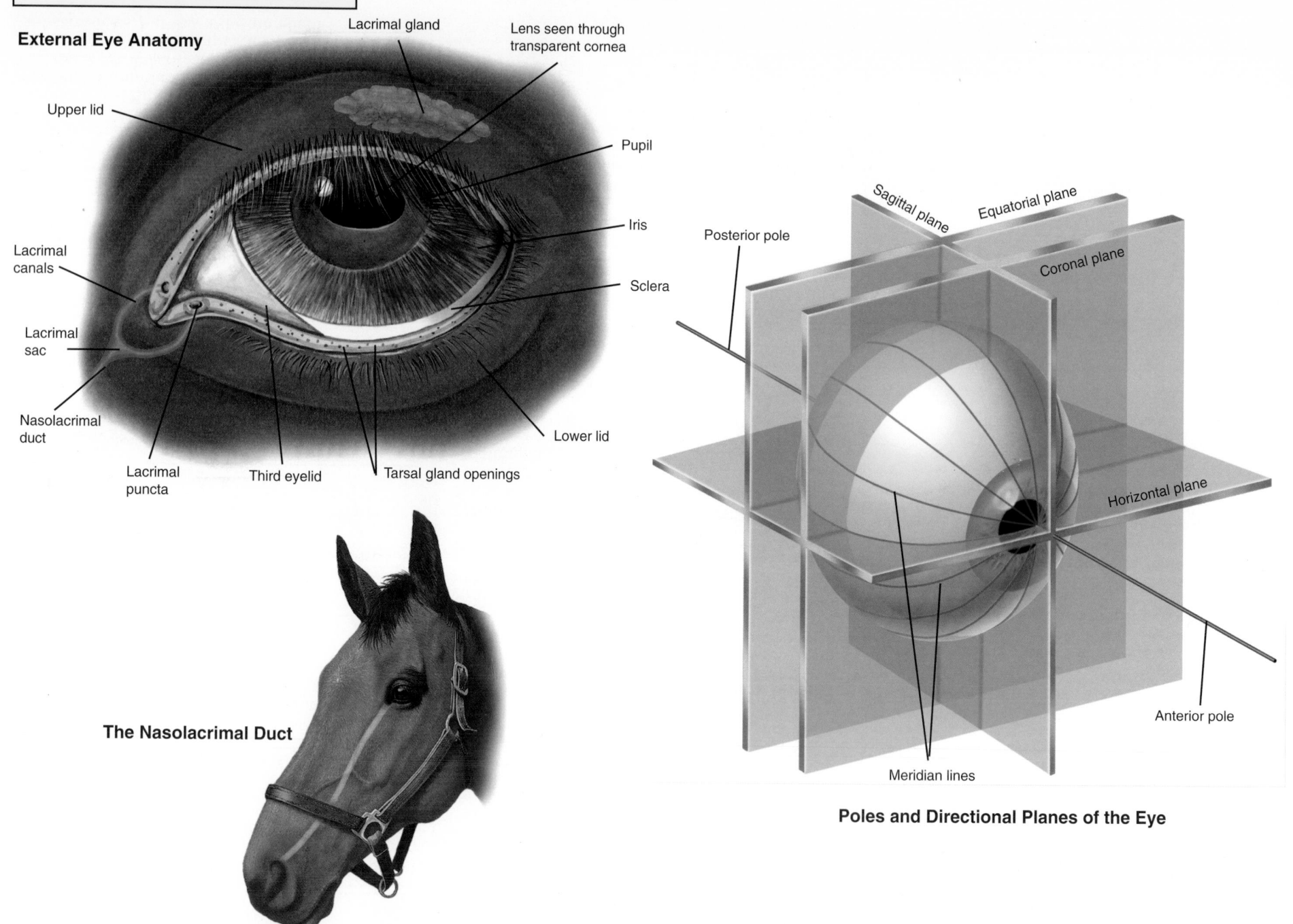

External Eye Anatomy

- Lacrimal gland
- Lens seen through transparent cornea
- Upper lid
- Pupil
- Iris
- Lacrimal canals
- Sclera
- Lacrimal sac
- Nasolacrimal duct
- Lower lid
- Lacrimal puncta
- Third eyelid
- Tarsal gland openings

The Nasolacrimal Duct

- Posterior pole
- Sagittal plane
- Equatorial plane
- Coronal plane
- Horizontal plane
- Anterior pole
- Meridian lines

Poles and Directional Planes of the Eye

9

The Eye

ANATOMY OF THE EYE AND ADNEXA

The organ of vision for the horse is the eye. It consists of the eyeball and all of the adnexa, or accessory structures, surrounding the eyeball. These accessory structures allow movement, provide protection, and moisten the eyeball. The adnexa includes the following: the ocular muscles, the eyelids, the conjunctiva, and the lacrimal apparatus. The eyes of the horse are positioned laterally on the skull which allows the horse to be constantly aware of its surrounding environment.

THE ADNEXA OF THE EYE

The muscles that provide movement to the eye arise deep within the orbit, originating in the vicinity of the optic foramen. The exception to this is the ventral oblique muscle which takes origin from a slight depression in the ventral medial wall of the orbit. There are four rectus muscles, two oblique muscles, and the retractor bulbi muscle. All but one of these muscles end on the sclera near or slightly anterior to the equator. The levator palpebrae muscle leaves the orbit and ends in the upper eyelid.

The four rectus muscles insert anterior to the equator of the eye via wide, but very thin tendons. These are the dorsal, the ventral, the medial, and the lateral rectus muscles. Attaching to the eyeball near the equator and aiding in the rotation of the eyeball are the dorsal and the ventral oblique muscles. The retractor bulbi muscle arises in the vicinity of the optic foramen and inserts on the eyeball posterior to the equator. This muscle is unique, and it forms a nearly complete muscular cone surrounding the optic nerve.

The eyelids are basically two musculofibrous folds which consist of three layers. The outermost layer is skin which is thin and covered with short hairs. There is a musculofibrous layer in the middle that includes the striated orbicularis oculi muscle, the orbital septum, the aponeurosis, and the smooth tarsal muscle. The deepest layer is that part of the eyelid which touches the eyeball and is termed the palpebral conjunctiva. The upper eyelid is more extensive and more mobile than the lower lid. The free margins of both eyelids meet at the medial and lateral angles of the eye and form an opening called the palpebral fissure.

The third eyelid is located between the lacrimal caruncle and the eyeball along the medial angle of the eye. Unlike the true eyelids, it consists of a T-shaped piece of cartilage whose bar lies in the free wedge of the fold, and whose stem points backward into the orbit medial to the eyeball. This cartilage is covered on both of its exposed surfaces with conjunctiva.

The lacrimal apparatus consists of a lacrimal gland that lies dorsal and lateral to the eyeball, an accessory lacrimal gland, which is the gland of the third eyelid, several other small accessory glands, and a duct system that conveys the lacrimal fluid from the eye down into the nasal cavity for evaporation. The lacrimal gland proper is a flat structure which lies between the eyeball and the dorsolateral wall of the orbit. Numerous minute ducts drain its secretion into the dorsal fornix of the conjunctival sac where it mixes with the secretions of the lesser glands. When the horse blinks, this lacrimal fluid is then distributed over the exposed part of the eye. This supplies moisture as well as some nutritional components to these tissues. The lacrimal secretions or tears also carry away any foreign material.

After the lacrimal fluid is spread over the cornea by blinking, it drains to the medial angle of the eye, where a complex duct system eventually allows it to flow to the floor of the nostril. The lacrimal lake is a shallow depression surrounding the prominent lacrimal caruncle. It allows a pooling of the lacrimal fluid which is then conveyed via the upper and lower lacrimal puncta, the lacrimal canaliculi, and the lacrimal sac to finally pass through the long nasolacrimal duct to the orifice which opens on the floor of the nostril. The lacrimal sac is actually a funnel-shaped fossa that occurs at the beginning of the nasolacrimal duct. The duct runs rostrally within the wall of the maxilla and then on the internal surface

THE EYE AND ADNEXA

Anatomy of the Eyeball

Artwork by S. Hakola / J. Dirig
Copyright Equistar Publications, Ltd.

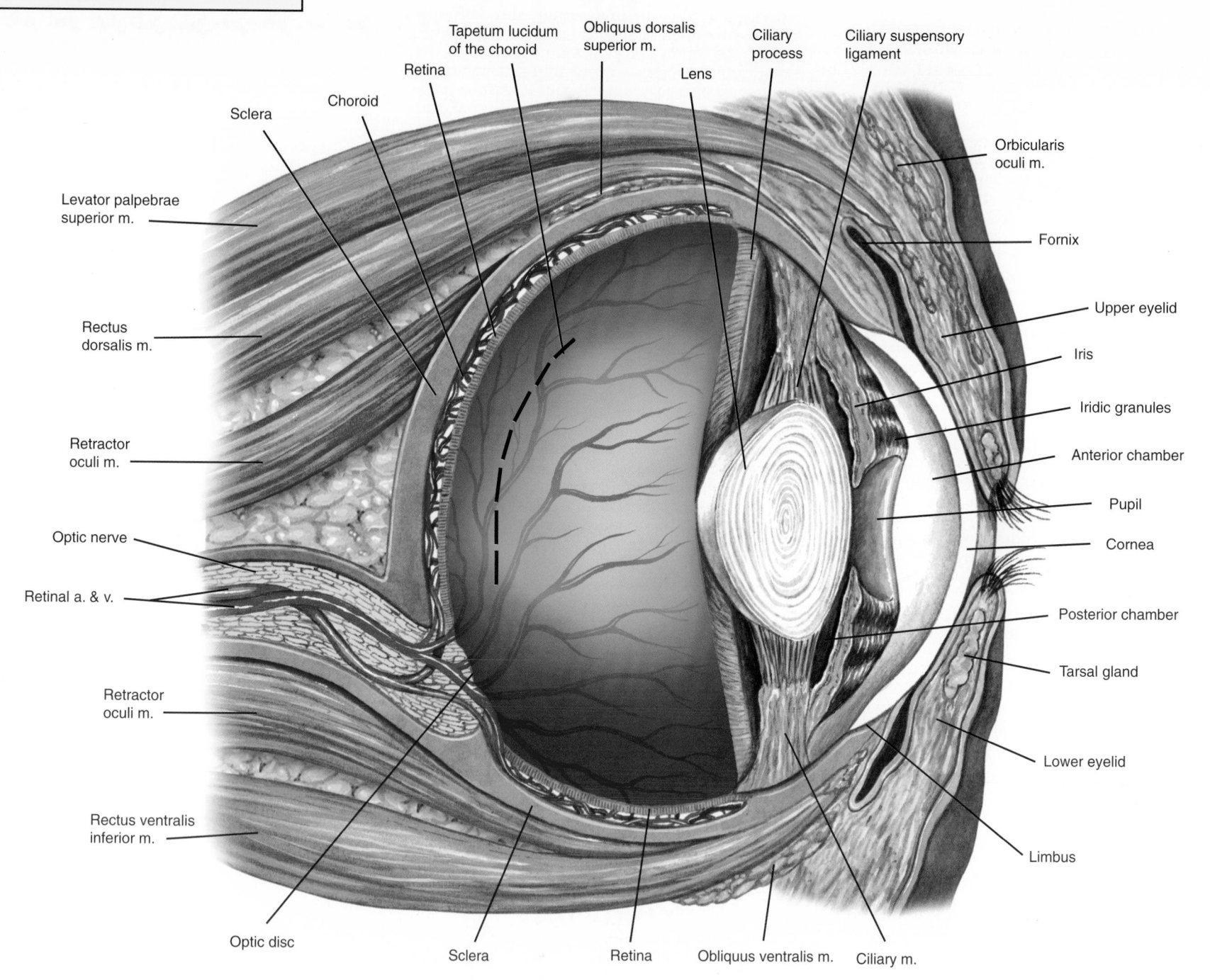

Tapetum lucidum of the choroid

Retina

Choroid

Sclera

Obliquus dorsalis superior m.

Lens

Ciliary process

Ciliary suspensory ligament

Orbicularis oculi m.

Levator palpebrae superior m.

Fornix

Upper eyelid

Rectus dorsalis m.

Iris

Iridic granules

Retractor oculi m.

Anterior chamber

Pupil

Cornea

Optic nerve

Retinal a. & v.

Posterior chamber

Retractor oculi m.

Tarsal gland

Lower eyelid

Rectus ventralis inferior m.

Limbus

Optic disc

Sclera

Retina

Obliquus ventralis m.

Ciliary m.

of the maxilla, where it is covered by nasal mucosa. This nasolacrimal duct terminates at the nasolacrimal orifice on the floor of the nostril.

THE EYEBALL

The eyeball of the horse is a nearly spherical structure which is slightly compressed anterior to posterior. The transparent portion of the eye, the cornea, bulges from the anterior surface. The anterior pole is located at the highest point on the cornea, whereas the posterior pole is the highest point on the posterior surface of the eyeball. The optic axis passes through both posterior and anterior poles of the globe. Just like its counter part on the planet Earth, the equator is that line about the eyeball which is equidistant from the poles. Meridian lines pass from pole to pole and intersect the equator at right angles.

The axes of both the horse's eyes diverge at an angle of about 90 degrees. In man, these axes are nearly parallel to each other. The smaller the angle between the axes, the larger the field of binocular vision, and the greater the perception of depth. These axes are positioned in the horse to permit a constant awareness of a large segment of its environment but little depth of field.

The eye consists of three layers that form a wall surrounding the liquid gelatinous center and include the following: the fibrous tunic, the vascular tunic, and the internal nervous tunic. The only complete layer of the eye is the fibrous tunic which functions to give form to the eye and provides protection. It consists of the sclera and the cornea. The area where these two structures meet is called the limbus.

The sclera is the white portion of the eye. It consists of both collagenous and elastic fibers. The optic nerve passes through the sclera ventral to the posterior pole of the eyeball and is surrounded by a sheath of connective tissue that is a continuation of the dura mater to the sclera. There are many small ciliary arteries, veins, and nerves which also penetrate the sclera. Along the area of the limbus, the sclera is covered by conjunctiva which functions as a connection to the inside of the eyelids.

The cornea is that translucent part of the fibrous tunic that bulges the anterior pole of the globe forward. The cornea is composed of special dense connective tissue arranged in lamellar form. The translucence of the cornea is not only a function of the arrangement of the connective tissue, but it is also due to the physiological phenomenon of the continuous pump of the interstitial fluids. The corneal tissue does not contain any vascular structures; therefore, nutrition for these cells arises from lacrimal fluid and aqueous humor.

Attached to the internal surface of the sclera is the vascular tunic of the eye, also known as the uvea. This vascular tunic consists of three zones: the choroid, the ciliary body, and the iris.

Lining the sclera from the optic nerve to the limbus is the choroid. It consists almost exclusively of blood vessels and is heavily pigmented. The tapetum lucidum is formed by the choroid over the dorsal portion of the fundus. This tapetum lucidum is an avascular, triangular fibrous layer that causes light to be reflected into a yellowish or bluish-green iridescence. This area is what makes the eyes "shine" when they look toward a light such as the headlights of an oncoming car.

The choroid thickens about half way between the equator and the limbus to form the ciliary body which is a raised ring of radical folds and processes radiating toward the lens in the center. Anteriorly, this ring is continued by the iris. The ciliary muscle is a smooth muscle that is located between the ciliary body and the sclera and functions during accommodation (the ability of the eye to change the curvature of the lens to focus on near or distant objects.)

The iris is located between the cornea and the lens. It is the smallest portion of the vascular tunic. The opening in the center is the pupil which allows light to enter the posterior portion of the eye. The iris divides the space between the lens and the cornea into anterior and posterior chambers. Both of these chambers are filled with aqueous humor which is a clear, watery gelatinous fluid.

The common term for the internal or nervous tunic of the eyeball is the retina which contains light-sensitive receptor cells that are an extension of the brain connected by the optic nerve. The retina lines the interior of the eyeball from the pupil to the optic disc. Only the posterior 2/3 of the retina can be reached by light entering the pupil. Therefore, only that portion of the retina contains receptor cells and is termed the pars-optica retinae. The remaining third of the retina is "blind" and termed the pars-ceaca retinae.

The optic disc contains no light-sensitive cells. It is commonly referred to as the blind spot and can easily be seen on an ophthalmic examination. This disc lies ventral to the tapetum lucidum and temporal posterior pole of the globe. It is within this structure that the axons of the pars-optica retinae pass through the sclera to form the optic nerve.

Suspended posterior to the iris is the lens. Anterior to the lens are both the anterior and posterior chambers which are filled with aqueous humor. Posterior to the lens is the vitreous body. The lens tissue itself is enclosed in a capsule and is composed of curved lens fibers whose ends are joined to neighboring fibers on the anterior and posterior surfaces. These fibers form concentric sheets that can be pealed off in layers just like an onion.

The external ophthalmic artery is the main blood supply of the eye and is a branch of the maxillary artery. The central retinal artery branches off the external ophthalmic artery and enters the optic nerve close to the globe. The external ophthalmic artery also gives rise to the long, the short, and the anterior ciliary arteries which supply the choroid, the ciliary body, and the iris. The external ophthalmic artery terminates by supplying the extraocular muscles, the lacrimal gland, and also portions of the eyelid.

Six of the cranial nerves innervate the eye and its accessory structures and include the following: the optic nerve (C.N. II), the oculomotor nerve (C.N. III), the trochlear nerve (C.N. IV), the trigeminal nerve (C.N. V), the abducent nerve (C.N. VI), and the facial nerve (C.N. VII). Dilation of the pupil and innervation of the orbital muscles arise from sympathetic nerve fibers, whereas

THE EYE AND ADNEXA

Examination of the Eye

A = Auriculopalpebral n. (a branch of the facial n.)
B = Palpebral n. (a branch of the facial n.)
C = Supraorbital branch of the frontal n.
D = Infratrochlear n. (a branch of the nasociliary n.)
E = Lacrimal n. (a branch of the ophthalmic n.)
F = Zygomatic n. (a branch of the maxillary n.)

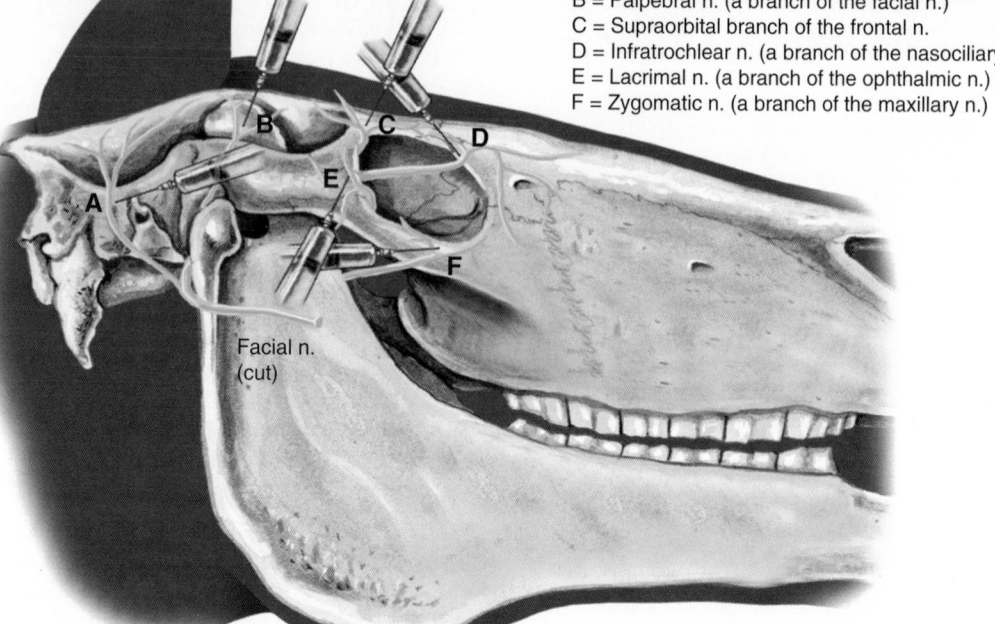

Facial n. (cut)

Sites for Regional Anesthesia With Local Nerve Blocks

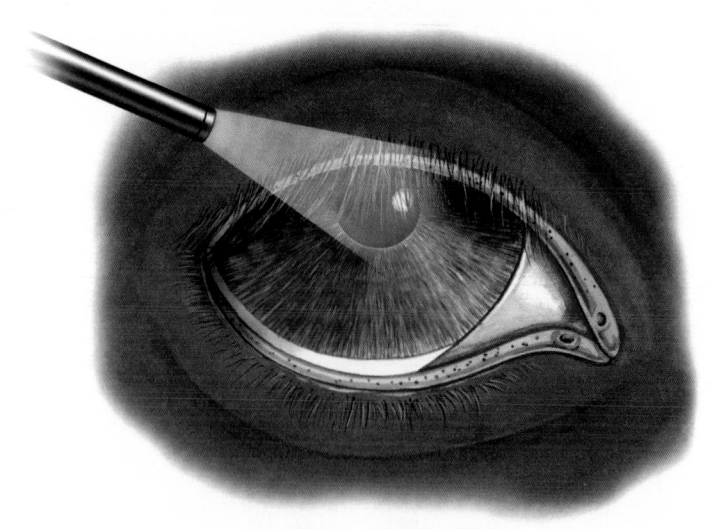

Pupillary Reflex Test

Close Direct Ophthalmoscopy

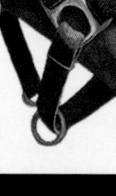
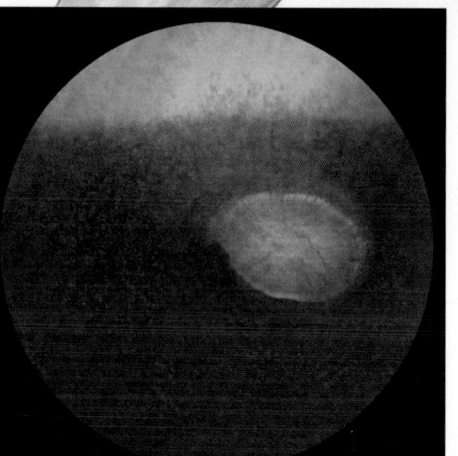

Normal fundus as seen in an ophthalmoscopic exam.

constriction of the pupil and innervation of the ciliary muscles are provided by parasympathetic presynaptic nerve fibers. These parasympathetic nerve fibers control both the accommodation of the lens and the pupillary constriction light response.

EXAMINATION OF THE EYE AND ADNEXA

History

The horse should undergo a general physical exam. The animal's age, breed, and previous illnesses should be noted. Information about the management procedures involved with the horse is important in the determination of its environment, stabling, and feeding program. A history of the present problem should be established. Questions to the owner should include the following: How fast has the problem occurred? Has the problem been present in the past? What treatments did it receive? Is the problem unilateral or bilateral in nature?

Examination

Control of the patient is essential in performing a detailed examination of the eye and adnexa. In most cases, a twitch is applied which provides control without chemical restraint. On certain occasions, sedation and analgesia are needed. Sedation is accomplished through the administration of detomidine hydrochloride. If analgesia is also required, a systemic analgesic such as butorphanol can be administered.

Local anesthesia can be provided topically or through the local infiltration of a nerve via a nerve block. When desensitization of the ocular surface is required, 0.5% proxymetacaine hydrochloride can be administered topically.

The auriculopalpebral nerve branches off the facial nerve to provide innervation to the adnexa. When blepharospasm occurs, this nerve can be blocked by injecting a local anesthetic near the base of the ear and caudal to the ramus of the mandible. A suitable small needle is used to administer 5 - 7 ml of a 1% prilocaine hydrochloride or 2% mepivacaine hydrochloride solution.

Sensory innervation to the middle 2/3 of the upper eyelid is supplied by the supraorbital branch of the ophthalmic division of the trigeminal nerve. A suitable needle is placed through the supraorbital foramen to a depth of approximately one half an inch. One to two milliliters of anesthetic solution is then administered through the foramen. This nerve block usually provides sufficient anesthesia for minor eyelid surgery.

External Examination

This part of the examination should be done outside or in a well lit area within the stable. A pen light, a magnifying loop, or magnifying spectacles may be used to enhance the eye and associated structures for evaluation.

Symmetry, eyelid function, abnormal discharges, signs of trauma, and swelling should be noted. The pupil should be examined for size, shape, and symmetry compared to the opposite eye. Careful examination and palpation should be used to determine the presence of any swelling within the periorbital region. An overflow of tears from the eye (epiphora) is quite common with most eye problems. This fluid should be examined for any evidence of exudate or inflammatory transudate. When the nasolacrimal duct is obstructed, it will produce a reflux of nasal lacrimal drainage which mimics other diseases of the eye and adnexa. The size of the globe should be evaluated by standing in front of the horse and noting symmetry and protrusion of the eye globe.

Ocular and Eyelid Reflexes

The pupillary light reflexes are usually conducted in a darkened room. A focal source of light is directed into each eye separately. A pupillary light reflex is present when the pupil constricts in response to light. An indirect pupillary reflex is present when a focal point of light is directed into the opposite eye causing constriction of the pupil in the examined eye.

The menace reflex is tested by threatening the eye with a hand or finger. The eyelids or cilia should not be contacted with the hand or finger, and care should be taken to ensure that wind currents are not generated which would cause the eye to blink. Corneal and palpebral reflexes are tested by gently touching each structure respectively. When these structures are contacted, a response should be elicited.

Vision can be tested by making the animal negotiate an unfamiliar obstacle course. Blindfolding each eye separately will also test the visual ability of the other eye.

Detailed Ocular and Adnexa Examination

A detailed examination of the eye should be conducted in a darkened room or stall. The animal should be adequately restrained and may have to be sedated. A focal light source, such as a pen light, a direct ophthalmoscope, an indirect ophthalmoscope, and a short-acting mydriatic solution may be useful in conducting this examination.

The anterior chamber and iris should be examined with a light source and some degree of magnification. Normal contents, the presence of foreign bodies, and any evidence of uveitis should be noted.

The equine cornea is large and prominent. There is an obvious gray line at the medial and lateral limbus which is caused by the insertion of the pectinate ligaments into the posterior cornea. This structure should be evaluated for foreign bodies, punctures, ulcers, lacerations, and edema.

Aqueous humor fills the anterior chamber of the eye. It should be clear with no opacities present. A slit beam rather than a diffuse beam of light should be used to examine this area.

The iris of the horse is heavily pigmented and can be present in a wide range of colors including dark brown, gold, blue, gray, white, and even pink. The distinctions between the pupillary and the ciliary zones at the collarette are not always precise.

Entropion

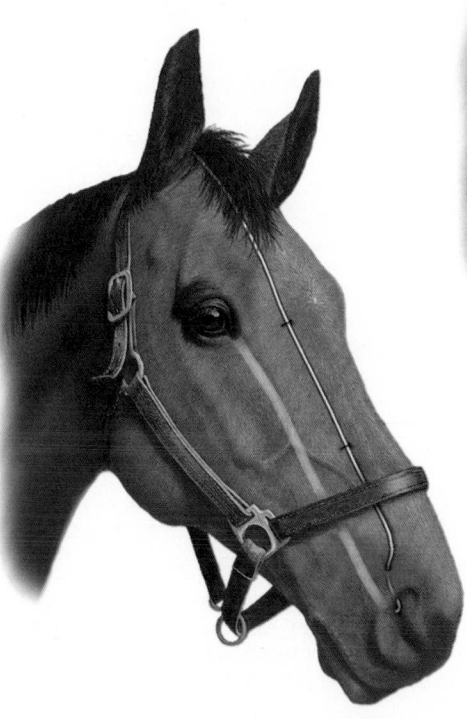

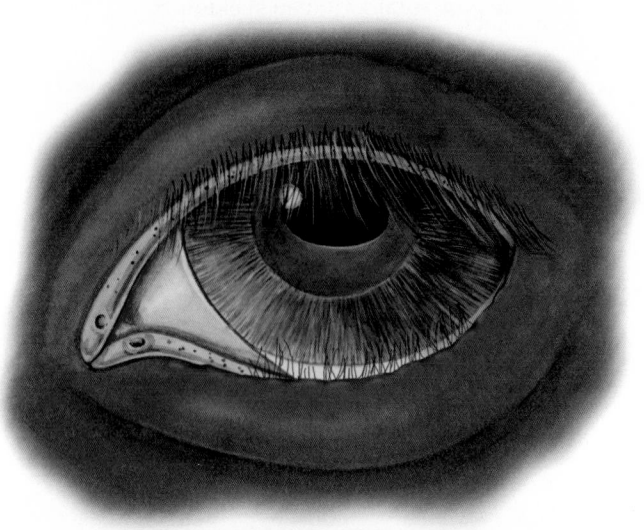

Eversion of the lower eyelid allows eyelashes to scrape against the cornea.

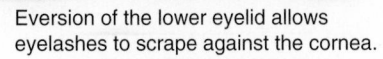

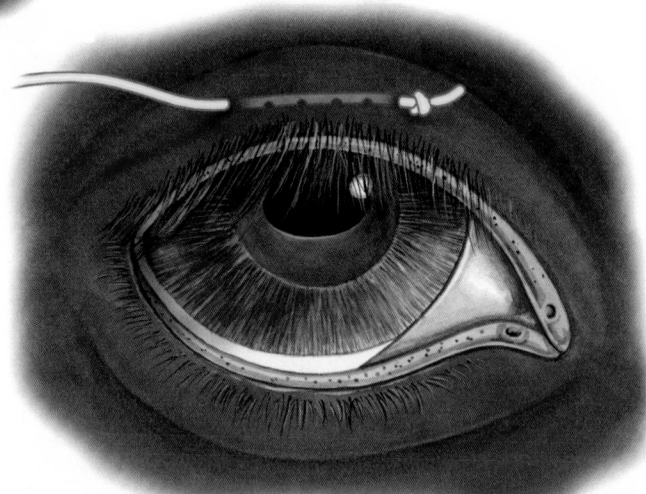

Application of topical ophthalmic ointment.

Silastic tubing placed into and beneath the upper eyelid.

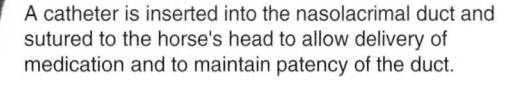

A catheter is inserted into the nasolacrimal duct and sutured to the horse's head to allow delivery of medication and to maintain patency of the duct.

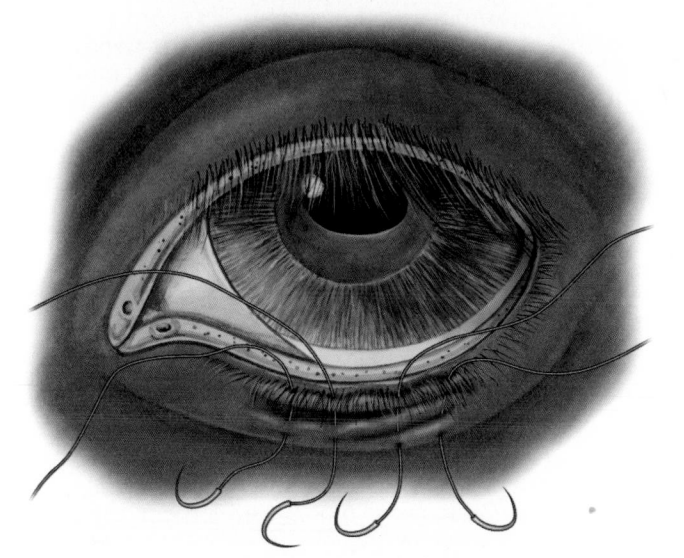

Sutures placed to pleat the lower eyelid prevent it from rolling inward.

Remnants of a persistent pupillary membrane are a common finding.

The corpora nigra, which are the darkly pigmented granula iridica along the pupillary borders of most horses, are prominent features of the borders. These are sometimes surprisingly large in structure but do not have any effect on vision.

Observations should be made as to the size and shape of the pupil. Using a focal light source, the pupillary light response, which is a subcortical reflex, is evaluated in a darkened stall. This light response is somewhat sluggish when compared to other species, unless the light is particularly bright.

In order to examine the entire lens, the pupil needs to be dilated, and the examination needs to be conducted in a darkened stall. The anterior and posterior surfaces of the lens should be examined for clarity. The anterior and posterior lens suture lines are a normal variation in lens opacity.

The internal structure of the globe beyond the lens can be examined using a light source, indirect ophthalmoscopy, distant direct ophthalmoscopy, and close direct ophthalmoscopy. The fundus can be examined using close direct ophthalmoscopy with a setting of -3 diopters within 12 -15 cm of the eye. Indirect ophthalmoscopy will allow visualization of a large area of the ocular fundus at a low power. The optic disc can be seen situated at the junction of the tapetal and nontapetal fundus. It should be examined for size, shape, and color. Retinal vasculature should be examined within all four quadrants of the ocular fundus.

The vitreous should be free of any opacities. Most remnants of the hyaloid system that are present at birth will have disappeared by nine months of age.

TOPICAL TREATMENT METHODS OF THE EYE

Topical treatments of the eye can often be difficult to administer due to the animal's temperament, the patient's size, the painful nature of the problem, and the frequency with which these topical treatments should be given. Medications can be administered manually, through subpalpebral lavage, or with the use of an indwelling nasolacrimal cannula.

Ophthalmologic liquids and ointments can be applied to the eye onto the lower conjunctival sac medial to the canthus. The hand that is holding the bottle, syringe, or tube should be rested against the animal's head. This steadies the hand which allows it to move when the horse moves suddenly. The treatment medium is then discharged with a moderate force directly onto the eye.

The placement of silastic tubing into the upper eyelid using a large needle will allow frequent topical therapy without the need to put pressure on an already painful eye. The animal is tranquilized, and a local anesthetic is administered dorsal to the upper eyelid. Using a 12 -14 gauge needle, a 20 cm piece of pliable polyethylene tubing is placed in the dorsal fornix parallel to or at 90 degrees to the upper eyelid margin. Several holes should be made toward the end of the tubing prior to placement underneath the eyelid. This tubing will emerge dorsal to the medial canthus. The end of the tube is blocked, and the tubing is sutured in place or fixed into position using Super-glue or Crazy-glue. To prevent further irritation or ulceration to the cornea, it is important to place this tubing as far dorsally as possible.

A fine gauge catheter can be inserted into the nasolacrimal duct via the nasal osteum. This cannula not only serves to deliver topical therapy to the eye but also retains patency within the nasolacrimal duct system.

The animal is sedated and the cannula is passed into the nasal osteum via a stab incision over the cranial aspect of the false nostril. The cannula is then advanced up the nasolacrimal duct until the moulded collar abuts against the osteum. Non-absorbable sutures are then used to maintain the cannula placement.

ENTROPION

Entropion can either be bilateral or unilateral in nature. This ocular irritation occurs more frequently in foals than it does in the adult. In foals, it may be due to a congenital problem or be predisposed through dehydration and debilitation.

Clinical Signs

This problem usually occurs in the lower eyelids. The eyelid is rolled inward which allows the eyelid hair to rub against the cornea. Initially, the cornea will appear swollen. Eventually an ulcer with increased vascularity of the corneal tissue will develop.

Differential Diagnosis

1.) Keratitis
2.) Conjunctivitis
3.) Trauma

Diagnosis

Diagnosis of this problem is based on a clinical examination revealing an inversion of the lower eyelid margin.

Treatment

Conservative treatment of entropion involves an eversion of the lower eyelid margin and topical application of antibacterial eye ointments. Manually repositioning the eyelid and frequent administration of topical therapy may interrupt the blepharospastic cycle within foals with this condition.

Placing staples or vertical mattress sutures in the eyelid will temporarily pleat the eyelid and prevent it from rolling inward. The sutures or staples can be removed within two weeks. During this period of time, frequent applications of topical antibacterial eye ointment should be administered.

THE EYE AND ADNEXA

Eyelid Trauma; Corneal Trauma

Eyelid Laceration

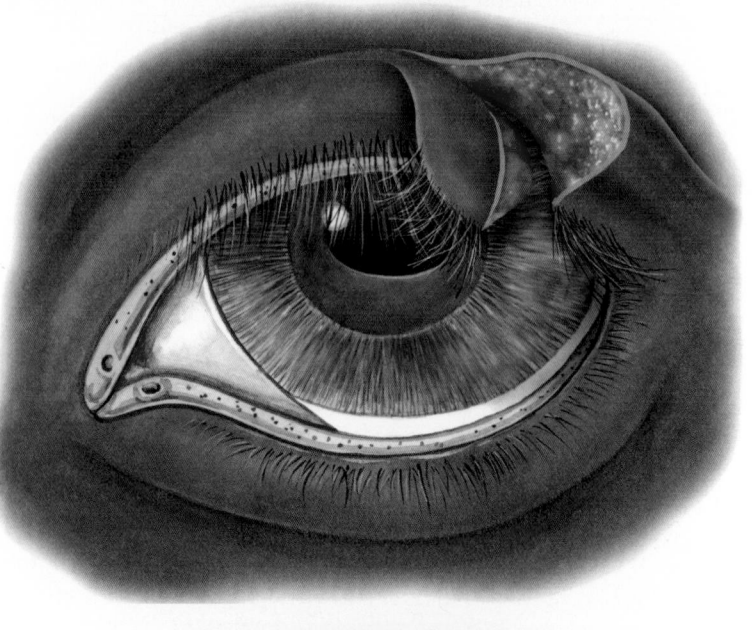

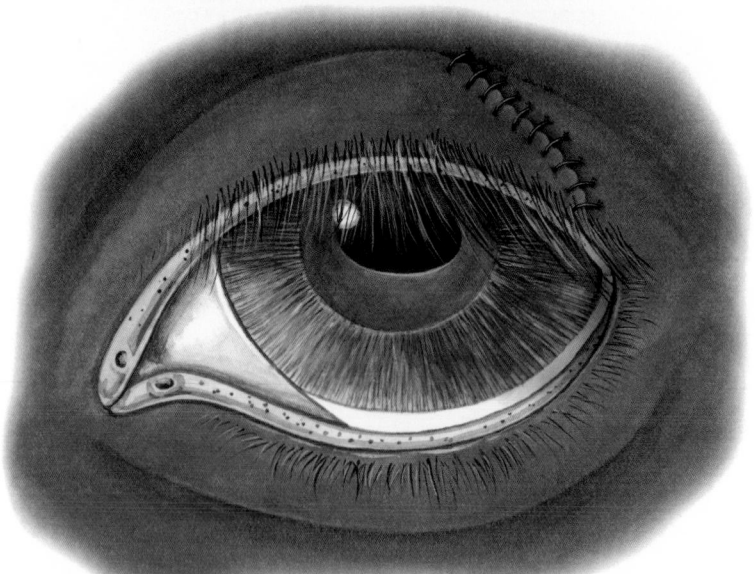

Surgical repair of eyelid laceration.

Corneal Trauma

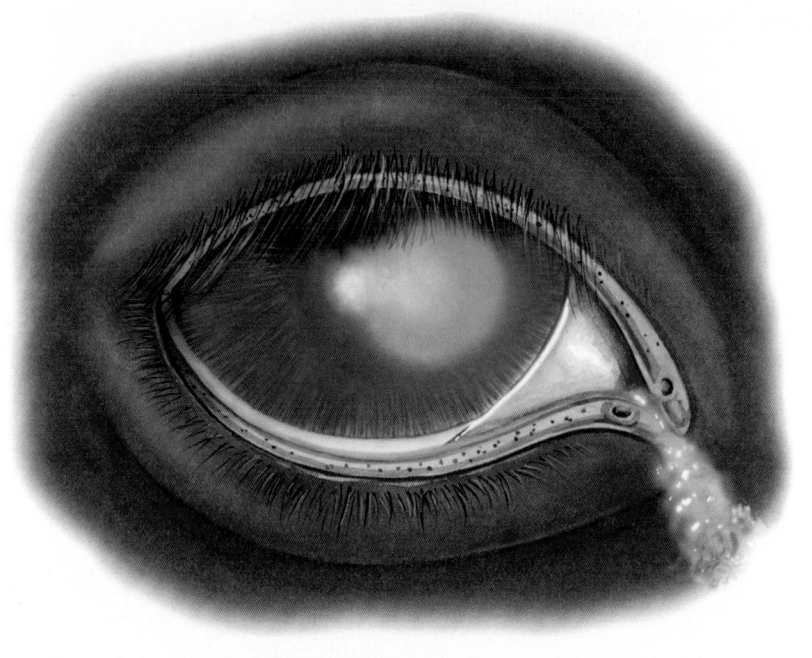

Corneal ulceration becomes very evident with the use of fluorescein stain.

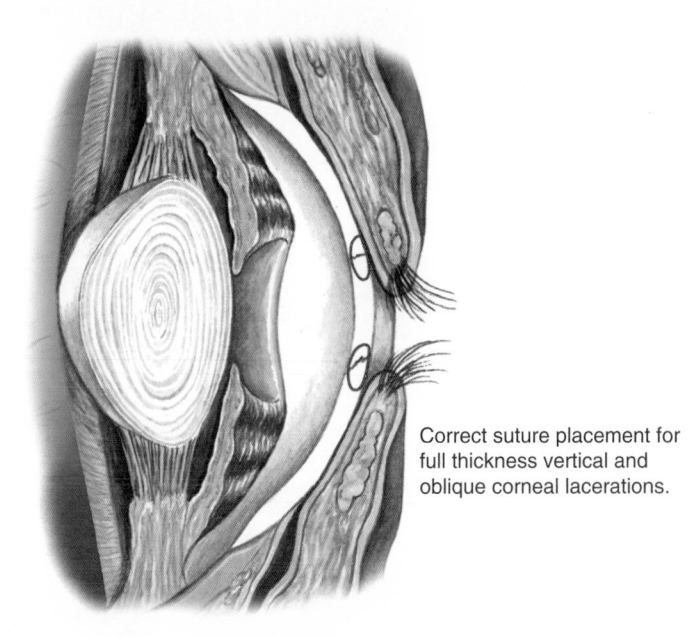

Correct suture placement for full thickness vertical and oblique corneal lacerations.

EYELID TRAUMA

Horses invariably rub their eyes on fences, feed bins, and stalls. This predisposes the animal to lacerations of the eyelid. Lacerations initially appear very severe, but because of the blood supply to this area, they usually heal with appropriate treatment. Vital tissue should be preserved whenever possible so that a cosmetic anatomical realignment of the lacerated tissues can be obtained.

Clinical Signs and Diagnosis

The diagnosis of an eyelid laceration is obvious. It is important to examine the eye for any other injuries that occured simultaneously. The cornea should be examined closely for the presence of an ulceration or laceration.

Treatment

Surgical repair should be performed promptly to avoid complications such as infection, conjunctivitis, and exposure keratopathy. The animal should be sedated. A nerve block may facilitate control over the patient for closure.

The affected area is cleaned using large quantities of saline mixed with povidine iodine solution. Ice can be applied to the injured area to help reduce swelling and allow for a more precise closure of the tissues. Debridement should be minimal and the edges of the laceration should merely be freshened to preserve as much of the tissue as possible.

Absorbable suture material should be used in a continuous or simple interrupted pattern through the deep layers of tissue. A nonabsorbable suture should be used to close the skin.

The tetanus innoculation history of the animal should be noted and tetanus toxoid administered if necessary. A 5 - 7 day course of topical and systemic antibiotics may also be needed. Systemic nonsteroidal antiinflammatories should be used to prevent extensive swelling. The skin sutures should be removed ten days after surgery.

CORNEAL TRAUMA

The horse has a large prominent cornea. Within the horse's environment are obvious hazards to this corneal tissue which include branches, nails, barbed wire, and fences. Bacterial infections can also produce deep abrasions and ulcerations.

Clinical Signs

The initial clinical sign is a loss of transparency to the cornea due to corneal edema. There may be deep or superficial vascularization. A deep red halo may appear surrounding the perilimbal episclera due to ciliary injection. Iris prolapse may be evident where the cornea has been penetrated. Ulceration of the cornea may be present, and a determination must be made as to whether it is superficial or deep, progressive or static. This can be done with fluorescein staining.

Differential Diagnosis

1.) Conjunctivitis
2.) Corneal Foreign Bodies
3.) Severe Uveitis

Diagnosis

Diagnosis is based on examination and a culture for bacterial organisms. Fluorescein staining will determine how deep the ulceration is and its extent within the corneal tissue. Bacterial cultures should be obtained from the eye, and sensitivity results should be the basis for treatment.

Treatment

Treatment involves topical antibiotic and anti-inflammatory therapy, systemic treatment, and possible surgery.

Topical antibiotic solutions, not ointments, are the conservative treatment of choice for corneal injuries. These solutions should be administered frequently and based on culture and sensitivity results when available. Anticollagenase therapy may also be added to this topical treatment regime

when the corneal erosion is complicated. Corticosteroids should never be used in acute phase treatment, because of the possibility of worsening the ulcer which could result in a rupture of the cornea. Topical nonsteroidal anti-inflammatories such as flurbiprofen sodium have value in treatment.

Systemic antiinflammatories and analgesics will help control pain for the patient. These medications also function to reduce any swelling within the surrounding structures.

If the cornea has been penetrated, reconstructive surgical repair should be considered. Simple interrupted sutures of 6-0 to 10-0 monofilament nylon or polygalction should be used to appose the edges of the cornea. Conjunctival flap and keratoplasty surgical techniques should also be considered when corneal damage is extensive. When the cornea has been severely damaged, enucleation of the eye may have to be considered.

Conjunctivitis

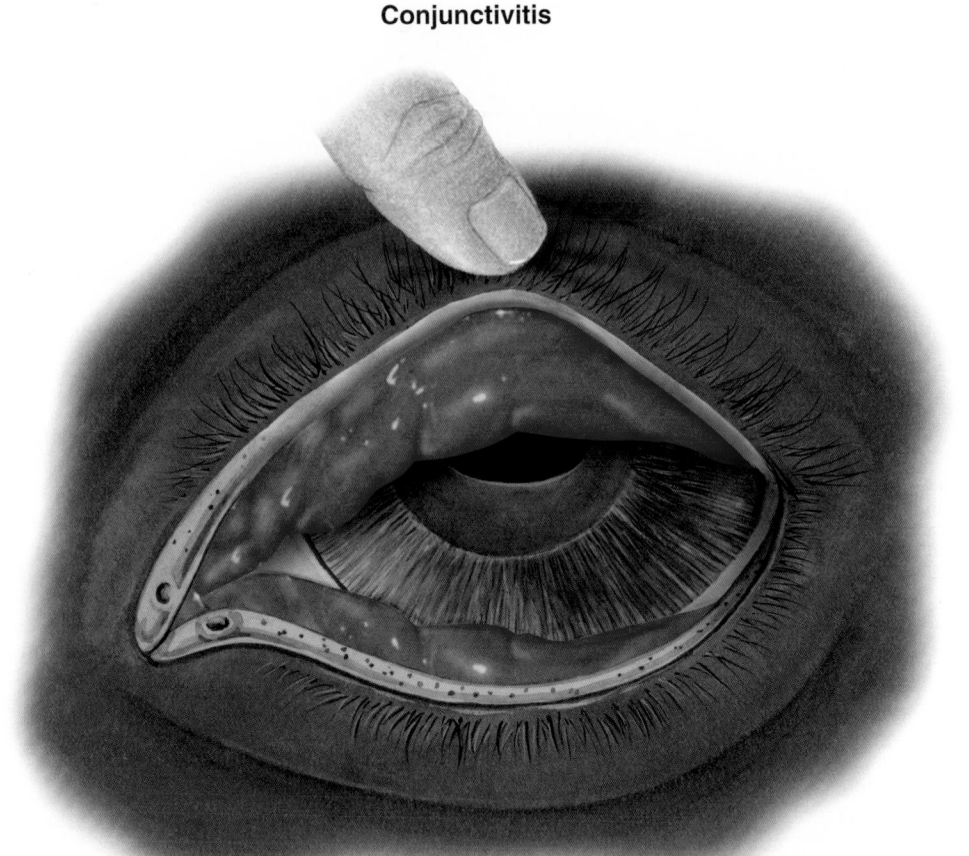

Severe inflammation of the conjunctival membranes.

Uveitis

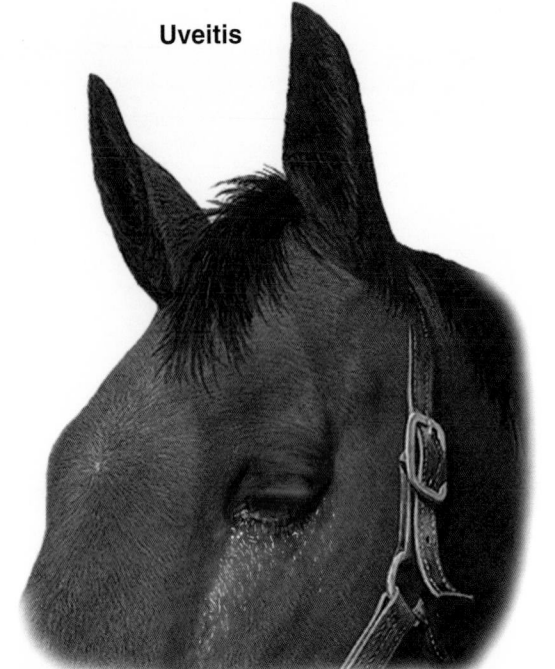

Blepharospasm and excessive tearing as seen in uveitis.

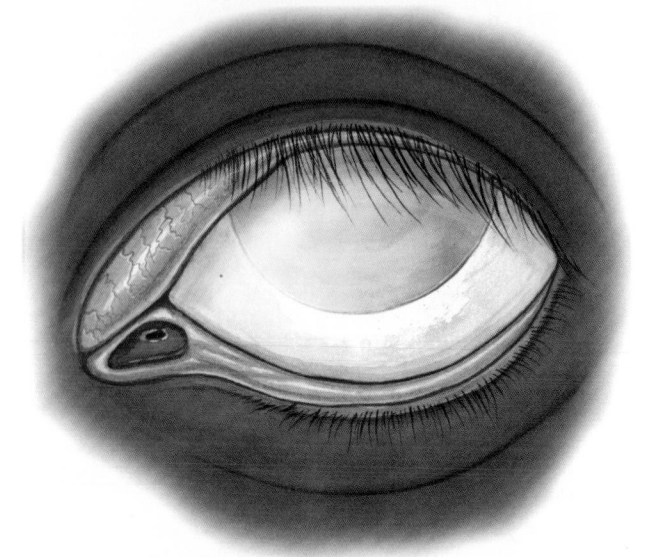

Moon blindness (periodic ophthalmia)

CONJUNCTIVITIS

Conjunctivitis is an inflammation of the conjunctival membranes. This condition may be a primary conjunctivitis such as that caused by infectious agents, or may be secondary to other ocular disorders such as keratitis. Primary causes of conjunctivitis are bacteria, mycotic agents, parasites, foreign objects, viral agents, trauma, and allergies. Secondary conjunctivitis can be a complication of lid problems, keratitis, or an intraocular inflammation such as endophthalmitis.

Clinical Signs

Inflammation is present within the conjunctival membranes either unilaterally or bilaterally. In the case of bacterial conjunctivitis, there is a mucopurulent ocular discharge. In the case of parasitic conjunctivitis, granulomatous reactions may be present.

Differential Diagnosis

1.) Habronemiasis
2.) Uveitis
3.) Keratitis

Diagnosis and Treatment

Diagnosis and treatment of the conjunctivitis is based on cytology, culture, and antibiotic sensitivity results. Ophthalmic ointments applied topically are the treatment of choice. Topical nonsteroidal antiinflammatory agents will also have some benefit. In the case of parasitic conjunctivitis, systemic therapy, including anti-inflammatory agents and parasiticides should be included with topical therapy. Fly control is also important in minimizing reinfection and irritation. Topical antihistimines and antiinflammatory medications should be utilized in the treatment of allergic conjunctivitis.

UVEITIS

Uveitis may be immune-mediated, such as that which occurs with recurrent uveitis, periodic ophthalmia (moon blindness,) be the result of trauma, or as a complication to a systemic disease.

Clinical Signs

Regardless of the etiology of the uveitis, the clinical signs are usually consistent and include the following:
1.) pain
2.) mild cornea edema
3.) conjunctival and episcleral injection
4.) excessive lacrimation
5.) blepharospasm
6.) cloudy eye
7.) cataracts

Differential Diagnosis

1.) Conjunctivitis
2.) Keratitis

Treatment

Systemic treatment of uveitis is based on the use of antiinflammatories and mydriatics. Cyclopegics should be applied to produce pupillary dilation. Topical applications of corticosteroids should be administered as often as possible for at least 10 - 14 days. In some cases, topical corticosteroids may have to be administered for up to 30 days. If this recurs, antiinflammatory therapy should be reinitiated until the clinical signs disappear.

Artwork by S. Hakola / J. Dirig
Copyright Equistar Publications, Ltd.

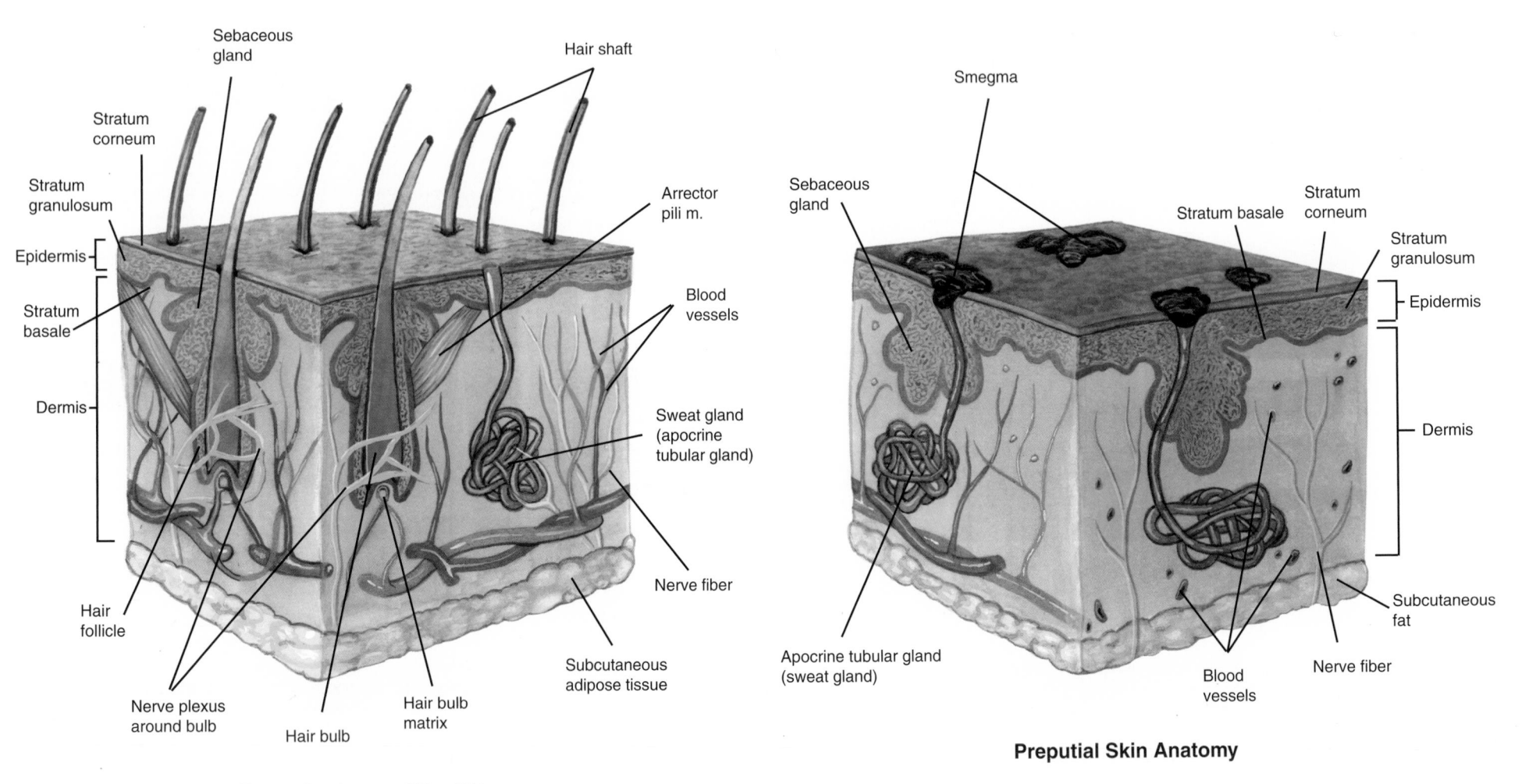

Sebaceous gland

Hair shaft

Stratum corneum

Stratum granulosum

Epidermis

Stratum basale

Dermis

Hair follicle

Nerve plexus around bulb

Hair bulb

Hair bulb matrix

Arrector pili m.

Blood vessels

Sweat gland (apocrine tubular gland)

Nerve fiber

Subcutaneous adipose tissue

Gross Anatomy of the Skin

Smegma

Sebaceous gland

Stratum basale

Stratum corneum

Stratum granulosum

Epidermis

Dermis

Subcutaneous fat

Nerve fiber

Blood vessels

Apocrine tubular gland (sweat gland)

Preputial Skin Anatomy

10

The Skin

SKIN FUNCTIONS

In terms of bulk, the skin is the largest body organ in the horse. It is continuous with the mucous membranes at all the body openings and varies in thickness over different anatomical areas. The chestnuts, ergots, and hooves originate from the epithelial layer and become structures unique to the horse. Present in the dermis, but continuous with the epidermis, are the specialized epithelial structures that include hair follicles, apocrine sweat glands, and sebaceous glands. Although the skin appears simple in structure, without it, an organism would cease to function.

The functions of the skin extend far beyond that of a mere protective barrier. They are as follows:
1.) A protective barrier from physical injury, poisonous substances, and microorganisms.
2.) The large surface area allows the skin to function in temperature regulation of the body through sweating, vasodilation, and the raising and lowering of the hair shafts.
3.) It allows communication with the environment through the sense of touch and allows interaction to the environment through responses to pain stimulations.
4.) Dehydration is prevented by not allowing the loss of essential body fluids.
5.) Glands that are associated with the hair follicles allow excretion of some waste products and are capable of producing pheromones for sexual attractiveness.
6.) Vitamin D is produced at the level of the skin.
7.) The immune system is represented in the skin since this is the main site of antigen presentation to T lymphocytes.

ANATOMY OF THE SKIN

The skin consists of two distinct layers: the epidermis and the dermis. The epidermis is a nonvascular, keratinized, stratified squamous epithelium that varies in thickness. The dermis consists of an intricately woven feltwork of collagen, elastic, and reticular connective tissue fibers.

The epidermis is the outermost protective layer of the skin. It actually provides structural, photoprotective, immunologic, and metabolic barrier protection. The epidermis can be divided into several layers according to the shape of the epithelial cells within that particular layer. The most superficial layer is termed the stratum corneum. This is the harder, dryer portion of the epidermis and consists of two to three layers of completely keratinized, flat, anucleate, and eosinophilic cells. In hairless areas of the skin, the stratum lucidum is present. This consists of several layers of fully keratinized and translucent cells in a tightly compact layer. The next layer is termed the stratum granulosum, and its thickness is dependent on whether or not the skin is haired. This flattened layer contains the basophilic keratohyaline granules. The stratum spinosum layer is produced directly from dividing basal cells. This layer consists of several layers of polyhedral spiny cells.

The stratum basale or basal cell layer is that layer closest to the dermis. It is composed of small, cuboidal-to-columnar cells and contains the germinal epithelial cells. This basal cell layer also produces the basement membrane which functions as the point of attachment for the epidermis to the dermis. This membrane consists of two layers: the lamina lucida layer, which is rich in glycoproteins and proteoglycans, and the lamina densa layer, which is composed of collagen. The basement membrane functions to attach the epidermis to the dermis and to provide a structural foundation for the attachment and polarity of the epidermal basal cells.

The dermis provides connection between the epidermis and the subcutaneous tissues. It is composed of collagen, elastin fibers, glycosaminoglycans, and glycoproteins. This layer functions to provide nutrition, tensile strength, and support to the epidermis.

The dermis is divided into the superficial and deep layers. The main difference between these two layers is the arrangement of the fibers. The superficial layer consists of finer, more loosely arranged collagen fibers, whereas the deep layer consists of dense, tightly arranged collagen fibers.

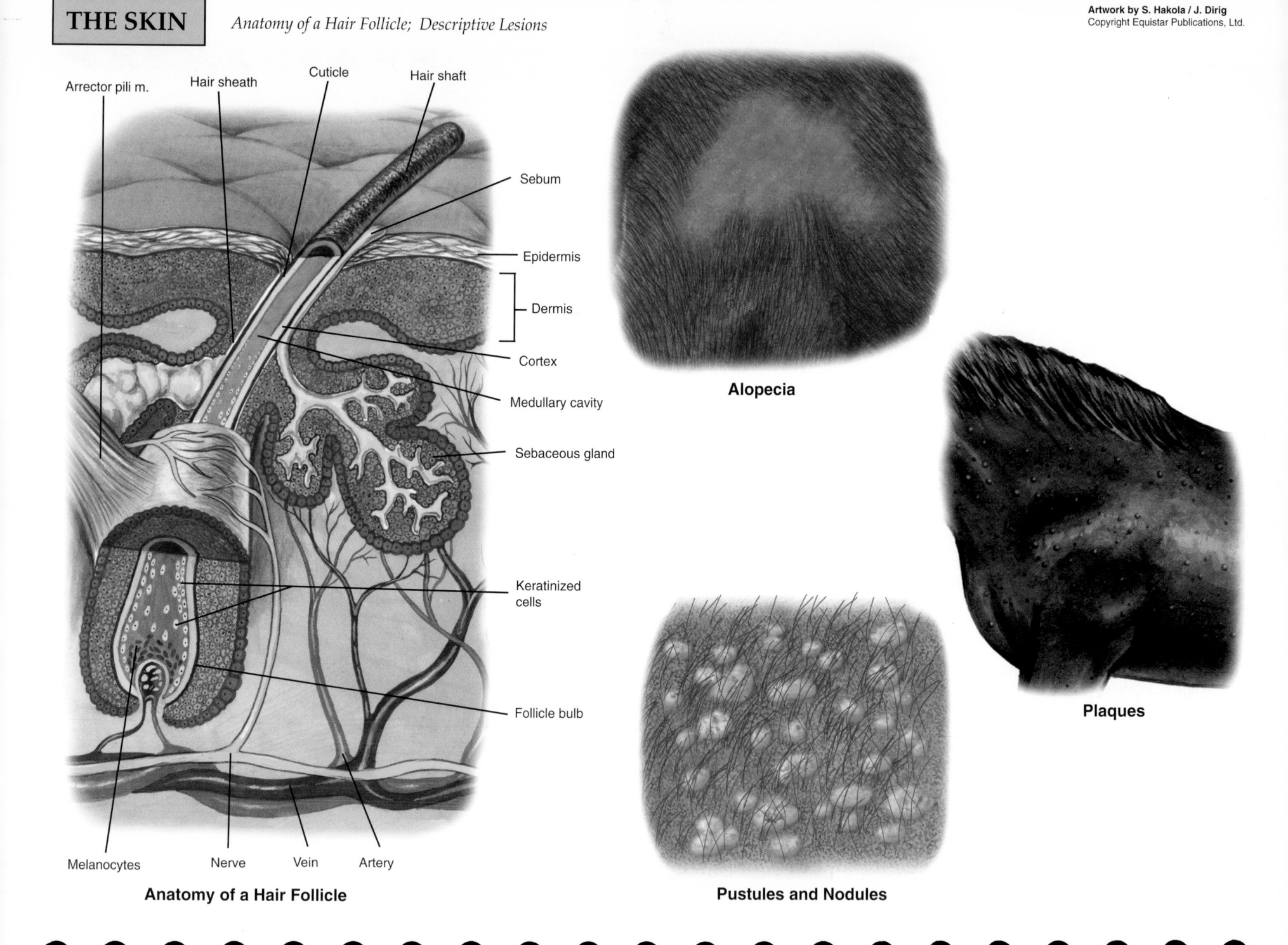

THE SKIN

Anatomy of a Hair Follicle; Descriptive Lesions

Arrector pili m.

Hair sheath

Cuticle

Hair shaft

Sebum

Epidermis

Dermis

Cortex

Medullary cavity

Sebaceous gland

Keratinized cells

Follicle bulb

Melanocytes

Nerve

Vein

Artery

Anatomy of a Hair Follicle

Alopecia

Plaques

Pustules and Nodules

The dermis includes the hair follicles, sweat and sebaceous glands, arrector pili muscles, blood vessels, lymphatics, and nerves. There are also additional components of the dermis which include collagen, elastin and reticular fibers, ground substance, and cellular elements such as fibroblasts.

THE ADNEXA OF THE SKIN

The adnexa are epidermal appendages that are specialized epithelial structures that lie within the dermis but remain connected to the epidermis. These include hair follicles, sebaceous and apocrine glands.

Hair has four main functions on the skin. It is a protective barrier, acts as a thermal insulator, supplies a source for keratinocytes in wound healing, and acts as a "wick" to allow emanation of apocrine gland secretions.

Hair is produced by a simple follicle. The visible portion of the hair is termed the shaft and the part within the follicle is termed the root. All follicles are primary in the horse, which means they are large in diameter, and their roots occur within the dermis. Most of the hair follicles have associated sebaceous and sweat gland structures and arrector pili muscle structures.

The root of a hair terminates in a hollow knob which is called the hair bulb. This is attached to a dermal papilla which is continuous with the dermis. The hair shaft is composed of an outermost cuticle which surrounds a cortex of densely pacted keratinized cells that contain the pigment which gives the hair its color. Loose cuboidal cells form an inner medullary layer. Sebaceous glands are alveolar glands which are associated with hair follicles and open into the upper part of the follicle. These glands secrete a substance known as sebum which consists of lipids, keratin, and proteins. These sebaceous glands are most numerous at mucocutaneous junctions, at the coronet, and over dorsal portions of the neck and rump.

Apocrine sweat glands are derived from the epidermis and are attached to the hair follicle by a long straight duct that empties near the skin surface. These glands are coiled and tubular in shape with the secretory portion located deep in the dermis. Apocrine glands are present throughout the skin but are more numerous and larger along the wings of the nostril, the flank, the mammary glands, and the free part of the penis.

DERMATOLOGICAL EXAMINATION

To ensure a proper diagnosis, a thorough and systematic examination should be conducted. This examination should begin with a complete history, a general physical examination, and the use of any ancillary diagnostic aids that are needed to reach a definitive diagnosis.

History

Information should be gathered that includes general information and the specific history of the skin disorder. General history should include the breed, color, age, sex, reproductive status, deworming history, vaccination status, and current medication adminstration. Questions should be asked concerning the animal's appetite, evidence of weight loss, or any behavioral changes. Environmental questions should include the type of housing, feed (including the date of the last delivery,) and the type of bedding that is currently being used. Questions regarding the tack and its cleanliness should also be answered. The type of grooming equipment and the frequency with which it is used should also be investigated. Insect problems within the barn or pasture need to be determined.

General Physical Examination

Skin disorders may be caused by infectious agents such as bacteria or fungi. Etiologies may also include: parasites, viruses, neoplasms, trauma, chemical irritation, immune-mediated disorders, and insect bites. Therefore, a general physical examination should be completed before specific attention is given to the skin disorder.

A thorough systematic examination of the skin should be conducted in a well-lit area. Examination should begin at the mucocutaneous junctions and continue in a systematic approach from the head to the tail. The character of the skin should be examined and recorded in all anatomical areas with particular attention being paid to any primary or secondary lesions that are in evidence. Records should be kept as to the thickness and pliability of the skin, the color, the odor, the sensitivity, and any evidence of pruritus. Excessive insects or external parasites should also be noted.

Several terms are used in the description of dermatological disorders which are as follows:
Abscess: The collection of pus within a cavity.
Pustule: A small circumscribed area of the skin that is filled with pus.
Cyst: An enclosed fluid-filled cavity that is not inflamed.
Vesicle: A circumscribed elevation of skin that is filled with serous fluid such as that found in a blister.
Sinus: A channel or fistule that results from the drainage of pus.
Macule: A well circumscribed flat area of color change in the skin usually less than 1 cm in diameter.
Nodule: An elevation of the skin greater than 1cm in diameter that extends into the deeper dermis.
Papule: Denotes a small solid elevation less than 1 cm in diameter.
Patch: A macule that is larger than 1 cm in diameter.
Plaque: A solid lesion greater than 1 cm in diameter that is elevated and flat on top.
Tumor: A swollen enlarged area that is usually neoplastic in origin.
Alopecia: Any loss of hair.
Crust: A general term describing a scab or dried exudate that occurs on the surface of a lesion.
Excoriation: The superficial loss of the epidermis that is the result of physical damage such as that from rubbing or an abrasion.
Erosion: Depicts a partial loss in thickness of the epidermis that does not penetrate the basal layer of the skin.
Fissure: Any split or crack in the skin due to dryness and a loss of pliability.
Hyperpigmentation: An increase in epidermal or

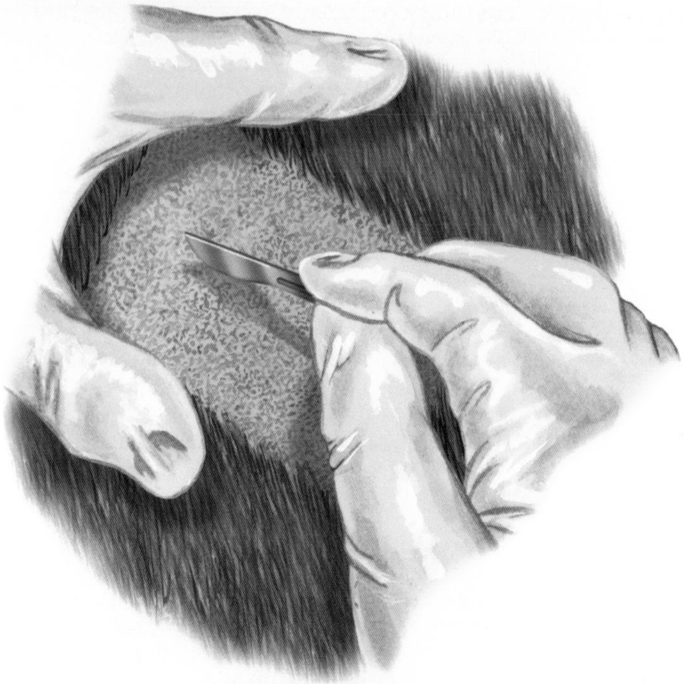

Skin Scraping

A

B

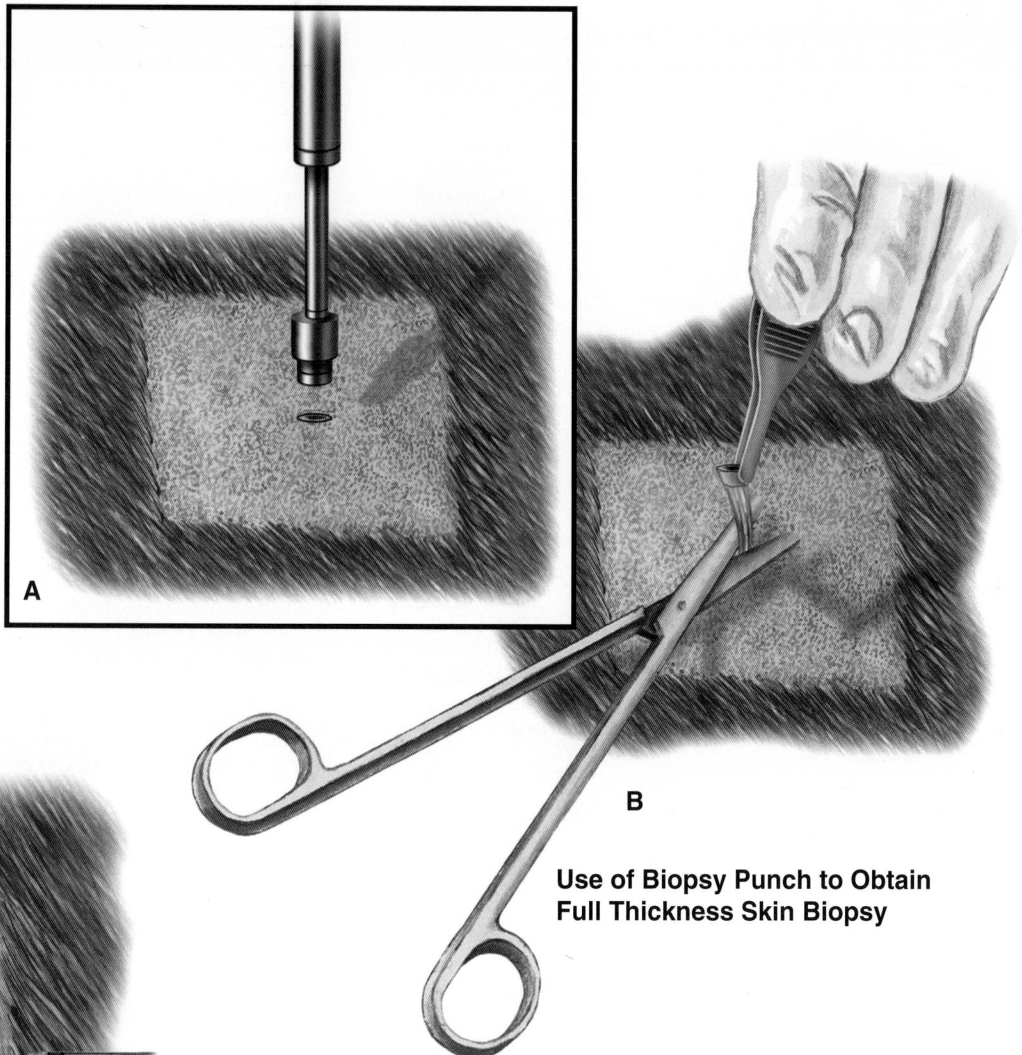

**Use of Biopsy Punch to Obtain
Full Thickness Skin Biopsy**

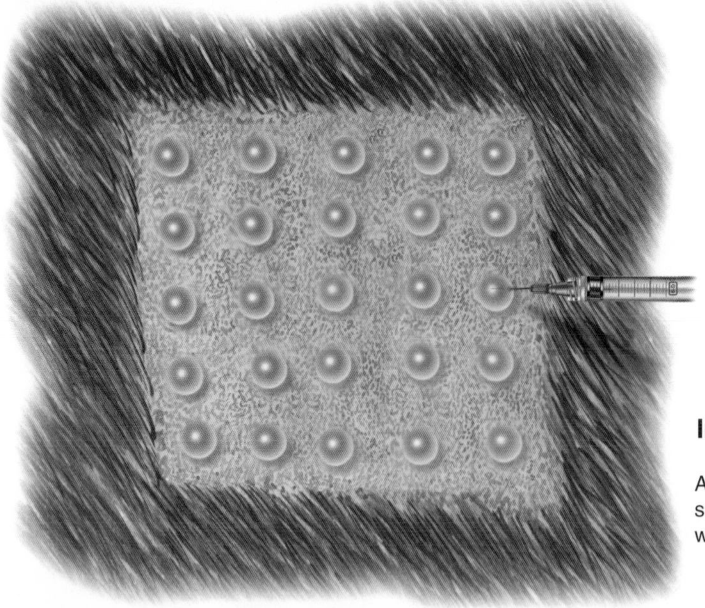

Intradermal Allergy Testing

Antigens are injected into the skin and reactions
such as redness, swelling, and irritation are noted
within 24 hours after the intradermal injection.

dermal melanin which in turn results in excessive darkening of the skin.

Hypopigmentation: A decrease in epidermal or dermal melanin which is manifested as a loss of pigmentation in the skin.

Hyperkeratosis: An increase in thickness within the horny layer.

Hyperhidrosis: A condition of excessive sweating.

Hypertrichosis: The presence of more hair than normal.

Scale: An accumulation of fragments of the horny layer commonly referred to as scurf or dandruff.

Scar: A lesion which is the result of fibrous tissue proliferation during the healing process.

Ulcer: This lesion occurs when the entire thickness of the epidermis is lost exposing the underlying dermis.

SPECIAL DERMATOLOGICAL EXAMINATION TECHNIQUES

Skin Scraping

Skin scraping is a very simple procedure and is the most common investigative sample taken for the diagnosis of skin disorders. All that is needed is a scalpel blade, mineral oil, microscope slides, and coverslips. The procedure is done by applying mineral oil directly on the skin to be scraped. The sample is collected by scraping the scapel blade across the area to be examined a number of times and with sufficient force to obtain a sample. The site should be squeezed, and the depth of scraping should be such that tissue fluid and a small amount of blood appear at the site.

Fungal Identification Techniques

The use of potassium hydroxide (KOH) is used in the preparation of a sample to dissolve keratin and bleach the hair so that fungal elements can be more easily identified.

Hair and skin samples should be collected from a number of different lesions by plucking with a forceps. Skin debris is then collected using a scalpel blade. A drop of KOH is placed on a microscope slide and the hair and skin samples are

added to the KOH. A cover slip is placed over the sample and the slide is warmed for a period of time before examination. DMSO solutions can be added to KOH which will allow a more rapid clearing of the sample. If this technique reveals the presence of any fungal hyphae, a sample should be submitted for culture.

Dermatophyte Test Medium or Sabouraud's agar with added pH indicator should be used to culture fungi. Samples are taken from a number of different lesions and pressed into the surface of the culture medium using sterile forceps. These samples should be left to incubate at room temperature for up to four weeks. A duplicate set of samples can also be incubated at 37 degrees centigrade, because some fungi grow better at this temperature.

Biopsy Techniques

Skin biopsies are indicated for most lesions in which a superficial scraping or culture has been nonrewarding in offering a diagnosis. This technique can be carried out with a needle, a scalpel blade, or a biopsy punch. If a deeper sample is required, an area can be excised in any size desirable. In most cases, the animal should be placed under sedation and a local anesthetic be administered.

The overlying skin should be clipped free of hair and covered with 70% alcohol when a needle biopsy is to be performed. Local anesthesia is usually unnecessary. A large bore needle with a syringe attached is used so that aspiration can be accomplished by applying negative pressure on the syringe plunger. The sample obtained from this technique can then be placed on a microscope slide and examined.

Punch biopsies are useful in obtaining a full-thickness section of a lesion. A 6 mm instrument is used to collect a sample that extends through the epidermis, dermis, and into the subcutaneous fat layer of the skin. In most cases, the animal should be sedated, and a local anesthetic agent should be injected beneath the lesion. The biopsy punch is placed over the lesion. The biopsy is cut by simultaneously rotating and applying pressure to

the punch. Subcutaneous tissue usually remains attached to the biopsy and must be severed with scissors. The wound created by this biopsy technique either can be left to heal by second intention or a single suture can facilitate closure.

Intradermal Testing

Intradermal testing allows the determination of the antigens that are responsible for certain allergic conditions. Different allergens are injected intradermally, and their response within the tissues is evaluated for up to 24 hours.

A large area, usually in the lateral cervical region, is clipped. The animal is then sedated or twitched. An amount of 0.1 ml is injected intradermally from each antigen solution. Each site is then identified to ensure accurate evaluation. Reactions must be determined at timed intervals and measured for size. Assessments should be noted as to whether these reactions are soft, firm, painful, or raised.

WOUND HEALING

One of the main functions of the skin is the protection of the underlying structures. The horse is predisposed to large traumatic injuries anywhere on its body. A great number of these injuries occur on the legs with the rear legs more commonly injured than the front limbs. This predispositon for injury is directly related to the animal and the environment in which it resides.

Traumatic wounds can be categorized as closed or open. Closed wounds do not penetrate all the layers of the skin and include abrasions, contusions, and hematomas. Open wounds penetrate through the skin into the subcutaneous and underlying tissues and include incisions, lacerations, avulsions, and punctures.

Abrasions commonly occur as a horse slides on concrete or while the horse is being loaded into a trailer. Only the superficial layers of the skin are removed, and bleeding is usually very minimal. These wounds are very sensitive to touch and must be taken care of properly, because the natural barrier of the skin is compromised.

THE SKIN   *Stages of Wound Healing*

Artwork by S. Hakola / J. Dirig
Copyright Equistar Publications, Ltd.

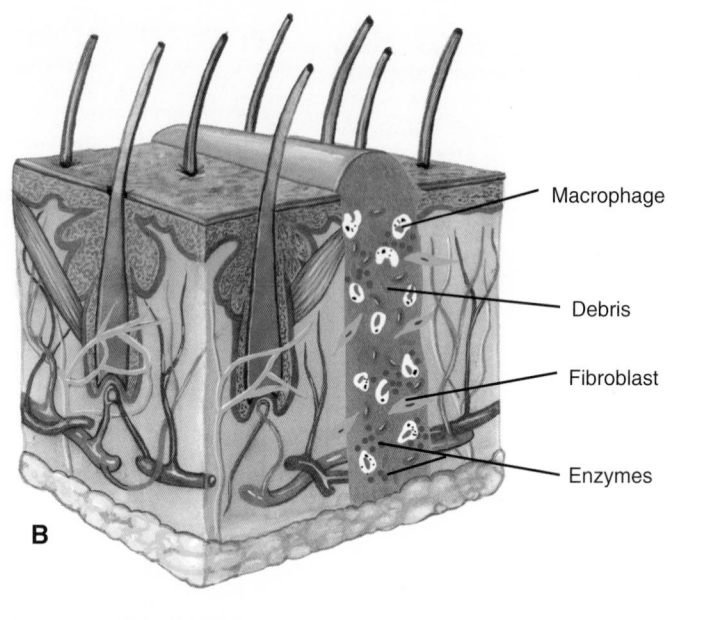

Hemorrhage

Neutrophil

Red blood cell

Platelets

A

**Inflammatory Stage: Hemorrhage and Infiltration
With Neutrophils and Platelets to Form Base for Clot**

Macrophage

Debris

Fibroblast

Enzymes

B

**Debridement Stage: Macrophages Ingest Debris; Enzymes Break
Down Foreign Matter; Fibroblasts Begin to Move into Wound**

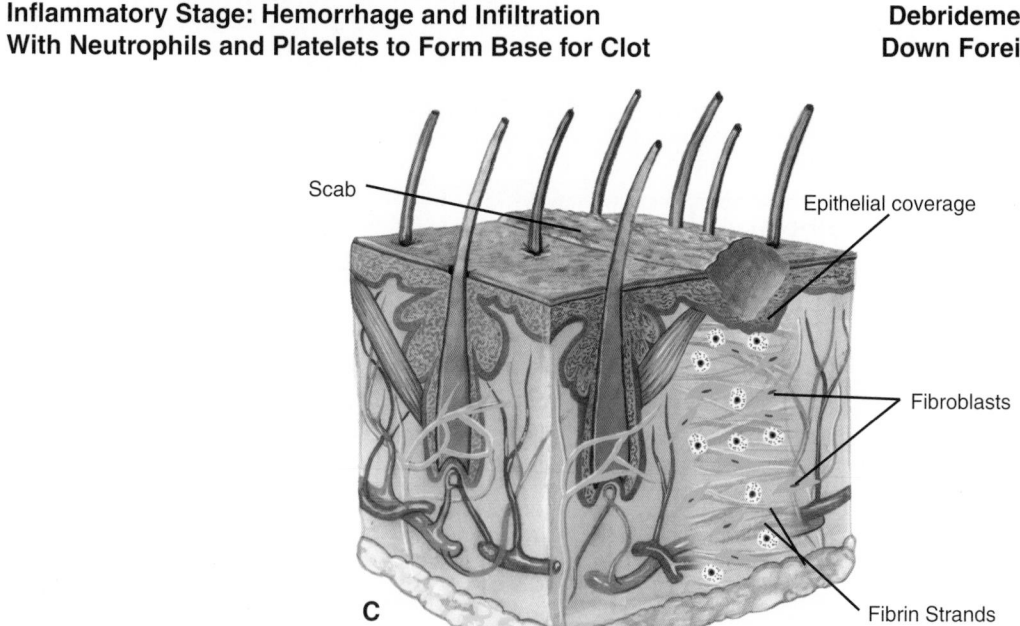

Scab

Epithelial coverage

Fibroblasts

Fibrin Strands

C

**Proliferation Stage: Fibroblasts Lay Down Strands of Fibrin;
Epithelialization of Surface Has Begun.**

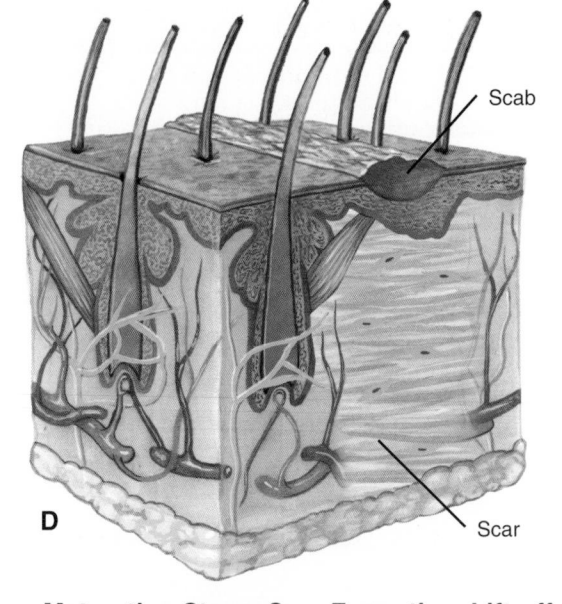

Scab

Scar

D

**Maturation Stage: Scar Formation, Lift-off
of Scab to New Epidermal Skin Layer.**

Contusions occur when there is direct trauma to the skin, but the skin is not broken. The tissues beneath the skin are bruised, swollen, and painful. Bleeding occurs beneath the skin which causes discoloration. This blood is usually absorbed, and this area typically heals through aggressive physical therapy techniques.

A hematoma usually results from blunt trauma which can occur during a kick or a fall. Blood accumulates under the skin and forms clots. Areas of contusions may surround the hematoma which results in two different kinds of wounds in one area.

Wounds from sharp objects such as scalpal blades, glass, or metal siding from a barn are categorized as incisions. The skin edges are precisely cut, and there is a minimum amount of trauma to the surrounding tissues. These wounds penetrate all layers of skin and are therefore termed open wounds. Damage must always be assessed to the underlying structures before treatment is initiated.

The most common wound sustained by horses is the laceration. These wound edges are irregular, and there is extensive trauma to the surrounding soft tissues. Lacerations are usually the result of barb wire, metal gates, nails, bites, or any sharp object within the horse's environment. These open wounds should all be considered contaminated, and aggressive treatment should be initiated immediately.

When tissue has been torn away from the body, the laceration is termed an avulsion. These are high energy wounds that result in extensive soft tissue damage to the underlying structures.

Any sharp object that penetrates the tissue results in a puncture wound. There may be minimal superficial damage to the skin, but the problem occurs with the inocculation of the underlying tissues with infectious agents. The most common causes of open wounds are nails, sticks, and splinters. Severe complications usually result from small superficial wounds that are not taken care of properly.

Wound healing is a series of events. The understanding of these events enables one to properly manage wounds and lacerations in horses. The process by which damaged skin repairs itself depends on the extent of the injury and its depth. Wound healing can then therefore be divided into four stages: **inflammatory**, **debridement**, **proliferation**, and **maturation**. These stages are continous processes and will always overlap.

Hemorrhage is the inital event in the inflammatory stage of wound healing. The animal's response to pain and trauma is vasoconstriction. This is initiated to control the hemorrhage. This vasoconstriction usually lasts 5 - 10 minutes and is followed by vasodilation of the vasculature, during which there is an increased capillary permeability. This allows cellular and noncellular blood compounds to enter the area of the wound. Initially, the components that escape from the blood vessels start to form a fibrous clot. The fibrin that accumulates in the area serves both as a framework for the clot and as a barrier to protect exposed subcutaneous tissue.

During the first 24 - 48 hours after the injury, the number of neutrophils entering the area of a wound is greatly increased. These cells release enzymes which break down tissue debris and kill microorganisms. Monocytes, immunoglobulins, and lymphocytes also accumulate during this time period to combat the microorganisms and begin the first stages of wound repair. Monocytes and macrophages begin the removal and transformation of the damaged tissue. The inflammatory stage results in the accumulation of these cells and fluids that results in heat, pain, swelling, and redness. The extent of the injury will govern the severity and the duration of this inflammatory response.

Because the inflammatory stage lasts 6 - 12 hours, the debridement stage usually begins 6 hours after the injury and is focused on the removal of any damaged tissue and the elimination of any infection. Enzymes are released from the leukocytes to aid in the breakdown of the injured tissues. Monocytes and macrophages phagocytize any cellular and extraneous debris along with

fibrin and bacteria. Immunoglobulins in the area aid in the removal of bacteria. Fibroblasts are attracted to the wound and speed the formation of granulation tissue and collogen. This influx of fibroblasts into the wound characterizes the end of the debridement stage and leads to the formation of granulation tissue which usually occurs 3 - 6 days after the injury.

The proliferation stage is characterized by the presence of fibroblasts, epithelialization, the formation of granulation tissue, and wound contraction. This stage is initiated when the blood forms clots, the necrotic debris has been removed, and any infection is under control. Fibroblasts begin synthesizing immature collagen which matures to strengthen the wound. This process occurs 5 - 15 days after injury. The epithelial cells at the wound edge begin to multiply and migrate across the wound deficit. In a sutured noninfected wound, new epithelium can actually form a bridge across the skin edges 48 hours after suturing.

Granulation tissue that forms during the proliferative stage is composed of capillaries, fibroblasts, macrophages, and mast cells. When a wound is sutured, there is a minimum amount of granulation tissue formed; however, in wounds that are healed by second intention, granulation tissue is vital to encourage wound contraction and epithelialization. Granulation tissue not only promotes wound contraction, but also protects the wound from infection.

When the collagen becomes mature, the maturation stage is initiated. The amount of vascularity and the number of fibroblasts and macrophages within the wound decreases. The wound gains tensile strength by intramolecular and intermolecular collagen cross-linking. This stage may take up to a year until the skin is remodeled and the tissue regains its tensile strength. The ideal end result is organized scar tissue that is covered with epithelium. Unfortunately, wounds never gain the appearance of normal tissue. Therefore, wound healing is a reparative process and not a regenerative process.

There are many ways to manage wounds. These techniques include aggressive physical therapy

Wound Healing

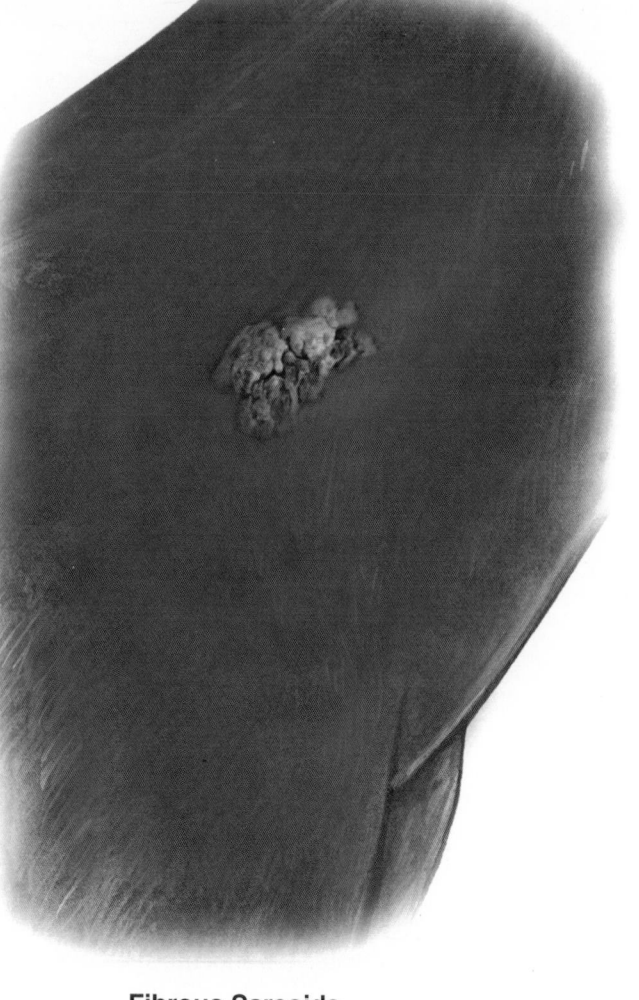

Fibrous Sarcoids

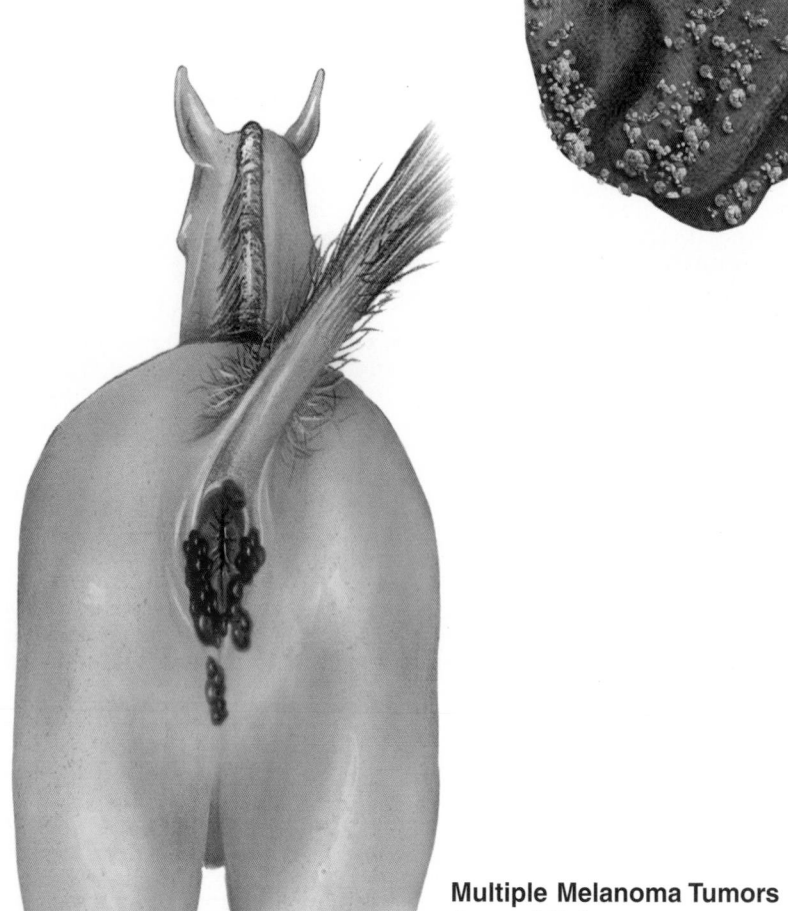

Multiple Melanoma Tumors Around Vulva

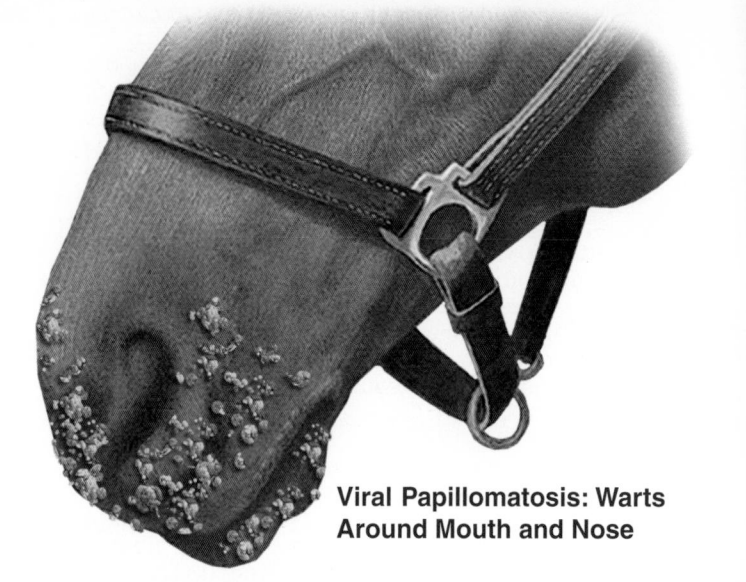

Viral Papillomatosis: Warts Around Mouth and Nose

protocols, surgery, and even skin grafting techniques. In all cases, wounds should be treated individually and managed in a way to return the tissues to a state as close to their normal function as possible.

SARCOIDS

Sarcoids are the most common tumor of the horse. They are nonmalignant aggressive fibroblastic tumors that arise spontaneously.

Etiology

It is suspected that sarcoids have a viral etiology. This is based on the evidence that papilloma virus DNA sequences have been found within the tumor cells. There is also genetic evidence of a hereditary predispostion or susceptibility. Literature has revealed that certain haplotypes of equine leukocyte antigens are associated with a higher frequency of sarcoid occurrence.

Clinical Signs

Sarcoids may appear to look like chronic granulation tissue. These are the common fibroblastic type of sarcoids. The verrucous or warty type sarcoids are usually less than 6 cm in diameter and are very slow growing. The fibroblastic type of sarcoid grows aggressively and occurs most frequently on the head, legs, and ventral abdomen.

An "occult" sarcoid appears as a flat, slightly raised lesion around the head. These lesions can even be found on the ears and eyelids. They can exhibit a variable degree of alopecia, crusting, and/or scaling. This occult sarcoid is slow growing and may eventually exhibit papules or nodules.

Differential Diagnosis

1.) Exuberant granulation tissue
2.) Viral papillomas
3.) Habronemiasis
4.) Other granulomas

Diagnosis

The histopathologic characteristics of the equine sarcoid are distinct from other lesions; therefore, it is necessary to biopsy these lesions or excise the entire mass for submission to the lab for diagnosis.

Treatment

Treatment of sarcoids involves surgical excision, electrocautery, cryosurgery, irradiation, or BCG therapy. The most commonly used treatment is a combination of surgical excision and electrocautery. Topical cytotoxic agents such as 5-fluorouracil ointment may be useful. The tumor is removed surgically, and the 5-fluorouracil is applied daily to the tumor base for 30 - 90 days until the lesion heals.

Cryosurgery is very successful in the treatment of sarcoids. The animal is sedated and the lesions are frozen 2 - 3 times to a temperature of minus 20 degrees centigrade. Between each freeze, the lesions are allowed to thaw to room temperature. Cryosurgery can also be used in combination with surgical excision. Complete healing of the tissue from this combination procedure may take at least two months.

When treating small lesions, like those surrounding the eye, injection of a *Mycobacterium bovis* extract may be of benefit. This injection consists of an extract called BCG (*Bacillus* Calmette-Gurein) which is a potent reticuloendothelial stimulant and a nonspecific immunostimulant that enhances the immune response to tumor specific antigens. This technique may require multiple injections of the lesion at 1 - 2 week intervals.

MELANOMA

There is a high incidence of melanomas in the Arabians and Percherons due to the gray color in those breeds. Melanomas may occur as a single nodule or may be multiple nodules occurring at multiple sites. A nodule is firm in texture, slow growing, but malignant. These nodules occur most frequently along the surface of the root of the tail, the perineum, and around the vulva.

Diagnosis

Physical examination of these nodules usually allows a diagnosis. If a biopsy is indicated to confirm the diagnosis, through cytologic and histopathologic examination, a complete excision should be done.

Treatment

There is a medical and surgical treatment protocol for handling melanomas. Surgical treatment involves complete excision or a combination of surgical excision and cryosurgery. Medical treatment involves the administration of cimetidine orally at a dose of 2.5 mg/kg every 8 hours. After a response to the lesion is noted, the dosage is then lowered to a maintenance level. This is an expensive medical treatment with variable results.

VIRAL PAPILLOMATOSIS (WARTS)

Warts usually occur in horses that are less than three years of age. These lesions are usually very characteristic and cannot be mistaken for any other skin disorders.

Etiology

The equine papilloma virus is the causative agent for warts which are spread through direct contact with other horses and through fomites. The incubation period after exposure is usually 30 - 60 days. After the warts appear, natural immunity develops, and the warts disappear spontaneously 60 - 100 days after development.

Clinical Signs

When first noticed, warts will appear as slightly raised smooth lesions. As they proliferate in number, they vary in size from 0.1 - 2.0 cm. A diagnosis can usually be made without any biopsy or other techniques due to the typical appearance of these lesions.

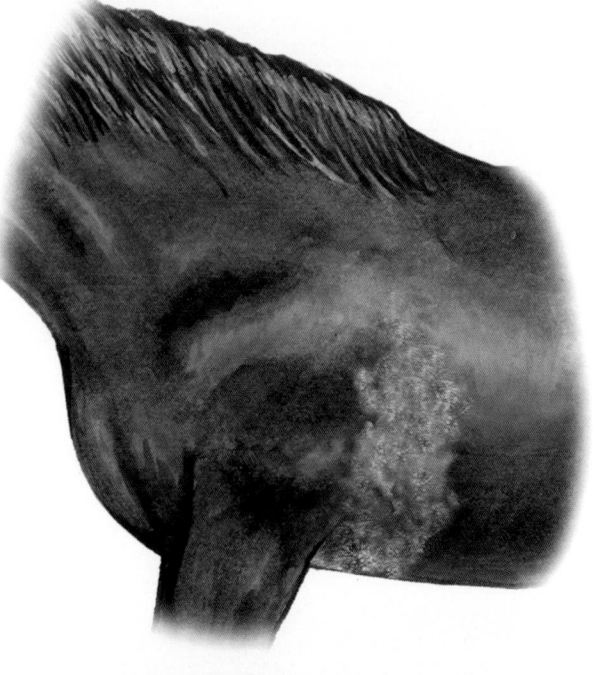

Cutaneous Onchocerciasis Lesions on the Anterior Chest and Ventral Midline

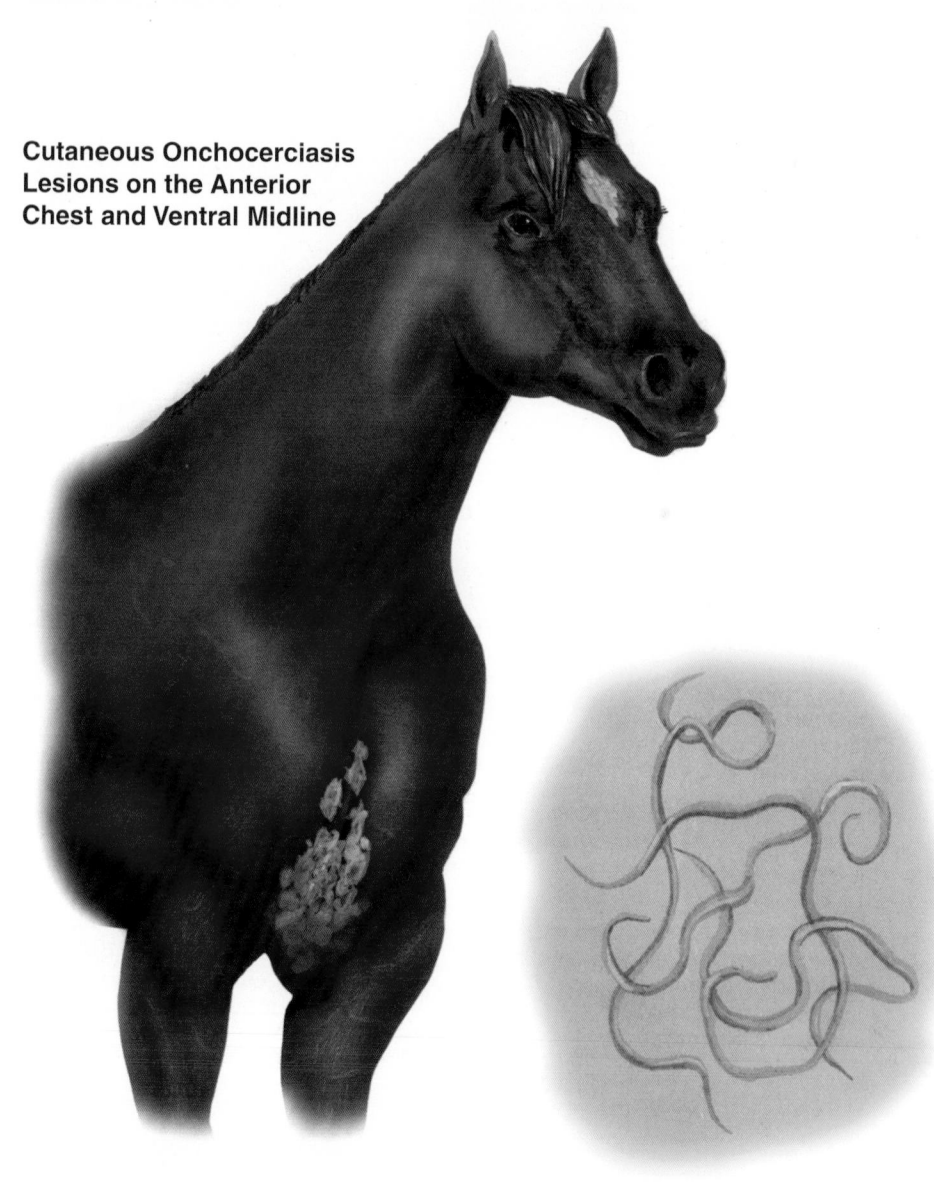

Cutaneous Onchocerciasis microfiliariae

Dermatophytosis ("Ringworm") Fungal Infection Creating Characteristic "Girth Itch" Lesions

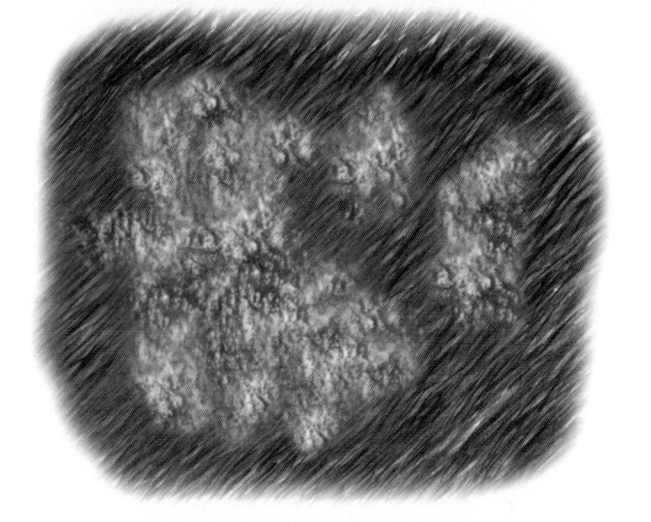

Close-up view of ringworm lesions

Treatment of Warts

Warts are a self-limiting disease. The horse develops natural immunity with the passage of time resulting in a regression of the lesions usually 60 - 100 days after their appearance. If warts must be removed for cosmetic reasons, cryosurgery is the treatment of choice. Surgical removal resulting in hemorrhage exposes the wart tissue to the circulation and may speed the natural immune process. Autotemnous vaccines are moderately to highly effective, whereas cattle wart vaccine is not efficacious at all.

Any affected animal should be isolated to prevent the spread of this virus. Disinfection of the premises should be done with formaldehyde.

CUTANEOUS ONCHOCERCIASIS

Etiology

Onchocerca cervicalis is the primary species of *Onchocerca* which causes a nonseasonal dermatitis in horses. The white adult nematode resides in the ligamentum nuchae and produces microfilariae that migrate to the dermis. The primary vector for this organism is the *Culicoides* gnat. In some locations, mosquitoes may also serve as a vector. Once these gnats ingest the microfilariae, they develop into infective larvae in about 25 days. The microfilariae occur more superficially and in greater numbers in the dermis during the spring and summer than they do in the winter.

Clincial Signs

The clinical signs of this disease are directly related to the hypersensitivity reaction within the skin. This reaction is most notable in the region of the ventral abdomen. The initial lesions consist of a thinning of hair or a mild scalding or crusting that occurs along the ventral midline or about the face, neck, chest, and withers. These lesions cause an intense pruritus.

Differential Diagnosis

1.) Fly and mosquito bites
2.) Dermatophilosis
3.) Ectoparasites

Diagnosis

A skin biopsy can demonstrate the presence of the microfilariae. This biopsy specimen can be chopped into fine pieces and placed into a Petri dish. The sample is then covered with physiological saline and incubated at 37 degrees centigrade for 10 - 30 minutes. Microscopic examination of this saline solution will reveal active microfilariae if they are present.

Treatment

Ivermectin should be administered orally at weekly intervals for 3 treatments and then again adminstered on a monthly basis for at least three more treatments. Ivermectin is lethal to the microfilariae, but is ineffective in killing the adult *Onchocerca* living in the ligamentum nuchae. Therefore, subsequent Ivermectin treatments are required to maintain these infected animals free of the skin disorder. As the microfilariae die, there is usually an intense period of pruritus. This should be addressed on an individual basis to prevent the animal from excessive rubbing which may lead to other skin disorders.

DERMATOPHYTOSIS (RINGWORM)

This is one of the most common skin disorders affecting stable horses. It is often referred to as "girth itch."

Etiology

Dermatophytosis is a superficial fungal infection of the skin caused by the fungi of the genera *Microsporum* and *Trichophyton*. Infection with this fungus is spread via direct contact between animals or more commonly by contaminated grooming equipment, blankets, and tack. The incubation for this fungal infection is very slow, and cases may take up to four weeks to exhibit clinical signs.

Clinical Signs

In the early stages, ringworm can mimic a wide range of other skin diseases. Eventually, these lesions develop into foci of scaling and crusting with circumscribed alopecia. In the early stages of the disorder, the animal may be sensitive to touch and exhibit pruritus. As this infection progresses, the pruritus usually disappears.

Differential Diagnosis

1.) Dermatophilosis
2.) Staphylococcal folliculitis
3.) Pemphigus
4.) Urticaria

Diagnosis

A KOH preparation is a rapid diagnostic test that may be useful. Samples can be collected and submitted for fungal culture that will confirm a definitive diagnosis.

Treatment

Treatment involves both a topical and systemic regime. Topical treatments include Thiabendazole in a 4% solution combined with DMSO, Captan in a 3% solution, iodine in a 1% available solution, and lime sulfur in a 3% solution. Systemic treatments of griseofulvin at a dosage of 10 mg/kg orally per day for thirty to sixty days have been found to be efficacious.

Artwork by S. Hakola / J. Dirig
Copyright Equistar Publications, Ltd.

Dermatophilosis

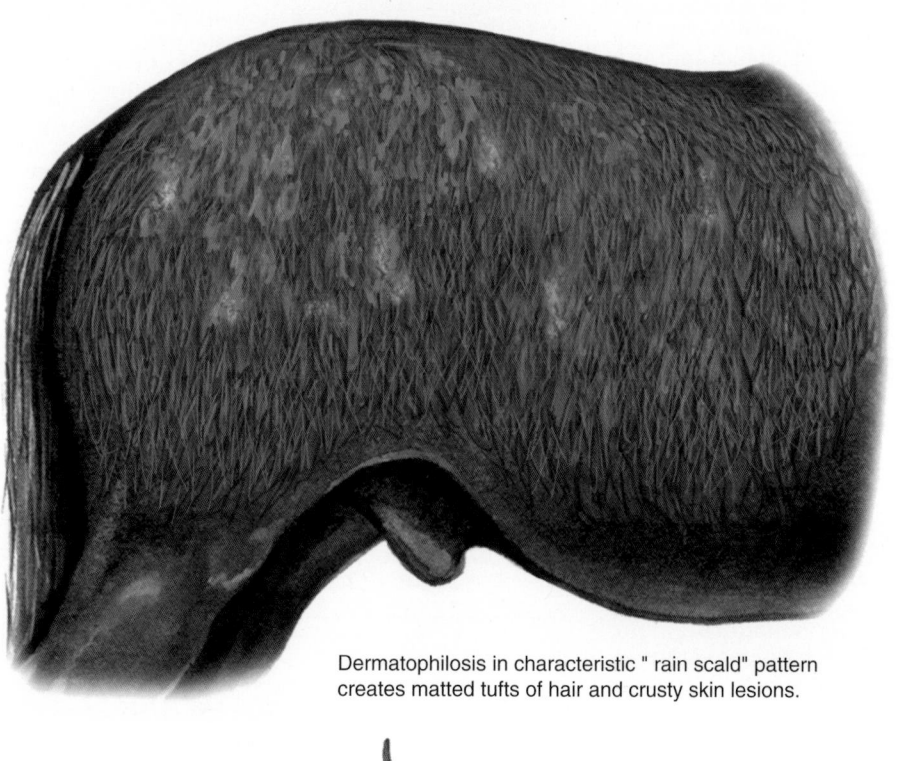

Dermatophilosis in characteristic " rain scald" pattern creates matted tufts of hair and crusty skin lesions.

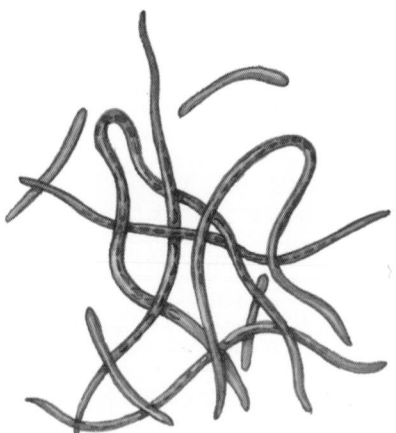

Filaments of coccoid cells as seen in dermatophilosis.

Pastern Dermatitis

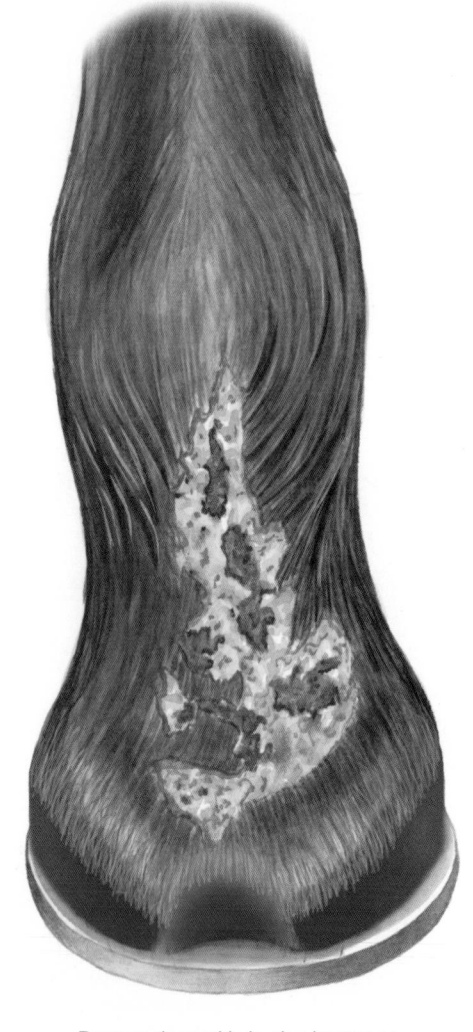

Pastern dermatitis is also known as grease heel, mud fever, or scratches.

DERMATOPHILOSIS (RAIN SCALD)

Etiology

This condition occurs during prolonged overcast and rainy weather. A gram-positive anaerobe, *Dermatophilus congolensis*, is the causative organsim.

Clinical Signs

This is an acute or chronic exudative dermatitis. These lesions appear as matted tufts of hair along the rump, loin, and saddle area. It gives the impression that large drops have scalded the skin. These lesions are usually less than 2 cm in diameter but may coalesce to cover a much larger area. Rain scald lesions are usually tender to the touch but are not pruritic. When the crust is removed, a moist pink bleeding lesion is revealed which is painful for the animal. These lesions are typically wet with varying amounts of exudate.

Differential Diagnosis

1.) The early stages of ringworm
2.) Seborrhea

Diagnosis

The diagnosis should be based on the history, a physical examination, and bacterial and fungal cultures. Bacterial cultures will hopefully isolate and identify the *Dermatophilus* organism, and fungal cultures will rule out ringworm. Microscopic examinations will reveal an organism that appears as branching filaments dividing both transversely and longitudinally to form 2 - 8 pairs of coccoid cells.

Treatment

Most horses recover spontaneously in approximately 3 - 4 weeks. These animals should be kept dry and groomed. Topical applications of chlorahexidine or 1% iodine solutions should be adminstered daily for ten days. Systemic treatment with penicillin G for five days will lead to a more rapid resolution of this infection.

PASTERN DERMATITIS

Pastern dermatitis is commonly referred to by horsemen as scratches, grease heel, or mud fever. It is a crusting and seborrheic dermatitis of the caudal heel and pastern regions.

Etiology

This disorder can occur in all breeds and is found most often within horses that have long fetlock hair or that are housed in unsanitary conditions. Grit particles from track surfaces may also cause the initial irritation predisposing this area to entry by a variety of microorganisms. Bacterial involvement of *Staphylococcus*, *Streptococcus*, or *Corynebacteria* are common findings. A number of other problems can result in this clinical condition and include: dermatophilosis, dermatophytosis, *Pelodera* dermatitis, contact dermatitis from irritants, horse pox, vasculitis, and photosensitization.

Clinical Signs

This condition tends to be bilateral with the rear limbs more commonly affected. These tissues exhibit pain, swelling, alopecia, exudation, and ulceration which usually begins at the heel and extends cranially. In chronic cases, these horses may become pruritic, give off a foul odor, and exhibit fissures within the tissue.

Differential Diagnosis

1.) Dermatophilosis
2.) Dermatophytosis
3.) Irritant Contact Dermatitis
4.) Chorioptic Mange
5.) Photosensitization

Diagnosis

Specific diagnosis can be obtained through skin scrapings, cytology, bacterial and fungal cultures.

Treatment

Treatment is dependent on the specific diagnosis reached. In general, the area should be clipped and cleaned. An astringent solution such as aluminum acetate or white lotion should be applied when the dermatitis is in the acute exudative stage. Antibiotic and antifungal creams and ointments can also be applied topically. Systemic treatment should include antiinflammatory agents, appropriate antibiotics, and the oral administration of griseofulvin when indicated. Treatment should always be combined with improved management procedures and better sanitary conditions.

REFERENCES

AANES, W.A.: Surgical management of foaling injuries. Vet. Clin. North Am. Equine Pract. Urogential Surg., 4:417-438, 1988.

ABRAMS, K.L., and BROOK, D. E.: Equine recurrent uveitis: Current concepts in diagnosis and treatment. Equine Pract. 12:27, 1990.

ADAMS, G.P., KASTELIC, J.P., BERGFELT, D.R., and GINTHER, O.J.: Effect of uterine inflammation and ultrasonically-detected uterine pathology on fertility in the mare. J. Reprod. Fertil. Suppl., 35:445-454, 1987.

ADAMS, O.R.: An improved method of diagnosis and castration of cryptorchid horses. J. Am. Vet. Med. Assoc. 145:439, 1964.

ADAMS, O.R.: Lameness in Horses. 3rd ed. Philadelphia, Lea & Febiger, 1974.

ADAMS, R.: Evaluation of the neurologic status of the newborn foal. Proc. 29th Ann. Conv. Am. Assoc. Equine Pract., 1983, p. 153.

ADAMS, S.B.: Diseases of the alimentary system. In Equine Medicine and Surgery — 4th edition. Colahan, P. T., Mayhew, I. G., Merritt, A. M. and Moore, J.N. (eds), Goleta, Calif.: American Veterinary Publications, 1991, pp. 473-489.

ADAMS, S.B.: Surgical approaches to the exploration of the equine abdomen. Vet. Clin. North Am. Large Anim. Pract. 4:89, 1982.

ALLEN, W.E., and NEWCOMBE, J.R.: Aspects of genital infection and swabbing techniques in the mare. Vet. Rec., 104:228-231, 1979.

ALLEN, W.E., and PYCOCK, J.F.: Current views on the pathogenesis of bacterial endometritis in mares. Vet. Rec., 125:298-301, 198.

ANDREWS, F.M., FENNER, W.R.: Indication and use of electrodiagnostic aids in neurologic diseases. In Neurologic Disease. Vet. Clin. North Am. Equine Pract. 1987; 3:293.

ANDREWS, F.M., and MATHEWS, H.K.: Localizing the source of neurologic problems in horses. Vet. Med. 85:1107, 1990.

ANDREWS, F.M., MATHEWS, H.K., and REED, S.M.: Medical, surgical, and physical therapy for horses with neurologic disease. Vet. Med. 85:1331, 1990.

ANSARI, M.M.: The Caslick operation in mares. Compend. Contin. Educ. Pract. Vet., 5:S107-S111, 1983.

ARNOLD, J.S., and MEAGHER, D.M.: Management of rectal tears in the horse. J. Equine Med. Surg., 2:64-71, 1978.

ARNOLD, J.S., MEAGHER, D.M., and LOHSE, C.L.: Rectal tears in horses. J. Equine Med. Surg., 2:55-61, 1978.

ARTHUR, G.H.: The cesarean operation in the mare. In Veterinary Reproduction and Obstetrics. 3rd ed. Baltimore, Willians & Wilkins, 1975, pp. 325-329.

ARTHUR, G.H., NOAKES, D.E., PEARSON, H., and PARKINSON, T.J.: Veterinary Preproduction and Obstetrics. London, W.B. Saunders, 1996.

ARTIFICIAL INSEMINATION (AI) OF MARES. In Technician's Manual for Artificial Insemination. American Breeders Service, DeForest, WI, 1972.

ASBURY, A.C.: Bacterial endometritis. In Current Therapy in Equine Medicine. Edited by N.E. Robinson. Philadelphia, W.B. Saunders, 1983.

ASBURY, A.C.: Large-volume uterine lavage in the management of endometritis and acute metritis in mares. Comp. Contin. Educ. Practicing Vet., 12:1477-1479, 1990.

ASBURY, A.C.: Management of the foaling mare. Proc. Am. Assoc. Equine Pract., 487-490, 1972.

ASBURY, A.C.: The reproductive system. In Equine Medicine and Surgery. Vol 2. 3rd ed. Edited by R.A. Mansmann, E.S. McAllister and P.W. Pratt. Santa Barbara, American Veterinary Publications, 1982, pp. 1305-1402.

ASHDOWN, R.R. and DONE, S.H.: Color Atlas of Veterinary Anatomy, Philadelphia, PA., J. B. Lippincott Co., 1987.

ASHDOWN, R.R., and HANCOCK, J.L.: Functional anatomy of male reproduction. In Reproduction in Farm Animals. 3rd ed. Edited by E.S.E. Hafez. Philadelphia, Lea & Febiger, 1974, pp. 3-23.

AUER, J.A.: Equine Surgery. Philadelphia, PA., W.B. Saunders, 1992.

BARBET, J.L., BAXTER, G.M., and MCMULLAN, W. C.: Diseases of the Skin. P. T. Colahan, I. G. Mayhew, A. M. Merritt, and J. N. Moore (Eds.), Equine Medicine and Surgery, 4th ed., Goleta, Calif.: American Veterinary Publications, 1991, p. 1569.

BACH, L.G., RICHETTS, S.W.: Paracentesis as an aid to the diagnosis of abdominal disease in the horse. Equine Vet. J. 6:116, 1974.

BACK, D.G., PICKETT, B.W., VOSS, J.L., and SEIDEL, G.E., Jr.: Observations on the sexual behavior of nonlactating mares. J. Am. Vet. Med. Assoc., 165:717-720, 1974.

BAKER, G.J.: Diseases of the pharynx and larynx. In Robinson E (Ed): Current Therapy in Equine Medicine. 2nd ed. Philadelphia, W. B. Saunders Company, 1987, p. 607.

BALL, B.A., LITTLE, T.V., HILLMAN, R.B., and WOODS, G.L.: Pregnancy rates at days 2 and 14 and estimated embryonic loss rates prior to day 14 in normal and subfertile mares. Theriogenology, 26:611-619, 1986.

BARBER, S.M.: Torsion of the uterus—a cause of colic in the mare. Can. Vet. J. 20:165, 1979.

BARNETT, K.C., CRISPEN, S.M., LAVACH, J.D., MATTHEWS, A.G.: Color Atlas and Text of Equine Ophthalmology, London, Great Britain, Mosby-Wolfe, 1995.

BECHT, J.L., RICHARDSON, D.W.: Ileus in the horse: Clinical significance and management. Proc. Am. Assoc. Equine Pract. 27:291, 1981.

BEECH, J.: Differential diagnosis of neurologic disease in the horse. Proc. 31st Annu. Conv. Am. Assoc. Equine Pract., 1985, p. 27.

BEECH, J.: Equine Respiratory Disease. Malvern, PA., Lea & Febiger, 1991.

BEECH, J.: Neurologic Diseases. In N. E. Robinson (Ed.): Current Therapy in Equine Medicine, Vol. 2. Philadelphia: W. B. Saunders , 1987.

BEECH, J.: Technique of tracheobronchial aspiration in the horse. Equine Vet. J. 1981; 13:136.

BELLING, T.H.: Surgery of the vulva: modification of the traditional Caslick operation. Vet. Med., 78:870-8, 1983.

BERGMAN, R.V.: Retained Meconium. In Robinson NE (Eds): Current Therapy in Equine Medicine. Philadelphia, W. B. Saunders Company, 1983, p. 260.

BERTONE, A.L., MCCLURE, J.J.: Therapy for sarcoids. Compend. Contin. Educ. Pract. Vet. 12:262, 1990.

BERTONE, J.J.: Pharynx. In Traub-Dargatz JL, Brown CM (eds): Equine Endoscopy. St Louis, Mosby, 1990, ch 4, p 33.

BLANCHARD, T.L., et al.: Comparison of two techniques for obtaining endometrial bacteriologic cultures in the mare. Theriogenology, 16:85-93, 1981.

BLANCHARD, T.L., et al.: Congenitally incompetent cervix in a mare. J. Am. Vet. Med. Assoc., 181:266, 1982.

BLANCHARD, T.L., et al.: Effects of postparturient uterine lavage on uterine involution in the mare. Theriogenology, 32:527-536, 1989.

BLANCHARD, T.L., MARTIN, M.T., VARNER, D.D., et al: Management of dystocia in mares: Examination, obstetrical equipment, and vaginal delivery. Comp. Cont. Educ. Pract. Vet. 11:745, 1989.

BLANCHARD, T.L., VARNER, D.D. and SCHUMACHER, J.: Manual of Equine Reproduction, St. Louis, Mosley-Year Book, Inc., 1998.

BLOOD, D.C., RADOSTITS, O.M.: Veterinary Medicine. Bailliere Tindall, London, 1989.

BLYTHE, L.: Neurologic examination of the horse. In Nerologic diseases. Vet Clin North Am. Equine Pract. 3:255, 1987.

BOENING, K.J., VON SALDERN F.C.H.: Nonsurgical treatment of left dorsal displacement of the large colon of horses under general anesthesia. Proc. Equine Colic Symp. 2:325, 1986.

BORROR, D.J., TRIPLEHORN, C.A., JOHNSON, N.A.: An Introduction to the Study of Insects, 6th Ed., Philadelphia, PA., Saunders College Publishing, 1989.

BORROR, D.J., and WHITE, R.E.: A Field Guide to Insects, Boston, MA., Houghton Mifflin Co., 1970.

BOWEN, J.M.: Venereal diseases of stallions. In Current Therapy in Equine Medicine 2. Edited by N.E. Robinson. Philadelphia, W.B. Saunders, 1987, pp. 567-571.

BOWMANN, D.D.: Equine protozoal myeloencephalitis: History and recent developments. Equine Pract. 13:28-33, 1991.

BRAMLAGE, L.R.: Examination in acute abdominal crisis. In: Equine Medicine and Surgery — 3rd edition. Mansmann R. A. and McAllister E. S. (eds), Santa Barbara: American Veterinary Publications, 1982, pp. 548-559.

BRAYTON, C.F.: Dimethyl sulfoxide (DMSO): A review. Cornell Vet. 76:61, 1986.

BRISTOL, F.: Studies on estrous synchronization in mares. Proc. Soc. Theriogenology, 258-264, 1981.

BROOK, D.: Further development of an indwelling nasolacrimal cannula for the administration of medication to the equine eye. Equine Pract. 9:12, 1987.

BURKI, F.: Equine rhinopneumonitis— An unsettled problem. J. Equine Vet. Sci., 8:65-69, 1988.

CAMPBELL, M.L., COLAHAN, P.L., BROWN, M.P., et al: Cecal impaction in the horse. J. Am. Vet. med. Assoc. 184:950, 1984.

CARON, J.P.: Guttural Pouch. In Traub-Dargatz JL, Brown CM (eds), Equine Endoscopy. St Louis, Mosby, 1990, ch 5, p 47.

CARR, J.P., HUGHES, J.P.: Penile paralysis in a quarter horse stallion. Calif. Vet. 5:13, 1984.

CASLICK, E.A.: The vulva and the vulvo-vaginal orifice and its relationship to genital health of the thoroughbred mare. Cornell Vet., 27:178-187, 1937.

CAUDLE, A.B., et al.: Endometrial levels of amikacin in the mare after intrauterine infusion of amikacin sulfate. Theriogenology, 19:433-439, 1983.

CHAFFIN, M.K., CARTER, G.K.: Equine bacterial pleuropneumonia. Part I. Epidemiology, pathophysiology, and bacterial isolates. Compend. Cont. Ed. Pract. Vet. 15:1642-1650, 1993.

CHAFFIN, M.K., CARTER, G.K., BYARS, T.D.: Equine bacterial pleuropneumonia. Part III. Treatment, sequelae, and prognosis. Comp. Cont. Ed. Pract. Vet. 16:1585-1589, 1994.

CHAK, R.M., and BRUSS, M.: The MIP test for diagnosis of pregnancy in mares. Proc. Am. Assoc. Equine Prac., 53-55, 1968.

CHURCH, S., WYN-JONES, G., PARK, A.H., RITCHIE, H.E.: Treatment of guttural pouch mycosis. Equine Vet. J. 18:362, 1986.

CLAY, C.M., SQUIRES, E.L., AMANN, R.P., and NETT, T.M.: Influences of season and artificial photoperiod on stallions: Pituitary and testicular responses to exogenous GnRH. J. Anim. Sci., 67:763-770,1988.

CLAY, C.M., SQUIRES, E.L., AMANN, R.P., and PICKETT, B.W.: Influences of season and artificial photoperiod on stallions: Lutenizing hormone, follicle-stimulating hormone and testosterone. J. Anim. Sci., 66:1246-1255, 1988.

CLEM, M.F., and DEBOWES, R.M.: Cryosurgical applications. In White, N.A., Moore, J.N. (eds): Current Practice of Equine Surgery. Philadelphia, J. B. Lippincott, 1990, pp. 12-16.

CLEM, M.F., and DEBOES, R.M.: Paraphimosis in horses—Part I. Compend. Contin. Educ. Practicing Vet., 11:72-75, 1989.

CLEM, M.F., and DEBOWES, R.M.: Paraphimosis in horses—Part II. Compend. Contin. Educ. Practicing Vet., 11:184-187, 1989.

COLAHAN, P.T., MAYHEW, I.G., MERRITT, A.M., and MOORE, J.N., Ed: Equine Medicine and Surgery. 4th ed., Goleta, CA., Am. Vet. Pub. Inc., 1991.

COLBERN, G.T., AANES, W.A., and STASHAK, T.S.: Surgical management of perineal lacerations and rectovestibular fisyulae in the mare: A retrospective study of 47 cases. J. Am. Vet. Med. Assoc., 186:265-269,1985.

COLE, J.R., et al.: Transmissibility and abortigenic effect of equine viral arteritis in mares. J. Am. Vet. Med. Assoc., 189:769-771, 1986.

THE COMPENDIUM COLLECTION: Abdominal Disease in Equine Practice, Trenton, N.J., Veterinary Learning Systems, 1994.

COOK, V.C., and SQUIRES, E.L.: Results from a commercial embryo transfer programme. Equine Vet. J. Suppl., 3:103, 1985.

COOK, W.R.: Some observations on form and function of the equine upper airway in health and disease. Proc. Am. Assoc. Equine Pract. 27:355, 1981.

COOK, W.R.: Specifications for speed in the racehorse. In The Airflow Factors. Menasha, WI, Russell Meerdink, 1989.

COSGROVE, J.S., SHEERAN, J.J., SAINTY, T.J.: Intussusception associated with infection with Anoplocephala perfoliate in a two year old thoroughbred. Irish Vet. J. 40:35, 1986.

COUTO, M.A., and HUGHES, J.P.: Intrauterine inoculation of a bacteria-free filtrate of Strepococcus zooepidemicus in clinically normal and infected mares. J. Equine Vet. Sci., 7:265-273, 1985.

COX, J., and DEBOWES, R.: Neurology: Episodic weakness caused by hyperkalemic periodic paralysis in horses. Compend. Contin. Educ. Pract. Vet. 12:83, 1990.

COX, J.E.: Excessive retainment of the placenta in a mare. Vet. Rec., 89:252-253, 1971.

COX, J.H., MURRAY, R.C., DEBOWES, R.M.: Diseases of the spinal cord. In Kobluk CN, Ames TR, Geor RJ, eds: The Horse Diseases and Clinical Management. Philadelphia, W. B. Saunders, 1995, pp. 443-472.

CRAWFORD, T.B.: Diagnostic virology in equine practice. In Proceedings of the 24th Annual Convention of the American Association of Equine Practitioners, 1978, p. 49.

CROWE, M.W., and SWERCZEK, T.W.: Equine congenital defects. Am. J. Vet. Res., 46:353-358, 1985.

CRUMP, J., Jr., and CRUMP, J.: Stallion ejaculation induced by manual stimulation of the penis. Theriogenology, 31:341-346, 1989.

CUPPS, P.T.: Reproduction in Domestic Animals, New York, N.Y., Academic Press, 1991.

DARIEN, B.: Duodenum. In Traub-Dagatz J.L., Brown C.M. (eds), Equine Endoscopy. St Louis, Mosby, 1990, ch. 11, p. 139.

DAVIDSON, M.G.: Equine ophthalmology. In Gelatt, KN (ed): Veterinary Ophthalmology. 2nd ed. Lea & Febiger, Philadelphia, 1991.

DE LAHUNTA, A.: Veterinary Neuroanatomy and Clinical Neurology, 2nd Ed., Philadelphia, PA., W. B. Saunders CO., 1993.

DIVERS, T.J., and PALMER, J.E.: Antimicrobial therapy in equine gastrointestinal disease. Proc. 32nd Annu. Conv. Am. Assoc. Equine Pract., 1986, p. 223.

DOLL, E.R., and BRYANS, J.T.: Incubation periods for abortion in equine viral rhinopneumonitis. J. Am. Vet. Med. Assoc., 141:351-354, 1962.

DORAN, R.E., WHITE, N.A., ALLEN, D.: Clinical aspects of ileal impaction in the horse. proc. Equine Colic Res. Symp. 2:182, 1986.

DOUGLAS-HAMILTON, D.H., et al.: A field study of the fertility of transported equine semen. Theriogenology, 22:291-304, 1984

DOWSETT, K.F., WOODWARD, R.A., and BODERO, D.A.V.: A study of nonsurgical embryo transfer in the mare. Theriogenology, 31:631-642, 1989.

DUBEY, J.P., DAVIS, S.W., SPEER, C.A., et al.: Sarcocystis neurona n. sp. (Protozoa: Apicomplexa), the etiologic agent of equine protozoal myeloencephalitis. J. Parasitol. 77:212-218, 1991.

DYCE, K.M., SACK, W. O., and WENSING, C.J.G.: Textbook of Veterinary Anatomy. Philadelphia, W. B. Saunders, 1987.

EHRHARDT, E.E., LOWE, J.E.: Observer variation in equine abdominal auscultation. Equine Vet. J. 1990; 22:182.

EMBERTSON, R.H.: Perineal lacerations. In Current Practice of Equine Surgery. Edited by N.A. White and J.N. Moore. Philadelphia, J.B. Lippincott, 1990, pp. 669-704.

ENGLAND, G.C.W.: Allen's Fertility and Obstetrics in the Horse. 2nd ed., Cambridge, MA., Blackwell Science, Ltd., 1996.

EVANS, A. G., and STANNARD, A. A.: Diagnostic approach to equine skin disease. Compend. Contin. Educ. Pract. Vet. 8(9):652, 1986.

EVANS, J.W., and TORBECK, R.L.: Breeding Management and Foal Development. Tyler, TX, Equine Research, Inc., 1982.

FADOK, V.A., and MULLOWNEY, P.C.: Dermatologic diseases of horses: I. Parasitic dermatoses of the horse. Compend. Contin. Educ. Pract. Vet. 5:5615, 1983.

FARROW, C.S.: Radiography of the equine thorax: Anatomy and technique. Vet. Radiol. 1981, 22:62.

FAULKNER, L.C., PINEDA, M.H.: Male reproduction. In McDonald LE (Ed): Veterinary Endocrinology and Reproduction, 2nd ed. Philadelphia, Lea & Febiger, 1975, p. 212.

FAYER, R., MAYHEW, I., BAIRD, J., et al.: Epidemiology of equine protozoal myeloencephalitis in North America based on histologically confirmed cases: A report. J. Vet. Intern. med. 4:54-57, 1990.

FENGER, C.K., GRANSTROM, D.E., LANGEMEIR, J.L., et al.: Identification of the opossum (Didelphus virginiana) as the definitive host of Sarcocystis neurona. J. Parasitol. 81:916-919, 1995.

FERRARO, G.L., EVANS, D.R., TRUNK, D.A., et al: Medical and surgical management of enteroliths in the equine. J. Am. Vet. Med. Assoc. 162:208, 1973.

FINOCCHIO, E.: A practical approach to the treatment of corneal ulcers in horses. Proc. 35th Annu. Conv. Am. Assoc. Equine Pract., 1989, p. 531.

FLOOD, P.F.: The development of the conceptus and its relationship to the uterus. In Reproduction in Domestic Animals. Edited by P.T. Cupps. New York, Academic Press, 1991, pp. 315-360.

FOERNER, J.J.: Diseases of the large intestine, differential dignosis and surgical management. Vet. Clin. North Am. Equine Pract. 4:130, 1982.

FOIL, C.S.: Cutaneous onchocerciasis. In Robinson NE (ed): Current Therapy in Equine Medicine. 2nd Ed. W. B. Saunders, Philadelphia, p. 627, 1987.

FRANDSON, R.D.: Anatomy and Physiology of Farm Animals. 4th ed. Philadelphia, Lea &Febiger, 1986.

FRANK, E.R.: Veterinary Surgery, 7th ed. Minneapolis: Burgess Publishing Company, 1964, p. 231.

FRANK, L.A.: Dermatophytosis. In Robinson, N.E. (ed): Current Therapy in Equine Medicine, ed 3. Philadelphia, W. B. Saunders, 1992, pp. 698-700.

FRAUNFELDER, H.C.: Cervical abnormalities. In Robinson NE (Ed): Current Therapy in Equine Medicine 2. Philadelphia. W. B. Saunders Company, 1987, p. 516.

FREEMAN, D.E., ORSINI, J.A., HARRISON, I.W., et al: Complications of umbilical hernias in horses: 13 cases (1972-1986). J. Am. Vet. Med. Assoc. 192:804, 1988.

FRETZ, P.B., BARBER, S.M.: Prospective analysis of cryosurgery as the sole treatment of equine sarcoids. Vet. Clin. North Am. 10:847, 1980.

FREW, D.G., and WRIGHT, I.M.: Supernumerary digits in the horse. Equine Pract., 12:21-26, 1990.

GEBAUER, M.R., PICKETTT, B.W., VOSS, J.L., and SWIERSTRA, E.E.: Reproductive physiology of the stallion: Daily sperm output and testicular measurements. J. Am. Vet. Med. Assoc., 165:711-714, 1974.

GELATT, K.N.: Veterinary Ophthalmology. 2nd ed. Lea & Febiger, Philadelphia, 1991.

GEORGI, J.R.: Parasitology for Veterinarians. 2nd ed. Philadelphia, W.B. Saunders, 1974.

GINTHER, O.J., GARCIA, M.C., SQUIRES, E.L., and STEFFENHAGEN, W.P.: Anatomy of the vasculature of the uterus and ovaries in the mare. Am. J. Vet. Res., 33:1561-1568, 1972.

GINTHER, O.J.: Reproductive Biology of the Mare: Basic and Applied Aspects. Ann Arbor, MI., McNaughton, Gunn, Inc., 1979.

GINTHER, O.J.: Sexual behavior following introduction of a stallion into a group of mares. Theriogenology, 19:877-887, 1983.

GINTHER, O.J.: The twinning problem: From breeding to day 16. Proc. Am. Assoc. Equine Pract., 11-26, 1983.

GINTHER, O.J.: Ultrasonic evaluation of the reproductive tract of the mare: The single embryo. J. Equine Vet. Sci., 4:75-81, 1984.

GINTHER, O.J., WHITMORE, H.L., and SQUIRES, E.L.: Characteristics of estrus, diestrus, and ovulation in mares and effects of season and nursing. Am. J. Vet. Res., 33:1935-1939, 1972

GOETZ, T.E., BOULTON, C.H., COFFMAN, J.R.: Inguinal and scrotal hernias in colts and stallions. Comp. Cont. Educ. Pract. Vet. 3:S272, 1981.

GOETZ, T.E., OGILVIE, G.K., KEEGAN, K.G., JOHNSON, P.J.: Cimetidine for treatment of melanomas in three horses. J. Am. Vet. Med. Assoc. 196:449-452, 1990

GUTHRIE, R.G.: Rolling for correction of uterine torsion in a mare. J. Am. Vet. Med. Assoc., 181:66-67, 1982.

HABEL, R.E.: Applied Veterinary Anatomy, 2nd ed. Ithaca, NY, R.E. Habel, 1981, p. 290.

HABEL, R.: The perineum of the mare. Cornell Vet., 43:249-278, 1953.

HACKETT, R.P., DUCHARME, N.G. (eds): Upper airway diseases. In Robinson N.E. (ed): Current Therapy in Equine Medicine, ed 3. Philadelphia, W. B. Saunders, 1992, pp. 265-297.

HAFEZ, E.S.E.: Reproduction in Farm Animals. 3rd ed. Philadelphia, PA., Lea & Febiger, 1974, p. 51.

HAFEZ, E.S.E.: Reproduction in Farm Animals. 5th ed. Philadelphia, Lea & Febiger, 1987.

HAKANSON, N.E., and MERIDETH, R. E.: Ocular examination and diagnostic techniques in the horse: 2. Assessment of vision and examination intraocular structures. Equine Pract. 9:6, 1987.

HANCE, R.S., DEBOWES, R.M., CLEM, M.F., and WELCH, R.D.: Umbilical, inguinal, and ventral hernias in horses. Compend. Contin. Educ. Practicing Vet., 12:862-871, 1990.

HAWCROFT, T.: The Complete Book of Horse Care, New York, N.Y., Howell Book House, 1983.

HAYES, H.M., JR.: Congenital umbilical and inguinal hernias in cattle, horses, swine, dogs and cats: Risk by breed and sex amoung hospital patients. Am. J. Vet. Res., 35:839-842, 1974.

HAYNES, P.F.: Arytenoid chondritis in the horse. Proc. Am. Assoc. Equine Pract. 27:63, 1981.

HAYNES, P.F.: Dorsal displacement of the soft palate and epiglottic entrapment: Diagnosis, management and interrelationship. Comp. Cont. Educ. Pract. Vet. 5:S379, 1983.

HAYNES, P.F.: Larynx. In Traub-Dargatz JL, Brown CM (eds): Equine Endoscopy. St Louis, Mosby, 1990, ch 6, p 59.

HAYNES, P.F.: Surgery of the equine respiratory tract. In Jennings PB (Ed): The Practice of Large Animal Surgery. Philadelphia, W. B. Saunders Company, 1984, pp. 388, 400, 410.

HERD, R.P.: Diagnosis of internal parasites. In Robinson N.E. (ed), Current Therapy in Equine Medicine, 2nd ed. Philadelphia, Saunders, 1987, p. 323.

HERD, R.P., DONHAM, J.C.: Efficacy of Ivermectin against cutaneous draschia and habronema infection in horses. Am. J. Vet. Res. 42:1953, 1981.

HERD, R.P., DOHAM, J.C.: Efficacy of Ivermectin against Onchocerca cervicalis microfilarial dermatitis in horses. Am. J. Vet. Res. 44:1102, 1983.

HILLMAN, R.B., and LESSER, S.A.: Induction of parturition. Vet. Clin. North Am. Large Anim. Pract., 2:333-344, 1980.

HINRICHS, K., and WATSON, E.D.: Clinical report: Recovery of a degenerating 14-day embryo in the uterine flush of a mare seven days after ovulation. Theriogenology, 30:349-353, 1988.

HOLT, P.E: Hernias and ruptures in the horse. Equine Pract. 8:13, 1986.

GRAY, P.: Parasites and Skin Diseases, London, Great Britain, J. A. Allen & Co., Ltd., 1995.

GRAY, P.: Respiratory Disease, London, Great Britain, J. A. Allen & Co., Ltd., 1994.

HOLTAN, D.W., SQUIRES, E.L., LAPIN, D.R., and GINTHER, O.J.: Effect of ovariectomy on pregnancy in mares. J. Reprod. fertil. Suppl., 27:457-463, 1979.

HONNAS, C.M., PASCOE, J.R.: Diseases of the paranasal sinuses. In Smith, B.P. (ed): Large Animal Internal Medicine. St. Louis, C.V. Mosby, 1990, pp. 555-557.

HOOD, D.M. and STEPHENS, K.A.: Physiology of equine laminitis. Compend. Contin. Educ. Practicing Vet., 3:454-460, 1981.

HUGHES, J.P.: Clinical examination and abnormalities in the mare. In Current Therapy in Theriogenology. Edited by D.A. Morrow. Philadelphia, W.B. Saunders, 1980, pp. 706-719.

HUGHES, J.P., and LOY, R.G.: Artificial insemination in the equine. A comparison of natural breeding and artificial insemination of mares using semen from six stallions. Cornell Vet., 60:463-475, 1970.

HUGHES, J.P., and LOY, R.G.: Investigations on the effect of intrauterine inoculations of Streptococcus zooepidemicus in the mare. Proc. Am. Equine Pract., 289-292, 1969.

HUGHES, J.P., STABENFELDT, G.H., and EVANS, J.W.: Estrous cycle and ovulation in the mare. J. Am. Vet. med. Assoc., 161: 1367-1375, 1972.

HUNTER, R.H.F.: Differential transport of fertilized and unfertilized eggs in equine fallopian tubes: A straightforward explanation. Vet. Rec. 125:304, 1989.

HURTGEN, J.P.: Stallion genital abnormalities. In Current Therapy in Equine Medicine 2. Edited by N.E. Robinson. Philadelphia, W. B. Saunders, 1980, pp. 558-562.

HUSKAMP, B.: The diagnosis and treatment of acute abdominal conditions in the horse: The various types and frequency as seen at the animal hospital in Hochmoore. Proc. Equine Colic Res. Symp. 1:261, 1982.

HUSKAMP, B., KOPF, N.: Right dorsal displacement of the large colon in the horse. Equine Pract. 5:20, 1983.

HYLAND, J., and JEFFCOTT, L.B.: Abortion. In The Current Therapy in Equine Medicine 2. Edited by N. E. Robinson. Philadelphia, W. B. Saunders, 1987, pp. 520-525.

JACOBSON, N.L., and MCGILLIARD, A.D.: The mammary gland and lactation. In Dukes' Physiology of Domestic Animals. 10th ed. Edited by M. J. Swenson. Ithaca, Comstock Publishing Associates, 1984, p. 871.

JACKSON, S.A., SQUIRES, E.L., and NETT, T.M.: The effect of exogenous progesterone on endogenous progesterone secretion in pregnant mares. Theriogenology, 25:275-279, 1986.

JACOBS, D.E.: A Colour Atlas of Equine Parasites. London, U.K., Gower Medical Publishing, 1986.

JEFFREY, D.: Horse Dentistry, The Theory and Practice of Equine Dental Maintenance, Norfolk, NB, World Wide Equine, Inc., 1996.

JENNINGS, P.B.: The Practice of Large Animal Surgery, Philadelphia, PA., W. B. Saunders Co., 1984.

JOHNSTON, J.K.: Botulism. In Robinson NE (Ed): Current Therapy in Equine Medicine. 2nd ed. Philadelphia, W. B. Saunders Company, 1987, p. 367.

JONES, T.: Complete Foaling Manual. Grand Prairie, TX. Equine Research, Inc., 1996.

JONES, R.L., et al.: The effect of washing on the aerobic bacterial flora of the stallion's penis. Proc. Am. Assoc. Equine Pract., 9-16, 1984.

JUZWIAK, J.J., SLOAN, D.E., SANTSCHI, E.M., and MOLE, H.D.: Cesarean section in 19 mares: Results and postoperative fertility. Vet. Surg., 19:50-52, 1990.

KENNEY, R.M.: Clinical aspects of endometrial biopsy in fertility evaluation of the mare. Proc. Am. Assoc. Equine Pract., pp. 105-122, 1977.

KENNEY, R.M., and DOIG, P.A.: Equine endometrial biopsy. In Current Therapy in Theriogenology 2. Edited by D.A. Morrow. Philadelphia, W.B. Saunders, 1986, pp. 723-729.

KENNEY, R.M., et al.: Minimal contamination techniques for breeding mares: Technique and preliminary findings. Proc. Am. Assoc. Equine Pract., 327-336, 1975.

KNOTTENBELT, D.C., and PASCOE, R.R.: Color Atlas of Diseases and Disorders of the Horse. Barcelona, Spain. Mosby-Year Book Europe, Ltd., 1994.

KNUDSEN, O.: Endometrial cytology as a diagnostic aid in mares. Cornell Vet., 54:415-422, 1964.

KOBLUK, C.N., AMES, T.R., GEOR, R.J.: The Horse Diseases and Clinical Management, Philadelphia, PA., W. B. Saunders Co., 1995.

KOPF, N.: Rectal examination of the colic patient. In Robinson NE (Ed): Current Therapy in Equine Medicine, ed 2. Philadelphia, W. B. Saunders Company, 1987, p. 23.

KOPF, N.: Rectal examination of the colic patient. In Robinson NE (Ed): Current Therapy in Equine Medicine, ed 3. Philadelphia, W. B. Saunders Company, 1992, p. 196.

LAING, J.A., MORGAN, W.J., BRINLEY, and WAGNER, W.C.: Fertility and Infertility in Veterinary Practice. 4th ed., London, Balliere Tindall, 1988.

LAMB, C.R.: Aspects of diagnostic imaging in equine pulmonary disease. Vet. Ann. 1989; 29:127.

LATIMER, C.A.: Diseases of the adnexa and conjunctiva. In Robinson, N.E. (ed): Current Therapy in Equine Medicine, ed 2. Philadelphia, W. B. Saunders, pp. 440-445, 1987.

LAVACH, J.D.: Large Animal Ophthalmology. Vol. 1. C.V. Mosby, St. Louis, 1990.

LAVACH, J.D.: Periodic ophthalmia. In Large Animal Ophthalmology. St. Louis, MO, C.V. Mosby, 199, pp. 162-171.

LAVOIE, J.P.: Chronic diseases of the respiratory tract. Compend. Cont. Educ. Pract. Vet. 16:1597-1601, 1994.

LEBLANC, M., and ASBURY, A.C.: Rationale for uterine lavage after breeding in mares. Proc. Am. Assoc. Equine Pract., 623-628, 1987.

LEE, J.J., HUTNER, S.H., BOVEE, E.C.: An Illustrated Guide to the Protozoa, Lawrence, KS., 1985.

LEIPOLD, H.W., SAPERSTEIN, G., and WOOLLEN, N.: Congenital defects in foals. In Large Animal Internal Medicine. Edited by B.P. Smith. St. Louis, C.V. Mosby, 1990, pp. 1567-1597.

LENSCH, J.: The early clinical diagnosis of pregnancy in mares. Proc. Am. Assoc. Equine Pract., 197-200, 1967.

LEY, W.B., et al.: Daytime foaling management of the mare. 2nd ed. Induction of parturition. J. Equine Vet. Sci., 9:95-99, 1989.

LOFSTEDT, R.M.: Termination of unwanted pregnancy in the mare. In Current Therapy in Theriogenology. 2nd ed. Edited by D.A. Morrow. Philadelphia, W.B. Saunders, 1986, pp. 715-718.

LOWE, J.E., Dougherty, R.: Castration of horses and ponies by a primary closure method. J. Am. Vet. Med. Assoc. 160:183, 1972.

LOY, R.G.: Characteristics of postpartum reproduction in mares. Vet. Clin. N. Amer. Large Anim. Prac., 2:345-358, 1980.

MCDONALD, L.W.: Veterinary Endocrinology and Reproduction. 3rd ed. Philadelphia, Lea & Febiger, 1980.

MCDONNELL, S.M.: Spontaneous erection and masturbation in Equids. Proc. Am. Assoc. Equine Pract., 567-580, 1989.

MCDONNELL, S.M., and LOVE, C.C.: Manual stimulation collection of semen from stallions: Training time, sexual behavior and semen. Theriogenology, 33:1201-1210, 1990.

MCENTEEE, K.: Reproductive Pathology of Domestic Animals. San Diego, CA., Academic Press, Inc., 1990.

MCILWRAITH, C.W.: Equine digestive system. In Jennings P.B. (Ed): The Practice of Large Animal Surgery. Philadelphia, W.B. Saunders Company, 1984, p. 628.

MCILWRAITH, C.W.: In Jennings PB (Ed): The Practice of Large Animal Surgery. Philadelphia, W. B. Saunders Company, 1985, p. 602.

MCILWRAITH, C.W., TROTTER, G.W.: Joint Disease in the Horse. Philadelphia, W. B. Saunders Co., 1996.

MCILWRAITH, C.W., TURNER, A.S.: Equine Surgery: Advanced Techniques. Philadelphia, Lea & Febiger, 1987, pp. 228, 235.

MCKINNON, A.O., et. al.: Diagnostic ultrasonongraphy of uterine pathology in the mare. Proc. Am. Assoc. Equine Pract., 605-622, 1987.

MCKINNON, A.O., and SQUIRES, E.L.: Equine embryo transfer. Vet. Clin. North Am. Equine pract., 4:305-333, 1988.

MCKINNON, A.O., and SQUIRES, E.L.: Morphological assessment of equine embryo. J. Am. Vet. Med. Assoc. 192:401-406, 1988.

MCKINNON, A.O., SQUIRES, E.L., and VOSS, J.L.: Ultrasonic evaluation of the mare's reproductive tract. Part I. Compend. Contin. Education Practicing Vet., 9:336-345,1987.

MCKINNON, A.O., SQUIRES, E.L., and VOSS, J.L.: Ultrasound evaluation of the mare's reproductive tract: Part II. Compend. Contin. Educ. Practicing Vet., 9:472-482, 1987.

MCKINNON, A.O., and VOSS, J.L.: Equine Reproduction. Media, PA., Williams & Wilkins, 1993.

MCMULLAN, W.: Habronemiasis. Proc. Am. Assoc. Equine Pract. 22:295, 1976.

MACKEY, V.S., WHEAT, J.D.: Endoscopic examination of the equine thorax. Equine Vet. J. 1985; 17:140.

MADWELL, B.R., PRIESTER, W.A., GILLETTE, K.L.: Neoplasms of the nasal passages of the paranasal sinuses in domesticated animals as reported by 13 colleges. Am. J. Vet. Res. 37:851, 1976.

MANSMANN, R.A., MCALLISTER, E.S., PRATT, P.W., Eds.: Equine medicine and Surgery, Santa Barbara, CA, American Veterinary Publishers, 1982.

MARDEN, D.T.: Enterolithiasis: A practitioner's view of selected cases. Vet. Med. Small Anim. Clin. 63:611, 1968.

MARKEL, M.D., PASCOE, R., SAMS, A.E.: Strangulation umbilical hernias in horses: 13 cases (1974-1985). J. Am. Vet. Med. Assoc. 190:692, 1987.

MATTHEWS, J.K., and ANDREWS, F.: Performing a neurologic examination in a standing or recumbent horse. Vet. Med. 85:1229, 1990.

MAYHEW, I.G.: Large Animal Neurology. A Handbook for Veterinary Clinicians. Philadelphia, Lea & Febiger, 1989.

MAYHEW, I.G., BEAL, C.R.: Techniques of analysis of cerebrospinal fluid. Vet. Clin. North Am. Small Anim. Pract. 1980; 10:155.

MAYHEW, I.G., WHITLOCK, R., DE LAHUNTA, A.: Spinal cord disease in the horse. Cornell Vet. 78:68 Suppl 6:44.

MEAGHER, D.M.: Obstructive disease in the large intestine of the horse: Diagnosis and treatment. Proc. Am. Assoc. Equine Pract. 18:269, 1972.

MEAGHER, D.M.: Rectal surgery. In Current Practice of Equine Surgery. Edited by N.A. White and J.N. Moore. Philadelphia, J.B. Lippincott, 1990, pp. 357-365.

MILLER, R.I.: Equine phycomycosis. Compend. Contin. Educ. Pract. Vet. 5:S472, 1983.

MODRANSKY, P.D, REED, S.M., BARBEE, D.D.: Dysphagia associated with guttural pouch empyema and dorsal displacement of the soft palate. Equine Prac. 4:34, 1982.

MONIN, T.: Vaginoplasty: A surgical treatment for urine pooling in the mare. Proc. Am. Assoc. Equine Pract., 99-102, 1972.

MONTES, L.F., and VAUGHAN, J.T.: Atlas of Skin Diseases of the Horse. Philadelphia, W.B. Saunders, 1983.

MOORE, C.P.: Diseases of the cornea. In Robinson, N.E. (ed): Current Therapy in Equine Medicine, ed 2. Philadelphia, W. B. Saunders, pp. 450-456, 1987.

MOORE, J.N.: Management of pain and shock in equine colic. Comp. Cont. Educ. Pract. Vet. 7:S169, 1985.

MORRIS, E.: Dynamic evaluation of the equine upper respiratory tract. Vet. Clin. North Am. Equine Prac. 1991; 7:403.

MORROW, D.A.: Current Therapy in Theriogenology, Philadelphia, PA., W. B. Saunders, Co., 1980.

MULLOWNEY, P.C.: Dermalogic diseases of horses. Part IV. Environmental, congenital, and neoplastic diseases. Compend. Contin. Ed. Pract. Vet. 1985, 7:S22.

MULLOWNEY, P.C.: The Veterinary Clinics of North America, Large Animal Practice, Large Animal Dermatology, Vol. 6, Number 1, Philadelphia, PA., 1984.

MUNROE, G.A.: Cryosurgery in the horse. Equine Vet. J. 18(1):14-17, 1986.

MURRAY, M.J.: Gastric ulcers in adult horses. Compend. Cont. Ed. pract. Vet. 16:792-794, 1994.

MUYELLE, E., OYAERT, W., OOMS, L., DECRAEMERE, H.: Treatment of tetanus in the horse by injections of tetanus antitoxin into the subarachnoid space. J. Am. Vet. Med. Assoc. 167:47, 1975.

NEELY, D.P.: Equine gestation. In Equine Reproduction. Edited by D.P. Neely, I.K.M. Liu, and R.B. Hillman, Princeton Junction, NJ, Veterinary Learning Systems, 1983, pp. 57-70.

NEELY, D.P.: Evaluation and therapy of gential disease in the mare. In Equine Production. Edited by D.P. Neely, I.K.M. Liu, and R.B. Hillman. Lawrenceville, Veterinary Learning Systems, 1982, pp. 40-56.

NEELY, D.P.: Evaluation and therapy of genital disease in the mare. In Equine Production. Edited by J.P. Hughes. Nutley, Hoffman-LaRoche, Inc., 1983, pp. 40-56.

NEELY, D.P.: Physical examination and genital diseases of the stallion. In Current Therapy in Theriogenology. Edited by D.A. Morrow Philadelphia, W.B. Saunders, 1980, pp. 694-706.

NEELY, D.P.: Progesterone/progestin therapy in the brood-mare. Proc. Am. Assoc. Equine Pract., pp. 203-218, 1988.

NEELY, D.P., et al.: Prostaglandin release patterns in the mare: Physiological, pathophysiological, and therapeutic responses. J. Reprod. Fertil. Suppl., 27:181-189, 1979.

NEELY, D.P., LIU, I.K.M., HILLMAN, R.B., Eds.: Equine Production, Lawrenceville, KS, Veterinary Learning Systems, 1982.

NICKELS, F.A.: In Traub-Dargatz JL, Brown CM (eds), Equine Endoscopy. St Louis, Mosby, 1990, ch 3, p 25.

O'CALLAGHAN, M.W., GOULDEN, B.R.: Radiographic changes in the lungs of horses with exercise-induced epistaxis. N Z Vet. J. 1982; 30:117.

O'CALLAGHAN, M.W., HORNOF, W.J., FISHER, P.E., et al: Exercise-induced pulmonary hemorrhage in the horse: Results of a detailed clinical, post mortem and imaging study: VI. Ventilation/perfusion scintigraphy in horses with EIPH. Equine Vet. J. 1987; 19:423.

O'CONNOR, J.P.: Rectal examination of the cryptorchid horse. Ir. Vet. J. 25:129, 1971.

OEHME, F.W., PRIER, J.E.: Textbook of Large Animal Surgery, Baltimore, M.D., The Williams and Wilkens Co., 1974.

OSTLUND, E.N.: The equine herpesviruses. Vet. Clin. North Am. Equine Pract. 9:283-294, 1993.

OSTLUND, E.N., POWELL, D., BRYANS, J.T.: Equine herpesvirus 1: A review. Proc. Am. Assoc. Equine pract. 36:387-395, 1990.

PACCAMONTI, D.L.: Elective terminationn of pregnancy in mares. J. Am. Vet. Med. Assoc., 198:683-689, 1991

PARADIS, M.R.: Chronic obstructuive pulmonary disease. Compend. Cont. Educ. Pract. Vet. 12:1651-1654, 1990.

PARK, A.H., DORAN R.E., WHITE, N.A., et al: Ileal impaction in the horse: 75 cases. Cornell Vet. 79:83, 1989.

PARKER, J.: Examination of the equine eye as part of the examination of the horse for purchase. Equine Vet. J., suppl. 2:3, 1983.

PASCOE, R.R.: A Color Atlas of Equine Dermatology., London, England, Wolfe Publishing, Ltd., 1990.

PASCOE, R.R.: Methods for the treatments of twin pregnancy in the mare. Equine Vet. J., 15:40-42, 1983.

PASCOE, R.R., et al.: Management of twin pregnancy by manual embryonic reduction and comparison of two techniques and three hormonal therapies. J. Reprod. Tertil. Suppl., 35:701-702, 1987.

PASCOE, R.R., ELLENBURG, T.V., CULBERTSON, M.R., MEAGHER, D.M.: Torsion of the spermatic cord in a horse. J. Am. Vet. Med. Assoc. 178:242, 1981.

PASQUINI, C., REDDY, V.K., RATZLAFF, M.H.: Atlas of Equine Anatomy, Eureka, CA, Sudz Publishing, 1978.

PAVORD, T., and DRUMMOND, M.: Horse Breeding: A Practical Guide for Owners. New York, Howell Book House, 1990.

PEYTON, L.C.: Surgical correction of equine umbilical hernias. Vet. Med. Small Anim. Clin. 76:1212, 1981.

PICKETT, B.W., et al.: Management of the Stallion for Maximum Reproductive Efficiency. II. Animal Reproduction Laboratory Bulletin No. O5. Fort Collins, Colorado State University, 1989.

PICKETT, B.W., et al.: Reproductive physiology of the stallion . VI. Seminal and behavioral characteristics. J. Anim. Sci., 43:617-625, 1976.

PICKETT, B.W., SULLIVAN, J.J., and SEIDEL, G.E., Jr.: Reproductive physiology of the stallion. V. Effect of frequency of ejaculation on seminal characteristics and spermatozoal output. J. Anim. Sci., 40:917-923,1975.

PICKETT, B.W., SQUIRES, E.L., and MCKINNON, A.O.: Procedures for Collection, Evaluation and Utilization of Stallion Semen for Artificial Insemination. Animal Reproduction Laboratory Bulletin No. 03. Fort Collins, Colorado State University, 1987.

PICKETT, B.W., VOSS, J.L., and DEMICK, D.S.: Stallion seminal extenders. Proc. Am. Assoc. Equine Pract., 155-274, 1974.

PLATT, H.: Cecal rupture in parturient mares. J. Comp. Pathol. 93:343, 1983.

POPESKO, P.: Atlas of Topographical Anatomy of the Domestic Animals, 2nd Ed., Philadelphia, PA., W. B. Saunders Co., 1977.

POURET, E.J.M.: Surgical techniques for correction of pneumo- and urovagina. Equine Vet. J., 14:249-250, 1982.

PRICKETT, M.E., REEVES, J.T., and ZENT, W.W.: Tetralogy of Fallot in a Thoroughbred mare. J. Am. Vet. Med. Assoc., 162:552-555, 1973.

PROVINCE, C.A.: Cooling and storage of canine and equine spermatozoa. M.S. thesis. Colorado State University, 1984.

PURVIE, A.D.: Elective induction of labor and parturition in the mare. Proc. Am. Assoc. Equine Pract., 113-118, 1972.

RAGLE, C.A., MEAGHER, D.M.: Abdominal auscultation as aid to the diagnosis of sand colic. Proc. AM. Assoc. Equine Pract. 33:521, 1987.

RAGLE, C.A., MEAGHER, D.M., LACROIX, C.A., et al: Surgical treatment of sand colic: Results in 40 horses. Vet. Surg. 18:48, 1989.

RANTANEN, N.W.: Diseases of the thorax. In Diagnostic ultrasound. Vet. Clin. North Am. Equine Pract. 1986; 2:49.

REED, S.M., and BAYLY, W.M.: Equine Internal Medicine, Philadelphia, PA., W. B. Saunders CO., 1998.

REED, S.M., GRANSTROM, D.E.: Equine protozoal encephalomyelitis. Proc. Am. Coll. Vet. Intern. Med. Forum 11:591-592, 1993.

REEF, V.B.: Equine Diagnostic Ultrasound. Philadelphia, W.B. Saunders, 1998.

REEF, V.B.: Problems in Equine Medicine. Philadelphia, Lea & Febiger, 1989, pp. 122-137.

REIMER, J.M.: Atlas of Equine Ultrasonography, St. Louis, MO, Mosby-Year Book, 1998.

RICKETTS, S.W.: Bacteriological examinations of the mare's cervix: Techniques and interpretation of results. Vet. Rec., 108:46-51, 1981.

RICKETTS, S.W.: Perineal conformation abnormalities. In Current Therapy in Equine Medicine. 2nd ed. Edited by N.E. Robinson. Philadelphia, W.B. Saunders, 1987, pp. 518-520.

ROBERTS, S.J.: Gestation and pregnancy diagnosis in the mare. In Current Therapy in Theriogenology. Edited by D.A. Morrow. Philadelphia, W.B. Saunders, 1980, pp. 736-746.

ROBERTS, S.J.: Internal examination for pregnancy in the mare. In Veterinary Obstetrics and Genital Diseases (Theriogenology). 3rd ed. Woodstock, VT, S.J. Roberts, 1986, pp. 25-26.

ROBERTS, S.J.: Veterinary Obstetrics and Genital Diseases, 2nd ed. Ithaca, NY, S.J. Roberts, 1971, p. 49.

ROBERTSON, J.T.: Cervical lacerations. In Current Practice of Equine Surgery. Edited by N.A. White and J.N. Moore. Philadelphia, J.B. Lippincott, 1990, pp. 696-699.

ROBERTSON, J.T.: Impaction of the large intestine. In Mansmann, R.A., McAllister, E.S., Pratt, P.W. (Eds): Equine Medicine and Surgery. Santa Barbara, CA, American Veterinary Publishers, 1982, p. 561.

ROBERTSON, J.T.: Resection of intussuscepted large colon in a horse. J. Am. Vet. Med. Assoc. 181:927, 1982.

ROBINSON, N.E.: Current Therapy in Equine Medicine, 2nd Ed., Philadelphia, PA., W. B. Saunders Co., 1987.

ROOK, A., WILKINSON, D.S., EBLING, F.J.G., Ed.: Textbook of Dermatology, 3rd Ed., London, England, Blackwell Scientific Publications, 1979.

ROONEY, J.R., and FRANKS, W.C.: Congenital cardiac anomalies in horses. Pathol. Vet., 1:454-464, 1964.

ROONEY, J.R. and ROBERTSON, J.L.: Equine Pathology, Ames, Iowa, Iowa State University Press, 1996.

ROONEY, J.R., SACK, W.O., and HABEL, R.E.: Guide to the Dissection of the Horse. Ithaca, W.O. Sack, 1967, pp. 63-70.

ROSE, R.J.: Experiences with fluprostenol as an induction agent in thoroughbred mares. J. Reprod. Fertil. Suppl., 32:645, 1982.

ROSS, M.W.: Surgical diseases of the equine cecum. Vet. Clin. North Am. Equine Pract. 5:363, 1989.

ROSSDALE, P.D.: The Horse from Conception to Maturity. London, J.A. Allen, 1993.

ROSSDALE, P.D., and RICKETTS, S.W.: Equine Stud Farm Medicine. 2nd ed. Philadelphia, Lea & Febiger, 1980.

ROSSIER, Y., SWEENEY, C.R., ZIEMER, E.L.: Bronchoalveolar lavage fluid cytologic findings in horses with pneumonia or pleuropneumonia. J. Am. Vet. Med. Assoc. 1991; 198:1001.

RUGGLES, A.J., ROSS, M.W., FREEMAN, D.E.: Endoscopic examination of normal paranasal sinuses in horses. Vet. Surg. 1991; 20:418-423.

SCHEBITZ, H. and WILKENS, H.: Atlas of Radiographic Anatomy of the Horse, Berlin, Germany, Verlag Paul Pary, 1978.

SCHEIDT, V.J., LLOYD, D.H.: Dermatophilosis. In Robinson NE (ed): Current Therapy in Equine Medicine. 2nd Ed. W. B. Saunders, Philadelphia, p. 630, 1987.

SCHMIDT, A.R.: Transrectal ultrasonography of the caudal portion of the abdominal and pelvic cavities in horses. J. Am. Vet. Med. Assoc. 1989; 194:365.

SCHUMACHER, J., and VAUGHAN, J.T.: Surgery of the penis and prepuce. Vet. Clin. North Am. Equine Pract. 4:473-493, 1988.

SCOTT, D.W.: Large Animal Dermatology. Philadelphia: W.B. Saunders, 1988.

SCOTT, E.A., GALLAGHER, K., BOLES, C.L., et al: Dental disease in the horse: 5 case reports. J. Equine Med. Surg. 1:301, 1977.

SCOTT, P., et al.: The aerobic bacterial flora of the reproductive tract of the mare. Vet. Rec., 88:58-61, 1971.

SHAW, E.B., HOUPT, K.A., and HOLMES, D.F.: Body temperature and behavior of mares during the last two weeks of pregnancy. Equine Vet. J., 20:199-202, 1988.

SHIDELER, R.K., et al.: Endometrial biopsy in the mare. Proc. Am. Assoc. Equine Pract., pp. 97-104, 1977.

SHIDELER, R.K., MCCHESNEY, A.E., SQUIRES, E.L., and OSBORNE, M.: Effect of uterine lavage on clinical and laboratory parameters in postpartum mares. Equine Pract., 9:20-26,1987.

SHIPLEY, W.D., and BERGEN, W.C.: Care of the foaling mare and foal. Vet. Med., 64:63-70, 1969.

SHIRES, G.M., and KANEPS, A.J.: A practical and simple surgical technique for repair of urine pooling in the mare. Proc. Am. Assoc. Equine Pract., 51-56, 1986.

SHIRES, G.M.H.: Rectal tears. In Current Therapy in Equine Medicine. 2nd ed. Edited by N.E. Robinson. Philadelphia, W.B. Saunders, 1987, pp. 75-79.

SHOSTER, J.V.: Surgical repair of equine eyelid lacerations. Vet. Med. 83:1042, 1988.

SIMPSON, R.E., et al.: Use of ultrasound echography for early diagnosis of single and twin pregnancy in the mare. J. Reprod. Fertil. Suppl., 32:431-439, 1982.

SISSON, S., GROSSMAN, J.D.: The Anatomy of the Domestic Animals, 4th ed. Philadelphia, W. B. Saunders Company, 1953, p. 581.

SISSON, S.: The Anatomy of the Domestic Animals, 5th ed., Philadelphia, W. B. Saunders Company, 1975, p. 402.

SLATTER, D.: Fundmentals of Veterinary Opthalmology, Philadelphia, PA., W.B. Saunders Co., 1990.

SLEIGH, M.: Protozoa and Other Protists, London, England, Edward Arnold, 1989.

SLOAN, D.E.: Ovariectomy, ovariohysterectomy and cesarean section in mares. Bet. Clin. North Am. Large Anim. Pract., 4:451-459, 1988.

SMITH, H.A., JONES, T.C., HUNT, R.D.: Pathology, 4th ed. Philadelphia, Lea & Febiger, 1972, p..315.

SMITH, B.P.: Large Animal Internal Medicine, St. Louis, C. V. Mosby, 1990.

SOMMARDAHL, C.S., HENTON, J.E., and PETERSON, M.G.: Rabies in a horse. Equine Pract. 12:11, 1990.

SPECHT, T.E., COLAHAN, P.T.: Surgical treatment of sand colic in equids: 48 cases (1978-1985). J. Am. Vet. Med. Assoc. 193:1560, 1988.

SPEIRS, V.C.: Clinical Examination of Horses, Philadelphia, PA., W.B. Saunders Co., 1997.

SPEIRS, V.C.: The surgical treatment of laryngeal hemiplegia in horses. Habil Thesis Med. Vet. Bern 1985.

SPIER, S.J., CARLSON, G.P., HOLLIDAY, T. A., et al.: Hyperkalemic periodic paralysis in horses. J. Am. Vet. Med. Assoc. 197:1009, 1990.

SQUIRES, E.L., et. al.: Relationship of altrenogest to ovarian activity, hormone concentrations and fertility of mares. J. Anim. Sci., 56:901-910, 1983.

SQUIRES, E.L., IULIANO, M.F., and SHIDELER, R.K.: Factors affecting success of surgical and nonsurgical equine embryo transfer. Theriogenology, 17:631-642, 1989.

SQUIRES, E.L., TODTER, G.E., BERNDTSON, W.E., and PICKETT, B.W.: Effect of anabolic steroids on reproductive function in young stallions. J. Anim. Sci., 54:576-582, 1982.

SQUIRES, E.L., VOSS, J.L., and VILLAHOZ, M.D.: Immunological methods for pregnancy detection in mares. Proc. Am. Assoc. Equine Pract., 45-51, 1983.

STABENFELDT, G.H., et al.: Endogenous and exogenous manipulation of the corpus luteum of the mare. In Twenty-eighth International Congress of Physiological Sciences. Edited by G. Pethes and V.L. Frenyo. Budapest, Pergamon Press, pp. 133-139, 1981.

STABENFELDT, G.H., et al.: Physiologic and pathophysiologic aspects of Prostaglandin F2~ during the reproductive cycle. J. Am. Vet. Med. Assoc., 176: 1187-1194, 1980.

STASHAK, T.S.: Clnical evaluation of the equine colic patient. Vet. Clin. North Am. Large Anim. Pract. 1:275, 1979.

STASHAK, T.S.: Equine Wound Management, Malvern, PA., Lea & Febiger, 1991.

STEVEN, D.H., JEFFCOTT, L.B., and MALLON, K.A.: Ultrastructural studies of the equine uterus and placenta following parturition. J. Reprod. Fertil. Suppl., 27:579-586.

STICK, J.A.: Amputation of the equine urethral process affected with habronemiasis. Vet. Med. Small Anim. Clin., 74:1453-1457, 1979.

STICK, J.A.: Esophagus. In Traub-Dagatz J.L., Brown C.M. (eds), Equine Endoscopy. St. Louis, Mosby, 1990, ch. 9, p. 111.

SULLINS, K.E., ROBERST, S.M., LAVACH, J.D., SEVERIN, G.A.: Equine sarcoid. Equine Pract. 8:21, 1986.

SWENSON, M.J.: Duke's Physiology of Domestic Animals, 10th Ed., Ithaca, N.Y., Comstock Publishing Associates, 1984.

SWERCZEK, T.W.: Contagious equine metritis— Outbreak of the disease in Kentucky and laboratory methods for diagnosing the disease. J. Reprod. Fertil. Suppl., 27:361-365, 1979.

TAYLOR, F.G.R. and HILLYER, M.H.: Diagnostic Techniques in Equine Medicine, London, Great Britain, W.B. Saunders Co., 1997.

TENNANT, B.: Intestinal obstruction in the horse: Some aspects of differential diagnosis in equine colic. Proc. Am. Assoc. Equine Pract. 22:426, 1976.

THEON, A.P., PASCOE, J.R., CARLSON, G.P., KRAG, D.N.: Intratumoral chemotherapy with cisplatin in oily emulsion for treatment of tumors in horses. J. Am. Vet. Med. Assoc. 202(2):261-267, 1993.

THEILEN, G.H.: Papillomatosis (warts). In Robinson, N.E. (ed): Current Therapy in Equine Medicine. W. B. Saunders, Philadelphia, p. 536-537, 1983.

THRALL, D.F.: Textbook of Veterinary Diagnostic Radiology, Philadelphia, PA., W. B. Saunders Co., 1998.

THRELFALL, W.R.: Broodmare uterine therapy. Compend. Contin. Educ. Practicing Vet., 11:246-254, 1980.

THRELFALL, W.R.: Recurrent torsion of the spermatic cord and scrotal testis in a stallion. J. Am. Vet. Med. Assoc., 196:1641-1643, 1990.

THRELFALL, W.R., and CARLETON, C.L.: Treatment of uterine infections in the mare. In Current Therapy in Theriogenology. 2nd ed. Edited by D.A. Morrow. Philadelphia, W.B. Saunders, 1986, pp. 730-737.

TIMONEY, P.J., and MCCOLLUM, W.H.: The epidemiology of equine viral arteritis. Proc. Am. Assoc. Equine Pract., 545-551, 1986.

TODHUNTER, R.J., PARKER, J.E.: Surgical repair of urethral transection in a horse. J. Am. Vet. Med. Assoc. 193:1085, 1988.

TORBECK, R.L., and RANTANEN, N.W.: Early pregnancy detection in the mare with ultrasonography. J. Equine Vet. Sci., 2:204-207, 1982.

TRAUB-DARGATZ, J.L., Ed., and BROWN, C.M.: Equine Endoscopy, 2nd Ed., St. Louis, Missouri, Mosby-Year Book, Inc., 1997.

TROTTER, G.W.: Paranasal sinuses. Vet. Clin. North Am. Large Anim. Pract. 9(1):153-169, 1993.

TROTTER, G.W., AANES, W.A.: A complication of cryptorchid castration in three horses. J. Am. Vet. Med. Assoc. 178:246, 1981.

TROTTER, G.W., and MCKINNON, A.O.: Surgery for abnormal vulvar and perineal conformation in

TULLENERS, E.P.: Correlation of performance with endoscopic and radiographic assessment of epiglottic hypoplasia in racehorses with epiglottic entrapment corrected by use of contact neodymium:yttrium aluminum garnet laser. J. Am. Vet. Med. Assoc. 198:621, 1991.

TULLENERS, E.P.: Transendoscopic laser surgery of the respiratory tract. In Traub-Dargatz JL, Brown, C.M. (Eds): Equine Endoscopy. St. Louis, C. V. Mosby, 1990, p. 85.

TURNER, A.S., and MCILWRAITH, C.W.: Cesarean section in the mare. In Techniques in Large Animal Surgery. 2nd ed. Philadelphia, Lea & Febiger, 1989, pp. 200-203.

TURNER, A.S., MCILWRAITH, C.W.: Techniques in Large Animal Surgery. 2nd ed. Philadelphia, Lea & Febiger, 1989, p. 254.

TURNER, D.D., et al.: FSH and LH concentrations in periparturient mares. J. Reprod. Fertil. Suppl., 27:547-553, 1979.

UHLINGER, C.A.: Effects of three anthelmintic schedules on the incidence of colic in horses. Equine Vet. J. 22:251-254, 1990.

UHLINGER, C.A.: Equine small strongyles: Epidemiology, pathology, and control. Compend. Contin. Educ. Pract. Vet. 13:863, 1991.

UHLINGER, C.A.: New information on parasite control and the incidence of colic: Anthelmintic protocol for prevention of colic. Proc. 35th Annu. Conv. Am. Assoc. Equine pract., 1989, p. 99.

VANDEPLASSCHE, M.M.: The pathogenesis of dystocia and fetal malformation in the horse. J. Reprod. Fertil. Suppl. 35:547, 1987.

VANDEPLASSCHE, M.M., BOUTERS, R., SPINCEMAILLE, J., BONTE, P.: Caesarean section in the mare. Proc. Am. Assoc. Equine Pract. 23:75, 1977.

VARNER, D.D., SCHUMACHER, J., BLANCHARD, T., and JOHNSON, L.: Diseases and Management of Breeding Stallions. Goleta, CA., Am. Vet. Pub., 1997.

VASEY, J.R.: Equine cutaneous habronemiasis. Compend. Contin. Educ. Pract. Vet. 3:290, 1981.

VAUGHAN, J.T.: Equine urogenital system. In The Practice of Large Animal Surgery. Edited by P.B. Jennings, Philadelphia, W.B. Saunders, 1984, pp. 1122-1150.

VAUGHAN, J.T.: The male genital system (horse). In Textbook of Large Animal Surgery. 2nd ed. Edited by F.W. Oehme. Baltimore, Williams & Wilkins, 1974, pp. 511-526.

VAUGHAN, J.T.: The Practice of Large Animal Surgery, edited by P.B. Jennings. Philadelphia, W.B. Saunders, 1984, pp. 1122-1140.

VAUGHAN, J.T.: Surgery of the equine reproductive system. In Current Therapy in Theriogenology. Edited by D.A. Morrow. Philadelphia, W.B. Saunders, 1980, pp. 820-821.

VAUGHAN, J.T.: Surgery of the male equine reproductive system. In The Practice of Large Animal Surgery. Vol. 2. Edited by P.B. Jennings, Jr. Philadelphia, W.B. Saunders, 1984, pp. 1083-1105.

VAUGHAN, J.T.: Surgery of the male equine reproductive system. In Current Therapy in Theriogenology. 2nd ed. Edited by D.A. Morrow. Philadelphia, W.B. Saunders, 1986, pp. 740-745.

VAUGHAN, J.T.: Surgery of the prepuce and the penis. Proc. Am. Assoc. Equine Pract., 19-40, 1972.

THE VETERINARY CLINICS OF NORTH AMERICA, Equine Pract., Dermatoloty, April 1995, vol. 2.

VOGEL, C.: The Complete Horse Care Manual, New York, N.Y., Dorling Kindersley Publishing Inc., 1995.

VON TSCHARNER, C., Ed., HALLIWELL, R.E.W.: Advance in Veterinary Dermatology, Volume 1, London, England, Bailliere Tindall, W. B. Saunders Co., 1990.

VOSS, J.L., PICKETT, B.W., BACH, D.G., and BURWASH, L.D.: Effect of rectal palpation on pregnancy rate of nonlactating normally cycling mares. J. Anim. Sci., 41:829-834, 1975.

WALKER, D.F., and VAUGHAN, J.T.: Examination of the stallion. In Bovine and Equine Urogenital Surgery. Philadelphia, Lea & Febgier, 1980, pp. 105-114.

WATKINS, J.P., et al.: Elective cesarean section in mares. J. Am. Vet. Med. Assoc., 197:1639-1645, 1990.

WELSCH, B.B.: Update on equine therapeutics: Treatment of equine protozoal myeloencephalitis. Compend. Contin. Educ. Pract. Vet. 13:1599-1602, 1991.

WHEAT, J.D.: Sinus drainage and teeth repulsion in the horse. Proc. Am. Assoc. Equine Pract. 19:171, 1973.

WHEAT, J.D., and MEAGHER, D.M.: Uterine torsion and rupture in mares. J. Am. Vet. Med. Assoc., 160:881-884, 1972.

WHITE, N.A.: The Equine Acute Abdomen. Philadelphia, Lea and Febiger, 1990.

WHITE, N.A.: Examination and diagnosis of the acute abdomen. In: The Equine Accute Abdomen, N. A. White (ed.), Philadelphia: Lea and Febiger, 1990, pp. 102-142.

WHITE, N.A., MOORE, J.N.: Current Practice of Equine Surgery, Philadelphia, PA., J. B. Lippincott, 1990.

WICHTEL, J.J., REINERTSON, E.L., and CLARK, T.L.: Nonsurgical treatment of uterine torsion in seven mares. J. Am. Vet. Med. Assoc., 193:337-338, 1988.

WILSON, J.M., DREIDER, J.L., and POTTER, G.D.: Nonsurgical recovery of degenerative ova from the uterus of mares. Theriogenology, 23:236, 1985.

WOODS, G.L., et al.: A field study on early pregnancy loss in standardbred mares. J. Equine Vet. Sci., 5:264-267, 1985.

WOODS, J., BERGFELT, D.R., and GINTHER, O.J.: Effects of time of insemination relative to ovulation on pregnancy rate and embryonic-loss rate in mares. Equine Vet. J., 22:410-415, 1990.

YOUNGQUIST, R.S.: Current Therapy in Large Animal Theriogenology. Philadelphia, W.B. Saunders, 1997.

ZENT, W.W.: Postpartum complications. In Robinson NE (Ed): Current Therapy in Equine Medicine 2. Philadelphia, W. B. Saunders Company, 1987, p. 544.

PHARMACEUTICAL APPENDIX

Acepromazine Maleate - (Prom Ace™) A central nervous system tranquilizer. It is indicated whenever sedation is required.

Acetazoleamide - (Diamox™) This agent is effective in the treatment of certain convulsive disorders. It also promotes diuresis in instances of abnormal fluid retention.

Acetylsalicylic Acid - (Aspirin) This is a nonsteroidal anti-inflammatory that has analgesic and antipyretic activities.

Adequan™ - (Polysulfated Glycosaminoglycans) This drug, when administered systemically, works by binding with the lysosomal enzymes that destroy the joint cartilage; therefore, the destructive enzymatic activity is stopped. This drug also helps form the building blocks for the new cartilage matrix. In this way, it is actually a drug that heals the cartilage of the joint. A normal treatment regime requires this drug to be given at regular intervals over a long period of time. A lesion that one is trying to heal was not created in a short period of time; therefore, it should not be expected that healing will occur in a short period of time.

Altrenogest - (Progesterone) Progesterones are responsible for the maintenance of pregnancy and the suppression of follicular development within the ovarian tissue. Progesterone also decreases the male hormone testosterone, and affects the production of sperm.

Amikacin Sulfate™ - (Amiglyde-V Solution) This is an aminoglycocide antibiotic. This antibiotic is bacteriocidal in activity; primarily against the gram-negative class of organisms.

Amphotericin B - This is an antifungal medication that is used primarily to treat respiratory infections.

Amp-Equine™ - (Polyflex™, Ampicillin Sodium) This is an antibiotic that is effective against many of the organisms that cause disorders within the skin, respiratory tract, and other soft tissues.

Ampicillin Sodium - (Polyflex™, Amp-Equine™) This is an antibiotic that is effective against many of the organisms that cause disorders within the skin, respiratory tract, and other soft tissues.

Anased™ - (Rompun, Xylazine) Affects the brain and produces sedation and analgesia. There is also a muscle relaxant and is indicated in any condition where sedation is the goal of therapy.

Anthelcide EQ™ - (Oxibendazole) This is a safe broad spectrum anthelmintic.

Antihistamine Injection - (Pyrilamine Maleate) An antihistamine; i.e., it counteracts the effects of histamine associated with common allergic reactions.

Arquel™ - (Meclofenamic Acid) This is a nonsteroidal antiinflammatory agent that is related to phenylbutazone and aspirin. The main use of this drug is in the treatment of laminitis and musculoskeletal pain.

Aspirin - (Acetylsalicylic Acid) This is a nonsteroidal antiinflammatory that has analgesic and antipyretic activities.

Atropine - This medication is used to temporarily reverse spasms of the bronchi and to treat organophosphate poisoning from some worming preparations. It is also used topically on the eye to dilate the pupil and prevent spasms within the internal structures.

Banamine™ - (Flunixin Meglumine) A nonsteroidal anti-inflammatory drug not related to the corticosteroids. Indicated as an analgesic agent for both colic and as an antiinflammatory agent for the musculoskeletal system.

Benzelmin - (Oxfendazole™) This is a safe broad spectrum anethelmintic.

Betadine - This is a germicidal solution that is nonirritating and nonstaining for external use as a cleanser or surgical prep.

Betamethasone - (Betavet ™) An extremely potent corticosteroid. Used in the treatment of numerous musculoskeletal disorders. Can be used as an intraarticular injection.

Biotin - This is a B vitamin that is significant in its role in the functioning of key enzyme systems. Biotin supplementation will improve the strength of the hoof wall and increase the amount of growth within the hoof. It normally occurs in hay and grains, and there is an established level for normal supplementation.

Boldenone Undecylenate - (Equipose™) This is an anabolic steroid that produces an increased appetite, increased muscle mass, and, to some extent, masculinization. This is indicated to enhance the recovery of severely debilitated animals.

Butorphanol Tartrate - (Stadol™) This is a very potent analgesic agent. It is a narcotic and is commonly administered with a tranquilizer.

Calcium gluconate - This is a 23% solution prepared for intraveneous administration.

Capsaicin - An alkaloid derived from plants of the Solanaceae family. This alkaloid has several pharmacological actions, mainly that of causing repeated depolarization of the action potential of the neuron; therefore, pain stimuli cease to be transmitted.

Carafate - (Sucralfate™) This is a protective agent that is used in the treatment of gastric and duodenal ulcers. It coats the surface of these lesions to form a protective barrier against gastric acid.

Cephalosporin antibiotics - This is a semi-synthetic antibiotic utilized in many forms for the treatment of resistant microorganisms.

Cimetidine- (Tagamet™) This is a pharmcological agent that inhibits the secretion of acid in the stomach. It is used orally, intravenously, or intramuscularly for the treatment of gastrointestinal ulcers.

Drug Reference

Clenbuterol - This is a drug which causes relaxation within the muscles of the airways and aids in clearing out mucus. It is used in the treatment of heaves and other pulmonary disorders.

Combot™ - (Trichlorfon) This is an anthelmintic drug with particular efficacy against bots.

Corticosteroids - This group includes cortisol, cortisone, corticosterone, 11-dehydrocorticosterone, and 11-desoxycorticosterone. Synthetically, they appear as prednisolone, betamethasone, dexamethasone, alpha-fluorocortisol, and triamcinolone. Basically all of these compounds have an antiinflammatory activity. They are used to treat arthritis, bursitis, tendinitis, problems within the musculoskeletal system, skin conditions, and lung problems within the other systems. Care must always be taken when administering corticosteroids, because they have such a wide range of side affects, the most serious being laminitis.

Coumadin™ - (Warfarin) A synthetic chemical with potent antivitamin K activity. This results in anticoagulation.

Detomide Hydrochloride - (Dormosedan™) This is a sedative with analgesic properties. It is indicated whenever tranquilization is desired.

Dexamethasone - (Azium™ , Dexamethazone sodium phosphate injection, Voren) This is a corticosteroid that has anti-inflammatory properties. It is used to treat both acute and chronic cases of inflammation within the musculoskeletal system.

Diamox™ - (Acetazoleamide) This agent is effective in the treatment of certain convulsive disorders. It also promotes diuresis in instances of abnormal fluid retention.

Dichlorvos - This is a strong broad spectrum anthelmintic.

Dinoprost™ - (Lutalyse) This is a prostaglandin. Administration results in a regression of the corpus luteum. It is used to induce estrus in the mare.

Dipyrone - This is an antipyretic agent with analgesic properties.

Di-Trim™ - (Tribrissen™ , Trimethoprim) This is an antibiotic compound containing sulfadiazine and trimethoprim and is a bacteriocidal drug that is very effective against many of the bacteria that infect the equine.

DMSO - (Dimethyl Sulfoxide) Is a biproduct of the paper pulp industry and is actually a chemical solvent. In the pure form, it is a clear colorless liquid that readily mixes with any organic compound, will freeze at 62 degrees, and will become a solid crystalline mass. It has the ability to be rapidly absorbed through the skin, by oral, or intravenous roots. DMSO is commonly used in topical applications and is usually mixed with another compound.

Dopram -V™ - (Doxapram hydrochloride) This is a drug that increases respiration. It acts as a stimulant and effects the respiratory centers of the brain. It is useful to stimulate breathing in newborns after a difficult birth or a cesarean section.

Dormosedan™ - (Detomide Hydrochloride) This is a sedative with analgesic properties. It is indicated whenever tranquilization is desired.

Doxapram hydrochloride - (Dopram - V™) This is a drug that increases respiration. It acts as a stimulant and effects the respiratory centers of the brain. It is useful to stimulate breathing in newborns after a difficult birth or a cesarean section.

Equimate™- (Fluprostenol Sodium) This is a synthetic form of prostaglandin. It is utilized to induce estrus in a mare that has a functioning corpus luteum.

Equipoise™ - (Boldenone Undecylenate) This is an anabolic steroid that produces an increased appetite, increased muscle mass, and to some extent, masculinization. This is indicated to enhance the recovery of severely debilitated horses.

Equizole™ - (Thiabendazole) This is a potent general anthelmintic.

Eqvalan™ - (Ivermectin) This is a broad spectrum anthelmintic that is effective against all intestinal parasites in addition to the adult and larval forms and *Habronema.*

Estrogen - This comes in many forms and is utilized in the synchronization of estrus and ovulation. It is also indicated in the treatment of pulmonary hemorrhage.

Febantel - (Rintal™) This is a broad spectrum anthelmintic.

Fenbendazole - (Mebendazole , Panacur™) This is a safe broad spectrum anthelmintic.

Flucort™ - (Flumethasone) A corticosteroid with antiinflammatory properties. It is almost seven hundred times more potent than cortisol. It is used in the treatment of acute and chronic inflammation of articular structures.

Flumethesone - (Flucort™) Corticosteroid with antiinflammatory properties. It is almost seven hundred times more potent than cortisol.

Flunixin Meglumine - (Banamine™) A nonsteroidal antiinflammatory drug not related to the corticosteroids. Indicated as an analgesic agent for both colic and as an antiinflammatory for the musculoskeletal system.

Fluprostenol Sodium - (Equimate™) This is a synthetic form of prostaglandin. It is utilized to induce estrus in a mare that has a functioning corpus luteum.

Follicle Stimulating Hormone - (F. S. H. -P) This hormone is a natural product of the pituitary gland and is utilized in the treatment of specific reproductive disorders where the stimulation of follicles is desired.

F. S. H. - P - (Follicle Stimulating Hormone) This hormone is a natural product of the pituitary gland and is utilized in the treatment of specific reproductive disorders where the stimulation of follicles is desired.

Furosemide - (Lasix™) This is a potent diuretic that is utilized in the treatment of noninflammatory edema, allergic reactions, and cardiac conditions. It has been used extensively to help control "bleeding" in race horses.

Garamycin™ - (Gentamicin Sulfate) A member of the -mycin group of antibiotics, effective against a wide variety of bacteria, including gram-negative strains and the gram-positive staphylococci.

Gentamicin Sulfate - (Garamycin™) A member of the -mycin group of antibiotics, effective against a wide variety of bacteria, including gram-negative strains and the gram-positive staphylococci.

Griseofulvin - This is a fungistatic agent that is effective against various species of fungi. It has no effect on bacteria and is indicated primarily in the treatment of ringworm.

Heparin - This is a naturally occurring substance that prevents the formation of blood clotting. It is a potent anticoagulant.

Hesperidin - One of a group of substances known as flavonoids. These were discovered when it was noted that natural proparations of vitamin C made from fruits were more effective in controlling the capillary lesions associated with vitamin C deficiency than purified vitamin C alone.

Histavet™ - (Pyrilamine Maleate) An antihistamine; i.e., it counteracts the effects of histamine associated with common allergic reactions.

Hyaluronic Acid - This is a substance that is normally found within joints. It is very viscous and provides an increased lubrication to the joint. This normal joint compound then reduces pain and helps protect the cartilaginous surfaces. It can be administered either systemically or intraarticularly.

Imathal™ - (Pyrantel Pamoate , Strongid™) This is a broad spectrum anthelmintic.

Immunostimulants - (Nomagen™ , Regressin - V™, Ribigen - V™) These immunostimulants are used to treat equine sarcoid tumors. Cell walls of

mycrobacterial agents are used in the preparation of these drugs. These active ingredients have potent antitumor properties that stimulate the horse's own immune system.

Insulin - This is a hormone that is produced by the islet cells located in the pancreas. It plays an important role in regulating the glucose levels within the blood stream.

Isoxsuprine Hydrochloride - A synthetic chemical with epinephrine-like effects. Its action relates specifically to the walls of arteries which are located in the muscles, internal organs, and extremities. It also causes these arteries to dilate. It is usually used in the treatment of navicular syndrome.

Ivermectin - (Eqvalan™) This is a broad spectrum anthelmintic that is effective against all intestinal parasites in addition to adult and larval forms and *Habronema*.

Kaolin pectin - This is an oral preparation to be administered in the aid and treatment of non-infectious diarrhea.

Ketoconazole - (Nizoral™) This is a broad spectrum synthetic antifungal agent.

Ketofen™ - (Ketoprofen) An antiinflammatory agent not related to the corticosteriods, but pharmacologically related to phenylbutazone, aspirin, indomethacin or dipyrone, and the other NSAID agents. It is used in the treatment of tendinitis and musculoskeletal disorders such as arthritis.

Ketoprofen - (Ketofen™) An anti-inflammatory agent not related to the corticosteriods, but pharmacologically related to phenylbutazone, aspirin, indomethacin or dipyrone, and the other NSAID agents. It is used in the treatment of tendinitis and musculoskeletal disorders such as arthritis.

Lactated Ringers Sterile Solution - This is a sterile solution that is administered for the purposes of rehydration and the replacement of electrolytes within the horse.

Lasix™ - (Furosemide) This is a potent diuretic that is utilized in the treatment of non-inflammatory edema, allergic reactions, and cardiac conditions.

Lidocaine HCl 2% - This is a drug that is administered to achieve local anesthesia of a specific anatomical area.

Liquamycin™ - (Oxytetracylcine Hydrochloride) A naturally occurring antibiotic with a wide range of activity against both gram-negative and gram-positive bacteria.

Lutalyse - (Dinoprost™) This is a prostaglandin. After administration there is a regression of the corpus luteum. In this way, it is used to induce estrus in the mare.

Mebendazole™ - (Fenbendazole , Panacur™) This is a safe broad spectrum anthelmintic.

Meclofenamic Acid - (Arquel™) This is a nonsteroidal antiinflammatory agent that is related to phenylbutazone and aspirin.

Methocarbamol - (Robaxin™) This agent is used as a muscle relaxer and can be administered orally or systemically. It is used in the treatment of "tying-up" syndrome and for any cases of muscle soreness or strain.

Morphine Sulfate - This is a narcotic analgesic used in the treatment of severe pain in the horse that does not respond to other drugs.

Moxidectin - (Quest™) This is an effective anthelmintic that has particular efficacy directed toward the small strongyles.

Naloxone - (Narcan™) A pure narcotic antagonist, counteracting the effects of narcotics, arcotic agonists, and narcotic agonist-antagonist drugs.

Narcan™ - (Naloxone) A pure narcotic antagonist, counteracting the effects of narcotics, narcotic agonists, and narcotic agonist-antagonist drugs.

Niclosamide - This is an anthelmintic that is indicated for the treatment of tapeworm infections.

Nizoral™ - (Ketoconazole) This is a broad spectrum synthetic antifungal agent.

Nomagen™ - (Immunostimulants, Regressin - V™, Ribigen - V™) These immunostimulants are used to treat equine sarcoid tumors. Cell walls of mycobacterial agents are used in the preparation of these drugs. These active ingredients have potent antitumor properties that stimulate the horse's own immune system

Normal Equine Plasma - This is a product that contains plasma from normal horses containing high levels of antibodies. It is used in the treatment of foals with suboptimal or no intake of colostrum.

Oxfendazole - (Benzelmin ™) This is a safe broad spectrum anthelmintic.

Oxibendazole - (Anthelcide EQ™) This is a safe broad spectrum anthelmintic.

Oxytetracycline Hydrochloride - (Liquamycin™) A naturally occurring antibiotic with a wide range of activity against both gram-negative and gram-positive bacteria.

Oxytocin - This is a natural hormone that produces contractions within the muscles of the uterus. It is used during parturition and in the treatment of a retained placenta.

Panacur™ - (Fenbendazole, Mebendazole™) This is a safe broad spectrum anthelminthic.

Penicillin - (There are numerous tradenames for this antibiotic) This is a naturally occurring antibiotic that is primarily effective against gram-positive bacteria. It is used in the treatment of skin, soft tissue, and urinary tract disorders.

Phenylbutazone - A nonsteroidal anti-inflammatory drug. It also has analgesic and antipyretic activity. This is one of the most widely used treatments for musculoskeletal disorders. It does not cure the disorder, but by controlling the inflammation, there is a decrease in the amount of scar tissue and adhesions that would normally result.

Phenytoin Sodium - This is an anticonvulsant.

Piperazine - This is a mild general anthelmintic with efficacy towards roundworms.

Polyflex™ - (Amp-Equine™, Ampicillin Sodium) This is an antibiotic that is effective against many of the organisms that cause disorders within the skin, respiratory tract, and other soft tissues.

Polysulfated Glycosaminoglycans - (Adequan™) This drug, when administered systemically, works by binding with the lysosomal enzymes that destroy the joint cartilage; therefore, the destructive enzymatic activity is stopped. This drug also helps form the building blocks for the new cartilage matrix. In this way, it is actually a drug that heals the cartilage of the joint. A normal treatment regime requires this drug to be given at regular intervals over a long period of time. A lesion that one is trying to heal was not created in a short period of time; therefore, it should not be expected that healing will to occur in a short period of time.

Potassium Chloride - This is a supplemental source of potassium chloride.

Prednisone - (Depomedrol™, Solu-delta-cortef™) Potent corticosteroid with antiinflammatory and antishock properties. This is used as a very short acting antiinflammatory agent in acute cases.

Progesterone - (Altrenogest) Progesterones are responsible for the maintenance of pregnancy and the suppression of follicular development within the ovarian tissue. Progesterone also decreases the male hormone testosterone, and affects the production of sperm.

Prom Ace™ - (Acepromazine Maleate) A central nervous system tranquilizer. It is indicated whenever sedation is required.

Psyllium hydrophalic mucilloid - This is an equine laxative used as an aid in the elimination and the expelling of foreign material such as sand.

Pyrantel Pamoate - (Strongid™ , Imathal™) This is a broad spectrum anthelmintic.

Pyrantel Tartrate - (Strongid C™ and C2X™) This is a broad spectrum anthelmintic that can be administered daily as a feed additive.

Pyrilamine Maleate - (Histavet™) An antihistamine; i.e., it counteracts the effects of histamine associated with common allergic reactions.

Quest™ - (Moxidectin) This is an effective anthelmintic that has particular efficacy directed toward the small strongyles.

Ranitidine - (Zantac™) This is an agent that is used to block the secretion of acid in the stomach. It is used in the treatment of gastric or duodenal ulcers in foals.

Regressin - V™ - (Immunostimulants, Nomagen™, Ribigen - V™) These immuno-stimulants are used to treat equine sarcoid tumors. Cell walls of mycrobacterial agents are used in the preparation of these drugs. These active ingredients have potent antitumor properties that stimulate the horse's own immune system.

Ribigen - V™ - (Immunostimulants ,Nomagen™, Regressin -V™) These immunostimulants are used to treat equine sarcoid tumors. Cell walls of mycrobacterial agents are used in the preparation of these drugs. These active ingredients have potent antitumor properties that stimulate the horse's own immune system.

Rintal™ - (Febantel) This is a broad spectrum anthelmintic.

R.V.I. - (Rubeola Viral Immunodulator) This is an inactivated viral product that is used in the treatment of myositis in the horse.

Robaxin™ - (Methocarbamol) This agent is used as a muscle relaxer and can be administered orally or systemically. It is used in the treatment of "tying-up" syndrome and for any cases of muscle soreness or strain.

Rompun - (Anased™, Xylazine) Affects the brain, producing sedation and analgesia. There is also a muscle relaxing effect. This drug is indicated in any condition where sedation is the goal of therapy.

Sarapin - A natural product, distilled from *Sarracena iaceae* in water. This product is used in the treatment of neuromuscular pain.

Selenium - (E- Se) This is a mineral that is required by the horse in trace amounts. It is administered in combination with vitamin E.

Sodium Hyaluronate - This is commonly called Hyaluronic Acid. This compound contains viscoelastic and lubricating properties to synovial fluid. It can be administered intraarticularly or intravenously. It comes in different molecular weights with the higher Dalton weight compounds being more therapeutic. It is indicated whenever there is an intraarticular condition requiring this type of medication.

Strongid™ - (Imathal™, Pyrantel Pamoate) This is a broad spectrum anthelmintic.

Strongid C™ and C2x™ - (Pyrantel Tartrate) This is a broad spectrum anthelmintic that can be administered daily as a feed additive.

Sucralfate^MT - (Carafate) This is a protective agent that is used in the treatment of gastric and duodenal ulcers. It coats the surface of these lesions to form a protective barrier against gastric acid.

Tagamet™- (Cimetidine) This is a pharmcological agent that inhibits the secretion of acid in the stomach. It is used orally, intravenously, or intramuscularly for the treatment of gastrointestinal ulcers.

Tetanus Antitoxin - This product is prepared from the blood of healthy equines that have been hyperimmunized with repeated doses of *Colstridium tetani* toxin. It is for prophylactic use to confer short-term passive immunity against tetanus. It is also used in the treatment of animals affected with tetanus.

Tetanus Toxoid - This is a sterile suspension of highly purified precipitated tetanus toxoid. It is used to confer long-term active immunity against tetanus.

Thiabendazole - (Equizole™) This is a potent general anthelmintic.

Torbugesic - A potent analgesic available in injectable form. Indicated for the treatment of colic or minor surgical procedures.

Tribrissen™ - (Di-Trim™, Trimethoprim) This is an antibiotic compound containing sulfadiazine and trimethoprim. This is a bacteriocidal drug that is very effective against many of the bacteria that infect the equine.

Trichlorfon - (Combot™) This is an anthelmintic drug with particular efficacy against bots.

Warfarin - (Coumadin™) A synthetic chemical with potent antivitamin K activity. This results in anticoagulation. This synthetic chemical has been used in the treatment of navicular syndrome and laminitis.

Xylazine -(Anased™, Rompun) Affects the brain, producing sedation and analgesia. There is also a muscle relaxing effect. This drug is indicated in any condition where sedation is the goal of therapy.

Zantac™ - (Ranitidine) This is an agent that is used to block the secretion of acid in the stomach. It is used in the treatment of gastric or duodenal ulcers in foals.

MANUFACTURER'S APPENDIX

Compounding

Mortar and Pestle Veterinary Pharmacy
3701 Beaver Ave.
Des Moines, IA 50310

Wedgewood Pharmacy
373- Kegg Harbor Road
Sewell, NJ 08080

Dental Instrumentation

Alberts
336 Loudon Rd.
Loudonville, NY 12211

Dermatological Products

VetGenix Ltd.
Coral Gables, FL 33134
(888) 838-4364
Fax: (305) 443-3467

Endoscopes

Endoscopy Support Services, Inc.
Croton River Executive Park
Building 3
Route 22
Brewster, NY 10509

Olympus America Inc.
2 Corporate Center Drive
Melville, NY 11747

Laboratory Testing and Equipment

BET Laboratories, Inc.
6174 Jacks Creek Pike
Lexington, KY 40515

Difco Laboratories
P.O. Box 331058
Detroit, MI 48232

Equine Biodiagnostics Inc.
University of Kentucky
A165 Astecc Building
Lexington, KY 40506-0286

IDEXX Laboratories Inc.
One Idexx Dr.
Westbrook, ME 04092

Mallinckrodt Veterinary Inc.
421 E. Hawley St.
Mundelein, IL 60060

Neogen Corp.
628 E. Third St.
Lexington, KY 40505

Nutritional and Natural Supplements

Chamisa Ridge Inc.
P.O. Box 23294
Santa FE, NM 87502

Equilite, Inc.
20 Prospect Avenue
Ardsley, NY 10502

Noah's Ark
P.O. Box 168
Buzzard's Bay, MA 02532

Select The Best
P.O. Box 1968
Carson City, NV 89702

Uckele Animal Health Corp.
5600 Siberhorn Hwy.
Blissfield, MI 49228

Vetri-Science Laboratories
20 New England Dr.
Essex JUnction, VT 05453

Vita Flex Nutrition Co. Inc.
R.R. 3 Box 2086-6
Waterbury, VT 05676

Physical Therapy

Animal Therapy
143 Perrin Place
Charlotte, NC 28207

Bioscan
6 Walden Rd.
Corrales, NM 87048

CHI China Healthways Institute
115 N. El Camino Real
San Clemente, CA 92672

Equi-Light Therapy System
2100 S. Dayton St.
Denver, CO 80231-5733

HydroSurge Inc.
7919 Silverton Ave. #412
San Diego, CA 92126

Tempra Technology
5945 North Washington Boulevard
Sarasota, FL 34245

Radiology

Bowie Mfg., Inc.
313 South Hancock
Lake City, IA 51449

Fluoroscopic Imaging System
Equine Only, Inc.
1-800-809-4677

Minxray Inc.
3611 Commercial Ave.
Northbrook, IL 60062-1822

Thermography

Agema Infrared Systems
550 County Avenue
Secaucus, NJ 07094

eMerge VISION
Sebastian, Fl
1-800-945-5310

Veterinary Pharmaceutical & Equipment

Bayer Company
P.O. Box 390
Shawnee Mission, KS 66201

Bayer Corp.
Division of Animal Health
Building 8
9009 W. 67th St.
Merriam, KS 66202

Boehringer Ingelheim
2621 N. Belt Hwy.
Saint Joseph, MO 64506-2002

Burns Veterinary Supply Inc.
1900 Diplomat Dr.
Farmers Branch, TX 75234

Butler Co.
5000 Bradenton Ave.
Dublin, OH 43017

Columbus Serum Company
2025 S. High St.
Columbus, OH 43207

CryoSurgery Inc.
P.O. Box 50035
Nashville, TN 37205

El Medical
348 N. Jefferson
Loveland, CO 80537

Equine Sports Inc.
P.O. Box 653
Lake Forest, IL 60045

Fort Dodge Animal Health
800 5th St. NW
Fort Dodge, IA 50501

Hamilton Thorne Research
P.O. Box 2099
S. Hamilton, MA 01982

Henry Schein Inc.
135 Duryea Rd.
Melville, NY 11747

Jorgensen Laboratories
1450 N. Van Buren
Loveland, CO 80538

Lutipold Pharmaceutical, Inc.
Animal Health Division
One Luitpold Dr.
Shirley, NY 11967

Macleod Pharmaceuticals Inc.
2600 Canton Court, #C
Fort Collins, CO 80525

Merck Ag Vet
Division of Merck and Company
P.O. Box 2000
Rahway, N.J. 07065

Merial
4545 Oleatha Ave.
St. Louis, MO 63116

Midwest Veterinary Supply Inc.
11965 Larc Industrial Blvd.
Burnsville, MN 55337

Milburn Distributions Inc.
Suite 100
21609 North 12th Avenue
Phoenix, AZ 85027

Nutramax
2208 Lakeside Blvd.
Edgewood, MD 21040

Pfizer Animal Health
812 Springdale Dr.
Exton, PA 19341

Schering-Plough Animal Health
1095 Morris Ave.
Union, NJ 07083

Solvay Animal Health
1201 Northland Dr.
Mendota Heights, MN 55120-1139
The Upjohn Co.
Kalamazoo, MI 49001

Western Veterinary Supply, Inc.
625 Sherwood Drive
Paris, TX 75462

Ultrasound Equipment

Classic Medical Supply, Inc.
19900 Mona Road, Suite 105
Tequesta, FL 33469

E.I. Medical
348 N. Jefferson
Loveland, CO 80537

Universal Ultrasound
299 Adams Street
Bedford Hills, NY 1050

GLOSSARY

Abaxial - This is a term of anatomical nomenclature which means that the point described is not situated in the axis of the body or of a particular part or organ. It indicates a distancing of structures away from the main axis of the body.

Abaxial nerve blocks - Nerve blocks that are administered upon a peripheral nerve that is located proximal to the required area of desensitization and lateral or medial to the axis of the median plane of the limb.

Abdominal floor - The bottom wall of the abdomen.

Abrasion - Any area found on the surface of the body where the dermis is broken.

Acupressure - A manual massage technique utilized during physical therapy whereby pressure is applied to various points on the body causing a beneficial stimulatory effect to the tissues.

Acetabulum - The large cup-shaped cavity on the lateral surface of the os coxae in which the head of the femur articulates.

Actin - A protein that occurs in filaments which, acting along with myosin particles, are responsible for the contraction and relaxation of muscle tissue.

Acupuncture - The Chinese science of influencing the body system by stimulating certain points on and within the body. This is usually done with needles and facilitates treatment for various conditions.

Acupuncture point - The point that is stimulated, usually by needles, to cause an effect on the body systems.

Acute - This is a descriptive term for a condition having a very brief and/or a very severe development.

Adaxial - This is an anatomical nomenclature term which indicates that structures are located on the side of, or in the direction of, the main axis of the body.

Adduction - This is an anatomical nomenclature term which indicates that a structure is drawn towards the median plane of the body.

Adhesions - This is a fibrous band or structure by which parts abnormally adhere.

Aerobic - Any functions that occur where the presence of oxygen is necessary.

Afebrile - This is a state without symptoms of fever.

Alimentary canal - Literally, this is the tube or canal which receives food or nourishment; i.e.: the digestive tract.

Allantoic sac - This is a tubular diverticulum of the posterior part of the embryo.

Alveolar - This is the portion of the jaw into which the teeth are set. This also refers to the minute lung components where oxygen is exchanged.

Amniotic cavity - This is the sac-like structure produced by the amniotic membrane.

Amniotic fluid - This is the fluid which is produced by the amniotic membrane.

Amniotic membrane - This is the thin, transparent membrane lining the chorion which produces the amniotic fluid.

Ampulla - This is anatomical nomenclature description that is used to designate a flask-like dilatation of a tubular structure

Anabolic - Any substance or procedure that promotes growth and development within the body.

Anaerobic - These are functions that occur where the presence of oxygen is not essential.

Analgesia - That state in which there is an absence of sensitivity to pain; designating particularly the relief of pain without loss of consciousness.

Analgesic - Any substance that is administered which helps in the control of pain.

Anastomoses - A communication of one structure to another as in arterioles and venules.

Anatomical - Pertaining to anatomy, or to the structure of the organism.

Anatomy - The science of the structure of the animal body and the relation of its parts.

Anatomical area - An area of the body that is bounded by specific borders: i.e.: the shoulder.

Anechoic - This is an area, on the ultrasound image, that does not produce an echo.

Anesthesia (also spelled **anaesthesia**) **-** This is the state where consciousness or sensation is lost.

Anestrus - A specific stage of the estrus cycle when sexual activity has ceased.

Aneurysms - This is a sac formed by a dilatation of the wall of an artery or a vein that is filled with blood.

Angiography - This is a study of the blood vessels through their visualization utilizing radiographic techniques.

Ankylosis - Abnormal immobility and consolidation of a joint.

Annular - Shaped like a ring.

Anomalies - These occur when there is marked deviation from the normal standard.

Anosteitis - Defective development of bone.

Antagonist - A muscle that acts in opposition to the action of another muscle.

Anterior - Situated in front of, or in the forward part of, affecting the forward part of an organ, toward the head end of the body.

Anthelmintics - This is any agent that is destructive to parasitic worms.

Antibacterial - These are substances that are capable of killing bacteria.

Antibodies - These are modified types of serum globulins, synthesized by lymphoid tissue that are produced in response to antigenic stimuli.

Anticoagulant - Any substance, pharmaceutical or otherwise, that prevents the clotting of blood.

Antiinflammatory - An agent that counteracts or suppresses inflammation.

Antimicrobial - Any agent that destroys microorganisms or suppresses their growth.

Antiseptic - These are substances or pharmaceutical agents that prevent the multiplication of and control the development of microorganisms.

Antitoxin - This is an antibody to the toxin of a microorganism that combines with the specific toxins for the neutralization of the toxicity.

Aponeurosis - A white, flattened or ribbon-like tendinous expansion, serving mainly as an investment for muscle, or connecting a muscle with the parts that it moves.

Appendicular skeleton - Includes the bones of the limbs.

Arcades - The individual rows of teeth.

Areolar - This is the term that pertains to or contains minute interspaces.

Arm - The upper extremity from the shoulder to the radius and ulna. It contains the humerus and all of its associated structures.

Arterial - pertaining to an artery or to the arteries.

Artery - This is a blood vessel that is filled with cells, oxygen, and fuel. They function to allow passage of blood away from the heart.

Artificial insemination - This is an insemination by any other means except naturally.

Arthritis - Any inflammation within the structures found in the joint.

Arthrocentesis - Puncture and aspiration of a joint.

Articular cartilages - Any cartilaginous structures found in the joint.

Articular cavity - The cavity of a joint.

Articular wing fracture - A fracture of the coffin bone that travels through the wing of the coffin bone into the distal interphalangeal joint.

Articulation - The place of union or function between two or more bones of the skeleton; a joint.

Aspiration - This is the act of breathing, drawing in, or the removal of fluid or gases from a cavity.

Ataxia - Failure of muscular coordination; or an irregularity of muscular action.

Atlas - The first cervical vertebra, which articulates above with the occipital bone and below with the axis or second cervical vertebra.

Atony - This indicates a lack of normal tone or strength.

Atrophy - This is the state of wasting away or degeneration of normal cells, tissues, muscles, or organs due to any cause, such as lack of innervation or disuse.

Auscultation - The act of listening for sounds within the body.

Avascular - This is the state in which an area is not supplied with blood vessels.

Avulsion - This is the act of tearing away a part of a structure.

Axial skeleton - That part of the skeletal structure which comprises the vertebral column, ribs, sternum, and skull.

Axis - This is the second and longest cervical vertebra of the vertebral column.

Bacteremia - This is the presence of bacteria in the blood.

Bactericidal - A substance that is capable of destroying the bacteria.

Balanoposthitis - This is an inflammation of the glans penis and prepuce.

Bandage cord - The swelling that occurs over the area of the soft tissue, usually the superficial and deep digital flexor tendons, resulting from an improperly applied tight bandage.

Base narrow - The left and right forefeet are placed closer together than the proximal portions of these limbs.

Base wide - The left and right forefeet are placed further apart than the proximal portions of these limbs.

Bench knees - A conformation in which the cannon bone is offset to the lateral side and does not follow a straight line from the radius.

Benign - Not malignant. Having the property of being not malignant.

Bilateral - Having two sides, or pertaining to both sides.

Bicipital bursa - An inflammation of a bursa underneath the tendon of the biceps brachii on the lateral side of the shoulder joint.

Bifurcation - This is the site where a single structure divides into two branches.

Biochemical - This term depicts physiological chemistry. It is the chemistry of living organisms and of vital processes.

Biological - With references to the study of life.

Body pregnancy - This is a pregnancy that occurs in the largest part of the uterus and does not extend onto the uterine horns.

Bog spavin - A chronic synovial effusion of the tarsocrural (hock) joint capsule of uncertain pathogenesis not associated with lameness, tenderness, heat, or radiographic changes.

Bone spavin - An osteoarthritis that involves the distal intertarsal, tarsometatarsal, and occasionally the proximal intertarsal joints of the hock.

Borborygmi - These are the rumbling noises that are caused by the propulsion of gases through the intestinal contents.

Bowed tendon - This is a tendosynovitis involving the tendons of the superficial and/or deep digital flexor tendons.

Bow-legged - An outward curve of one or both legs at or below the knee.

Breech birth - A dystocia wherein the posterior end of the newborn is presented first.

Buccal - This term means pertaining to the cheek.

Buccal borders - These are the borders pertaining to or directed toward the cheek.

Buccal cavity - Is that cavity within the cheek.

BUN - This is the abbreviation for blood, urea, and nitrogen.

Bursa - A sac or sac-like cavity filled with viscous fluid and situated at places in the tissues at which friction would otherwise develop. Certain bursa are so consistently recognized as to be given official names in anatomical nomenclature.

Bursa podotrochlearis - This is a bursa interposed between the tendon and the fibrocartliage-covered flexor surface of the navicular bone, cushioning the movement of the tendon against the bone.

Bursitis - This is a condition of inflammation within the bursa which can lead to the formation of a calcium deposit.

Buttress foot - When viewed laterally in the area of the coronary band, the hoof exhibits a protuberance or bump.

Calculi - This is any abnormal concretions occurring within the animal's body. These are usually composed of mineral salts.

Calf knees - Backward deviation of the carpus or carpal joints.

Camped out behind - The entire hindlimb is placed too far caudally when viewed laterally.

Cancellous bone - That bone that is structured with a reticular sponge or lattice-like infrastructure.

Cancellous screw - These orthopedic screws are designed to provide rigid fixation to the soft cancellous bone. Often, they have a shaft and are not threaded the entire length.

Canines - These are the conical teeth that are found between the incisors and cheek teeth.

Cantharidin - This is the highly poisonous substance within the blister beetle.

Cap - This is the remanent of the deciduous tooth which is shed at a specific time.

Capillary - This is a very small vessel with walls that are only one cell thick enabling the exchange of all the components within the body's structure, such as oxygen, nutrients, and waste materials.

Capillary refill time - The time in which it takes the capillaries to refill after pressure is exerted on them.

Capped hock - This is actually a hygroma of the hock with fluid accumulating in the subcutaneous layer directly over the point of the hock.

Capsaicin-based - Any compound containing capsaicin.

Capsule - This is the tissue that surrounds a joint and assists in joint lubrication.

Carcinomas - This is a malignant growth arising within the epithelial cells that give rise to metastases.

Cardiac - Pertaining to the heart.

Cartilage - A dense connective tissue that is found on the articular ends of bones within a joint.

Caseous - This is a substance within the body that resembles cheese or curd.

Castration - Removal of the gonads.

Cataracts - This is an opacity of the eye lens or of its capsule.

Catecholamines - One of a group of similar compounds having a sympathomimetic action, the aromatic portion of whose molecule is catechol, and the aliphatic portion an amine. Such compounds include dopamine, norepinephirine, and epinephrine.

Catheterize - This is the introduction of a catheter into a body cavity.

Cartilaginous - Consisting of or of the nature of cartilage.

Caudal - This is an anatomical nomenclature term which means toward the tail.

Cautery - This is the application of heat, electric current, or caustic substance for the means of killing tissue and clotting blood to stop bleeding.

Cavity - This is a hollow place or space within the body or within a particular anatomical structure.

Cellulitis - This is the inflammation within cellular tissue.

Cementum - This is the bony material covering the root of a tooth. It enwraps the external enamel of the molars and premolars and fills the infundibulae of the molars, premolars, and incisors.

Centrifuge - This is the machine that is used to separate the lighter portions of a solution, mixture, or suspension from the heavier portions through the use of centrifugal force.

Cervical vertebrae - This is the first region of the vertebral column that consists of the first seven vertebrae in the neck.

Cervicitis - This is an inflammation within the tissues of the cervix.

Chromosome - This is one of several dark-staining bodies which appear in the nucleus of a cell at the time of cell division. These structures contain the genes for hereditary factors and are constant in number for each species.

Chronic - This is a term that applies to a condition or a state where there is a continued or long term affliction.

Cicatrix - This is the new tissue which is formed in the healing of a wound.

Cicatrization - Is the healing process which leaves a scar or cicatrix.

Closure - The act of shutting, or of bringing together two parts.

Club foot - This is a foot deformity that can be either congenital or acquired.

Coccygeal vertebrae - Is the fifth region of the vertebral column and consists of eighteen vertebrae.

Colic - This is a general term indicating acute abdominal pain.

Collagen - The main protein of skin, bone, tendon, cartilage, and connective tissue.

Colonization - Is the collection or grouping of bacteria in a culture derived from an increase of an isolated single or group of organisms.

Colostrum - It is the milky fluid secreted by the mammary gland a few days before and after parturition which contains many nutrients and antibodies necessary for the offspring's survival.

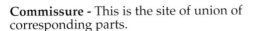

Commissure - This is the site of union of corresponding parts.

Compact bone - A bone that is dense in structure.

Concavity - A hollowed-out space on the surface of an organ or other structure; a hollow, depressed area on a curved surface, organ, or line.

Conception - This is theunion of the female ovum and the male sperm; fertilization.

Conceptus - This is the product of conception at any stage in development, from fertilization of the ovum to birth.

Concussion - A violent jar or shock, or the condition which results from such an injury.

Concussive forces - Those physical forces that result from the impact of bone against bone, cartilage against cartilage, or basically from the hoof hitting the ground with the weight of the animal being directed upon it.

Conformation - The shape or contour of the body or any particular body structure.

Congenital - This refers to conditions that are present usually before or at birth regardless of their cause.

Conjunctivitis - This is an inflammation of the conjunctiva.

Connective tissue - The tissue that binds other tissues into a functional unit.

Contracted heels - A condition in which the heels are narrower than normal. When viewed caudally, the palmar or plantar aspect of the foot appears narrow.

Contracture - This is the drawing together or shortening of a structure.

Contralateral - This term refers to a location that is situated on or pertaining to the opposite side

Coon footed - A conformational hoof characteristic where an axis drawn over the dorsal surface of the hoof is more vertical than that axis drawn through the proximal phalanx. The pastern slopes more than does the dorsal surface of the hoof wall highlighting this conformational fault.

Copulation - Sexual congress: coitus.

Corium - It is an especially modified vascular part of the hoof that furnishes the nutrition to the hoof.

Corium of the frog - This is the sensitive portion of the frog that supplies nutrition to it.

Corium of the sole - This corium supplies nutrition to the horny sole.

Cornua - A horn-like projection.

Coronary - Coronet or hair surface, the part of the hoof that is the farthest from the basal surface of the hoof at any given point.

Coronary band - Encircling in the manner of a crown: the term applies to vessels, nerves, ligaments, etc. contained within this structure.

Coronary corium - This structure is the thickest part of the corium and is found within the coronary groove. This corium provides nutrition to the bulk of the hoof wall.

Coronary dermis - A wider (up to 15 mm) raised band adjoining the periople dermis distally. It nourishes the production of the bulk of the hoof wall that grows down from it in the same way as a fingernail.

Corpus luteum - "Yellow body." This yellow glandular mass in the ovary formed by an ovarian follicle that has matured and discharged its ovum.

Cortical - Pertaining to or of the nature of a cortex.

Cortical bone - Pertaining to or the nature of the cortex of bone.

Cortical screw - An orthopedic device in which the screw is imbedded and held in place by the corticies of the bone. A cortical screw does not have a smooth shaft and is threaded through its entire length.

Costal surface - Pertaining to the surface of a rib or ribs.

Coupage - This is a massage technique utilized in physical therapy.

Cow hocks - This is a conformational characteristic where there is a medial deviation of the tarsal joints.

Coxofemoral luxation - A displacement or dislocation of the hip joint.

Crackles - These are small sharp sounds that can be heard when listening to the thoracic cavity.

Cranial - Pertaining to the cranium, or to the anterior surface (front) or superior end of the body.

Crepitation - The friction noise made by rubbing together tissue surfaces.

Crura - This is a general term describing a leg-like part.

Cryptorchidism - This is a developmental defect that is characterized by the failure of the testes to descend into the scrotum.

Culture - This is the propagation of microorganisms or of living tissue cells in special media that is conducive to their growth.

Cunean bursitis - An inflammation within the bursa sack that lies beneath the cunean tendon.

Cunean tendon - This is the median tendon of the cranial tibial muscle that travels in a medial oblique direction to insert onto the second metatarsal bone.

Cuneiform cartilage - These are two paired laryngeal elastic fibrocartilages found within the epiglottic folds.

Curb - An inflammation and thickening of the long plantar ligament of the tarsus, causing a swelling at the back of the hock joint which results in lameness.

Curettage - This is the removal of growth or other material from a wall of a cavity with a curette.

Curette - 1. An instrument for removing growths or other material from the walls of cavities. 2. To remove growths or other material from the wall of a cavity or other surface with a spoon-shaped instrument.

Curvature - This is a deviation from a rectilinear direction.

Cutaneous - This is a term meaning anything pertaining to the skin.

Cyanosis - This is any bluish discoloration of the skin and mucous membranes due to reduced hemoglobin and an excessive concentration of carbon dioxide within the blood.

Cystitis - This is a general term meaning inflammation of the urinary bladder. This can result from numerous etiologies.

Cytological - This pertains to any scientific study of cells, their origin, structure, and function.

Cytoplasm - This is the protoplasm of the cell exclusive of that of the nucleus.

Debilitated - This is a case where the animal lacks or has lost both strength and body condition.

Debridement - The removal of all foreign matter and devitalized tissue in or about a traumatic or other lesion.

Deciduous - This is a term that is used to describe the teeth of the first dentition. These are not permanent teeth but are cast off when the permanent teeth erupt.

Deferent Ducts - These are ducts that convey anything away from a center.

Deformity - This is a distortion of any part or general disfigurement of any portion of the body.

Degeneration - This is the change from a higher to a lower form. An example of this is a change of tissue to a lower or less functionally active form.

Dehiscence - This is the act or process of splitting apart.

Dehydration - This is a condition of the body which results from a loss of water.

Demineralized - This is an excessive elimination of minerals or inorganic salts.

Dentin - This is the chief substance or tissue of the teeth which surrounds the tooth pulp and is covered by enamel on the crown and by cementum on the roots of the teeth.

Denuded - This is the physical act of laying bare or the removal from the surface of its epithelial covering.

Depression - This is a hollow area.

Dermal papillae - Those papillae found in the dermal layer.

Dermatitis - This is any inflammation of the skin.

Dermatone - This is an instrument of incising the skin or cutting the skin into thin layers for transplantation.

Dermatone patterns - The thermographic pattern depicted on the dermis corresponding to the amount of heat being emitted from those tissues. There is a direct correlation to the innervation within these tissues.

Desensitization - A condition in which the tissues react to a specific stimulus to a lesser degree than they would normally.

Desiccated - This is an area of extreme dryness.

Desmitis - This is the inflammation of any ligament.

Desmotomy - The cutting or division of ligaments.

Detumescent - An indicating of swelling or turgidity within the tissues.

Diagnosis - The identification of a disease or injury that is identified through the use of tests, examinations, or observations.

Diaphysis - That portion of a long bone that consists of a tube of compact bone enclosing the medullary cavity and located between the ends or extremities of the bone.

Diastema - This is a space or cleft.

Diestrus - This is a period of sexual quiescence.

Digital cushion - This is a wedge-shaped mass that overlies the frog.

Dilatation - That physical state of being dilated or stretched beyond normal.

Dilation - This is a stretching or expansion of an object.

Discharge - An excretion or substance is liberated and evacuated.

Disinfection - This is the destruction of pathogenic germs or other disease causing agents.

Dissection - This is a separation of a part or the entire organism by incising tissues with either a blunt or sharp edge.

Distal - Remote; farther from any point of reference; opposite of proximal.

Distention - That physical state of being swollen or enlarged due to pressure originating internally.

Diuretics - This is an agent that increases the excretion of urine.

Diverticulum - This is a circumcised pouch or sac of variable size created within another structure.

Dorsal - This is a anatomical nomenclature term which means that the structure or point in reference pertains to the back or towards the back of the animal.

Dremel drill - A common household tool that provides a cordless way of boring holes and providing abrasive discs to be utilized in farrier work.

Duct - This is a tubal structure with well-defined walls for the passage of excretions or secretions.

Dysfunctional - This is the abnormal functioning or impairment of an organ.

Dysphagia - This is difficulty in swallowing.

Dysphasia - The impairment of vocal capability.

Dysplasia - Is an abnormality of development.

Dystocia - This is any abnormal labor or birth.

Echocardiography - An evaluation of different anatomical and pathological changes within the heart can be examined through the use of ultrasonography.

Edema - This is the presence of an abnormally large amount of fluid in the intercellular tissue spaces.

Edematous - This describes any area that is affected by edema.

Effleurage - This is a type of massage technique.

Efficacious - Having or showing an effect as a means, measure, or remedy.

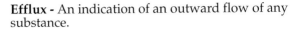

Efflux - An indication of an outward flow of any substance.

Ejaculate - The act of expelling suddenly.

Electrocardiogram - This is a graphic tracing of the electric currents produced through the contractions of heart muscles.

Electrolytes - This is any solution of ions.

Electromyography - The recording of the changes in electric potential of muscles.

Emasculator - This is an instrument that is used primarily for castrations in the removal of the male gonads.

Embolic colic - This is abdominal pain that results from an obstruction within the circulation of the bowel caused by an embolus.

Embolus - This is a blood clot that is brought from another vessel and forced in a smaller one so that it obstructs the circulation.

Embryonic - This is any description that pertains to the embryo.

Enamel - This is the white, compact, and very hard substance that covers and protects the tooth.

Encyst - Enclosed in a sac.

Endemic - Disease that is constantly present within a particular area.

Endocrine - Those organs that function to secrete a substance internally that has a specific effect on another organ or part of the body.

Endometritis - This is an inflammation within the endometrium.

Endometrium - This is the innermost layer of the uterus.

Endorphins - These are pain relieving substances that are naturally produced by the body's own nervous system.

Endoscope - This is an instrument that is used for an examination of the interior of a hollow area.

Endosteum - The tissue lining the medullary cavity of the bone.

Endotoxin - This is a toxin that is present in the bacterial cell, is pyrogenic, and increases capillary permeability. It is found primarily in enteric bacilli but also in certain gram-negative cocci and other microorganisms.

Engorged - This is the state where a specific tissue or area is distended or swollen with fluids.

Enteritis - This is an inflammation within the intestine.

Entercolitis - This is inflammation that involves both the small intestine and colon.

Enterogastric reflux - This is an efflux of fluid from both the stomach and small intestine.

Enterogastritis - This is an inflammation of both the small intestine and stomach.

Enterolith - This is any calculus or concretion found within the intestine.

Entropion - This is the turning inward of an edge of the margin of the eyelid towards the eyeball.

Enzyme - These are the catalysts within a biochemical reaction.

Epidermis - This is the outer most layer, usually referring to the skin, typically not supplied with blood vessels.

Epidural - This term means to be placed upon or outside of the dura.

Epidural anesthesia - This is any anesthetic that is situated upon or outside the dura.

Epilepsy - This is a disease that has several forms. It is usually characterized by recurring impairment or loss of conciousness. There may be involuntary excess or cessation of muscle movements or sensorary disturbances. Epilepsy can be genetic in origin or aquired.

Epiphysis - That portion of the long bone which occurs on the end. It can be entirely cartilaginous or separated from the shaft by a cartilaginous disc.

Epistaxis - This is any hemorrhage from the nares.

Epithelium - This is the covering of the internal and external surfaces of the body.

Erection - The condition by which a structure is made rigid and extended.

Esophagostomy - This is the creation of an artificial opening into the esophagus.

Estrus - Period of sexual receptivity in the female, "heat."

Etiology - This is the study or theory of the cause of the disease or disorder.

Euthanasia - The putting to death of an animal suffering from an incurable disease or injury.

Evisceration - Is the removal of the viscera or internal organs.

Exfoliation - This is the shedding or falling off in scales or layers.

Exocrine - The opposite of endocrine. It is the external secretion of any gland.

Extension - The movement that brings a limb into a straight line.

Extensor - Any muscle that extends a joint.

External - Situated or occurring on the outside.

Exotoxin - This is a toxin or toxic substance that is formed by the bacteria and is found outside of the bacterial cell.

Expulsion - To drive or force out.

Extraction - This is the process or act of pulling or drawing out.

Exudate - This is material which has escaped from the blood vessels and is then deposited in tissues or on tissue surfaces as a result of inflammation.

Fascia - A sheet or band of fibrous tissue that lies deep to the skin or forms an investment for muscles and various organs of the body.

Fascicle - A small bundle of fibers within a nerve or the central nervous system.

Fascicular - Pertaining to or forming a fascicle.

Fasciculation - This is a small localized contraction of the muscles that is visible through the skin. This contraction represents a spontaneous discharge of a number of fibers innervated by a single motor nerve neuron.

Femoropatellar joint - This is one of the two articulations that comprise the stifle. This articular joint is between the femur and the patella.

Femorotibial joint - This is one of the two articulations that make up the stifle. This is an articular joint between the femur and the tibia.

Fermentation - This is the enzymatic decomposititon of food stuffs.

Fetid - This is the quality of having a rank or disagreeable smell.

Fetus - This is the unborn offspring of any animal.

Fibrin - This is the whitish insoluable protein formed from fibrinogen by the action of thrombin in the clotting of blood.

Fibrocartilage - This is present in synovial joints at the junction of the articular cartilages, synovial membrane, periosteum, and within the menisci.

Fibrosis - This is the formation of fibrous tissue.

Fistula - This is an abnormal passage or communication usually between two internal organs or leading from an internal structure to the surface of the body.

Flaccid - This term means weak, lax, or soft.

Flexion - The act of bending or condition of being bent.

Floating teeth - This is the method that is used to remove the buccal and lingual edges of the arcades along the protuberant portions of the surface of cheek teeth and incisors in an effort to create a more perfect occlusion.

Fluoroscope - Diagnostic instrumentation whereas radiographic images are taken in a continuous sequence. This allows 360 degree radiographic examination of a specific area.

Fluoroscopy - An examination utilizing the fluoroscope.

Follicle - This term depicts a very small excretory or secretory sac or gland. An ovarian follicle is the egg and its encasing cells at any stage of its development.

Foot axis - This is the inclination of the hoof as it is in reference to the ground surface.

Foramen - A natural opening or passage; used as a general term in anatomical nomenclature to designate such a passage, especially one into or through a bone.

Foramina - Plural of foramen.

Forearm - The part of the upper member of the body between the elbow and the wrist.

Fornix - This is a general term depicting an arch-like structure or the vault-like space created by an arch-like structure.

Fossa - A trench or channel; used in anatomical nomenclature as a general term to denote a hollow or depressed area.

Founder - Laminitis; inflammation of the sensitive or live tissues of the hoof.

Fracture - This literally means break or the parting of two structures. This is especially significant in relation to bone tissue.

Friction - This is a type of massage stroke; the rubbing of two surfaces together.

Frog - The band of horny substance in the middle of the sole of a horse's foot, dividing into two branches and running towards the heel in the form of a fork.

Fungiform papillae - These are papillae that are shaped like a fungus or mushroom.

Gait - This is the way or manner of the horse's movement performed in sequence.

Gastric - This is a term that refers to anything pertaining to the stomach.

Gastric reflux - This refers to the fluid that can be evacuated from the stomach via a stomach tube.

Gastritis - This is any inflammation of the stomach.

Gastroduodenal - Pertaining to or communicating with the stomach and duodenum.

Genitalia - The reproductive organs.

Geriatric - This term describes anything relating to an older animal.

Gestation - This is the time period of development from fertilization of the ovum to the termination of the pregnancy.

Gingiva - The mucous membrane and fibrous tissue that covers the alveolar processes aroung the teeth.

Gingivitis - This is an inflammation that involves only the gingival tissue.

Ginglymus joint - A type of synovial joint that allows movement in but one plane, forward and backward, as the hinge of a door.

Glenoid cavity - A cavity resembling a pit or socket.

Granulation tissue - This is the formation of abnormal masses of highly vascularized tissue in wounds.

Granuloma - This is a tumor or neoplasm made up of granulation tissue.

Halitosis - This is the condition of having offensive or bad breath.

Haploid - This is the state of having a single set of chromosomes.

Heel - An anatomic term which is used to designate the palmar portion of the hoof wall medially or laterally.

Hematoma - This is an accumulation of blood within the tissue which clots to form a solid swelling.

Hemoconcentration - This is a decrease of the fluid content of the blood which results in an increase in its concentration.

Hemoglobin - This is the oxygen carrying pigment of the erythrocytes.

Hemorrhage - Literally, this is bleeding. It is the escape of blood from the vessels.

Hemostasis - This is any means or agent that arrests the flow of blood.

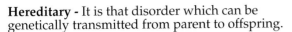

Hereditary - It is that disorder which can be genetically transmitted from parent to offspring.

Hernia - In general, this is the protrusion of a loop or knuckle of an organ or tissue through an abnormal opening.

Herniation - This is the abnormal protrusion of an organ or other body structure through a defect or natural opening.

Hilus - (Also spelled **Hylus.**) This is the depression or pit at that part of an organ where the vessels and nerves enter.

Histology - That study of anatomy which deals with the minute structure, composition, and function of the tissues on a cellular level.

Histopathological - This is the study of diseased tissues in minute structure, composition, and function.

Hock - The tarsal joint or region of the tarsus in the hind leg of the horse.

Holosystolic - Pertaining to the entire systole.

Homeopathy - This is the treatment of any disease or state by the use of natural substances in minute doses.

Homogeneous - This is the state by which the structure consists of, or is composed of similar elements or ingredients of a uniform quality throughout the tissue.

Homologue - Any organ or part that is similar in structure, position and origin to another organ.

Hoof/Pastern axis - An imaginary line passing through the center of the pastern.

Humerus - The bone that extends from the shoulder to the elbow.

Hunters' Bumps - This is a condition that is caused by the bony prominences on the dorsal midline of the caudal lumbar area or on top of the hindquarters.

Hyaline cartilage - That cartilage that is the most common type of cartilage which lines most of the articular surfaces in the horse. It is nonvascular,

and nourishment must diffuse into its cells from outside its substances.

Hydrocele - This is a circumscribed collection of fluid.

Hydrocephalus - This is a condition that is characterized by an abnormal accumulation of fluid in the cranial vault.

Hydroexercise - This is any exercise or exertion which involves or takes place in water.

Hyperemia - This is an excess of blood in a particular part.

Hyperextend - The state in which there is an extreme or excessive extension of a limb.

Hyperflexion - The state of forcible over-flexion of a limb.

Hypermotile - This is an excessive or abnormally increased motility.

Hyperperistalsis - This an excessive active movement in the musculature of the bowel.

Hypertrophy - This is an abnormal enlargement or overgrowth of an organ or part do to an increase in the size of its constituent cells.

Hypoalbuminemia - This is an abnormally low albumin content of the blood.

Hypoglycemia - This is an abnormally diminished content of glucose within the blood.

Hypokalemia - This is the state where there is an abnormally low potassium content within the blood.

Hypomotile - This indicates a lack of movement or motion within a specific part.

Hyponatremia - This is when there is a deficency of sodium within the blood.

Hypoplasia - This depicts a state of defective or incomplete development.

Hypoxia - There is a low oxygen content or deficiency of oxygen within tissue.

Hypoxemia - This is a low oxygen content of the blood.

Iatrogenic - This term means the creation of a disorder or problem that results from a man-made activity.

Icterus - This is a description of a jaundiced condition.

Idiopathic - This is a condition that is created spontaneously.

Ileum - The last portion of the small intestine.

Ilium - The largest of the three bones of the pelvis.

Immobilize - To render something that is incapable of being moved.

Immune - This is protection against any particular disease either by inoculation or natural antibody production.

Immunitiy - This is the state or condition of being immune.

Impacted teeth - These are teeth which have been prevented from erupting by some mechanical obstacle.

Impaction - This is the condition of being firmly lodged or wedged.

Impar ligament - A fibrous sheet attaching the distal border of the bone to the flexor surface of the distal phalanx, palmar to the insertion of the deep digital flexor tendon.

Implantation - This is the insertion of a part or tissue such as skin, nerve, or tissue into a new site.

Incision - This is to produce a cut or wound by surgical intervention.

Induce parturition - This is the initiation of the birth process by unnatural or artificial means.

Inelastic - Not able to be stretched or manipulated in any way.

Infarction - This is an area of coagulation necrosis within a tissue due to a local anemia resulting from the obstruction of circulation to that area.

Infective - The abiltity to produce an infection.

Inferior - Situated below, or directed downward; in official anatomical nomenclature, used in reference to the lower surface of an organ or other structure.

Infertility - This is the absence or the lack of ability to conceive or induce inception.

Infiltrate - This is the act of penetration through the interstices of a tissue or substance.

Inflammation - This is a reaction of the tissues when injured that results in a redness to the dermis, the production of heat, swelling of the tissues, and pain.

Infrared thermography - This is a noninvasive diagnostic technique which converts the skin's radiated thermal energy to electrical energy that can be amplified and displayed on a video screen. This results in two dimensional graphical and quantitative information regarding the precise skin temperature of the horse. This then can be interpreted to depict inflammation, atrophy, neoplasia, and neurological disorders.

Infundibulum - This term depicts a funnel-shaped passage.

Ingesta - This is any food or water that is taken into the stomach.

Innervation - This is the distribution or supply of nerves to a specific anatomical part.

Insemination - This is the deposition of seminal fluid within the vagina.

Insertion - This is the point of attachment of the muscle to the bone.

Integument - This is the covering of the body or skin.

Interference - This the striking of a limb by the contralateral foot which usually results in trauma to this limb.

Internal - situated or occurring within a structure.

Internal fixation - The surgical technique whereas through the use of pins, plates, and screws, there is a compression of the fracture fragments through rigid fixation.

Interosseous Ligament - Two separate ligaments attaching the 2nd to the 3rd metacarpal, the 4th to the 3rd metacarpal in the forelimb. In the hindlimb, the ligaments connect the 2nd and the 3rd metatarsals and also the 4th to the 3rd metatarsal.

Interstitial - This is a location that is situated in the interstices of a tissue.

Intraarticular - Anything within a joint.

Intraarticular fracture - This is a fracture that occurs within a joint.

Intranasal - Within the nose.

Intranuclear - Within the nucleus.

Intrasynovial block - The administration of a local anesthetic within the synovial cavity.

Intrauterine - Within the uterus.

Intravenous - The administration of any substance within a vein.

Intussusception - This is the prolapse of one part of intestinal tract into the lumen of an immediately adjoining part.

Inversion - This is a reversal of a normal relation of a part. It is the turning inward, inside out, upside down or other position that is not normal.

In vitro - Within a glass or observable container.

In vivo - Within the living body.

Involution - This is the rolling or turning inward over a rim.

Ischemia - Deficiency of blood in a part, due to functional constriction or actual obstuction of a blood vessel.

Ischemic - Pertaining to, or affected with ischemia.

Ischemic necrosis - The death of any tissues or cells due to a deficiency of blood caused by a constiction or actual obstruction of a blood vessel.

Ischium - One of the pelvic bones. It is triangular in outline and much smaller than the ilium. It joins the ilium anteriorly and along its dorsal border, except around the sciatic foramen.

Isothermal gradient - a specific infrared temperature measurement in relationship to other thermal readings within a specific area.

Isthmus - This is the narrow connection that is found between two larger bodies or parts.

Jaundice - This the condition that is characterized by hyperbilirubinemia and the deposition of bile pigment in the skin and mucous membranes which results in a yellow appearance.

Joint - This is an articulation: it is the union or junction between two or more bones of the skeleton.

Joint lavage - This technique is where fluid is infused and drained from the joint for therapeutic reasons.

Keratinize - This is the process by which tissue will become horny.

Keratitis - This is an inflammation of the cornea.

Knock knees - This is a conformation that refers to a deformity in which the metacarpus deviates laterally, and the distal radius deviates medially.

Labium - This is an anatomical description meaning a fleshy border or edge.

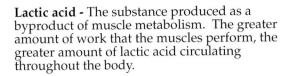

Lactic acid - The substance produced as a byproduct of muscle metabolism. The greater amount of work that the muscles perform, the greater amount of lactic acid circulating throughout the body.

Lactobacillus - A genus of microorganisms of the tribe Lactobacilleae, family Lactobacillaceae, order Eubacteriales, occurring as large gram-positive, anaerobic or microaerophilic bacilli.

Lacuna - This is a descriptive term indicating a small pit or hallow cavity. It can also be used to designate a compartment within or between other body structures.

Lag screw - A basic orthopedic technique used routinely to privide fixation within bony structures.

Lamellae - Thin leaves or plates, as of bone.

Lamina - This is an anatomical term to indicate a structure or layer of specific tissues.

Laminar corium - This primary and secondary laminar layer is interdigitated with the horny laminae of the hoof wall. This corium supplies nutrition to the horny lamina and to the interlaminar horn of the white line.

Laminitis - Inflammation within the lamina of the horses hoof: referred to as "founder."

Lampas - This is the swelling and hardening of the mucosa of the hard palate. This usually occurs immediately behind the upper incisors.

Laparotomy - This is a surgical incision through the flank. In general, it means an abdominal incision along any area.

Larvicidal - This is any agent that is destructive to parasitic larva.

Laser - A high energy beam of intensive light.

Lateral - This is an anatomical term denoting a position further away from the median plane or the mid line of the body.

Lavage - This is the procedure where an organ or cavity is irrigated.

Laxative - This is any agent that acts to promote evacuation of the bowel.

Legumes - The pod or fruit of a leguminous plant, such as peas or beans.

Lesion - It is a change in texture or structure of tissue due to an injury or disease process.

Leukocyte - This applies to one of the formed elements of blood consisting of a colorless granular mass of protoplasm having ameboid movements. There are several varieties of leukocytes found in normal blood.

Leukocytosis - This is an increase in the number of leukocytes in the blood.

Leukopenia - This is reduction in the number of leukocytes in the blood.

Libido - This is sexual desire.

Ligaments - A band of tissue that connects bones or supports viscera.

Ligated - This is to tie or bind the vessel or structure strangulating it at a particular point.

Lingual - Anything pertaining to the tongue.

Lipemia - This is the presence of any abnormally high concentration of fat or lipid in the blood.

Lobulated - This indicates that the structure is made up of or divided into lobules.

Low level light therapy - This is a form of therapeutic treatment utilizing photo energy on a regular basis to enhance the healing process.

Lucencies - Areas on a radiograph that appear more transparent since the tissues being penetrated are less dense.

Lumbar vertebrae - Is the third region of the vertebral column that consists of six vertebrae and is noted by the characteristic transverse processes.

Lumen - This is the cavity or channel within a tube or tubular organ.

Luteolysis - This is the destruction of the luteal tissue.

Luxation - Involves the loss of integrity to one or more of the joint ligaments (as in a severe sprain), as well as damage to other joint structures such as the fibrous joint capsule and surrounding tendons.

Lymphocyte - This is a variety of white blood corpuscles which arises in the reticular tissue of the lymph glands.

Macrophage - This is a large mononuclear wondering phagocytic cell which originates in the tissues.

Malnourished - A state of being underfed or undernourished.

Malocclusions - This is a state in which the contact of the maxillary and mandibular teeth are not positioned at a point where they will have their highest efficiency during mastication.

Manipulated - A manual examination or treatment of any part of the body.

Marrow - The soft material that fills the cavities of bones.

Massage - The systemic therapeutical friction, stroking, and kneading of the muscles of the body to stimulate their action and relieve strain.

Mastication - This is the act of chewing food.

Meatus - This is an anatomical term that designates an opening or passageway in the body.

Meconium - This is the dark green mucilaginous material in the intestine of the full term fetus.

Meconium retention - This is when the foal is unable to pass the meconium after birth.

Medial - This is an anatomical term pertaining to structures or points that lay close to the mid line or median plane of the body.

Median plane - This anatomical plane divides the animal symmetrically into right and left halves with any plane parallel to the median plane being referred to as a sagittal plane.

Medullary - Pertaining to the marrow or to any part of the medulla.

Melanocytes - This is the cell that is responsible for the synthesis of melanin.

Membrane - This is the thin layer of tissue which covers a surface or divides a space or organ.

Meningitis - This is an inflammation within the meninges.

Mesosalpinx - This is a portion of the broad ligament of the uterus above the mesovarium composed of layers that enclose the uterine tube.

Mesovarium - This is the portion of the broad ligament of the uterus between the mesometrium and mesososalpinx.

Metabolic - This indicates a reference to metabolism.

Metabolism - This is all of the physical and chemical processes by which all living organized substance is produced and maintained. It is also the transformation by which energy is made available for the use of the organism.

Metatarsals - These are the bones of the hind limb that extend from the hock to the fetlock.

Microaerophilic - This is the condition where growth is enhanced when only a small amount of atmospheric oxygen is present.

Microfractures - Microscopic fractures that are very difficult to diagnose utilizing normal radiographic techniques. Their presence is usually dignosed by nuclear scintigraphy.

Microvasculature - Microscopic blood vessels. Many times these are small enough to only allow one or two cells to pass through at any given time.

Micturition - This is the passage of urine; urination.

Mitochondria - A filamentous or granular component (organelle) of cytoplasm; the principle site of oxidation reactions by which the energy in foodstuff is made available for processes which occur in the cell.

Mobility - This is the ability to move.

Morphology - This is the science of form and structure of an organism.

Motor unit - This is the motor neuron plus the muscle fiber it innervates.

Mucopurulent - Indicates a state where both mucous and pus are present.

Mucosa - A mucous membrane, or tunic mucosa.

Multiparous - This is the state where an animal has had two or more pregnancies that have resulted in viable offspring.

Mummification - Conversion into a state resembling that of a mummy. An example of this would be the shriveling and drying up of a dead fetus.

Murmur - This is a gentle flowing ausculatory sound.

Muscle atrophy - Is the visible wasting away of any muscle tissue.

Muscle tremor - This is an involuntary trembling or fasciculation of a muscle.

Musculoskeletal - This is the anatomical term given to structures made up of bones, joints, ligaments, muscles, and tendons.

Mutation - This is the change in form, quality or some other characteristic.

Myofibrils - These are the bundles of very fine fibers that almost fill the sarcoplasm of a muscle cell.

Myofilament - These are the ultra-microscopic structures that are found in myofibrils.

Myoglobinurea - This is the presence of myloglobin within the urine.

Myometrium - This is the smooth muscle coat of the uterus.

Myopathy - Any disease of a muscle.

Myosin - A globin which is the most abundant protein (68 percent) in muscle. Along with actin, it is responsible for the contraction and relaxation of muscle.

Nares - This is the external orifice of the nose.

Nasogastric tube - This is the synthetic tube that is passed from the nose down through the esophagus and into the stomach.

Natural gait - These gaits are the walk, trot, and gallop; whereas an artificial gait is one that is taught to the horse by man.

Nebulization - This is a treatment modality where the liquid treatment or medication is converted into a spray that is inhaled.

Necropsy - An examination of the dead.

Necrosis - This is the general term for the death of tissue.

Neonatal - This is anything that pertains to the first four weeks after birth.

Neoplasia - This is the formation of a neoplasm.

Nephrosis - This is any disease or disorder of the kidney.

Nerves - These are specialized structures that provide pathways which carry messages to and from the brain.

Nervous system - This is the system which coordinates all activities of the body.

Neurectomy - This is the surgical or chemical excision of a part of a nerve.

Neurogenic muscle atrophy - A localized phenomenon characteristic of a few well recognized syndromes in the horse, the best known of which is denervation atrophy due to paralysis of the suprascapular nerve, refered to as "sweeny."

Neuromas - A tumor or new growth largely made up of nerve cells and nerve fibers; a tumor growing from a nerve.

Neuromuscular junction - This is the anatomical area where a motor neuron connects to the sarcolemma at the motor end point.

Neuropathy - A general term denoting functional disturbances and/or pathological changes in the peripheral nervous system.

Neurosis - A disorder of the psychic or mental constitution.

Neutropenia - This is a decrease in the neutrophilic leukocytes in the blood.

Neutrophils - This is a cell or structural element, in particular a lymphocyte which is stainable by neutral dyes.

Neutrophilia - Increased number of neutrophil leukocytes in the blood.

Nidus - This is the point of origin or focus of a morbid process.

Nodules - A small node or mass which is solid and can be detected by touch.

Nomenclature - Terminology; specifically a classified system of names.

Nonsteroidal - Any pharmaceutical compound that does not contain corticosteroids.

Nuchal bursa - Is located above the dorsal arch of the atlas.

Nuchal ligament - This is a ligament that divides the dorsal cervical muscles into right and left groups. It supports much of the burden of the head and allows the head to be raised and lowered.

Nystagmus - Involuntary rapid movement of the eyeball.

Oblique - This indicates a slanting or inclination between a horizontal and a perpendicular plane.

Obturator foramen - Is situated between the pubis and the ischium. It is oval in outline, the longer axis being directed forward and outward. Its margin is grooved anterolaterally for the obturator nerve and vessels.

Occlusal - This pertains to closure as applied to the masticating surfaces of the teeth.

Occult - This indicates that something is concealed from observation or obscure.

Ocular - This is anything that pertains to the eye.

Oliguria - This is the excretion of a diminished amount of urinein relation to the amount of fluid intake.

Omentum - This is the fold of the peritoneum that extends from the stomach to adjacent organs in the abdominal cavity.

Oocyte - This is a growing or full grown oogonial cell, or ovum, that has not yet completed its maturation process.

Opacification - This is the development of an opacity within the cornea or lens.

Open knees - When viewed laterally, the carpal joint appears irregular as a result from the lack of closure of the distal radial epiphysis.

Orchiectomy - This is the excision of one or both testes.

Orchiopexy - This is surgical fixation within the scrotum of an undescended testis.

Orifice - This is the entrance or outlet of any body cavity.

Os coxae - Consists of the ilium, ishium, and pubis, commonly referred to as the pelvis or pelvic bone.

Osselets - An exostosis within the fetlock joint. This is commonly referred to as traumatic arthritis of the metacarpophalangeal joint.

Osseous - Of the nature or quality of bone; bony.

Ossification - The formation of bone or of a bony substance; the conversion of fibrous tissue or of cartilage into bone or a bony substance.

Ossify - This is process in which there is a change of the tissue or development into bone.

Osteoarthritis - Chronic multiple degenerative joint disease.

Osteoblasts - A cell which arises from a fibroblast and which, as it matures, is associated with the production of bone.

Osteochrondritis Dissecans - A degenerative condition of the articular cartilage with loose bodies of cartilage and flaps visibly attached to the articular cartilage.

Osteoclasts - A large multinuclear cell associated with the absorption and removal of bone.

Osteoid - 1. Resembling bone. 2. The organic matrix of bone; young bone which has not undergone calcification.

Osteomyelitis - Inflammation of bone caused by a pyrogenic organism. It may remain localized or may spread through the bone to involve the marrow, cortex, cancellous tissue, and periosteum.

Osteophytes - An abnormal bony extension or osseous outgrowth.

Osteoporosis - A condition in which there are band-like areas of condensed bone at the epiphyseal lines of long bones and condensation of the edges of smaller bones.

Ovariectomy - This is a surgical removal of the ovaries.

Over in the knees - This is a conformational fault in which there is a forward deviation of the carpus.

Ovulation - This is the discharge of a mature unimpregnated ovum from a follicle or the ovary.

Paddle - An outward deviation of the foot during flight.

Paddling - This is a movement of the foot during flight where the foot moves away from, then back, at the beginning and at the end of the stride.

Palmar - Pertaining to the palm and refers to the back of the forelimb.

Palpable - Perceptible to touch.

Palpation - The act of feeling with the hand; the application of the fingers with light pressure to the surface of the body for the purpose of determining the consistence of the parts beneath the surface to obtain a physical diagnosis.

Papilla - This is a small nipple-like projection of elevated tissue within or on a structure.

Papilloma - This is a branching or lobulated benign tumor derived from the epithelium.

Paracentesis - This is the surgical puncture of a cavity for the purpose of aspirating fluid.

Paralysis - Loss or impairment of motor function due in a part to a lesion of the neural or muscular mechanism; by analogy, impairment of sensory function.

Parasitic - This is a term pertaining to, or of the nature of a parasite.

Parenchyma - This is the functional element of an organ.

Parturition - This is the act or process of giving birth.

Passive movements - These are gentle movements made by a handler to anatomical structures rather than having the animal move these structures on its own accord.

Pastern - The portion of a horse's foot occupied by the first and second phalanges.

Pastern axis - This is the inclination of the pastern with references to the growing surface observed from both the dorsal and the lateral views.

Pastern joint - Formed by two convex areas on the distal extremity of the proximal phalanx and two shallow concave areas expanded by a palmar fibrocartilaginous plate on the proximal extremity of the middle phalanx.

Patella - This is a long and narrow bone located in the interior portion of the stifle joint. The free surface is convex from side to side and slightly concave proximally to distally.

Patent - This indicates open and unobstructed.

Pathogen - This is any disease-producing microorganism or agent.

Pathogenic - This is the ability to give rise to a disease or disorder.

Pathological - This is any process or aspect of disease. The effects of which occurs on cells, tissues, body structures, and organs.

Pathology - This is the study of the nature of disease.

Pedal osteitis - A demineralization of the distal phalanx resulting from inflammation. It usually manifests itself radiographically as a roughening of the solar borders of the distal phalanx.

Pediatric - Any reference to young animals.

Pendulous - Literally means to hang loosely or be dependent.

Perforation - The act of boring or piercing through a part.

Periarticular - Those structures that are situated adjacent to a joint.

Perineal - Pertaining to that area or space between the associated structures occupying the pelvic inlet.

Perioplic corium - This corium supplies nutrition to the periople and lies in the perioplic groove above the coronary border of the hoof wall.

Periosteum - A specialized connective tissue covering all bones of the body, which possesses bone-forming characteristics.

Peritoneum - This is the serous membrane lining the abdominal cavity.

Peritonitis - This is an inflammation within the peritoneum.

Petrissage - This is a type of massage stroke.

Phalangeal - Having to do with the bones of the digit.

Phallectomy - This is an amputation of the penis.

Physical therapy - The restoration of function and promotion of tissue healing by assisting normal physiologic processes.

Physiological - This is anything that pertains to the science which treats the functions of a living organism and its parts.

Physis - This is the segment of tubular bone which is concerned mainly with growth.

Physitis - This is an inflammation within the growth area of bone.

Pigeon toed - A conformation fault in which the toe of the hooves point medially, usually resulting in a paddling motion during movement.

Pigmentation - This is the deposition of coloration within an area.

Placentitis - This is an inflammation within the placenta.

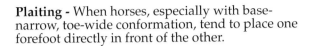

Plaiting - When horses, especially with base-narrow, toe-wide conformation, tend to place one forefoot directly in front of the other.

Plantar - Pertaining to the sole of the foot and to the back of the hind limb.

Platelet - This is the blood component that is concerned with coagulation of the blood and contraction of a blood clot. It is a circular or oval disc that is 2 - 3 microns in diameter and found in the blood of all animals.

Plexus - A network or tangle; used in anatomical nomenclature as a general term to designate a network of lymphatic vessels, nerves, or veins.

Pneumonia - This is a general term indicating any inflammation of the lung tissue.

Pneumovagina - This is a conformational defect which allows air within the anterior portion of the vagina.

Podotrochleosis - Inflammation of the navicular bone within the horse's foot.

Polypnea - This is a condition in which the rate of respiration is increased.

Porous - Penetrated by pores and open spaces.

Posterior - Situated in the back of, or in the back part of, or affecting the back part of an organ; in official anatomical nomenclature, used in reference to the back or dorsal side of the body.

Posthitis - This is an inflammation within the prepuce.

Post Legged - This is a conformational characteristic where there is an excessively straight pelvic limb.

Postpartum - This is any event or change that occurs after delivery.

Poultices - A soft, moist, hot mass applied to the surface of a part for the purpose of supplying heat and moisture.

Prepatent - This is the period of time that elapses between infection and the appearance of the parasites within a diagnostic test.

Prepubertal - This pertains to a period of time of accelerated growth preceding gonadal maturity.

Prepuce - This the covering fold of skin surrounding the penis.

Priapism - This is a constant state of persistent, abnormal erection of the penis.

Proglottis - This is any one of the joints of a tapeworm.

Prognosis - This is the prospect of recovery from a disease or an injury.

Prolapse - This is falling down or sinking of a part.

Proliferation - This is to grow through multiplication: i.e. a rapid increase in cells.

Prophylaxis - This is the prevention or preventive treatment of a disease or disorder.

Protrusion - This is the state of being thrust forward or laterally.

Proud flesh - This is the accumulation of excessive granulation tissue.

Proximal - Nearest, closer to any point of reference: opposed to distal.

Pruritus - This is any condition that is characterized by itching.

Pulse - The rhythmic throbbing of an artery which can be palpated digitally.

Purulent - Consisting of or associated with the formation of pus.

Pus - Substance that is produced through the inflammatory action which contains cells, bacteria, and fluid.

Quarter - This an unofficial anatomic term which is used to designate the medial or lateral portion of the hoof wall.

Quidding - This is a term used to describe the eating habits of a horse whereas the food dribbles out of the mouth uncontrollably.

Quittor - This an infection of the lateral cartilage of the foot.

Radiography - This is the act of making a record or photograph by means of the action of actinic rays on a sensitive film surface.

Ramify - To branch or diverge in different directions.

Raphe - This is an anatomical term that is used to designate a line of union of the halves of various symmetrical parts.

Recumbent - This is a term that means lying down.

Reflux - A backward or return flow.

Regeneration - To produce, or bring to life. The natural renewal of a substance, such as a lost tissue part.

Regression - This is a return to a former or earlier state. An example of this would be the subsidence of symptoms of a disease process or disorder.

Remodeling - The process in which bone or other tissue structures undergo reconstruction.

Renal - This is a term that means anything pertaining to the kidney.

Repulsion - This is the forcing apart of two bodies, or the forcing of two structures away from each other.

Resection - This is the surgical excision of a considerable portion of an organ or structure.

Respiration - This includes inspiration and expiration. It is the physical act of breathing by which air is drawn in and expelled from the lungs.

Ringbone - (Phalangeal exostosis) Osteophytosis from periosteitis from the proximal, middle, and distal phalanges.

Rotation - The process of turning on an axis.

Roughage - This is the portion of the diet that contains fiber and cellulose.

Rupture - This is tissue which has been torn or parted.

Sacculated - This is a structure that is characterized by little bags or sacs.

Sacral vertebrae - the fourth region of the vertebral column that is comprised of the fusion of five vertebrae.

Salivation - This is the discharge of saliva.

Sarcolemma - This is the plasma membrane of a muscle fiber.

Sarcomere - This is the contractile unit of the myofibrils.

Sarcoplasma - This is the cytoplasm of a muscle fiber.

Sarcoplasmic reticulum - The structure is the analog of the endoplasmic reticulum of other animal cells. It is composed of a network of tubules and sacs within the muscle fiber.

Scapula - The flat, triangular bone comprising the shoulder.

Scapulohumeral joint - This is the articular surface between the scapula and the humerus.

Scar tissue - This is tissue that remains after healing has occurred within the wound or injury.

Scoliosis - Is a deviation of the spine laterally off the median plane.

Scratches - Eczematous inflammation usually located in the heel of a horse's foot.

Scrotum - This is the pouch which contains the testes and their accessory organs.

Sedation - The calming or allaying of excitement by any agent.

Seedy toe - This is a separation of the dermal and epidermal lamina. It usually occurs as a sequela to chronic laminitis.

Semen - The thick whitish excretory liquid of the reproductive organs in the male composed of spermatozoa and various secretions from the accessory sex glands.

Semilunar crest - The large rough curved line that divides the volar surface of the third phalanx into two unequal parts.

Septicemia - Presence in the blood of bacterial toxins.

Septically - Produced by or due to putrefaction and decomposition.

Sequela - Any lesion or affliction following or caused by another disorder.

Serology - The study of antigen/antibody reactions in vitro.

Serosanguineous - This is any fluid that contains both serum and blood.

Serous - This is any structure or cyst that produces or contains serum.

Serum - The clear portion of any animal liquid separated from its more solid elements.

Sesamoid bones - A paired set of bones which are located behind the distal end of the large metacarpal bone. These bones are held in place to the first phalanx by several large ligaments.

Shoulder - The junction of the arm and the trunk.

Sickle hocks - Conformational fault characteristic of the tarsal joint that laterally depicts an excessive angulation.

Smegma - This is the thick, cheesy, foul-smelling secretion that is found chiefly around the external genitals.

Sole - The bottom of the foot.

Somatic - This term indicates anything that pertains to or is characteristic of the body.

Spasm - These are unwilling contractions of muscle tissue which usually result in pain.

Spavin test - A test that occurs during a lameness exam which includes an observation of the gait after forced flexion of the hock for a period of time.

Spermatid - This is a cell derived from a secondary spermatocyte.

Spermatocyte - This is the mother cell of a spermatid.

Spermatozoa - This is a mature male sperm cell that serves to impregnate the ovum.

Spermicidal - Any agent that kills sperm.

Sphincter - This is a ring-like band of muscle fibers that constricts a passage or closes a natural orifice.

Spongy bone - Bone with a sponge-like appearance or texture.

Sprain - This is a disorder that results from an abnormal stretching of a limb causing a partial or full ligament rupture.

Squamous cells - Cells that are scaly, or plate-like.

Standing under - A deviation in which the entire forelimb from the elbow down is placed in back of the perpendicular and too far under the body when the animal is viewed from the side.

Stasis - This is the act of stopping a flow of blood or any other body fluid from any part.

Sternum - A longitudinal unpaired plate of bone forming the middle of the ventral wall of the thorax.

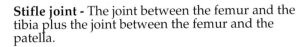

Stifle joint - The joint between the femur and the tibia plus the joint between the femur and the patella.

Strain - This is a disorder that results from the over work of the horse's musculature.

Strangulation - This is the occlusion of a specific anatomical area that arrests any circulation or air passage through that area.

Stratified - This term depicts deposition in layers.

Stratum externum - A thin layer of horn extending distally from the periople whose variable distance decreases with age.

Stratum germinativum - This epithelial layer of the hoof proliferates and maintains the constant growth of the hoof.

Stratum internum - (stratum lamellatum) The layer of the hoof wall containing the interdigitation of corial and epidermal laminae.

Stratum medium - The bulk of the hoof wall consisting of horn tubules and intertubular horn.

Stratum tectorium - See stratum externum.

Stress - This is forcibly exerted weight or pressure.

Stride - The measured distance between hoof prints originating from the same limb.

Stringhalt - This is an involuntary flexion of the tarsal joint during motion which usually involves the lateral digital extensor muscle on the hind limb.

Stroma - This is a term describing the structural elements of an organ. This can be the framework or matrix of an organ and is different from its functional elements or parenchyma.

Subacute - This is stage that occurs between acute and chronic.

Subcutaneous - Under the skin.

Subluxation - An incomplete or partial dislocation.

Sulci - Plural of sulcus.

Sulcus - A groove, or furrow; used in anatomical nomenclature as a general term to designate such a depression. These are located between the frog and the sole of the foot and also in the cerebral hemispheres of the brain.

Superficial - Pertaining to or situated near the surface.

Superior - Situated above, or directed upward; in official anatomical nomenclature, used in reference to the upper surface of an organ or other structure, or to a structure occupying a higher position.

Supernumerary - This is an extra tooth which is not a normal part of the dentition.

Surgical arthrodesis - A surgical technique where a given joint is made immobile.

Suspensory ligament - A ligament that serves to hold up a part of the body or an organ.

Sweeny - This is a neurogenic atrophy of a muscle or muscle group, specifically that caused by the paralysis of the suprascapular nerve.

Synovial cavity - The cavity created by the joint which contains the synovial fluid.

Synovial fluid - The viscous fluid produced by the synovial membrane that is contained within the joint.

Synovial membrane - Membrane that lines the joint and produces the synovial fluid.

Systemic - This indicates an affect on the body as a whole.

Systemic antibiotics - Those medications that combat infections which are administered parenterally either intravenously, intramuscularly, or subcutaneously.

Systolic - This is the contraction or period of contractions of the heart that mainly involves the ventricles.

T-tubules - These are transverse tubules that allow electrical impulses traveling along the sarcolemma to move deeper into the cell structures.

Technetium 99 - The metallic chemical element of atomic number 43; atomic weight 99; symbol, Tc, the pharmacological component used in nuclear scintigraphy.

Tendon - A fibrous cord by which a muscle is attached to the bone.

Tendonitis - This is the inflammation of any tendon.

Tendosynovitis - This is the inflammation of both the tendon and its synovial sheath.

Tenosynovitis - This is an inflammation of a synovial sheath around a tendon.

Tenotomy - The surgical cutting of a tendon.

T.E.N.S. - Transcutaneous Electrical Nerve Stimulators} This is a type of therapeutic machine used in treating muscular disorders.

Therapy - This is the treatment of any illness, injury, or disorder.

Thermal gradient - That temperature radiating from a specific area of the dermis in relationship to other temperatures radiating from within the area.

Thermography - This is a diagnostic technique where the heat emitted from the body surfaces is recorded and analyzed.

Testis - This is a male gonad.

Testosterone - This is the hormone produced by the testis in the male.

Thoracic vertebrae - The second region of the vertebral column that consists of eighteen vertebrae which articulate with the ribs.

Thoroughpin - This is the common term used to describe the condition of the tenosynovitis within the deep flexor tendon sheath.

Thrombosis - The formation, development, or presence of a thrombus.

Thrombus - This is a plug or clot in a blood vessel or in one of the cavities of the heart formed by the coagulation of blood and remaining at its point of formation.

Thrush - A common disease of the foot caused by a bacteria (*Spherophorus necrophorus* or *Fusobacterium necrophorum*) which can live only in an anaerobic environment.

Toe - An anatomic term which focuses on the dorsal part of the hoof wall.

Toed-in - A position of the feet in which the toes point toward one another when viewed from the front.

Toed-out - The toes point away from one another when viewed from the front.

Topical - This is anything that pertains to a particular spot or localized area on the surface.

Topographical - Pertaining to topography.

Topography - The description of an anatomical region or of a specific part.

Torsion - This is the act of twisting.

Tortuous - A structure that is twisted and full of turns in numerous places.

Toxemia - This is a general intoxication due to the absorption of bacterial toxins formed from an infection.

Toxicosis - This is any disease condition that is due to a poisoning.

Toxin - A poisonous, harmful substance. This term is frequently used to refer specifically to a protein or conjugated protein substance produced by either a plant, animal or pathogenic bacteria.

Toxoid - A "tamed" version of a toxin that is injected into the animal to stimulate its immune system to produce antibodies that will be ready to guard against a specific poison.

Trabeculae - A small beam, used in anatomical nomenclature as a general term to designate a supporting or anchoring strand of connective tissue, such as strand extending from a capsule into the substance of the enclosed organ.

Tranquilization - The administration of an agent that acts upon the animal to produce a quiet or calm sedation.

Transmission - Transfer of a disease through the communication of inheritable qualities to an offspring.

Transudate - This is a fluid substance which has passed through a membrane or been extruded from a tissue. This usually involves the inflammatory reaction.

Transverse plane - These transect any anatomical part, i.e. the neck or a limb, perpendicularly to its own long axis.

Trauma - Any injury or insult to the tissues.

Trephine - An act of perforating with a cylindrical saw to allow the cutting of a circular piece of bone out of a skull.

Tubular - Shaped like a tube; of or pertaining to a tubule.

Tumescence - This is a condition of swelling or of being swollen.

Tumor - A neoplasm or a mass of new tissue which persists and grows independently of its surrounding tissues.

Turgid - In general this means swollen and congested.

Typing-up - A syndrome of muscular cramping, pain, and varying degrees of muscle breakdown associated with exercise or overexertion.

Udder - This is the mammary gland of the horse.

Ulceration - The formation or development of an ulcer.

Umbilicus - This is the site of attachment of the umbilical cord in the fetus.

Unilateral - Affecting only one side.

Ultrasound - This is a diagnostic and therapeutic instrument that emits radiant energy at different frequencies.

Urethra - The membranous canal that conveys urine from the bladder to the exterior of the body.

Urethritis - This is an inflammation of the urethra.

Urinalysis - Chemical and microscopic analysis of urine.

Urogenital - Anything that pertains to the urinary system and genitalia.

Urticaria - A vascular reaction of the skin marked by the transient appearance of smooth slightly elevated patches.

Vaccine - This is a suspension of attenuated or killed microorganisms that is administered for the prevention or treatment of infectious diseases.

Vaginitis - Any inflammation of the vagina.

Varicocele - A varicose condition of the veins, typically used in relation to the tortuous enlargement of the pampiniform plexus of veins in the spermatic cord.

Vascularization - The process of becoming vascular, or the development of vessels in a part or tissue.

Vasoconstriction - The diminution of the caliber of vessels, especially constriction of arterioles leading to a decreased blood flow to a part.

Vector - This is a carrier which transfers an infectious agent from one host to another.

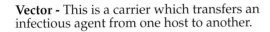

Vector - This is a carrier which transfers an infectious agent from one host to another.

Veins - These are vessels which carry deoxygenated blood back to the heart.

Ventral - This is an anatomical term which refers to structures that lay toward the belly of the animal.

Vesicle - This is a small structure or sac containing liquid. This can also refer to a small blister or a small circumscribed elevation of the epidermis containing a serous fluid.

Vestibule - This is the space or cavity at the entrance to a canal.

Vestigial - This pertains to a remnant of a structure which functioned in a previous stage of a species or individual during their development.

Viable - This is the ability to live.

Vice - A bad habit.

Villi - This is the small vascular process or protrusion from a free surface of a membrane.

Viral - Pertaining to, or caused by a virus.

Virus - One group of minute infectious agents, with certain exceptions (i.e. poxviruses, psittacosis group) not resolved in the light microscope, and characterized by lack of independent metabolism and by the ability to replicate only within living host cells.

Viscera - Any large interior organ.

Viscous - The description characterized by a high degree of friction between component molecules as they slide by each other.

Voluntary - these are actions that are accomplished through the command of the animal's own nervous system.

Wind puff - This is a cosmetic blemish caused by the synovial swelling of a tendon or tendon sheath.

Winging - This is the movement of the foot through flight toward, and then away from, a medial plane at the beginning and the end of a stride.

Zygote - This is the cell that results from the fusion of two gametes.

INDEX

G

Gasterophilus haemorrhoidalis 210
Gasterophilus intestinalis 209, 210
Gasterophilus nasalis 210
Gastric arteries 172
Gastric dilation 183, 184
Gastric rupture 184, 188
Gastric veins 174
Gastrocnemius muscle 262, 273; *See also Volume 1*
Gastroduodenal ulcers 130, 133, 134, 183, 184
Gastroendoscopy 134
Gastroenterostomy 186
Gelding 12, 14, 16
Genioglossus muscle 155
Geniohyoideus muscle 155
Gingivitis 166, 168, 169, 170
Girth itch 303, 304
Glossopharyngeal nerve 256, 258, 266
Gluteus medius muscle 273; *See also Volume 1*
Gonadotropin-releasing hormone 24, 56
Graafian follicle 47, 55, 57
Granulosa-theca cell tumor 71, 72
Great colon 174, 175, 176, 178, 187, 189
Greater petrosal nerve 256
Guttural pouch 155, 216, 217, 218, 220, 226, 228, 232, 234, 236, 237, 238, 239, 240, 242, 244, 258
Guttural pouch disorders 216, 228, 237, 238
Guttural pouch tympany 238, 239, 240, 242
Guttural pouch infections 226, 232

H

Habronema majus 214
Habronema microstoma 22
Habronema muscae 22, 44, 214
Habronemiasis 21, 22, 32, 43, 44, 202, 213, 214, 292, 302
Hair 25, 71, 72, 100, 102, 190, 202, 204, 210, 228, 282, 288, 293, 294, 295, 296, 298, 304, 305, 306
Hair follicle 294, 295, 296

Hand breeding 86, 87, 88, 90
Hard palate 155, 156, 158, 168, 216
Heart 118, 126, 128, 130, 134, 135, 136, 172, 173, 186, 188, 192, 198, 222, 223, 224, 228, 264
Heat stroke 272
Heaves 250
Hematomas 22, 40, 64, 72, 73, 74, 228, 229
Hemorrhage 15, 16, 18, 20, 22, 24, 26,32, 40, 74, 108, 112, 116, 117, 118, 124, 144, 204, 216, 218, 226, 230, 234, 240, 246, 251, 252
Hernia 14, 16, 20, 24, 29, 30, 130, 141, 142, 226
Hernia clamps 142
High flanker 16
Hilus of lung 222, 224
Hydrocele 14, 15, 16, 27, 28
Hyoepiglottic muscle 219
Hyoid bone 155, 158, 217, 220
Hyperkalemic periodic paralysis 254, 274, 277, 278, 308
Hypoalbuminemia 204
Hypocalcemia 146
Hypochloremia 194
Hypoglossal nerve 158, 256, 258, 265, 266
Hypoglycemia 144,146
Hypokalemia 194
Hyponatremia 194
Hypophysis 255
HYPP 254, 274, 277, 278, 308

I

Ileum 174, 175, 176, 185
Iliohypogastric nerve 262
Iliopsoas muscle 262; *See also Volume 1*
Ilium 5, 51; *See also Volume 1*
Immunoglobulin G (IgG) 128
Impaction 126, 180, 182, 184, 186, 187, 188, 189, 190, 192, 202
Impaction colic 187, 188
Incisors 157, 158, 159, 160, 162, 164, 166, 168, 170
Induction of parturition 109, 110, 112
Infectious arthritis 148

Inferior alveolar artery 155
Inferior buccal glands 156
Inferior palatolabial arteries 156
Influenza virus 138, 140, 234
Infraorbital artery 155
Infraorbital nerve 216, 256
Infrared thermography 20, 268; *See also Volume 1*
Infraspinatus muscles 262; *See also Volume 1*
Inguinal cryptorchid 18
Inguinal hernia 14, 16, 29
Inguinal ring 2, 14, 15, 16, 18, 20, 28, 29, 30, 50, 182
Inhibin 57, 58
Interarcuate ligament 268
Intercostal muscles 224, 262; *See also Volume 1*
Intercostal nerves 262
Internal abdominal oblique muscle 17, 18, 29
Internal and external pudic arteries and veins 8
Internal auricular nerve 256
Internal carotid artery 155, 218, 237, 240, 255
Internal iliac artery 262
Internal inguinal ring 2, 15, 29
Internal pudic artery 8, 178
Internal pudic vein 8, 178
Intestinal clostridiosis 195, 196
Intradermal testing 298
Intussusception 130, 182, 186, 195, 196
Irradiation 302
Ischiocavernosus muscle 1, 5, 7

J

Jejunum 139, 174, 175, 176, 202, 208
Joint IU 148
Jugular vein 222

K

Keratitis 288, 292
Kidney 1, 47, 48, 115, 117, 133, 135, 140, 173, 174, 176, 178, 182, 191, 192
Klebsiella pneumoniae 30, 42
Klebsiella spp. 72, 78, 138